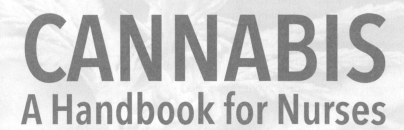

CANNABIS
A Handbook for Nurses

Carey S. Clark, PhD, RN, AHN-BC, RYT, FAAN
Past President
American Cannabis Nurses Association
Albany, New York
Professor, Director of Nursing, and Chair of the Medical
Cannabis Certificate Program
Pacific College of Health and Science
San Diego, California

T0176371

Philadelphia • Baltimore • New York • London
Buenos Aires • Hong Kong • Sydney • Tokyo

Not authorised for sale in United States, Canada, Australia, New Zealand, Puerto Rico, and U.S. Virgin Islands.

Acquisitions Editor: Nicole Dernoski
Development Editor: Maria M. McAvey
Editorial Coordinator: Anthony Gonzalez
Production Project Manager: Kim Cox
Design Coordinator: Teresa Mallon
Manufacturing Coordinator: Kathleen Brown
Marketing Manager: Linda Wetmore
Prepress Vendor: S4Carlisle Publishing Services

Copyright © 2021

9 8 7 6 5 4 3 2 1

Printed in China

Library of Congress Cataloging-in-Publication Data

Names: Clark, Carey S., editor.
Title: Cannabis: a handbook for nurses / editor, Carey S. Clark.
Other titles: Cannabis (Clark)
Description: First edition. | Philadelphia : Wolters Kluwer Health, [2021]
 | Includes bibliographical references and index.
Identifiers: LCCN 2020028446 | ISBN 9781975144265 (paperback)
Subjects: MESH: Medical Marijuana | Nurse's Role | United States
Classification: LCC RC568.C2 | NLM WB 925 | DDC 616.86/35—dc23
LC record available at https://lccn.loc.gov/2020028446

CCS1220

Dedicated with loving kindness to all who have suffered and sacrificed through the cannabis prohibition era, including the Mother-Earth; the Black, Indigenous and People of Color populations who have experienced disproportionate suffering; the patients in need of healing and palliation; the law-breakers; the advocates and activists; and the prisoners. May we move forward in harmony as this plant is emancipated.

Carey S. Clark, PhD, RN, AHN-BC, RYT, FAAN

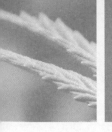

Contributors

Jodi Chapin, RN
Liaison and Educator
Green Nurse Group
Rockland, Massachusetts

Carey S. Clark, PhD, RN, AHN-BC,
  RYT, FAAN
Past President
American Cannabis Nurses Association
Albany, New York
Professor, Director of Nursing, and
  Chair of the Medical Cannabis
  Certificate Program
Pacific College of Health and Science
San Diego, California

Denise A. Foster, PhD, MSN, RN, CNE
Adjunct Associate Professor
School of Nursing,
University of Maryland Global Campus
Adelphi, Maryland

Marissa Fratoni, BSN, RN, LMT,
  RYT, INHC
Founder
HolisticNurseMama.com
Editor/Content Writer
Yoga Teacher
Green Nurse Group
Leominster, Massachusetts

Eileen Konieczny, RN, BCPA
Author
Cannabis Nurse Expert
Past President, American Cannabis
  Nurses Association
Albany, New York
Founder and Director
Olive's Branch
New York, New York

Barbara J. Ochester, MSN, BSN, RN
Professor
Aspen University
Denver, Colorado
Cannabis Nurse Educator
Philadelphia, Pennsylvania
Faculty
Pacific College of Health and Science
San Diego, California

Rachel A. Parmelee, MSN, RN, CRRN
Secretary
American Cannabis Nurses Association
Albany, New York
Faculty
Pacific College of Health and Science
San Diego, California

Llewellyn Dawn Smith, MSN, RN
Board of Director
American Cannabis Nurses Association
Albany, New York
Smith Cannabis, LLC
Portsmouth, Virginia
Endoscopy Nurse
Sentara Obici Hospital
Staff Nurse, Ambulatory Surgery
Sentara BelleHarbour
Suffolk, Virginia
Nursing Instructor
Sentara College of Health Sciences
Portsmouth, Virginia

Deanna M. Sommers, PhD, MSN, RN,
  CPNP-PC
Assistant Dean and Director
College of Nursing and Health Science
Lewis University
Chicago, Illinois

Eloise Theisen, MSN, RN,
   AGPCNP-BC
Cofounder and Chief Visionary Officer
Radicle Health
Walnut Creek, California
Faculty
Pacific College of Health and Science
San Diego, California
President
American Cannabis Nurses Association
Albany, New York

Sherri Tutkus, BSN, RN
CEO and Founder, GreenNurse Group
Director of Nursing at Irie Bliss
   Wellness
Rockland, Massachusetts
Founding Member of the Cannabis
   Nurses Network
San Diego, California
Founding Member of the International
   Association of Psychedelic Nursing
Dadeville, Alabama
Member of American Cannabis Nurses
   Association
Albany, New York

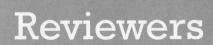

Reviewers

Karen Bean, DNP, FNP-c, CNE
Clinical Assistant Professor
Oregon Health and Science University
School of Nursing-La Grande Campus,
    FNP Program
La Grande, Oregon

Tammy Bryant, MSN, RN
Program Chair Nursing
Associate of Science Nursing Faculty
Southern Regional Technical College
Thomasville Campus
Thomasville, Georgia

Timothy Byars, MS
President, Radicle Health
Walnut Creek, California

Erla Champ-Gibson, PhD, MDiv, RN
Assistant Professor
Undergraduate Nursing Program
    Coordinator
School of Nursing
Pacific Lutheran University
Tacoma, Washington

Lori A. Cook, MS, RN, CNE
Associate Dean of Health Sciences
Emily Griffith High School
Denver, Colorado

Claire DeCristofaro, MD
Clinical Assistant Professor
DNP Program, College of Nursing
Medical University of South Carolina
Charleston, South Carolina

Brian Essenter, RPh
Owner
MM Consult CT
Shelton, Connecticut
Dispensary Manager
Affinity Health and Wellness
New Haven, Connecticut

Jessie Gill, RN
CEO and Founder of Marijuana
    Mommy
Woodbridge, New Jersey
Director of Nursing at Cannabis
    Education Group
Board of Director of the American
    Cannabis Nurses Association
Albany, New York
Member of the Cannabis Nurses
    Network
Founding Member of the International
    Association of Psychedelic Nursing
Dadeville, Alabama

Jeffrey Y. Hergenrather, MD
Founding Member
President
Society of Cannabis Clinicians
Cannabis Consultant
Sebastopol, California

Laura Bevlock Kanavy, MSN, RN
Director
Career Technology Center of
    Lackawanna County Practical
    Nursing Program
Scranton, Pennsylvania
Lawrence Township, New Jersey

Martha Kershaw, EdD, RN
Assistant Professor of Nursing
Daemen College
Amherst, New York

Loretta A. Moreno, DNP, RN
Program Director Licensed Vocational
    Nursing Program
Faculty, RN-BSN Program
Schreiner University
Kerrville, Texas

Tamara S. Pehrson, MS, RN
Associate Professor
Practical Nursing
Health Science and Human Services
College of Southern Idaho
Twin Falls, Idaho

Christina Pendrak Pepin, PhD,
RN, CNE
Assistant Professor
Leighton School of Nursing
Marian University
Indianapolis, Indiana

Regina Prosser, DNP, RN-BC,
CNE, LNHA
Assistant Professor of Nursing
Ursuline College
Pepper Pike, Ohio

Lu Ann Reed, DNP, CRRN, BC-RN,
LNHA, WCC, DWC
Assistant Dean of Nursing
Fortis College
Lawrence Township, New Jersey

Donna De Silva, MSN, APRN, FNP-C
Assistant Professor of Nursing
Southern Utah University
Cedar City, Utah

Eloise Theisen, MSN, RN, AGPCNP-BC
Cofounder and Chief Visionary Officer
Radicle Health
Walnut Creek, California
Faculty, Pacific College of Health and
    Science
San Diego, California
President
American Cannabis Nurses Association
Albany, New York

Shena Williams-Harrison, MSN, RN
Assistant Professor
School of Nursing and Allied Health
Southern University and A&M College
Baton Rouge, Louisiana

Lauren Winters, BSN, RN
Assistant Professor
Practical Nursing 2nd Level
    Coordinator
Nunez Community College
Chalmette, Louisiana

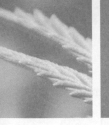

Nurse Interviews, Contributors

Janna Champagne, BSN, RN
Founder, Integrated Holistic Care
Founder, Cannabis Nurse Approved,
    LLC
Medford, Oregon
Founding Member, Cannabis Nurses
    Network
Cannabis Nurses Network Education
    Project Manager
San Diego, California
Medical Correspondent, Walk 4 Change
    Media
Member, Cannabis Nurses Network
    Speaker's Bureau
San Diego, California
Member, Oregon Cannabis Clinician's
    Group
Member, Oregon Cannabis
    Commission, Patient Care
    Subcommittee
Awarded Leader of Nursing Cannabis
    Nurses Network
Awarded Outstanding Author, Cannabis
    Nurses Media

Melanie C. Dreher, RN, MPhil, PhD
Dean Emeritus
Rush University College of Nursing
Chicago, Illinois

Bryan Krumm, MSN, CNP, RN, BC
Director, Harmony Psychiatric
Albuquerque, New Mexico

Mary Lynn Mathre, MSN, RN, CARN
Cannabis Nurse Educator and
    Consultant
Independent Legal Consultant
President and Cofounder, Patients Out
    of Time
Howardsville, Virginia
Past President and Cofounder,
    American Cannabis Nurses
    Association
Albany, New York

Alice O'Leary-Randall, LPN
Editor-in-Chief, *Mary's Cannabis Primer*
    and *Mary's Prime Time*
Denver, Colorado
Past Treasurer, American Cannabis
    Nurses Association
Albany, New York
Member, Scientific Advisory Council,
    United in Compassion (Australia)
Author, *Medical Marijuana in America:
    Memoir of a Pioneer*

Nique Pichette, MSN, RN
CEO, Founder, Cannabis Nurse
    Navigator
Fall Rover, Massachusetts
Founding Member, Cannabis Nurses
    Network
San Diego, California
Member, American Cannabis Nursing
    Association
Albany, New York
DNP Candidate 2022, Salve Regina
    University
Newport, Rhode Island

Ethan Russo, MD
Board-Certified Neurologist,
    Psychopharmacology Researcher,
    and Author
Founder/CEO of CReDO Science
Vashon, Washington

Inbal Sikorin, RN
Clinical Nursing Director
Tikun-Olam, Israel

Heather Sobel-Manus, RN
Founder, Nature Nurse
Founding Member, Cannabis Nurse
    Network
President, Genesis International
    Cannabis Solutions
San Diego, California

Ken Wolski, RN, MPA
Executive Director
Coalition for Medical Marijuana—New
    Jersey, Inc.
Trenton, New Jersey

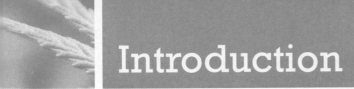

Introduction

WELCOME TO CANNABIS CARE NURSING

This handbook is intended to give the readers an overview of the art and science of cannabis care nursing. Cannabis care nurses work in a variety of settings, and they have specialized areas of knowledge, skill, and experience related to supporting patients' safe and effective use of cannabinoid medicines. Cannabis care nurses also use holistic approaches to ensure that patients are maximizing their health potential via homeostasis that emerges from the patients' enhanced endocannabinoid system (ECS) tone and health. Most importantly, cannabis care nurses care deeply for the patients that they help to educate and coach toward their best life and greatest health status.

The reality is that many patients use cannabis for palliation and healing; therefore, whether we call ourselves cannabis care nurses or not, all nurses must have a knowledge base of how to care for patients using cannabinoid medicines for healing. The motivation to write this book stemmed from a growing need in nursing academia and nursing practice for nurses to be able to provide informed and evidence-based care for their patients who use cannabis for healing. Medicinal use of cannabis has been a possibility for many citizens for over two decades; however, nurses have not been adequately prepared to provide evidence-based or theory-driven care for these patients, and due to the issue of the federal prohibition of cannabis, the matter of patient use of medicinal cannabis was often condemned, ignored, or silently accepted within our health care systems.

As more states legalize cannabis for medicinal or legal adult use, the call to be able to proficiently care for this population has emerged. In response to this phenomenon, the National Council of State Boards of Nursing (NCSBN, 2018) defined six essential areas of knowledge and skill acquisition for all nursing students working with medical cannabis patients; the resultant intention of the book is to support nurses' cannabis care educational process and act as a resource for all nurses interested in cannabis care. It is no longer acceptable to leave patients in the dark around the best practices and body of evidence related to medicinal cannabis use, and nurses are now obligated to be knowledgeable and confident in their support of patients' autonomous decisions to use cannabis for palliation and healing (NCSBN).

NATIONAL COUNCIL OF STATE BOARDS OF NURSING SIX PRINCIPLES OF ESSENTIAL KNOWLEDGE

The NCSBN (2018) six principles of essential nursing knowledge to support patient's medical use of cannabis include the following:

1. The nurse shall have a working knowledge of the current state of legalization of medical and recreational cannabis use.

2. The nurse shall have a working knowledge of the jurisdiction's medical marijuana program.
3. The nurse shall have an understanding of the endocannabinoid system, cannabinoid receptors, cannabinoids, and the interactions between them.
4. The nurse shall have an understanding of cannabis pharmacology and the research associated with the medical use of cannabis.
5. The nurse shall be able to identify the safety considerations for patient use of cannabis.
6. The nurse shall approach the patient without judgment regarding the patient's choice of treatment or preferences in managing pain and other distressing symptoms.

The purpose of this book is to provide a medical cannabis foundational resource for nursing faculty/educators, nursing students, and practicing nurses. It is a book that can be used across levels of curricula to meet the NCSBN (2018) educational recommendations, as well as in practice to guide nurse-driven coaching and educational interventions with medicinal cannabis patients.

Purpose

Ideally, the book is used continuously across the nursing curriculum, as medical cannabis care and the patient's need to achieve homeostasis cross over all specialty areas of nursing, impacting human life from preconception through death. Once the nurse understands that the human ECS is the largest receptor system in the body and that it interacts with all body systems with its role in supporting homeostasis, they will understand the importance of knowledge acquisition in this area. Unfortunately, most of our anatomy and physiology, and pathophysiology textbooks and courses do not have content around this vital body system, though ideally, nursing students would be introduced to this system when taking these prerequisite courses. Until nursing faculty request or demand that this body system is included in the essential science textbooks, they will need to strive to support nurses in gaining this knowledge. Hence, the foundational science around this body system is provided here, and it may be shared with biology faculty to encourage the inclusion of the ECS in their course offerings.

Likewise, as the cannabinoid pharmacology content is missing from most nursing pharmacology textbooks, it is included here. Faculty may weave this fundamental information throughout both pre- and post-licensure pharmacology courses. Current cannabis science evidence-based research is provided throughout the book so that the learner has a foundational knowledge base of the current state of the evidence around cannabis effectiveness and specific disease processes. With the rapid evolution of cannabis science, the reader will also need to use resources like the Cannabis Health Index's cannakeys website (https://cannakeys.com) to stay abreast of the current body of cannabis science knowledge.

This textbook is also different from other nursing textbooks in that it explores the applied art and lived experiences of cannabis care nurses, making it useful or inspiring for students who are learning about politics, policy, and advocacy. Through the humanistic approach to sharing cannabis care nurses' stories of pioneering and advocacy efforts, the emerging history of cannabis care nursing is revealed. Nurses have contributed greatly to ending cannabis prohibition, and their stories should be heard. It is hoped that new nurse leaders will be inspired to take on advocacy roles, whether these efforts be cannabis care or other related health care or population-based needs.

When considering the roles of both the cannabis care nurse and advanced practice nurse, this book takes a holistic perspective. Exploring tools like motivational interviewing, ethics, coaching techniques, and use of holistic/integrative modalities to upregulate the patient's ECS, this book also provides the readers with concepts they can apply across their nursing practice, inclusive of patients who are not actively using cannabinoid therapeutics. The ultimate goal of the cannabis care nurse is to coach patients toward maximal health and potentiation of the ECS so that the least amount of cannabis can be used to support homeostasis. Ideally, this book is a much-utilized resource shared among colleagues, and it should not end up in the resale, yard sale, or thrift store bookshelves where so many textbooks go to die.

I urge nurses to begin to notice and change their vocabulary when it comes to the name of the plant *Cannabis* L (hemp) and *Cannabis sativa* L (commonly known as marijuana). Note that calling the plant cannabis instead of marijuana, weed, pot, dope, etc., helps to move us away from derogatory and racist terms ("marijuana" was used as a slanderous term aimed at migrants from Mexico who brought the plant with them) and into a place of science and professionalism when nurses discuss this herbal plant. The term "marijuana" is used at times in this text, mostly to refer to state medical marijuana programs (MMPs), as that is what most states still call these programs, or for historical purposes.

CHAPTER OUTLINE

This textbook is designed to be used by nurses both in academia and in practice settings. The chapters take different approaches to support learning in a variety of ways: some may have case studies, while others may have applied and verify learning points or nursing implications highlighted. All chapters have NCLEX-style questions at the end to support and verify learning. The first five chapters are foundational for the nurse's learning, as they provide an overview of the history of cannabis prohibition and regulation, information on the ECS, and pharmacodynamics and pharmacokinetics. The next four chapters focus on the nurse's role in cannabis care.

Chapter 1: History of Cannabis and Prohibition

This chapter explores the history of the cannabis plant from ancient times through prohibition. This chapter also highlights some of the work done by cannabis care nurse pioneers who have worked to help end prohibition. As learners delve into growing their knowledge base around the medicinal use of cannabis, it will become important to reflect on any prohibition-era biases one may have toward this medicine and how these biases might interfere with the ability to support patients' autonomous decision-making process around the use of medical cannabis. Over 100 years ago, the prohibition movement began to traverse across the United States, state by state, despite the medical establishment's stance against prohibition of cannabis and the American Medical Association's call for more research around the medicinal use of cannabis. Prior to prohibition, cannabis was a first-line medication that was produced by companies like Eli Lily and Pfizer, and cannabis tinctures could be purchased at the corner drug store. Knowing the history of this medicinal herb is an essential aspect of understanding the current political climate of prohibition.

Chapter 2: The Human Endocannabinoid System (ECS): Physiology

This chapter walks the reader through the complexities of the largest receptor system in the body, the ECS. The reader will grow in their understanding of how we produce our human cannabis–like substances, called endocannabinoids. The endocannabinoids support the body's ability to remain in homeostasis; they are made on demand and are broken down versus being stored in the body. With a strong foundation around the physiology of this system, the reader will be prepared to consider how cannabis moves in the body (pharmacokinetics), the mechanisms and effects of cannabis in the body (pharmacodynamics), and the need for patients to have access to safe, tested cannabinoid medicines. For many nurses and students, once they understand the physiology of the ECS, they begin to question their previous stance about this medicine and move toward greater acceptance of cannabis as medicine.

Chapter 3: Cannabis Pharmacology: From the Whole Plant to Pharmaceutical Applications

This chapter was written by nurses, for nurses. The authors discuss the pharmacokinetics of the cannabis plant, from phytocannabinoids to terpenes. An exploration of other cannabinoid plants and synthetic cannabinoid drugs is also included. This chapter explores the effects, side effects, dosing, delivery methods, safety, and substance use disorders. Unlike many other prescribed allopathic medicines, patients generally self-titrate their medicine to find the lowest effective dose to palliate their symptoms. This chapter supports the reader in their preparation to coach and guide patients through this cannabis titration process, which consists of sharing with patients evidence-based approaches that support the safe and effective use of cannabis.

Chapter 4: Cannabidiol

Due to the grand popularity of cannabidiol or CBD, this one phytocannabinoid has been singled out for special consideration in this textbook. CBD is now available in every product from soap to lip balm, but we must not assume that CBD's wide availability ensures that safe products are being used. Many patients use CBD without knowing the potential drug–drug interactions or how to ascertain the quality of the product they are using. This chapter explores all things CBD, including dose, drug–drug interactions, CBD from hemp versus CBD from cannabis, and the body of evidence related to CBD's effectiveness. With the inclusion of case studies and dosing considerations, the nurse explores how CBD can be used to potentiate the ECS.

Chapter 5: Cannabis Science: Reviewing Trends

This chapter provides the reader with a review of some of the recent cannabis science evidence. Since the National Academies of Science, Engineering, and Medicine

(NASEM, 2017) issued a report on levels of evidence related to cannabis science effectiveness, the science continues to emerge. This chapter provides some highlights around promising cannabinoid research findings and helps the reader to build a foundation of knowledge related to particular medical issues and cannabis effectiveness. The findings shared here expand upon the NASEM report and point the reader toward a more in-depth exploration of the evidence base. Cannabis is the most studied plant on the planet, and new findings emerge daily. The reader is invited to also begin their own evidence-based exploration of the current findings.

Chapter 6: The Nurse's Role: Providing Cannabis Care

This chapter provides an overview of the role of the nurse when providing care for cannabis patients. A summary of how nursing theory guides the cannabis care nurse's practice is provided. Additionally, skills such as motivational interviewing, coaching, spiritual care, ethics, use of holistic modalities to upregulate the ECS, and the applied nursing process with cannabis care patients are offered. With advocacy techniques and a review of how to critique cannabis science findings, the reader is prepared with the knowledge to enact the role of the nurse with patients using medical cannabis. Many of these holistic skills can also be used with the nurse's other patient care efforts beyond caring for medical cannabis patients.

Chapter 7: Advanced Practice Nursing Considerations

Currently, APRNs in some medical cannabis states can support potential medical cannabis patients in receiving their medical recommendation or certification to use cannabis. For APRN nurses, this chapter reviews the process of assessing patients for medical cannabis qualification. Training, the role of the APRN, educating patients and other providers, and how to best support patients with the titration process are reviewed. The APRN should define the legal, ethical, and complex practice issue considerations that come with providing direct patient cannabis care.

Chapter 8: Legal, Ethical, and Advocacy Concerns: Cannabis From the Federal to State Level

Readers will learn about the current federal status of cannabis in the United States, how to review their state cannabis laws, advocacy approaches, and the grand ethical considerations related to cannabis prohibition. Social justice issues related to the long cannabis prohibition era are discussed. Nurse advocacy pioneers are highlighted. Ideally, the nurse is inspired to integrate their role of patient advocacy with cannabis care or other social justice issues.

Chapter 9: The Cannabis Care Nurse's Experience

This final chapter explores the lived experience of the cannabis care nurse. Expert cannabis care nurses share their approaches, challenges, and successes with providing patients with cannabis care. Highlights from nurses who work directly with cannabis care patients are provided as they explore telemedicine, documentation, entrepreneurship, and professionalism.

INTO THE FUTURE: BEYOND CANNABIS PROHIBITION

In the United States, we are gradually, state by state, leaving the prohibition era and entering an era of cannabis regulation. There is hope that the United States can begin to contribute more to the emerging science that supports the high safety profile of the plant. Meanwhile, other countries that have ended prohibition already are at the forefront of enacting high-quality research and human trials that remain, at the time of the writing of this chapter, federally illegal in the United States.

While this book is slated to be published in 2021, cannabis care nursing is an evolving field of practice and will continue to change until (and then likely beyond) the next edition of this textbook is published. The *Scope and Standards of Practice for Cannabis Nurses* (American Cannabis Nurses Association) was developed in 2017 and revised in 2019 to include the APRN role. However, it is a long process to develop nursing specialty areas and certifications to be officially recognized by groups like the American Nurses Credentialing Center. The scope and standards document remains in an evolving state, with the role of the cannabis care nurse continuing to emerge as the *who*, *what*, *where*, *why*, *when*, and *how* of cannabis care nursing grows and is further defined.

As laws shift and research emerges, nurses may find themselves in a unique place to be the leaders in coaching and educating patients around how to safely and effectively use cannabis and also upregulate the human ECS through lifestyle changes and use of holistic modalities to potentiate the body toward homeostasis. There is still much work to be done to define our role in this specialty medical area, particularly around the need for advocacy in support of patients and populations. As we find our way out of the federal cannabis prohibition era and into an era of regulation, there is the real risk that medicinal cannabis use could be even more challenging for patients in need if cost, access, and quality are not adequately addressed. While it would be nice to think of cannabis potentially being deregulated and sold in ways that are similar to how other herbal supplements are sold, while maintaining patients' rights to grow their own medicine, it is more likely that cannabis regulation will create new challenges around patient access. Nurses must therefore be prepared to continually advocate for patients' rights to access safe, tested, affordable cannabinoid therapeutics.

References

National Council of States Boards of Nursing. (2018). THE NCSBN national nursing guidelines for medical marijuana. *Journal of Nursing Regulation, 9*(2), S5-S46. https://doi.org/10.1016/S2155-8256(18)30098-X
National Academies of Science, Engineering, and Medicine. (2017). *The health effects of cannabis and cannabinoids: The current state of evidence and recommendations for research.* National Academies Press.

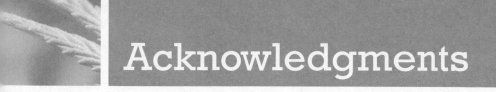

Acknowledgments

This book was inspired by many of the authors of the chapters and the other nurses featured throughout it. During an era of cannabis prohibition, these nurses' commitment to bringing cannabis care nursing into the mainstream allopathic care settings is commendable, as many of them risked ridicule and loss of income to do the right thing to end the prohibition of a herbal plant that has evolved to support human health and homeostasis. These nurses have become my friends, and they understand the challenges of being a leader in the face of stigmatization. The American Cannabis Nurses Association (ACNA) is a 501c3 nonprofit organization that created a safe haven and connected community for those nurses who are committed to patients having access to safe, tested, and affordable cannabinoid therapeutics.

I also can't express enough gratitude to the mentors I have had along my nursing journey including Dr. Kathleen O'Conner, Dr. Alfonso Montuori, Dr. Jean Watson, and Dr. Peggy Chinn. Cannabis care medical doctors have also taught me about cannabis and the endocannabinoid system including Dr. Dustin Sulak and Dr. Ethan Russo. And of course a legion of great caring nurses have supported my healing journey, from my friends at ACNA to the amazing members of the American Holistic Nurses Association: both organizations have become my family. Many thanks to my colleagues at Pacific College of Health and Science who believed in medical cannabis care so much that they created the platform for us to develop the first academic Medical Cannabis Certificate for health care professionals. And lastly and most importantly, I offer unending gratitude and all of my love to my family, Brackett Clark, Kacey-Jane Clark, and Brackett-Anne Clark, for creating a home-space filled with love, care, and encouragement that allowed for this work to emerge in a very short period of time: you made this book possible!

Contents

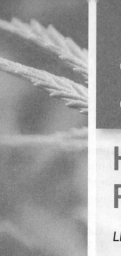

1

History of Cannabis and Prohibition

Llewellyn Dawn Smith, MSN, RN

CONCEPTS AND CONSIDERATIONS

Historical perspectives related to cannabis medicine may help nurses to understand how the past influences the current societal context of medical cannabis and healthcare. Learning this historical knowledge is foundational for all nurses who are managing complex medicinal cannabis patient issues and working with interprofessional healthcare providers. Current cannabis perspectives are often shrouded in misinformation, and knowing the history behind cannabis and prohibition helps the nurse to best address these issues. This chapter explores the historical roots of cannabis and the societal impact prohibition has made. As we move from an era of prohibition to that of regulation, it is clear that we must know where we came from to continue the journey toward cannabis emancipation.

Learning Outcomes

Upon completion of this chapter, the learners will:

- Understand the cultural significance of cannabis consumption throughout history.
- Develop a working historical foundation for understanding the current state of legalization of medical and recreational use of cannabis.
- Understand social justice implications for patients utilizing medical cannabis.
- Identify significant cannabis care nurse pioneers.

Cannabis has in the past been considered by some to be "just a weed," yet it has a long and interesting history. The cannabis plant carries with it a story that is full of wonder, excitement, mystery, enchantment, adventure, danger, benevolence, and redemption. This chapter covers an essential historical knowledge regarding cannabis therapeutics so that the nurse will understand the medicinal evolution of the cannabis plant's origins and how American society now finds itself in the confusing situation of conflicting legal, social justice, and regulatory issues surrounding its use, both medically and recreationally. Cannabis prohibition is a global issue that impacts patients and their ability to palliate symptoms and move toward healing.

Nursing standards and curriculum dictate that nursing practice be carried out with compassion and respect for the dignity, worth, and unique attributes of all people (American Nurses Association [ANA], 2018). Nurses are educated to help patients by taking on the roles of advocacy, providing patients with opportunities for informed decision-making and seeking guidance when individual rights conflict with that of the public health guidelines. The nurse identifies and advocates for vulnerable populations suffering from issues related to social injustice, racial inequality, and health disparities. Utilizing evidence, science, and collaboration, the nurse "advances policies, programs services and practice that reflect respect, equality, and values for diversity and inclusion" (ANA, 2018, p. 70). Access to safe cannabis medicine is a political cause that is worthy of the nurse's advocacy: we are called to support and advocate for suffering patients who are not able to obtain legal medicinal cannabis, a relatively safe herbal medication.

The ethical and legal dilemmas surrounding the therapeutic use of cannabis and cannabinoids have been rightfully supported by the ANA since 2016. The ANA Center for Ethics and Human Rights developed a position statement in support of the removal of cannabis from federal Schedule I to facilitate clinical research about the efficacy of cannabis in the context of healthcare (ANA, 2016). This position statement accurately reflects that cannabis and cannabinoids "alleviate disease-related symptoms and side effects" and it encourages research and development of evidence-based approaches related to its use as a treatment modality.

Cannabis care nursing should be based on nursing philosophies, models, and theories. As a moral undertaking, nurses are responsible for providing vital services to society that address needs associated with human functioning (Alligood, 2013). The use of nursing philosophies during the nurse's cannabis care practice is appropriate. The concept of pairing nursing theory with cannabis therapeutics could be an extensive topic of its own, and it is now ripe for introduction in this text.

For example, Nightingale's environmental philosophy might serve to support the natural alteration in milieu created by individual consumption of the cannabis plant, allowing nature to improve health and spirits within one's perceived environment. Dorothy Johnson's Behavioral System Model, focusing on common human needs, care and comfort, stress, and tension reduction, would pair well when developing a unique body of cannabis care nursing evidence. Another excellent model to use for furthering cannabis nursing research might be Martha Rogers' Science of Unitary Human Beings, which rejected the idea of causality and considers the "pan-dimensional view of people with their world" (Alligood, 2013, p. 23). Doretha Orem's three-part model of self-care could prove useful in forming a framework for nursing curricula regarding cannabis nursing principles. The current Scope and Standards of Practice for Cannabis Nurses (Clark et al., 2019) utilized Jean Watson's theory of human caring and holistic theory to support how the nurse best cares for their cannabis care patients.

Cannabis therapeutic evidence-based nursing practices should also be developed, utilizing proven nursing theory and models to further support guidelines and standards of care that may fall within the scope of practice for this emerging nursing subspecialty. Modern-day perspectives about cannabis are generally not based on collective historical literature, science, or recent discovery. The nurse learner should have a realistic understanding surrounding the evolution of cannabis therapeutics to appreciate current trends in this controversial practice involving a reemerging plant medicine. Important historical events related to cannabis as medicine will be covered in this chapter first by global location, followed by exploring the more recent historical timelines covering the 18th, 19th, 20th, and 21st centuries. Because of the controversial nature of the topic, pro-cannabis bias may be evident within the chapter and should be acknowledged and recognized by the learner. This chapter provides the foundational historical basis from which cannabis care nursing must evolve, as we strive to meld nursing theory and emerging evidence to further define this specialty area in nursing.

ANCIENT ORIGINS AND LEGENDS

Historical perspectives of cannabis therapeutics span centuries, beginning with antiquity (Holland, 2010; Lee, 2012). It is unknown exactly how long the cannabis plant has been on earth or how it emerged, although humans have coevolved in the presence of the cannabis plant. Mankind has questioned if the cannabis plant is a biologic wonder that developed and evolved or was it a "gift from the Gods"? According to an ancient historical legend, the Dogon tribe of West Africa believed that inhabitants of the large stars Sirius A and Sirius B descended to earth from the sky and gifted the "two-dog plant" to humans (Conley, 2017). Native American Indian legends exist that described "star people" who brought cannabis to the planet. Cherokee tribes called the plant "gatunlati," honoring the name of the planet where the cannabis plant is thought to have been gifted to earth by extraterrestrials (Conley, 2017). The oldest surviving documentation for cannabis usage arises from an archaeological dig site, where 10,000-year-old clay jars from the Japanese Jōmon era were discovered to contain dried cannabis flower, confirming that cannabis has been cultivated for more than 10,000 years (Lee, 2012). Other well-preserved archaeological cannabis specimens from 2,500-year-old Chinese Yanghai Tombs have also been preserved (Holland, 2010). It is thought that many of these specimens of cannabis were used during ceremonial rituals.

A plant that is native to Central Asia since prehistoric times, the qualities and utility for cannabis quickly became well known as it traveled west with various populations. Originating in the Kush Himalayan foothills, the cannabis herb's role as a fiber and psychoactive flower migrated across the globe. Neolithic peoples had many uses for cannabis during ancient times, including fiber provision, food sources, medicinal concoctions, and ritual preparations. Lee (2012) stated that cannabis's historical path diverged into two separate roles: one path as a textile and food plant, and the other path as a psychoactive flower for medicine or a spiritual crop.

EARLY HISTORY

Cannabis plants have comingled with humans perhaps since the beginning of time (Holland, 2010). Cannabis was distributed along an essential channel of trade associated with ancient China, Central Asia, and southwest Asia to the Western world (Ren et al., 2019). It is hypothesized that the practice of smoking flower began during the

5th century BCE, as recorded by Herodotus, in the *Histories*. Ren et al. (2019) discovered a site in western China where rituals were conducted utilizing inhalation of high-dose psychoactive cannabis plants as part of burial ceremonies. Examination of the wooden smoking bowls known as a "brazier" suggested that the cannabis was smoked or orally consumed after grinding the plant matter in mortars. Chemical analysis revealed the possibility that ancient people may have hybridized and cultivated the cannabis plant for its stronger psychoactive properties through human selection and dispersal (Ren et al., 2019). Perhaps because of climate differences, western regions cultivated cannabis primarily for food and textiles, as opposed to psychoactive and medicinal purposes (Ren et al., 2019). Cannabis migrated to the West via the ancient trade route beginning with China and concluding with the Americas (Holland, 2010).

The notion of cannabis as a spiritual tool is further validated by Herodotus in the *Histories*, where he recorded that Central Asians known as the Scythians, who were warrior nomads, used the psychoactive botanical for "cleansing" during burial rites to connect with the divine and the deceased spirits. Herodotus described the funeral ceremonies of the Scythian kings where tribal members created tents and burned hemp seeds and blooms on red-hot stones, causing the Scythians to "howl for joy" after entering the tents and inhaling the vapors. These accounts were later verified by the discovery of cannabis charred kettles located within the Scythian tombs in the Altai Mountains (Mathre, 1997). A mobile society of people who utilized horse-power as a means of transportation, Scythians were also responsible for the spread of cannabis knowledge throughout the ancient civilizations (Holland, 2010; Lee, 2012). Scythian influence may have introduced these ceremonial rituals to other parts of the world (Mathre, 1997). Herodotus also wrote in the *Histories* about Araxes river island inhabitants who would get "drunk" by inhaling fumes from an unidentified fruit thrown on an open fire.

In another recent find, a 2,500-year-old well-preserved mummy was buried with cannabis. She was known as the "Siberian Ice Princess" and was discovered in 1993 from a tomb in the Altai Mountains in Russia. Newer technology reveals that the "Siberian Ice Princess" suffered from metastatic breast cancer and other ailments, and it is believed that she was medicating with cannabis as a form of comfort (IFLScience, 2019).

Cannabis History: China

O'Leary-Randall (2014, p. 20) noted in her memoir that Chinese people used medicinal "cannabis twenty-eight centuries before the birth of Christ, recommending it for a variety of disorders including rheumatic pain and constipation." China was once known as the epicenter of hemp cultivation of both textile and medicinal varieties. Documented Chinese cannabis medicine practices began about 1,800 years ago and emerged into a unique specialty specifically utilizing the seeds of the flower, also known as the "achenes" (Brand & Zhao, 2017). Achene (pronounced a-ken) means a one-seeded indehiscent dry fruit ovary that does not split at maturity (Ohio Plants Organization, 2019). Cannabis seeds were consumed as food during ancient Chinese times. Chinese legends suggested that a Chinese Buddha existed for 6 years off a daily solitary cannabis seed while awaiting enlightenment from the Gods (Mathre, 1997).

Cannabis is an annual, dioecious plant in the family of Cannabaceae (Mathre, 1997). *Cannabis sativa*, *Cannabis indica*, and *Cannabis ruderalis* are different species within the *Cannabis* genus. They originally grew in different climate zones, and they differ in appearance, growth patterns, and effect. The time of this split designation of biotypes is not well defined and there is a complicated taxonomic history (Brand & Zhao, 2017). *C. sativa* is known to produce a thin, narrow leaf and grows tall. *C. indica* produces a broad, wide, short leaf and does not grow as tall (Figure 1.1). *C. ruderalis* is a very small plant with a short flowering period. The varieties change along with the environment they are grown in, and most cannabis plants today are hybrids of these three varieties. Varieties cultivated nearer the equator, in warmer regions with more intense sunlight, tended to become more psychoactive in nature. This might explain how different regions utilized the plant for various purposes depending on how close to the equator the plant was grown.

There is some confusion among Chinese translators regarding the naming of the cannabis plant parts. The terms *mafen*, *mahua*, and *mabo* refer to the flowering tops of the plant bud or the spike-shaped inflorescence, making it difficult for scholars to translate ancient Chinese text (Brand & Zhao, 2017). Therefore, it is not known which part of the plant might have been used in ancient Chinese medicinal recipes. However, because of the psychoactive description of some concoction's effects on individuals, it is widely assumed that the flower with its seeds was used in medicinal

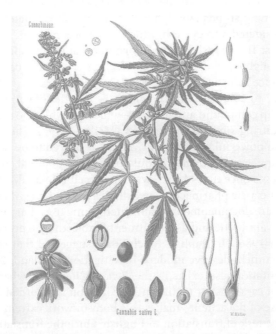

Figure 1.1: *Cannabis sativa* by Koehler. (Adapted from Franz Eugen Köhler's Medizinal-Pflantzen. Published and copyrighted by Gera-Untermhaus, FE Köhler in 1887 [1883-1914]. Open access article distributed under the terms and conditions of the Creative Commons Attribution [CC BY] license.)

recipes. The Chinese prepared cannabis elixirs, pellets, wines, and extracts to treat pain, malaria, mental illness, hysteria, cough, convulsions, and insomnia; as anesthetics; and to create happiness.

For millennia, the Chinese have used *C. sativa* (L.) as a fiber and for food and fabrics, dividing the plant's parts for differing purposes. Both medicinal and textile traditions were passed down to generations of Chinese verbally for over 2,000 years. The earliest known usage of cannabis as a medication began in China circa 2,800 BC. However, evidence of cannabis cultivation exists as far back as 4,000 BC. Known as one of the "top grains," cannabis was farmed for various purposes, including food, textiles, and oils. Chinese ancestors included cannabis as part of the "oral generation-to-generation transmission of plant lore," reaching as far back as the legendary Emperor Shen-Nung (circa 2,700 BC), a Chinese emperor and medicine man, who prescribed cannabis for his patients to address more than 100 ailments (Backes, 2014). Emperor Shen-Nung was considered a patron deity of agriculture. Legend states that his celestial nature allowed the deity to visualize his translucent abdomen and experience the effects of absorption, distribution, and synthesis of the medicine within his own body (Mathre, 1997).

Chinese oral cannabis traditions numbered more than 100 and were included in the first Chinese pharmacopoeia, *Pen-ts'ao Ching* (Backes, 2014). The *Pen-ts'ao Ching* was compiled between 0 and AD 100 and cited hundreds of Shen-Nung's cannabis treatments for conditions like rheumatic pain, gout, and malaria, with cannabis being declared the "Superior Elixirs of Immortality" (Hand et al., 2016). The oldest pharmacopoeia notes the psychoactive effects of cannabis calling it "ma-fen" or "fruit of cannabis," conveying that the plant lightens the body and facilitates spiritual effects. "Ma-fen" was considered a spicy herb, which could become toxic, and it was useful in wasting diseases. The *Pen-ts'ao Ching* informs us that when cannabis is consumed for long periods it lightens the body; the book also warns that if cannabis is taken in excess it will produce hallucinations (Backes, 2014).

Around AD 117 to 207, *Hua T'o*, known as the founder of Chinese surgery, created a boiling hemp compound and mixed it with wine, which he then used to anesthetize patients during surgical procedures (Mathre, 1997). The ancient surgeon *Hua T'o* called the powerful concoction "Ma-yo." It proved to be rather effective as an anesthetic, so much so that *Hua T'o* could perform abdominal and other invasive surgeries on patients once the "Ma-yo" was consumed (Holland, 2010). In another published ancient classic pharmacopoeia called *Pen ts'ao Kang Mu of Li Shih-Chen* in AD 1578, there are documented cannabis therapeutic uses that include efficacy as an antiemetic and antibiotic and as a treatment for bleeding, leprosy, and parasites. Centuries later in 1986, Dr. Raphael Mechoulam suggested that conditions listed in this classic document deserve modern investigation (Holland, 2010). Extensive Chinese documentation also exists in the *Bencao Literature*, where the country's long cultivation of cannabis for textile and medication is recorded (Brand & Zhao, 2017). Chinese use of the achenes makes this body of work extremely valuable and worth the arduous task of translation to English. Once the translation of the enormous resource to English occurs, these 1,800 years of documented evidence might reveal even more potential options for therapeutic applications related to today's medical cannabis market.

Cannabis History: India

Chinese use of the cannabis plant migrated toward India by 1,000 BC. Hindu Indians consumed cannabis while worshiping, and the plant was utilized for medicinal, recreational, and spiritual purposes (Hand et al., 2016). Indians consumed cannabis for many conditions: as an analgesic, anticonvulsant, anesthetic, antibiotic, and anti-inflammatory. Cannabis treated epilepsy, rabies, anxiety, rheumatism, and respiratory conditions. The prominent physician Sushruta of ancient India recommended cannabis as an antiphlegmatic because it caused the mucous membranes to dry out and created relief from congestion.

Indian culture used cannabis flowers as a religious sacrament, a household health remedy, and a recreational substance. There were more than 50 names for the plant, reflecting the many attributes within. Folk healers treated anxiety, fevers, fatigue, and insomnia with "ganja." Cannabis was even thought to improve intellect and creativity (Lee, 2012). Used during rituals to overcome enemies and evil forces, cannabis provided relief from distress and was associated with magic, medicine, religion, and cultural customs in India for centuries (Mathre, 1997). Ayurvedic medicine denotes thousands of uses for cannabis as a remedy for many ailments, including as an appetite stimulant, digestive aid, analgesic, aphrodisiac, and intoxicant.

Bhang, as cannabis was called in India, was one of five sacred plants. Cannabis was known as a "gift to the world from the god Shiva," contributing to longevity and good health (Lee, 2012). It was consumed as a tradition in Hindu worship practices. Cannabis was utilized daily during these religious activities: hashish and bhang were ingested to improve meditation and devotion (Lee, 2012), and this spiritual use also facilitated medicinal benefits (Mathre, 1997). An old Hindu Vedic scripture mentions cannabis as a sacred plant conveying that an angel lives in the leaves and is responsible for happiness, joy, and freedom (Mathre, 1997).

As late as the 1890s, India was investigating native testimony touting the therapeutic effects of cannabis. The Indian Hemp Drugs Commission of 1893 to 1894 listened to numerous accounts of the effects of cannabis upon conditions, and they noted that *C. indica* was one of the most important drugs in the Indian *Materia Medica* (Mathre, 1997).

Cannabis History: Ancient Middle East

Scythian tribes brought cannabis to the Mideast as they migrated away from their Asian tribal roots near Russia and China. Ancient Assyria Egypt recorded medicinal uses of cannabis as part of the Assyrian tablets created in the 17th century BC. Many uses for cannabis were identified including assisting with symptoms of depression and treating arthritis by using topical applications. In Judea, evidence exists of 4th-century use of cannabis to facilitate childbirth, with the case of a 14-year-old girl who died while delivering her infant. Her remains were found in a tomb along with cannabis containing delta-9-tetrahydrocannabinol (Δ9-THC), burned in a bowl and perhaps administered for labor pains or as a ritual following her untimely death (Mathre, 1997).

Cannabis oil was included in the sacred anointing oil used during the biblical era: the holy anointing oil was considered to have healing powers. Sula Benet, a Polish anthropologist, found the recipe for holy anointing oil in the Hebrew Old Testament book of Exodus and determined that the key ingredient was *q-neh bosm*, or cannabis (Backes, 2014). Researchers have cited multiple other references to religious rituals that include cannabis in the Hebrew Scriptures and the Old Testament (Holland, 2010). One use was to control convulsions, whereas another use was to encourage visionary experiences (Holland, 2010). It is hypothesized from the scripture that Jesus consumed cannabis with his disciples and that cannabis anointing oils were used during the time of Moses. Researchers theorize that Jesus and other priests used anointing oils for their healing properties in addition to their spiritual and ritual purposes (Holland, 2010). Anointing oils were to be used only by priests, this perhaps being one of the first and oldest restrictions placed on the usage of the cannabis plant.

About 900 BC, the Assyrians were aware of cannabis's psychotropic effects, and by 450 BC, cannabis usage spread throughout the Mediterranean. Cannabis was first recorded as an effective treatment for epilepsy in Arabic medicine as early as AD 1,000 and again in the 1,300 AD and 1,400 AD. There are references to cannabis medicinal use as cited in Egyptian medical texts from 1,300 BC to 1,700 BC. Arabic traders carried cannabis from India to Africa, where the leaves were used to treat malaria and dysentery symptoms (Hand et al., 2016). Medicinal use was well known in Persian medicine, where the biphasic effect of cannabis was recorded by Avicenna. Avicenna published *Avicenna's Canon of Medicine*, influencing Western medicine development from the 13th until the 19th centuries. Assyrians recorded the use of topical cannabis rubs and lotions on medical tablets, with documentation of this being found in a Louvre collection in Paris, France. Further ritualistic cannabis recipes known as *gunabu* have been documented in the Cuneiform Library and include the legendary Assyrian king Ashurbanipal and his father Esarhaddon. In ancient Mesopotamia, *gunabu* was used medicinally and spiritually in the form of oils and incense. The smell was considered a favorite of the gods during the first millennium. *Gunabu* was also a source of oil and fiber. Documentation on an Assyrian medical tablet described the use of cannabis topicals and lotions promoting "good rapport for god and man" (Holland, 2010).

Muslims have little documentation to support hashish consumption in the 13th to 16th centuries, and Muslim cultures issued severe punishment for using hashish as an intoxicant. Because medicinal cannabis usage was not excluded in the Koran, Muslim society found benefits in its therapeutic value. There is Muslim documentation to support hashish's usefulness as an antiepileptic, a diuretic, and also for "cleansing" the brain. Muslims established hemp paper–making mills, introducing this art to Europeans beginning in 1,150 AD (Mathre, 1997).

Cannabis History: Central Asia

Cannabis plants likely originated near the Shan mountains in Central Asia. This origin is the basis for today's medicinal cultivars (Grotenhermen & Russo, 2012). The Chinese and Indians first cultivated the herb for its euphoric effects, and easterners in Europe preferred the fiber and food sources cannabis provides. Most mentions of *Kannabis* in Greek and Roman literature are related to its usage as a fiber, rather than that of a medication, or in spiritual and ceremonial traditions. However, several notations are recorded documenting cannabis's multiple uses.

Pliny the Elder noted around 23 to 79 AD that boiled cannabis roots were effective for burns and gout. He was also among the first to note that cannabis was not miscible in water. Dioscorides, a doctor in AD 1st century, considered that fresh hemp seed oil was helpful for earaches and joint pain. Galen, a doctor in the 2nd century, documented euphoria resulting from oral consumption of cannabis preparations (Mathre, 1997).

Cannabis History: Africa

Africa was introduced to cannabis by land and sea traders from the Middle East, Portugal, Egypt, and India at least six centuries ago (Lee, 2012). Evidence of ancient pollen samples was found to contain traces of cannabis dating back about two millennia. The Africans developed many tools for consuming cannabis, otherwise known as *dogga*, by tribesmen. The South African *dogga* pipe was effectively shared to relieve the symptoms of asthma in humans (Mathre, 1997). Africans claimed that cannabis was medicine and recognized the plant's value for gaining insight and wisdom (Lee, 2012).

Africans have cultivated cannabis as a source of fiber, resin, and medication for centuries. Afghani Indica chemovars were known for their medicinal and intoxicant values (Brand & Zhao, 2017). In Africa, the botanical was used as a poisonous snake bite remedy, to facilitate childbirth, and as a treatment for malaria and dysentery (Mathre, 1997). Many conditions such as diarrhea, typhus, and rheumatism were treated with cannabis concoctions. West Africans burned marijuana leaves and flowers during rituals for healing in conjunction with drum circles, dancing, and singing. These ceremonies celebrated the spirit of their ancestors, thanking them for providing the botanical wonder (Lee, 2012).

Cannabis History: Europe and Americas

During the Middle Ages in Europe, there were few references to hemp. Near the 10th century, a single medicinal reference about hemp as an ingredient of a "holy salve" was recorded (Mathre, 1997). Despite the existence of consistent and extensive literature recordings about medicinal cannabis utilization in multiple pharmacopoeias (from China and India), this knowledge was poorly translated to English, creating a deficient historical background understanding for Westerners about medicinal cannabis plant sources and therapeutic purposes (Brand & Zhao, 2017). Fifteenth-century physicians discovered that cannabis effectively kills vermin and specified its use as an antibiotic. This usage spread through Western medicine in Europe and North America. This was later documented to be effective by Czech scientists in some 1,950 experiments, along with verification of cannabis as a treatment of burns and earaches (Mathre, 1997).

In the 1500s, the slave trade facilitated the migration of cannabis plants to the Americas (Hand et al., 2016). Europeans arrived at the New World in the 16th century and brought slaves and cannabis. Both slaves and ethnic Europeans carried seeds aboard the ships that landed in the Americas. English, Dutch, French, Spanish, and Portuguese vessels transporting the Europeans and their slaves had their fleets outfitted with hemp products. Slaves also utilized the cannabis flower for spiritual and euphoric purposes. Native American people were already using psychoactive plants in their religious and spiritual ceremonies and for therapeutic purposes. Slaves shared their cannabis flowers with the natives, and it was easily adopted within their culture.

Recreational and therapeutic consumption spread steadily across the continents of North and South America (Lee, 2012).

Europeans cultivated hemp primarily for its industrial purposes (Brand & Zhao, 2017). They depended on hemp to maintain their ships. The hemp plant is long and slender, and it lacks the high concentrations of the psychoactive Δ9-THC cannabinoid. Hemp was necessary for maintaining fleets of ships: rope, sails, fabric, and netting were crafted out of the plant because of its strength and durability (Lee, 2012). Hemp was considered a valuable textile at the time. Colonial-era settlers were required to grow hemp for personal purposes and to meet production needs in England as the royal establishments required. During the 1600s, the Virginia Assembly passed a law requiring all households in Jamestown to cultivate the plant for its many beneficial uses (Lee, 2012). Rather than depend on other nations for this important supply, both North and South Americans were able to grow their own hemp.

European military demand for hemp and cannabis products used for ship rigging, sails, rope, and textiles was enormous. In 1764, King George III paid 8 pounds sterling for every bale of raw hemp delivered to London. In the late 1700s, settlers prepared for the revolutionary war by having their slaves grow and process hemp. As a result of the work of slaves, hemp materials provided paper, clothing, ropes, linens, oil, and other products. Hemp's strength contributed to the founding father's decision to declare U.S. independence from Great Britain (Lee, 2012), and the Declaration of Independence was drafted on hemp paper. Soldiers' uniforms and the U.S. flag were also made from hemp cloth (Lee, 2012).

CANNABIS IN THE 1800s

During the 1800s, hemp was well established as a fiber crop in the Americas. Hemp was very difficult to process and labor intensive. Other textiles such as cotton and new machines such as the cotton gin decreased the demand for hemp products. It was during this century that medicinal cannabis consumption developed a reputation as a curative (Mathre, 1997). Indian, African, and Middle Eastern cannabis was very different from hemp grown in Europe. The psychoactive component Δ9-THC was much less potent in the European variety of cannabis, thus making it more hemp-like.

Dr. William B. O'Shaughnessy

Dr. William B. O'Shaughnessy was an extraordinarily successful Irish scientist and doctor who conducted studies on Indian cannabis while serving the British East India Company around 1830 (Lee, 2012). His research culminated in a monograph publication depicting the various applications for cannabinoid therapy. In his clinical trials, Dr. O'Shaughnessy treated many conditions with cannabis, including rabies, cholera, tetanus, epilepsy, and rheumatism. He was one of the first to note the biphasic effects of cannabis (Lee, 2012), where a small dose causes the desired effect, but a higher dose might induce unpleasant side effects. Collaborating with German founder of homeopathy, Dr. Samuel Hahnemann, they suggested that microdosing be recommended for nervous disorders.

Upon Dr. O'Shaughnessy's return to England, he partnered with pharmacist Peter Squire and developed an alcohol-based cannabis tincture that was broadly prescribed to treat a variety of conditions and ailments (Lee, 2012). Dr. O'Shaughnessy prescribed this safe medication to treat muscle spasms, tetanus, and rabies. His extensive medicinal results provided material for well-documented literature on the various uses of the cannabis plant. Dr. O'Shaughnessy is responsible for reintroducing cannabis therapeutics into Europe and America in 1839 by authoring *On the preparations of the Indian hemp, or gunjah*. Filling a void for its medical application in Europe and America, Dr. O'Shaughnessy shared his cannabis knowledge that demonstrated usefulness in treating convulsions, muscle spasms, and as an analgesic (O'Leary-Randall, 2014).

In 1839, Dr. O'Shaughnessy recalled that a Napoleon expedition to Egypt in 1798 observed that the emperor's legendary assassins used hashish. This observation set the stage for ushering in the French literary society establishment, *Club des Hashischins*. In France, "Hashish Clubs" existed where hash was the product of choice for cannabis consumers, despite the potential for hallucinogenic effects; perhaps the hallucinogenic effect was part of hashish's therapeutic appeal (Lee, 2012). Dr. Jacques-Joseph Moreau (de Tours) of France, one of the hash club's founders, based his studies of psychotomimetic psychopharmacology on the premise that cannabis intoxication might provide some insights into the origin of mental illness (Mathre, 1997).

Dr. O'Shaughnessy is also credited with testing cannabis resin in animals, validating its safety, before treating humans with cannabis extract. He was able to provide relief for rheumatism, convulsions, muscle spasms, and rabies with the concoction. Dr. O'Shaughnessy successfully treated the symptoms of vomiting and diarrhea from cholera with cannabis drops. Supported by Dr. O'Shaughnessy's research, cannabis medication demonstrated successful treatment for many diseases and conditions in the 19th century. Around 1840, the doctor brought his precious life's work from India back to London with samples for the Royal Botanical Gardens.

During the next 60 years, over 100 articles on the value of cannabis medicine were published (Mathre, 1997). Sir William Brooke O'Shaughnessy (1809-1889) was knighted by Queen Victoria in 1856 for his distinguished services. Sir William possessed a broad range of interests beyond cannabis. His talents included a passion for biochemistry, implementation of intravenous therapy, and authoring a standard chemistry textbook. In another significant humanitarian act, Dr. O'Shaughnessy introduced the telegraph service to India while he was conducting cannabis research on animals and humans (Backes, 2014).

Dr. J. R. Reynolds

One of the most famous accounts of cannabis recommendation in the 1800s was for menstrual cramps suffered by Queen Victoria of England, prescribed by Dr. J. R. Reynolds (O'Leary-Randall, 2014). It was rumored that during the Victorian era a famous doctor to the Crown, Sir John Russell Reynolds, prescribed Queen Victoria a hemp tincture to relieve painful menstrual cramps and help with sleep. Sir John suggested administering it carefully as he felt it was one of the most valuable medications (Lee, 2012).

Without the burden of modern stigmatization, in 1890, Dr. Reynolds went on to publish a paper, "Therapeutic uses and toxic effects of *Cannabis Indica*." In the British medical journal, *The Lancet*, Sir John wrote about cannabis's efficacy in treating elderly delirium (now called dementia). Dr. Reynolds recommended what he considered a moderate dosage of one-quarter to one-third grain of cannabis extract at bedtime to induce sound sleep and prevent senile insomnia and wandering (Backes, 2014). Dr. Reynolds once wrote that Indian hemp was useful for stopping so-called fits in adults, but described that he had not found it helpful in genuine chronic epilepsy. Sir Reynolds prescribed cannabis products for more than 30 years as an effective treatment for insomnia, dysmenorrhea, neuralgias, tics, and spasms. Sir Reynolds avoided the toxic effects of cannabis preparations by advising patients to start tinctures and extracts with very small doses and increase gradually until relief was obtained (Mathre, 1997).

CANNABIS HISTORY: LATE 1800s

By the latter half of the 1800s, more than 100 research articles about cannabis and hemp appeared in medical and scientific journals. Cannabis concoctions were abundantly prescribed and could be purchased from a pharmacy. Indian hemp appeared in the U.S. Pharmacopoeia in 1854 and many described it as a wonder drug (Lee, 2012). By 1860, the Ohio State Medical Society (OSMS) was doing research and literature reviews about the many conditions physicians had successfully treated with cannabis. OSMS noted enormous success in treating multiple ailments with cannabis as over-the-counter preparations grew in abundance, treating ailments from migraines, cough, inflammation, bronchitis, and postpartum depression (Backes, 2014). The British government conducted and published the 1893 to 1894 "Indian Hemp Drugs Commission" report. This report was the culmination of extensive testimonies and interviews conducted in India regarding the effects of hemp drugs with a summary of conclusions. The commission concluded that cannabis may have a medicinal effect and be helpful when used in moderation (Backes, 2014).

Eighteenth-century botanists confused the two sexes of the cannabis plant for many years, with old textbooks showing inaccurate pictures of the male and female versions of the plant, mixing up the male and female cultivar. This mistake was corrected by Linnaeus when he classified *C. sativa* L. in 1753 by separating the male and female plants in various stages of development. Linnaeus also described *C. indica* as a potentially different species (Mathre, 1997).

Some of the U.S. founding fathers were procannabis. George Washington attempted to grow and separate hemp at Mount Vernon to provide adequate hemp supplies for early Americans. Thomas Jefferson contributed to the cause by designing a hemp rake to break down the strong raw hemp stalk and fibers. The slave population in early America might have been aware of cannabis's intoxicating effects, but there is no evidence that plantation owners were using it for medicinal or euphoric purposes (Mathre, 1997). Medicinal usage continued to grow rapidly until the early 1900s when more modern drugs such as aspirin and vaccines reduced the demand for cannabis medicine (Hand et al., 2016).

CANNABIS HISTORY: 1900s AND FREEDOM

In Europe and the Americas, the early 19th century was a period where individuals could autonomously consume cannabis products and psychedelic entheogens simply by entering an apothecary and purchasing substances of choice. No medical prescriptions were needed. Folk medicine and herbal remedies prevailed for much of the century (Lee, 2012). Cannabis consumption was deemed as essential for both medical and recreational purposes. The cannabis plant was frequently eaten. Inhalation and smoking emerged later as a delivery method. There was no stigma attached to cannabis, and its usage was considered stylish. All of the drugs that were later considered to be illicit were available to the average consumer until the early 20th century: even cocaine and heroin were available through Sears (Lee, 2012). Abuse of opium was problematic for some and, unfortunately, cannabis was inaccurately associated with "narcotics." Usage of these drugs was loosely tied to vulnerable and disparaged populations, who were feared, setting the stage for the prohibition era (Lee, 2012).

CANNABIS HISTORY: THE 20TH CENTURY AND THE PROHIBITION ERA

The Pure Food and Drug Act of 1906 and the Harrison Narcotics Tax Act of 1914 became the foundation for narcotics control and drug prohibition, preventing or hindering physicians from prescribing these substances to their patients.

Massachusetts took the first steps to restrict the sale of cannabis in 1911, allowing only pharmacists and physicians to sell it, with the plant being outlawed in the state in 1914. In the late 1920s, congress enacted the Narcotic Farms Act, which misclassified "Indian Hemp" as a "Habit-forming narcotic," establishing a moral obligation for protecting the citizens (Lee, 2012). In 1925, the League of Nations supported the International Opium Convention, with their language limiting "marijuana" and its derivatives in any manner except for medical and scientific use. The United Kingdom completely banned cannabis in 1928 (Backes, 2014).

As the industrial age began in the early 1900s, the demand for medications moved from the use of folk remedies to uniform and repeatable standardization (O'Leary-Randall, 2014). Before modern cultivation techniques, cannabis plants were grown in so many varieties that producing consistent results to align with this demand for repeatable and uniform expectations was difficult. Common botanical medications such as morphine from poppies, digitalis from foxglove, and aspirin from birch bark were being synthesized; however, pharmacists were not yet able to synthesize cannabis. Therefore, consumers and healthcare providers were trading their powders, tinctures, and elixirs for pills and injectables, which were more predictable in providing consistent results (O'Leary-Randall, 2014). Concurrently, folk and herbal medicine fell out of favor. The development of modern drug companies was prominent. Modern medications began to replace traditional and historic treatment methods (Lee, 2012).

In good faith, the U.S. government created the Pure Food and Drug Act of 1906, designed to protect the public from misrepresentation in the medication industry (Lee, 2012). Cannabis was mentioned in this legislation as an intoxicant that must be identified on the medication label. Other intoxicants included alcohol, opiates, cocaine, and chloral hydrate. This legislation was the beginning of government regulation regarding which substances people could legally consume or ingest (Lee, 2012). Cannabis, once a food, fiber, and textile, was now considered a medication and all other purposes were prohibited from importation. This effort was followed by another legislative action, the Harrison Narcotics Tax Act of 1914, which gave the government control over narcotics and held physicians accountable for recreational drug use (Lee, 2012). As a result of these legislative acts, doctors were arrested by the thousands on narcotic charges and had their medical licenses revoked. In an extreme measure of governmental control, many doctors were sent to jail to keep them from prescribing opiates.

Cultural Use in America

Cannabis consumption in America has long been a cultural tradition. People of color have historically utilized cannabis for spirituality and pleasure. African American slaves celebrated with songs and dance to drumbeat rhythms while consuming herbal cannabis in America. During the second half of the 1800s, people from Mexico were known for smoking the rampant cannabis "weed" that had become more potent as a result of the hot sun's influence over several centuries (Lee, 2012). Many poor Mexican people consumed cannabis for social purposes or to combat boredom. As Mexican refugees migrated into the United States, cannabis use endured, and it became a racial issue. The term "marijuana" was used as a racial slur against migrants and refugees from Mexico, and Mexican refugees were called "loco" when they smoked cannabis. Cannabis prohibition became a means by which to control various ethnic and minority populations, furthering racism and racial stigma associated with its use (Lee, 2012).

Around 1929, congress erroneously declared "Indian hemp" as a "habit-forming narcotic" and began treating soldiers for "marijuana addition" (Lee, 2012). Members of the armed services openly consumed cannabis until complaints about their usage surfaced and became a concern in the Panama Canal Zone. Soldiers popularized smoking during the Mexican-American war of 1910 to 1920. Pancho Villa's army inspired the ballad *La Cucaracha*, forever dubbing the butt of a marijuana cigarette a "roach" (Lee, 2012). American soldiers adopted the habit of smoking cannabis, even mixing cannabis with tobacco to create the first version of a "blunt." To control some of this activity, congress passed the Narcotic Farms Act criminalizing cannabis, claiming a moral obligation to protect people from themselves and addiction. This type of legislation also served to draw lines between society, separating races, the poverty-stricken, and foreigners (Lee, 2012), thereby enhancing stigma and racial connotations related to cannabis use. Once the Great Depression became a reality in the 1930s, societal lines became further separated.

Cannabis Prohibition: The Federal Bureau of Narcotics

The Eighteenth Constitutional Amendment became law on January 16, 1920, making alcohol consumption illegal for approximately the next 13 years. The Federal Bureau of Narcotics (FBN) was created in the 1930s and employed an alcohol prohibitionist enforcer, the imposing Harry J. Anslinger, as director. In 1933, when the eighteenth amendment was repealed, the FBN needed a new reason to continue to exist. The Great Depression affected the FBN financially and almost closed the office, which would have put Anslinger and his employees out of business and out of jobs. Although more than half the states prohibited cannabis, there was no organized governmental effort to criminalize the plant. Cannabis prohibition became the new reason for continuing to run the FBN, as the director seized an opportunity to criminalize cannabis.

The reader should be aware that some bias concerning governmental actions victimizing the cannabis plant may be evident in the following sections and care should be taken to perceive the information in an appropriate context of historical significance.

In a true entrepreneurial spirit, Anslinger recognized an opportunity to keep his bureau open and his staff employed by seeking to control cannabis. He changed the name of cannabis to "marijuana" through media publications and promoted false myths about the effects of cannabis on people, creating a smear campaign commonly known as "Reefer Madness." Governmental agencies reinforced embellished horror stories about marijuana-induced mayhem, murders, drug dens, and reefer babies, which were published by newspapers. The Reefer Madness campaign was the "fake news" of this era.

Anslinger's strategy was supported by his friend, William Randolph Hearst. Hearst was a wealthy media and newspaper mogul who hated immigrants from Mexico because of the occupation of his home during the Mexican-American war. William Randolph Hearst possessed a skilled understanding of mass psychology, which allowed him to use yellow journalism techniques to launch a propaganda campaign against people of color including Mexican refugees and migrants, "negros," and foreigners who consumed cannabis (Lee, 2012). Through the joint effort of both men, this era of Reefer Madness grew and stories were fabricated to villainize the plant. Yellow journalism techniques took advantage of white American's feelings that they were sacrificing jobs and economic wealth to people of color who were migrating into the United States. Anslinger and Hearst utilized this societal vulnerability to promote their Reefer Madness campaign. Movies were made demonstrating immoral behaviors when using "marijuana" and stigmatizing those who smoked it (Lee, 2012). Violent crime was depicted as deliberately being committed by minorities using cannabis. Interracial relationships were also depicted to be a result of cannabis use and these relationships were not only looked down upon and not accepted by society during the mid-20th century, they were also forbidden by law. Sloman (1979) suggested that one of Anslinger's primary motivations for promoting his smear campaign and yellow journalism about cannabis was the prejudicial fear that white women might comingle with people of color. Prejudicial views of the time often assumed that males of color frequently smoked the "weed" to entice young white females to join them in the fun.

Past American Cannabis Nurses Association (ACNA) president Eileen Konieczny, RN, and Wilson (2018, p. 26) keenly summarized cannabis prohibition in their best-selling book *Healing with CBD* stating: "The early 20th century was not cannabis or hemp friendly, providing a perfect storm for cannabis prohibition, with the mingling of unstable medicine, racism, greed, and power." Economic depression, poverty, and racial disparity created a political frenzy for members of congress, who responded by outlawing cannabis with the Marijuana Tax Act (MTA) of 1937 (Lee, 2012). Unlike modern 21st-century standards, the mid-1900s was not a time when society relied on scientific information to make decisions. Congress heard testimony from stakeholders before passing the MTA. Armed with a large graphic scrapbook of Hearst's articles, Anslinger testified before congress with outrageous lies about cannabis's negative effects on society as propagated by the FBN, yellow journalism, and Hollywood's tainted scripts.

The American Medical Association (AMA) testified on behalf of the medical efficacy of cannabis and supported the medicinal use of marijuana. Dr. William C. Woodward, legal counsel for the AMA, testified to congress that prohibition would prevent researchers from discovering potential future benefits from the cannabis plant. His prediction was accurate, as medical research related to cannabis efficacy is currently deficient because of the prohibition effect (Mathre, 2017; O'Leary-Randall, 2014).

Congress validated these Reefer Madness claims and took less than 2 hours to consider the bill before passing the MTA. President Franklin D. Roosevelt signed this bill into effect on October 1, 1937, effectively outlawing cannabis. It did not take long for the judicial system to convict sellers and consumers, sentencing vulnerable populations to severely unfair labor and confinement. Medical use and access were virtually eliminated by the FBN following the passing of the MTA. The FBN failed to arrest any drug cartels and only arrested a few Hollywood idols and musicians. Hemp production suffered significantly as a result of the MTA because of the excessive additional cost to farmers and importers. The MTA was successful in wiping out the domestic hemp industry. A 1942 movie called *Hemp for Victory* encouraged farmers to grow hemp to support war efforts (Lee, 2012). However, in later governmental efforts to subdue genuine uses of hemp, this patriotic film was "lost down the memory hole" (O'Leary-Randall, 2014, p. 20) by the U.S. Department of Agriculture National Archives from the Library of Congress. Fortunately, because of the diligent efforts of cannabis advocate and writer Jack Herer, another copy was located and donated to the Library of Congress replacing the lost *Hemp for Victory* movie (Mathre, 1997).

Musicians and Cannabis

Cannabis consumption and listening to music often facilitate some delightful insights within the minds of human beings. These feelings, visions, and revelations are a result of synergy that might not otherwise occur without the combination of cannabis and music. Sloman stated in *Reefer Madness* about great musicians who consume cannabis that "it always made its devotees feel good" (Sloman, 1998, p. 85). Cannabis culture and jazz music grew in popularity and spread from its origins in New Orleans northward to Chicago and New York in the 1930s. Jazz musicians were generally African Americans and, as such, they suffered stereotypes and stigma as "marijuana users." Jazz musicians adopted, utilized, and ritualized cannabis consumption from within their subculture (Sloman, 1998). Participants enjoyed the euphoria associated with the substance in conjunction with the harmonic jazz sounds. Celebrity partakers included Errol Flynn, the Marx Brothers, and many of the jazz bands of the times (Lee, 2012). These celebrities touted the medicinal effects of cannabis as therapeutic. Famous African American trumpet player, singer, and actor Louis Armstrong used cannabis daily. Many of his songs were written touting the euphoric effects of the "southern weed."

Jazz songs and cannabis consumption blurred social boundaries (Lee, 2012). Viper mythology evolved in the jazz era and was derived from black cultures: the stereotype involved smokers who knew how to select the right clothes and the right music and also understood a different language. These vipers returned to their home neighborhoods dressed as "hipsters" and were considered to have a higher social status, above the average person (Sloman, 1998). A well-known Harlem cannabis dealer, Milton "Mezz Mezzrow," sold cannabis to many of the jazz musicians and club members. An oddball viper in the jazz crowd, Milton was a white trumpet player. His cannabis solicitation was so successful that at one time the slang for marijuana was "Mezz." The mighty Mezz ran jazz clubs or "tea pads," as they were called. Tea pads were apartments in New York where consumers would gather to enjoy the herb while listening to music and socializing with others. Eventually, the mighty Mezz was arrested following the passage of the MTA in 1937, ending his career as a cannabis salesman (Konieczny & Wilson, 2018).

Cannabis Prohibition: The Marijuana Tax Act of 1937 to 1969

With the emergence of many modern pharmaceuticals in the early to mid-1900s, there was a resultant decreased demand for cannabis as a medicine. Concurrently, recreational use became prevalent in the United States among marginalized populations, those who immigrated to the country, and black, indigenous, and people of color (BIPOC) populations. These social circumstances ripened the stage for a perfect political storm, resulting in decades-long cannabis prohibition beginning in the 1930s (Konieczny & Wilson, 2018). By the mid-1930s, access to cannabis was almost impossible, even though it was still included in the U.S. Pharmacopoeia as a medication, along with the endorsement from the AMA (Backes, 2014). As the "marijuana menace" and Reefer Madness campaigns of the 1900s waged on, American folk medications were being replaced with pharmaceutical-grade synthetic medications. The MTA of 1937 made it very inconvenient for manufacturers to include cannabis in their products (Mathre, 1997).

Cannabis Prohibition: Removal from the U.S. Pharmacopoeia and National Formulary

Even though the AMA supported the medicinal use of cannabis, congress passed the MTA. Dr. William C. Woodward, legal counsel for the AMA, testified to congress that "The prevention of the use of the drug for medical purposes can accomplish no good end whatsoever. How far it may serve to deprive the public of the benefits of a drug that on further research may prove to be of substantial value, it is impossible to say" (as cited in Mathre, 1997). The only other dissenting voice before the congressional hearings was from the birdseed industry that was successful in winning some concessions for hemp seeds (O'Leary-Randall, 2014). However, Dr. Woodward did succeed in preventing absolute prohibition until Mr. Anslinger interfered by making FBN regulations so difficult for doctors to follow that it was easier to prescribe the popularized synthesized medications than it was for them to prescribe cannabis. Mr. Anslinger's and the government's unreasonable regulations led to the removal of cannabis from the U.S. Pharmacopeia and National Formulary in 1941. This created a gap in the use of cannabis as medicine, until a revival of medical interest in cannabis during the 1970s (Hand et al., 2016). Dr. Woodward was insightful with his prediction about the lack of further research involving cannabis therapeutics.

One positive result of the MTA was the agreement from governmental agencies to investigate cannabis usage. As a result, they created the LaGuardia Committee to perform this research. New York City Mayor Fiorello La Guardia was concerned about cannabis usage spreading throughout New York. He suggested the need for more investigation of cannabis use to verify skeptical reports (Konieczny & Wilson, 2018). In 1944, owing to his call for more knowledge, Mr. La Guardia (the commissioner of the New York Academy of Medicine) was selected by Anslinger to investigate the effects of cannabis. "The Marihuana Problem in the City of New York" publication studied the psychological, physical, and sociologic effects of cannabis use and concluded that the drug had no addictive qualities and was not a route to other forms of addiction, such as narcotics. It was essentially concluded that cannabis consumption was not a huge problem for youth or crime in New York City. Unfortunately, Anslinger and the FBN dismissed the report and continued to threaten and arrest medical investigators using cannabis in their research projects. The La Guardia Committee evaluated the "marijuana" issue in New York and suggested that law enforcement officials' assumptions about "marijuana" causing criminal problems were unsubstantiated. The commission even proposed that euphoria caused by cannabis might have some useful purpose in treating mental illnesses (Mathre, 1997). Despite the La Guardia report in 1951, the Boggs Act was passed and included mandated minimum sentencing for drug possession. It was subsequently followed by the Narcotics Control Act of 1956, which called for even harsher sentences (Konieczny & Wilson, 2018).

Cannabis Prohibition: The 1940s and 1950s

Cannabis's status loomed in the background during the 1940s world wars and the 1950s obsessional fear with communism. Precipitated by studies conducted by the Nazis regarding the use of drugs for mind control during warfare, a different political opinion about controlling psychedelic substances emerged. In April 1953, the CIA was working on a large budget project with the code name MKULTRA, also known as MKDELTA (O'Leary-Randall, 2014). This project was developed for army use of large-scale chemical and biologic warfare, designed to alter mind control by creating a "truth serum" to influence political outcomes. Cannabis was part of this research effort too. Anticipating fallout, all MKDELTA files were destroyed before the 1973 Watergate crisis (O'Leary-Randall, 2014). As a result of government processes, the research on cannabis completed during this MKULTRA/MKDELTA project was also flushed down the memory hole, creating yet another block for scientists and lawmakers surrounding the potential known benefits of cannabis (O'Leary-Randall, 2014).

In 1927, between World Wars I and II, three German addiction specialists, Walter Benjamin, Dr. Ernst Joel, and Dr. Fritz Frankel, began researching hashish products. These scientists held great hope for hashish as an effective treatment for mankind. Unfortunately, their research was interrupted by the Nazi regime and never completed (Lee, 2012).

Cannabis Prohibition: The 1960s and Social Issues

As the 1960s approached, there was a need for the reorganization of drug laws. The nation was involved in horrendous wars during the 1940s through the 1970s, including World War II and the Korean and Vietnam wars. Drug problems were fueled by wartime activities and heroin synthesis became abundant in parts of Asia. Southern Vietnam officials were profiting as they smuggled heroin into the United States within the body bags of war veterans (Lee, 2012). As more soldiers developed heroin addictions, the Nixon administration recognized the crisis and decided to get tough on the drug trafficking situation.

Cannabis legalization was just one of the social causes led by 1960s activist and social transformation mentor, Allen Ginsberg. Ginsberg became a trusted spokesman for the younger generation and the counterculture leading the antiprohibition movement during the civil rights era. Ironically, the American people's antiwar demonstrations were often manifested with flagrant cannabis consumption, which was associated with a grassroots effort questioning governmental and/or political policies, both nationally and internationally (Lee, 2012). Military soldiers consumed cannabis as a means of coping and protesting wartime activities. During the Vietnam War, scared military troops created a political statement and developed coping mechanisms by smoking cannabis. Soldiers bonded by participating in cannabis rituals of sharing joints, water pipes, and rifle butts among themselves. The soldiers discovered cannabis's effectiveness to maintain peacefulness, inhibit nightmares, and create calm in an otherwise chaotic and horrendous environment of war (Lee, 2012). Many troops transported Asian cannabis home in their bags when they returned from deployment in Vietnam. Perhaps this consumption was one of the first known uses of cannabis as a self-treatment for posttraumatic stress disorder (PTSD), a debilitating condition common in war-ravaged troops.

Cannabis Prohibition: The Tidal Shift Begins, 1970s to 1990s

Social justice issues involving global wars and civil rights movements during the 1960s ripened the emergence of recreational cannabis use by the counterculture in the following decade across the United States (Hand et al., 2016). This cultural phenomenon developed as a result of frustration with government, politics, and world events. The counterculture population began as large groups of young adults, mostly students, who valued antiestablishment viewpoints. The counterculture advocated for democracy through demonstrations. The use of cannabis during these protests was common. Illegal cannabis was defiantly used by protestors to demonstrate their antiwar and antiprejudice values during organized political demonstrations. Civil rights efforts in combination with the emerging counterculture during the 1960s and 1970s manifested a massive increase in consumption of cannabis for recreational purposes, bringing the use of the plant back into vogue. Prejudice against blacks and musicians was not exclusive, as an emerging group of cannabis consuming people included white, middle-class college students and "hippies" who developed a comradery of liberal ideals. This counterculture population suffered through several awful wars, and the moral injury inflicted by complicated and unimaginable cataclysmic events spawned a change in attitudes about the future. Hippies were just another subset of vulnerable groups that governmental administrations, like Nixon's, felt could be managed with societal control mechanisms in favor of cannabis prohibition (O'Leary-Randall, 2014).

With recreational cannabis use spotlighted by the counterculture, governmental agencies engaged in studies to discover the active components of cannabis. Dr. Raphael Mechoulam originally conducted cannabis research in Israel until the U.S. government hired him at the National Institutes of Health (NIH; Backes, 2014). Dr. Mechoulam began studying cannabinoids, including cannabidiol (CBD). On the basis of this research, he and his colleagues were able to isolate Δ9-THC shortly thereafter. The CBD and Δ9-THC cannabinoid molecules provided the foundation for Dr. Machoulam's discovery of the endocannabinoid system (ECS) in 1964. The human ECS has evolved over thousands of years. In 1964, Gaoni and Mechoulam isolated Δ9-THC, the psychoactive cannabinoid found in the plant's cola. Scientists could now study cannabis compounds' effects on people. Later, in 1988, scientists discovered the cannabinoid receptors CB1 and then CB2 (Konieczny & Wilson, 2018).

Lyndon Johnson drafted legislation, signed by President Richard Nixon in 1969, called the Comprehensive Drug Abuse Prevention and Control Act of 1970. It divided illicit drugs into four schedules, separating the medications by its potential for abuse. This was the beginning of the Controlled Substances Act passed in 1970 and established five drug schedules. In an effort not to confuse legal medications with illicit ones, pharmaceutical interest insisted that a Schedule I be created, outlining certain substances as having "no medical value" and as unsafe for physicians to prescribe. Proponents of this Schedule I felt that this separation would eliminate public confusion about legal and illegal substances while creating a hard stance against drug abuse (O'Leary-Randall, 2014).

Senator Ted Kennedy and other congressmen objected to the assumption that cannabis was as dangerous as LSD and heroin, and they asked for scientific proof. The lawmakers were able to access over 5,000 years of past medical usage; however, the evidence trail came to a halt beginning with the 1937 Medical MTA, falling into the emptiness of what was called the "Memory Hole" (O'Leary-Randall, 2014). Prohibitionists insisted that ancient uses of cannabis medication were mere "folklore," and the black hole prompted Kennedy and others to request research to determine just how dangerous cannabis was. The Nixon administration compromised and authorized a government-financed research effort designed to scientifically evaluate cannabis to fill in the knowledge gaps: the National Institute on Drug Abuse (NIDA).

Following an inquiry by lawmakers, the National Commission on Marihuana and Drug Abuse, otherwise called the Shafer Commission, penned a report to President Nixon concluding that cannabis was not a priority, it was not addictive, and it did not lead to consumption of more intoxicating substances (Brand & Zhao, 2017). The Shafer Commission led by Pennsylvania Governor Raymond P. Shafer recommended in March 1972 that cannabis should be rescheduled and decriminalized (O'Leary-Randall, 2014), yet President Nixon ignored the findings from the "White Paper on Drug Abuse: A Report to the President." The report included evidence of cannabis treatments for glaucoma, migraines, alcoholism, and terminal cancer. Nixon dismissed the Commission's recommendation during the reelection time. "In many parts of the world marijuana has been and still is, used as a folk medicine"—the NIDA report to congress dismissed the plant's vast history of medical use with a single line, reducing 5,000 years of use to nothing more than "folklore" (O'Leary-Randall, 2014, p. 26).

When Ronald Reagan took office in 1981, he promised to crack down on substance abuse and continue to rebuild the war on drugs that President Nixon started in the early 1970s. In 1982, President Reagan's wife, the First Lady Nancy Reagan, went on to launch the "Just Say No" campaign. In 1986, President Reagan signed the Anti-Drug Act. He then procured 1.7 billion dollars to continue this war on drugs, while also creating minimum sentencing for specific drug offenses. These events led to an increase in arrests and incarceration, particularly among vulnerable minorities (Konieczny & Wilson, 2018). In 1980, fewer than 50,000 people were incarcerated for drug offenses; by the late 1990s, that number had leaped up to over 400,000 people.

FROM PROHIBITION TO REGULATION: CURRENT CANNABIS AFFAIRS

Cannabis remains a Schedule I narcotic on the Controlled Substance Act, even as the U.S. government's NIH holds a patent for cannabinoids as healing substances, the same controlled substances it lists as dangerous. Patent no. 6630507 designates cannabinoids as powerful antioxidants and neuroprotectants that are safe for human consumption (Konieczny & Wilson, 2018). The patent's abstract summarizes that cannabinoids are neuroprotectants that limit brain damage following ischemia, stroke, and trauma; in addition, the patent states that cannabinoids act as free radical scavengers that repair many pathologic conditions. Cannabis may assist in the treatment of neurodegenerative diseases such as Alzheimer's, Parkinson's, and human immunodeficiency virus dementia. CBD is most useful in treating neurodegenerative diseases because the psychoactive effects are avoided if Δ9-THC is not included in treatment. Many other comprehensive disease processes can be potentially treated with the powerful antioxidant properties of cannabinoids. However, because of cannabis's status as a Schedule I drug, scientists in the United States are unable to perform clinical investigations to confirm efficacy claimed by this patent. Luckily, other countries such as Israel, China, and Iran are leading the charge of studying the healing powers of cannabinoids and their interactions with the ECS (Figure 1.2).

The medical cannabis movement has taken several decades to create a presence in modern medicine. There are multiple states in the nation that are asserting their state's rights to provide medical access to cannabis for their citizens. The state of California led the way in cannabis law reform by passing the Compassionate Use Act of 1996, which was filed on September 29, 1995, in the city of Sacramento (Lee, 2012).

US006630507B1

(12) **United States Patent**   (10) **Patent No.:**   **US 6,630,507 B1**
Hampson et al.   (45) **Date of Patent:**   Oct. 7, 2003

Figure 1.2: **U.S. patent no: 6,630,507 B1.**

Under the leadership of activist Dennis Peron, the golden state was responding to the AIDS epidemic with Proposition 215. In San Francisco, during the 1990s, amid the AIDS epidemic, 80% of voters on a San Francisco ballot item Proposition recommended that cannabis be available legally for those in medical need. Proposition 215, a California statewide ballot initiative, was crafted with language that stated seriously ill Californians had the right to use, obtain, and cultivate cannabis on the recommendation of a doctor to treat cancer, anorexia, AIDS, pain, spasticity, glaucoma, arthritis, migraines, or any other illness where cannabis might provide relief. The passing of this historic legislation opened the door for other states to reform their medical cannabis laws (Mathre, 1997). Acting on this initiative, in 1992, the San Francisco board of supervisors approved therapeutic cannabis for AIDS, glaucoma, cancer, spastic-and-convulsive diseases, and chronic pain.

Cannabis use or possession in California was designated a low arrest priority. The statewide ballot initiative was the brainchild of Denis Peron, a gay veteran who founded the Cannabis Buyers Club in the early 1990s. He established a medical registry of more than 10,000 patients and named it the "Cannabis Buyers Club" (Mathre, 1997). Peron, otherwise known as the "Prince of Pot," and his colleagues risked federal arrest and launched the cannabis club as an avenue for AIDS patients and other medical consumers to obtain medical cannabis with support from San Francisco city officials (Lee, 2012). Peron's colleagues were other well-known advocates for cannabis reform, including Robert Randall, the first recognized medical cannabis patient in the United States and the cannabis nurse activist Alice O'Leary-Randall's husband.

Through his nonprofit Alliance for Cannabis Therapeutics (ACT), Randall supported AIDS patients by helping them to get their medicine from the government by assisting patients with completing their compassionate investigational new drug program applications (Sloman, 1979). The Randalls created "MARS, the Marijuana/AIDS Research Service," which assisted at least 50 people to obtain government marijuana by petitioning the Food and Drug Administration (FDA) for legal access. Other supporters for Dennis Peron and Proposition 215 included prominent wealthy businessmen like George Soros, Peter Lewis, Ethan Nadelmann, Jack Herer, Dr. Todd Mikuriya, Laurance Rockefeller, George Zimmerman, Gail Zappa, and Larry Flynt. "Brownie Mary" Rathbun popularized her potent pot brownies among cancer and AIDS patients in San Francisco at Peron's Buyers Club (Sloman, 1979).

Talented author Jack Herer wrote the book *The Emperor Wears No Clothes* in 1985, and it became the bible of the hemp movement. Herer shared that hemp could replace many other textile substances to make paper, clothing, and building materials; furthermore, it was naturally pest repellent, could be used as a medicine and a food source, and just might save the world from environmental disaster (Sloman, 1979). Unfortunately for the San Francisco Cannabis Buyers Club, the medical cannabis movement angered the U.S. Attorney General, and he ordered the Bureau of Narcotic Enforcement agency to raid Peron's business, confiscating money and medication, essentially closing the cannabis refuge. In response to the situation, the comic strip Doonesbury, created by Garry Trudeau, helped the cause by running 2 weeks of comic strips dealing with the medical cannabis movement. During the Proposition 215 campaign, Doonesbury characters criticized Attorney General Dan Lungren for "raiding a sanctuary for dying AIDS and cancer patients." This both angered the administration and called the public's attention to the medical use of cannabis in California (Figure 1.3).

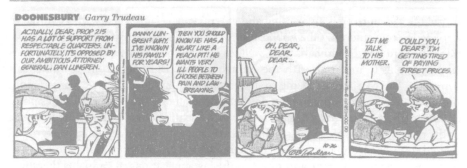

Figure 1.3: **Doonesbury cartoon by Garry Trudeau.**

In addition to displaying positive influence for cannabis consumers, the group was able to raise the financial capital to run a successful ballot campaign. Political supporters included Congressman Newt Gingrich, who sponsored H.R. bill 4498 providing for the therapeutic use and supply of cannabis to patients with the threatening illness. Peron also had monetary and legal support from the National Organization for the Reform of Marijuana Laws (NORML). Not being the best strategic planner or rule follower, Peron was assisted by associate rule monger Scott Imler, a seizure sufferer who managed his symptoms with cannabis. The collaborative efforts of this group of medical cannabis advocates were so effective in the late 1980s that the Drug Enforcement Administration's (DEA's) own chief administrative law judge, Francis L. Young, declared in 1988 that cannabis is safe and should be rescheduled (Lee, 2012). Despite progress in cannabis reform during the early 1990s in California, DEA officials and President George H. W. Bush ignored Judge Young's recommendation and declared an escalation of the war on drugs later in 1989, further complicating the efforts of Peron and his colleagues on the federal level (Lee, 2012).

Thanks to the effort with Proposition 215 in California, the medical movement established a positive momentum across the nation. As a result, many states have exercised their rights by creating policies and laws that support consumers who find the effects of cannabis therapeutics beneficial for their medical conditions. Society is beginning to see some support for reform on the federal level. At the time of this writing, federal legislation has been introduced, calling for the removal of cannabis from Schedule I status and the end to prohibition. In addition, laws for adult-use cannabis were enacted in more than 11 pioneering states and Washington, DC. These actions are paving the way for other states to assert their rights regarding recreational cannabis regulation. The cannabis industry is becoming a driving financial force in today's economy, contributing to employment opportunities, free consumer choice, and economic success. And finally, the budding cannabis industry is eagerly beginning to support research and clinical human trials to determine both the benefits and limitations of cannabis therapeutics, both medically and recreationally.

With a solid background in the historical implications of cannabis, from medicine to prohibition and back to medicine again, the reader is now prepared to explore some of the implications of cannabis nursing, the end of the prohibition era, and the movement toward cannabis care as a specialty in nursing.

CANNABIS NURSING AND NURSING PIONEERS

Cannabis care nursing is an exciting and emerging new subspecialty where in-depth knowledge implementing the application of medical cannabis processes guides patients toward improved health and wellness. Numerous states are supporting consumers' rights to medicate with the cannabis plant. The population of individuals across the United States choosing to utilize cannabis therapeutics is growing rapidly. Inconsistency in our cannabis laws nationally and among the individual states poses a barrier that requires diligent navigation, for which the nurse is duly suited. As one of the most trusted professionals in healthcare, and with our educational background related to wellness and disease processes, nurses are uniquely positioned to help patients navigate the complex and often confusing applications of cannabis therapeutics. Medical cannabis is a useful adjunctive therapy for many conditions and disease processes.

Being natural educators, nurses teach patients principles for achieving healthcare goals. Nurses who practice with cannabis patients should possess intimate knowledge of the ECS and understand cannabinoid therapeutics. Cannabis care nurses can assist patients as they treat conditions, primarily through education and coaching. A care plan that identifies treatable conditions according to desired outcomes should be developed and implemented. Nurse coaches might educate patients regarding appropriate cultivar/chemovar selection, on the basis of a cannabinoid profile, and provide coaching about the initiation of cannabis medication. Education about possible methods of titration to determine the right dosage to produce desired effects should also be provided. Directing patients toward cannabis science evidence related to their condition is another action that nurses can take. Cannabis nurse leaders propose that perhaps all "budtenders" working in medical cannabis dispensaries should collaborate with cannabis care nurses who have the education, knowledge, experience, and skills necessary to properly guide patient usage of medicinal cannabis.

With such a wide array of potential benefits, cannabis therapeutics should be properly implemented on the basis of nursing theory and the nursing process. The profession of nursing is an academic discipline based on science and artful practice. The nursing process is an excellent tool for assisting patients' achievement of their healthcare goals, regardless of their current state of wellness. When developing a nursing care plan for the cannabis consumer, the nurse must consider which nursing theories, philosophies, and models are the most appropriate to base the individual's goals of care upon. Theory utilization facilitates change by influencing and developing nursing's knowledge and restructuring the current practice of applying medical cannabis recommendations. Specialty nursing is based on the praxis of related knowledge development. As an emerging subspecialty, cannabis nursing leaders are in the preliminary phases of collecting theory-based nursing research data to create a solid foundation for scope and standards of practicing as a cannabis nurse consultant. The National Council of State Board of Nursing Guidelines for Medical Marijuana of 2018 outlines the foundational knowledge about cannabis therapeutics all nurses should know. Later chapters in this text expand on the contents of this important document.

Florence Nightingale

Florence Nightingale, the founder of modern nursing, referenced cannabis in one of her many written letters (Nightingale, 1882). Miss Nightingale's archived collection is housed at the Wellcome Library in London, England. Although little is recorded about her personal experiences utilizing cannabis therapeutics in practice, there is some evidence that implies her support of such medical usage. In a letter to her niece, Margaret Varney, Nightingale refers to Florence's ill sister Parthenope Verney. She conveys her gratitude that Margaret is coming to provide some care for Parthenope and writes about her desire to discuss her sister's state of health with the niece before a visit from Parthenope's doctor. Within the letter dated St. Thomas' Day, December 21, 1882, Nightingale shared with Margaret her concern that she was "very anxious to hear what the doctor says [about Parthenope's condition]. And, he must change the 'bhang' [hashish] pill, must he not?"

Some conclusions might be drawn about this recorded letter regarding Ms. Nightingale's insights surrounding cannabis therapeutics. Undoubtedly, the founder of nursing is aware of cannabis's therapeutic usage for her sister. There also appears to be an acceptance of the usage, as it was commonly prescribed in the late 1800s. Furthermore, she is interested in considering the dosage because she suggests hearing what the doctor thinks about the effects the cannabis medication may be having on her sister and wonders if the pill must be changed. One must wonder what change in dosage Ms. Nightingale was seeking and why. What were Parthenope's manifestations on the hashish pill? And, how were the medicines prepared, and were the results consistent between prescriptions? Or perhaps, the dosages were strain and preparation dependent, causing the effects to vary. Regardless of all the potential insights of Ms. Nightingale's stance regarding cannabis therapeutics, the fact remains that Florence Nightingale was aware of the therapeutic purposes found in the cannabis plant and she appears to support its usage for her sister's health issues.

This section has provided the reader with a broad overview of the history of cannabis as medicine. The section ensures that the reader is aware of the long medicinal nature of the herb and the challenges prohibition brought forth in humans accessing it for healing.

The next section reviews some of the more contemporary cannabis nursing history, identifying some of the key players in the movement and sharing their knowledge for all nurses to consider. The reader should consider that cannabis care nursing is intertwined with the social justice issues related to prohibition and the human right to use medicinal cannabis as a healing and palliative supplement that supports human homeostasis.

Mary Lynn Mathre, MSN, RN, CARN

As one might imagine, the "Mother of Cannabis Nursing" is a fierce military maverick who defiantly challenged drug prohibition during the 1980s by researching cannabis usage and demonstrating that cannabis consumption has a legitimate role as a therapeutic medicine, thereby creating the cannabis nursing movement. The title certainly belongs to such a staunch advocator and cannabis nurse educator such as Mary Lynn Mathre, MSN, RN, CARN (Figure 1.4). When others were "just saying no," Ms. Mathre was saying "yes" to medical cannabis. For decades, Ms. Mathre has passionately demonstrated significant professional nursing contributions on behalf of medical cannabis patients, developing public education and supporting veterans' rights regarding cannabis reform.

Mary Lynn (aka "ML") graduated from the College of Saint Teresa in Winona, Minnesota, in 1975, and she began her nursing career in the U.S. Navy Nurse Corps. She earned her master's degree from Case Western Reserve University in 1985 and her thesis was on "Marijuana Disclosure to Health Care Professionals." Originally a medical-surgical nurse, Ms. Mathre changed specialties in 1987 and has been a certified addictions registered nurse (CARN) since 1989. She practiced as the charge nurse in the Addiction Treatment Unit at the University of Virginia (UVA) Health System. Later as an expert clinician, she was the Addictions Consult Nurse for UVA Health System until 2002. Following her UVA experience, Ms. Mathre was executive director for an opioid dependence treatment center in Charlottesville, Virginia.

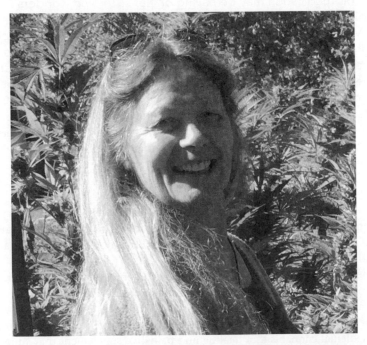

Figure 1.4: **Picture of Mary Lynn Mathre, MSN, RN, CARN.** (Photo provided by Mary Lynn Mathre, MSN, RN, CARN. Used with permission.)

Ms. Mathre wed fellow serviceman and Notre Dame rugby player Al Byrne, who was from New England. Mr. Byrne is currently a retired navy officer, Vietnam veteran, and Agent Orange victim. Following his service in Vietnam, Lieutenant Commander (LCDR) Byrne returned home in the 1980s very much aware of the struggles of his fellow troops (Lee, 2012). He became a peer counselor seeking out disillusioned, disabled, and broken veterans haunted by PTSD who were hiding in the Appalachian Mountains. The officer discovered that many of these veterans were self-medicating with cannabis to treat their symptoms of postwar trauma. Often, prescribed medications were traded for illegal cannabis products to obtain appropriate symptom relief. Many disabled veterans preferred cannabis's effects to that of prescription medications or alcohol. Cannabis use enables the veterans to achieve sleep, something that can be difficult for those with PTSD. One of the rights a veteran is entitled to receive is appropriate treatment for PTSD, including therapeutic cannabis (Lee, 2012). Mr. Byrne is a long-term cannabis reform advocate having worked with organizations like NORML and contributed to documentaries. He is also considered to be a medical cannabis expert by the DEA, and he remains active in political circles by influencing legislation (Lee, 2012).

Together, Ms. Mathre and Mr. Byrne have had an enormous impact on society by establishing several volunteer nonprofit organizations that support veterans' rights, including Patients Out of Time (POT). POT is a charity organization created in 1995 to educate healthcare professionals about the benefits of cannabis therapeutics. Mary Lynn Mathre remains the president of POT. She has served on the planning committee for POT's accredited National Clinical Conference on Cannabis Therapeutics educational series since it began in 2000. Located in the Commonwealth of Virginia, POT might be considered a humorous acronym for one of the oldest nonprofit medical cannabis advocacy organizations in existence. The name was chosen to signify the urgency faced by many sick Americans who were dying, literally running out of time for treatment, and could no longer wait for the system to complete the political process of ending prohibition. The patients needed cannabis immediately. POT's mission is:

> *To educate all disciplines of health care professionals; their specialty and professional organizations; the legal profession; and the public at large, about medical cannabis (marijuana) … Patients Out of Time focuses its power on re-instituting cannabis as a legitimate medicine for use within the United States … Patients Out of Time seeks people who are members of professional health care organizations or other social/ professional organizations who are willing to take the lead in urging their organizations to formally support patient access to therapeutic cannabis … Patients Out of Time has no other interest, nor does the organization have any opinion, stated or unstated, about any issue other than therapeutic cannabis. All educating, lobbying, communication or any other endeavor of Patients Out of Time is limited to the sole subject Marijuana as Medicine. (Patients Out of Time, 2019)*

POT seeks to provide a compassionate, science-based education forum for the restoration of medical cannabis knowledge. A pioneer organization ahead of its time, POT paved the way as the earliest organization to focus on cannabis science education for healthcare professionals, including the ECS and therapeutic consumption.

POT is an avid advocate for the medical cannabis population, with a special focus on military veterans who consume cannabis as a treatment for various disorders commonly shared among U.S. military troops.

POT is a trailblazer in cannabis reform, whose existence spawned the birth of several other professional organizations dedicated to improving safe access and therapeutic usage. Most importantly, as the "Mother of Cannabis Nursing," Ms. Mathre formed the ACNA in conjunction with other cannabis nurse pioneers. The ACNA was conceived by Julia (Ed) Glick in 2006 during the POT's Fourth National Clinical Conference on Cannabis Therapeutics in Santa Barbara, California. The ACNA was envisioned as a nursing organization that would represent the emerging field of endocannabinoid therapeutics for professional nurses, providing scientific, patient, and educational opportunities to assist nurses in understanding, and advocating for, their patients' needs. The ACNA was officially born in 2010 when the nurse pioneers Glick, Mathre, Bryan Krumm, Ken Wolski, Sharon Palmer, and advocates such as Vincent Shelzi and Stacie Boilard became the first members of ACNA's board of directors. Other significant pioneers helping to grow ACNA in the following years included Dr. Melanie Dreher, Heather Manus-Sobel, Marcie Cooper, Leslie Reyes, and Dawn Marie-Merrill.

Ms. Mathre is also an accomplished published author, having written several chapters on the topic of medical cannabis, numerous peer-reviewed articles on the topic, and resolutions for several professional organizations in support of patient access to medical cannabis, including those of the Virginia Nurses Society on Addictions, the Virginia Nurses Association, the National Nurses Society on Addictions, and the American Public Health Association. She is editor of *Cannabis in Medical Practice: A Legal, Historical Pharmacological Overview of the Therapeutic Use of Cannabis* (1997) and coeditor of *Women and Cannabis: Medicine, Science, and Sociology* (2003). Ms. Mathre is a cohost on two weekly radio programs on medical cannabis and she has testified before multiple state legislative committees. She speaks frequently on the topic of medical cannabis at many local, regional, national, and international conferences. Ms. Mathre contributed to the development of the National Council of State Boards of Nursing (NCSBN, 2018) National Nursing Guidelines for Medical Marijuana by presenting *A Historical, Legal and Evidence-Based Review of Medical Cannabis* during the NCSBN's Annual Institute of Regulatory Excellence Conference at Clearwater Beach in Florida in 2017.

When considering recommending cannabis therapeutics for patients, Ms. Mathre supports using the public health model of harm reduction. The author of *Cannabis and Harm Reduction: A Nursing Perspective* (2002), Ms. Mathre suggested that nurses consider cannabis's potential to decrease harm associated with drug addiction from other substances. In hindsight of the opioid addiction crisis, once again Mary Lynn was ahead of her time, suggesting that other substances pose greater harm to patients than therapeutic use of medical marijuana would. Mary Lynn views harm reduction models from a nursing perspective, stating that cannabis has a high benefit–low risk ratio when compared with standard pharmaceuticals and illicit substances. Ms. Mathre noted that cannabis has a high therapeutic potential, with few side effects and adverse reactions. She accurately pointed out that the greatest harm from recreational marijuana usage is the potential for legal consequences stemming from prohibition, rather than adverse reactions or side effects from the plant itself. Another suggested consequence of prohibition is the compromise of therapeutic relationships with healthcare providers because many patients are reluctant to discuss their cannabis consumption out of fear of retribution. However, as medical acceptance is adopted by most states and social stigma softens, patients are becoming more confident in confiding their usage and asking their practitioners about cannabis therapeutics.

Interview with Mary Lynn Mathre, MSN, RN, CARN

(Interview used with permission from Mary Lynn Mathre, MSN, RN, CARN)

In a personal interview with the nursing pioneer, Ms. Mathre explained that:

> *The medical marijuana movement was initially led by patients. As patient advocates, nurses who have listened to their patients and looked to history and cannabis research, readily understand the harm of the cannabis prohibition. This is a strong example of the professional responsibility of all health care clinicians to educate legislators about good health practices and work to change laws/regulations that have no supporting evidence and cause harm. It's been a long and difficult effort to advocate for a healing plant when our federal government has declared it to be a forbidden drug with harsh penalties for growing, possessing or distributing any portion of it. Manuscripts to nursing journals were rejected, which meant that nurses' education on cannabis was limited to lies & myths. With science and history to back me, I felt my primary role was to speak openly about cannabis therapeutics and advocate for patients' rights to this plant and to work towards ending the prohibition. I think nurses are key to helping patients understand how to incorporate cannabis/hemp into their daily lives as an essential nutrient and how to use it therapeutically when needed. We are the most trusted profession and we earn that trust by being caring and honest with our patients and by relying on science and experience to guide us—not politics. As for the future goal of ACNA, it should include recognition as a specialty organization in nursing and a resource to other nursing specialties to help them incorporate cannabis therapeutics into their practice. ACNA should act as a resource for hospitals and clinics to find expert cannabis clinicians and to help incorporate cannabis therapeutics into hospitals/clinics' policies and practice.*

Alice O'Leary-Randall, LPN

Perhaps one of the most famous and enduring advocates for cannabis therapeutics and cannabis care nursing is the "First Lady of Medical Marijuana" Ms. Alice O'Leary-Randall (Figure 1.5). She was there at the start of the antiprohibition movement, as for two decades, she and her husband, Robert C. Randall, were advocates for medical access to cannabis. As the "First Lady of the medical marijuana movement," Alice O'Leary-Randall has consistently communicated her singular perspective on the emotional and long-running movement to legalize cannabis as medicine. Alice became a Licensed Practical Nurse (LPN) following the death of her husband, who was the first "medical marijuana patient" and "Father" of the "medical marijuana movement," Robert Randall. In 1976, he became the first U.S. citizen to have cannabis prescribed for a medical condition.

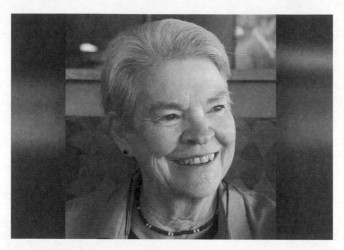

Figure 1.5: **Picture of Alice O'Leary-Randall, LPN.** (Photo provided by Alice O'Leary-Randall, LPN. Used with permission.)

Following a diagnosis of juvenile glaucoma, Robert keenly observed that his eyesight improved after consuming cannabis. Initially, Miss O'Leary doubted him, but as his symptoms progressed, she observed his visual improvements under the influence of cannabis and supported Robert's choice to consume cannabis to improve his health despite the illicit nature of the Schedule I drug. Needing a safe and dependable method to maintain Robert's cannabis supply, the couple successfully grew their medication on their apartment balcony in Washington, DC. While away on vacation in August 1975, looking on from a neighbor's porch, police officers stumbled upon several cannabis plants growing on the Randalls' sundeck. Robert and Alice arrived home to a ransacked house and a note on the table from the authorities instructing them to turn themselves in. Thus, they began the convoluted legal processes of a series of criminal and civil proceedings, where Robert Randall was ultimately victorious and declared to be the first medical cannabis patient in the United States.

Alice O'Leary-Randall was a senior spokesperson for the medical cannabis movement beginning in 1976 with her late husband. In 1980, the Randalls founded the ACT, the first nonprofit organization dedicated solely to resolving the medical cannabis issue. They drafted national legislation that was introduced in the U.S. House of Representatives with 110 cosponsors. ACT served as the primary plaintiff in the historic DEA hearing on marijuana's medical utility in the mid-1980s. In the 1990s, Alice and Robert secured funding from a Chicago-based backer and took the medical movement to new heights, paving the way for state ballot initiatives that have secured legal medical access to cannabis for citizens of 17 states.

Ms. O'Leary-Randall has a solid background in association leadership and management. She served as director for the ACT from 1980 to 1995 and on the Society for Scholarly Publishing as Administrative Officer from 1981 to 1989. In addition, Ms. O'Leary volunteered with the NORML. She also severed as coordinator for a Medical Reclassification Project from 1978 to 1980, and she was on the National Women's Health Network as membership coordinator from 1976 to 1977. In addition,

Ms. O'Leary founded Galen Press, a publishing company that compiled and released five massive volumes of information collected between 1986 and 1987 during cannabis rescheduling hearings conducted by the DEA. These court-ordered hearings, spearheaded by ACT, constituted the most complete investigation of cannabis's medical utility in the 20th century. Galen Press has a second imprint, Looking Glass Publications, for noncannabis-related titles.

In 2001, Alice took a well-earned break from the frontlines of the medical movement and embarked on a nursing career as an LPN, and she practiced nursing professionally for 10 years. From 2006 to 2012, O'Leary-Randall worked as a grief specialist and nurse for Tidewell Hospice; she also worked in oncology and emergency rooms in Southwest Florida. In addition, she has utilized her nursing skills on medical missions to Haiti, Peru, Uganda, and India.

Alice is the author of *Medical Marijuana in America: Memoir of a Pioneer*. Originally written by Robert Randall in 1998 entitled *Marijuana Rx: The Patients' Fight for Medicinal Pot*, Alice revised the book in 2014 with an update on the nation's progress toward legalizing cannabis medication in this historical account, including her own experiences as Robert's wife, medical cannabis advocate, and nurse.

Interview with Alice O'Leary-Randall, LPN

(Interview used with permission from Alice O'Leary-Randall, LPN)

In an interview with Ms. Alice O'Leary-Randall, she shares what it was like facing challenges as a medical marijuana movement founder and later as a nurse:

> *My family has always been two things: teachers and revolutionaries. From both my parents I inherited an appreciation of knowledge and the importance of always growing your mind. On my mother's side, I can trace my ancestors back through the American Revolution and even to Plymouth Rock. My father's Irish heritage is, I expect, equally rich but the records are harder to find. My point is that I was born with a keen sense of righting wrongs and both Robert and I firmly believed that if we just kept slogging away at getting out the truth about medical cannabis then things would change. And they have.*
>
> *After Robert died in 2001, I was sort of lost for a while. Robert and I had worked together closely for more than 25 years and I just didn't think I could carry on without him because medical cannabis, particularly in those early years, was a damn hard fight. We dealt with so many patients who had no options left, patients who knew cannabis was giving them a better quality of life than they might otherwise have. Many of them died and some spent the last good days of their lives lobbying and pushing for medical cannabis. I just didn't think I could carry that burden on my own. But what to do? My sister asked what I would do if I could do anything at all and my answer was "work with hospice." I knew I would need credentialing of some sort—nurse, social worker—to work with the patients and their families. I was fairly certain I did not want to be a social worker and I learned I could become an LPN with just a year of schooling. I was 54 years old at this point and I thought becoming an RN would take me about three years. I just wasn't prepared to go back to school for that long. And becoming an LPN was great because I really got to do patient care. I didn't have a lot of paperwork to do like Plans of Care and what not.*

After graduating I "paid my dues" before joining hospice by working first in the ER, which I loved, and then with an oncology practice. Being a nurse opened all sorts of doors for me. I went on some extraordinary medical missions including going to India just one month after the terrible tsunami of 2004. Nursing was a wonderful path for me and contributed significantly to my continued growth as a human being. Everything was a challenge in the early days because medical cannabis was unheard of and so we had to convince everyone we met, starting with our lawyers. They laughed when Robert told them why we were growing marijuana. The prohibition of marijuana had been a spectacular failure on every level except for medical use. In that area, the government had completely wiped clean the memory of medical use, and doctors knew nothing about it. Similarly, the public was sure it must be a joke. So, everyone had to be educated.

Ms. O'Leary "feels that nursing can gain immeasurably from the end of prohibition, because medical cannabis is unlike conventional medicine and most doctors, frankly, do not want to take the time either to learn or to treat their patients with the time and respect that it takes. Nurses are taught to listen and that is what a medical cannabis patient requires, particularly at the start of cannabis therapy. I hope to see cannabis clinics across the country that are operated almost entirely by nurses."

Regarding her service to the ACNA, Alice stated that:

Throughout my life, I have been fortunate to be in a position to help establish new associations. My husband I founded the Alliance for Cannabis Therapeutics in 1980, and I worked at a small association of publishers in the 1980s that was just getting started. I seem to have a facility for the work that is needed at the start of an organization's life. ACNA was no different. It takes a certain amount of basic, managerial work to get a group going and I feel I was able to help define those areas of ACNA that required basic organization such as a website, member database and correspondence processes, association financial accounting, etc. Those areas improved while I was on the Board and I am proud of that. ACNA continues to need volunteers who are willing to work hard, and I hope the foundation established by the early Board will give them plenty with which to work.

Nurse Heather Sobel-Manus, RN

Heather Sobel-Manus, RN (Figure 1.6), is a native New Mexican and registered nurse specializing in all aspects of medical cannabis care. "Nurse Heather" began her career as a registered nurse providing psychiatric home healthcare to patients in New Mexico. Nurse Heather graduated from San Juan College in New Mexico with an associate degree in nursing and then continued her education, working on a bachelor of science in psychology from New Mexico Highlands University. Interestingly, in 2002, Ms. Manus became a Certified Master Grower, holding a horticulture degree from New Mexico State University. Nurse Heather has an extensive background and experience in natural healing modalities and herbal remedies, some of which she obtained from her close association with Hispanic and Native American healers in New Mexico. Her vast knowledge, and holistic approach to individualized patient care, has been the cornerstone of her success as a nurse, educator, entrepreneur, and promoter of health. As a reiki master and horticulturist utilizing Native American

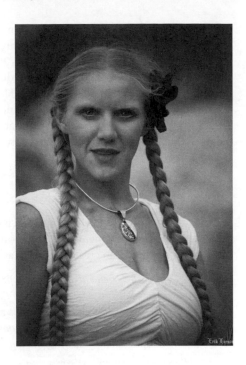

Figure 1.6: **Picture of Heather Sobel-Manus, RN.** (Photo provided by Heather Sobel-Manus, RN. Used with permission.)

healing techniques, it is appropriate that Nurse Heather's trademarks are her signature 5-foot braids and a floral arrangement tucked neatly behind her ear.

Nurse Heather served on the board of directors of the ACNA as one of its earliest members. She later went on to establish the Arizona Cannabis Nurses Association, where she served as president. As the founder of the Arizona Cannabis Nurses Association and a fierce advocate for veterans and mental health, Nurse Heather was responsible for supporting the addition of PTSD as a debilitating condition under Arizona's Medical Marijuana Act. In 2015, Heather recognized a deep gap in cannabis nursing resources that exist surrounding cannabis therapeutics and launched Cannabis Nurses Network (CNN), a for-profit professional nursing organization. CNN's mission to support nursing is dedicated to the four cornerstones: education, opportunity, recognition, and advocacy. The organization has a poignant 2019 conference slogan "Rooted in science and nourished by nature." Part of Heather's philosophy for the CNN model is providing a safe organization for cannabis nurses to gather, network, and develop within their specialty.

An intelligent businesswoman and leader, Nurse Heather seeks to bridge the gap and bring cannabis nursing and cannabis industry participants together for the benefit of patients. As a "Cannabis Nurse Entrepreneur," Nurse Heather established herself in both New Mexico (2010) and Arizona (2013), where she opened the first licensed medical cannabis infusion facilities to provide cannabis patients with smokeless alternative products. As a public figure, Nurse Heather has shared knowledge nationally and internationally. Nurse Heather has been a beloved presenter in the educational, medical, and cannabis industry conference speaking circuits since 2010, and she has a history of providing information related to the ECS, cannabinoid therapeutics, mental health, plant medicine education, and cannabis industry assistance. Nurse Heather was awarded the 2015 CannAwards "Best Charitable/Community Outreach Program" and Cannabis Business Awards 2015 and 2017 "Activist of the Year." She has been featured and published in several videos, films, and magazines, and she hosts an online podcast "Good News with Nurse Heather." Nurse Heather was honored to receive the Cannabis Business Awards "Educational Achievement" Award in 2016 and a "Leader of Nursing" Award from Cannabis Nurses Magazine in 2016 and 2017. She believes that knowledge is power and strives to empower as many people as possible.

Interview with Heather Sobel-Manus, RN

(Interview used with permission from Heather Manus, RN)

Ms. Manus shares in an interview the challenges she faced as an advocate for the medical cannabis movement, participation with ACNA, and how those experiences influenced her choice to create CNN. Heather stated that:

> Lack of knowledge and access were the first barriers to providing cannabis patient care. Helping patients navigate through the legal aspects of becoming an approved patient under the state medical cannabis program was the first step. I began asking the question "Do you use medical marijuana/cannabis?" I found that by asking this additional question, in a nonjudgmental manner, patients were much more willing to disclose their cannabis use.
>
> The next challenge arose once patients received their legal cannabis patient cards: Where and how to safely access legal cannabis products became the next question. Patients would report that they were unable to access cannabis from any legal entity in our rural area of New Mexico. After doing some investigation, I was offered a position as the Medical Board Member for a state-licensed medical cannabis producer. The position and legal status allowed my involvement to cultivate, process, transport, and distribute cannabis products legally to qualified patients in New Mexico.
>
> The work I engaged in helped to shape the future of ACNA by establishing groundbreaking ideas that manifested into widespread recognition for the organization and cannabis nursing as a professionally recognized subspecialty. For example, by expressing the importance of an official up to date ACNA website to serve as a public presence, membership was able to grow much more rapidly. As the conference committee chair, my role included management of educational content developed for the ACNA cannabis nursing core and advanced curricula presented live in 2014 and 2015 during the Patients Out of Time conference. Planting seeds of knowledge that continue to grow and advance the profession of cannabis nursing through continued education is the work I am most proud of. In 2013, I established the Arizona Cannabis Nurses Association to serve as a local presence for the legal advocacy work needing to be conducted in Arizona at the time. In 2015, a group of cannabis nurses gathered in Nevada to celebrate progress and continue to educate others. The gathering, now known as the Cannabis Nurses Network Conference (CNNC) became an annual continued nursing education event; dedicated to educating nurses, providing professional networking opportunities, and celebrating individual and collective successes by recognizing outstanding leaders of nursing. Cannabis Nurses Network's mission is to empower nurses through education, opportunity, recognition, and advocacy.

Melanie C. Dreher, RN, MPhil, PhD

Melanie C. Dreher, RN, MPhil, PhD (Figure 1.7), had a distinguished career in research and academic leadership, including publishing several books, reports, and many articles. She received her bachelor's degree in nursing from Long Island University in Brooklyn, New York, and her PhD in anthropology from Columbia University. In addition to her research studies—which have been quoted widely by *The New York Times*, *The Wall Street Journal*, and *The Chronicle of Higher Education*—Dr. Dreher served as a charter member of the National Institute for Nursing Research and the NIH's Director's Council of Public Representatives. Her four decades of leadership in nursing education include deanships at the University of Miami, the University of Massachusetts at Amherst, the University of Iowa, and Rush University College of Nursing, where she is now dean emeritus.

Most recently, Dr. Dreher's focus has shifted from education administration to healthcare governance. She serves as a member of the Chicago Board of Health, a member of the Wellmark Blue Cross/Blue Shield Board of Directors, a trustee of Loyola University Chicago, and chair of Trinity Health Board of Directors. After serving as president of Sigma Theta Tau International, Dr. Dreher was honored by the Nursing Honor Society through the establishment of the Melanie Dreher Dean's Award given annually to a dean who has most embraced the values of Sigma Theta Tau. She is also a fellow in the American Academy of Nursing and was recently named among the 40 smartest people in healthcare in Becker's Hospital Review. Dr. Dreher's favorite accomplishment consists of the students and faculty whom she has taught and mentored in an academic nursing career spanning 40 years. That work

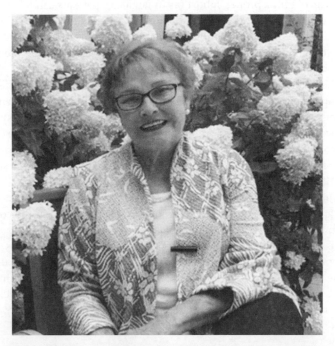

Figure 1.7: **Picture of Melanie C. Dreher, RN, MPhil, PhD.** (Photo provided by Melanie C. Dreher, RN, MPhil, PhD. Used with permission.)

has generated the greatest meaning in her career, her greatest contribution to society, and her most worthwhile legacy to the academy in the magi's spirit of doing more for others.

Dr. Dreher has maintained a subtle role as a pioneering cannabis nurse researcher. Her anthropology efforts in rural Jamaica studying "ganja" consumption among working men, youths, pregnant women, and newborns have been widely shared (Mathre, 1997). Jamaican culture favors the use of the ganja plant and associated stigma is not displayed against consumers, including mothers and children. Dr. Dreher's research reviewed pregnant women's cannabis use and evaluated risks associated with its consumption for both the women and her baby. Her work failed to confirm the negative effects associated with cannabis consuming mothers upon their newborns (Mathre, 1997). Unfortunately, Dr. Dreher's decades-long body of work researching cannabis therapeutics had been largely ignored until recently.

In Mathre's (1997) book, *Cannabis in Medical Practice*, Dr. Dreher summarized her research about pregnancy, childbirth, motherhood, infancy, and cannabis use. Unfortunately, cannabis studies have been conducted within a negative connotation focusing on possible adverse effects and complications. One of the most significant reasons Dr. Dreher was able to perform effective research surrounding maternal use of cannabis in Jamaica is because of the country's unique political and spiritual culture accepting the sacred ganja plant consumption as part of Rastafarianism. Many studies have focused on research linking prenatal cannabis consumption to neurologic abnormalities, inadequate maternal weight gain, fetal distress, and malformations. Recruiting subjects for these types of studies proves to be a difficult task given the legal and social sanctions against marijuana usage during maternal functions. Even when researchers can obtain a proper cohort (as in Jamaica), patients can be unreliable and tend to inaccurately report their true consumption habits out of fear of retribution. Regardless, in 1980, Fried found no relationship between cannabis use during pregnancy and the amount of weight a mother gained, the length of the pregnancy and duration of labor, or differences in APGAR scores (as cited in Mathre, 1997).

Dr. Dreher's Jamaican studies demonstrated that 1-month-old breastfed cannabis newborns appeared to show better physiologic stability. The heaviest cannabis consuming mothers had the most adaptable babies, where the autonomic systems were robust, appeared more organized, and required less stimulation from the examiner to elicit a response. Dr. Dreher recommended that health officials place more emphasis on health benefits associated with maternal cannabis usage instead of stigmatizing the population for seeking the pleasures derived from recreational use.

In addition to its routine use, the contribution of the Jamaican project was its ethnographic approach, in which, for 2 years, field workers resided in the communities from which the women were selected, developed trusting relationships, and directly observed usage. In 1980, Jamaican studies demonstrated that cannabis use during pregnancy posed no harm to the neonate. Given its benefits to the pregnancy, including appetite stimulation, reduction of fatigue, and alleviation of morning sickness, Dr. Dreher's research suggests that healthcare and law enforcement officials discontinue the penalties placed on women who use cannabis during pregnancy. (Used with permission from Melanie C. Dreher, RN, MPhil, PhD.)

Bryan Krumm, MSN, CNP, RN, BC

Bryan Krumm, MSN, CNP, RN, BC (Figure 1.8), is a psychiatric nurse practitioner at Sage Neuroscience Center in Albuquerque, New Mexico. He provides comprehensive evidence-based psychiatric care, treating a variety of disorders. He is also the director of New Mexicans for Compassionate Use and Bishop of Medicine for the Zen Zion Coptic Orthodox Church. He helped author New Mexico's Medical Cannabis law and is one of the leading referral sources to New Mexico's Medical Cannabis Program. He maintains hundreds of patients in the program, the majority of whom have been referred for PTSD.

Mr. Krumm is a nationally recognized expert on the use of cannabis for treating PTSD. He helped write New Mexico's Medical Cannabis law and is actively working to force the DEA to end the prohibition of medical cannabis at the federal level. He has presented at numerous medical conferences across the country and is the author of "Cannabis for Posttraumatic Stress Disorder: A Neurobiological Approach to Treatment," a peer-reviewed article explaining what PTSD is and why cannabis is the only medication effective in treating PTSD (Krumm, 2016). Krumm's most significant contributions as a nurse pioneer and advocate are seizing opportunities to directly influence policies involving cannabis as medication by taking local legal action. To read all the documents, please visit the following sources:

- United States Court of Appeals, Case #18-1058, Bryan A. Krumm, CNP (Petitioner) v. Drug Enforcement Administration (Respondent), Document #1752176, Filed: 09/24/2018. http://www.harmonypsych.org/wp-content/uploads/2019/06/appendix-pdf.pdf

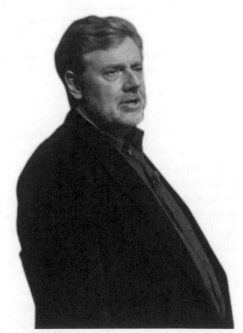

Figure 1.8: **Picture of Bryan Krumm, MSN, CNP, RN, BC.** (Photo provided by Bryan Krumm, MSN, CNP, RN, BC. Used with permission.)

- *The Health Effects of Cannabis and Cannabinoids: Committee's Conclusions,* January 2017. The National Academies of Sciences, Engineering, and Medicine. To read the full report and view related resources, please visit https://www.nap .edu/resource/24625/Cannabis_committee_conclusions.pdf
- *Recommendation to Maintain Marijuana in Schedule I of the Controlled Substances Act.* Department of Health & Human Services, Food and Drug Administration, Silver Spring, MD. May 20, 2015. https://www.fda.gov/files/ Marijuana%20Schedule%20I%20Recommendation.pdf
- Letter to Honorable Chuck Rosenberg, U.S. Department of Justice, Drug Enforcement Administration, Springfield, VA. Letter from Karen B. DeSalvo, MD, MPH, MSc. June 3, 2015. https://www.deadiversion.usdoj.gov/schedules/ marijuana/Incoming_Letter_Department%20_HHS.pdf
- Letter to Honorable Gina M. Raimondo (Governor of Rhode Island), U.S. Department of Justice, Honorable Jay R. Inslee (Governor of Washington), U.S. Department of Justice, and Mr. Bryan A. Krumm. Letter from Honorable Chuck Rosenberg, U.S. Department of Justice. August 11, 2016. https://www .deadiversion.usdoj.gov/schedules/marijuana/Acting_Adminstrator_Rosenberg_ Response_to_Request_Marijuana_Rescheduling.pdf
- *Appendix H*, Federal Register/Vol. 81, No. 156/Friday, August 12, 2016/Proposed Rules. https://www.govinfo.gov/content/pkg/FR-2016-08-12/pdf/FR-2016-08-12.pdf
- DEA Announces Actions Related to Marijuana and Industrial Hemp. Drug Enforcement Administration. August 11, 2016. https://www.dea.gov/press-releases/2016/08/11/dea-announces-actions-related-marijuana-and-industrial-hemp
- Cannabis for posttraumatic stress disorder: A neurobiological approach to treatment, by Bryan A. Krumm, MSN, RN, CNP, BC. *The Nurse Practitioner*, Vol. 41, No. 1, 50–54, January 2016, Wolters Kluwer Health, Inc. https://journals.lww .com/tnpj/Fulltext/2016/01000/Cannabis_for_posttraumatic_stress_disorder__ A.6.aspx (Used with permission from Bryan Krumm, MSN, RN, CNP.)

Inbal Sikorin, RN

Inbal Sikorin (Figure 1.9) is an international nurse pioneer establishing therapeutic cannabis medications for geriatric patients residing in Israel. She is the cofounder and head nurse of Niamedic Healthcare and Research Clinics Ltd., a multidisciplinary medicinal research clinic with locations all over the world. Ms. Sikorin implements revolutionary work that integrates superior conventional medicine with proprietary medical cannabis treatments. Before cofounding Niamedic, Inbal Sikorin was the head nurse of the "Hadarim" nursing home at Kibbutz Na'an. There, Inbal Sikorin founded a groundbreaking medical cannabis program for the elderly. In 2010, Ms. Sikorin collaborated with Tikun Olam and established its cannabis nursing clinic.

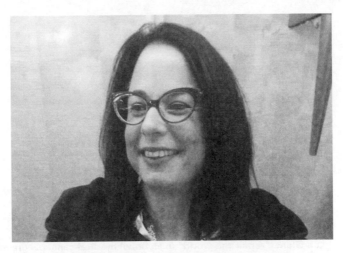

Figure 1.9: **Picture of Inbal Sikorin, RN.** (Photo provided by Inbal Sikorin, RN. Used with permission.)

Hadarim nursing home piloted with its residents a project to develop strategies and methods to make cannabis treatments comfortably accessible. The nursing home staff and medical team were directly involved in the implementation and adjustments necessary to provide outstanding results, thus pioneering a new model of geriatric cannabis treatment implementation (Tikun Olam, 2019).

For almost a decade, Ms. Sikorin has been a world-renowned pioneer and expert in the medical cannabis field, treating and counseling thousands of patients over the years, with a special focus on exceptional treatment methods, and developing treatment protocols and data analyses. In addition, Ms. Sikorin helped develop a palliative care course for medical staff, a rich and comprehensive curriculum that has changed the world view of patient care and accessibility of medical cannabis as a treatment option in nursing homes. Inbal is a popular speaker at medical cannabis conferences. Inbal Sikorin collaborated with Tikun Olam to run their most recognized achievement, the first professional cannabis nursing clinic. They provide services to more than 20,000 patients ranging from pediatric populations to the elderly. Tikun Olam and Inbal Sikorin are pioneers in establishing a nursing model demonstrating the implementation of the cannabis nursing process. Tikun Olam's patient education and treatment adjustments are performed by certified nurses, whose recommendations are based on a decade of research that has been investigated and analyzed (Figure 1.10). (Used with permission from Inbal Sikorin, RN.)

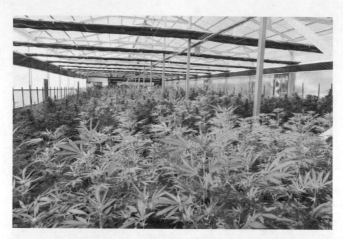

Figure 1.10: **Tikun Olam ("repair the world" in Hebrew) medical cannabis greenhouse.** (Tikun-Olam.org.il)

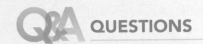 **QUESTIONS**

1. Ancient historical records indicate that cannabis was used for which purposes?
   A. Spiritual rituals and as a therapeutic medication
   B. As a cure-all for modern ailments in the 1800s
   C. To treat victims of the AIDS virus
   D. There are no historical indicated usages for cannabis

2. Where does extensive medical documentation for cannabis therapeutics exist?
   A. The Congressional Library of Congress in Washington, DC
   B. The Controlled Substances Act of 1970
   C. Healthcare curricula
   D. Multiple pharmacopoeias from ancient times through the early 20th century

3. Why is the practicing cannabis nurse responsible for understanding federal, state, and local laws surrounding cannabis therapeutics?
   A. CBD is considered legal in the United States.
   B. Marijuana has no medical value and is listed as a Schedule I narcotic.
   C. Cannabis laws vary federally and from state to state.
   D. Hemp laws allow for the cultivation of Δ9-THC products.

4. Cannabis is currently a federally illegal substance and consumers risk suffering potential legal consequences from its use. True or False?

5. Which marginal or vulnerable patient populations have suffered prejudicial consequences and stigma of laws regarding cannabis consumption? Select all that apply:
   A. Caucasians
   B. Mexicans and/or Latinos
   C. Musicians
   D. Artists
   E. African Americans
   F. Veterans
   G. AIDS victims
   H. Cancer patients
   I. Politicians and/or bureaucrats
   J. LBGTQ populations

6. Laws prohibiting cannabis were instituted as a result of "Reefer Madness" campaigns as a tool for?
   A. Controlling immigrants, people of color, and vulnerable/marginal populations.
   B. Preventing crimes as a result of people's marijuana use.
   C. Preventing the movement of jazz musicians from New Orleans to Northern cities.
   D. Creating jobs for bureaucratic agencies.

7. Matching question: Match the title to the pioneering individual: (mix up the answers for the test)

A. Dennis Peron   "Father of the Medical Marijuana Movement"
B. Mary Lynn Mathre   "Mother of Cannabis Nursing"
C. Robert Randall   "Grandfather of Cannabis Science"
D. Raphael Mechoulam   "Commissioner of the FBN"
E. Alice O'Leary-Randall   "First Lady of Medical Marijuana"
F. Harry Jacob Anslinger   "Prince of Pot"

ANSWERS

1. **Answer: A.** Spiritual rituals and as a therapeutic medication

2. **Answer: D.** Multiple pharmacopoeias from ancient times through the early 20th century

3. **Answer: C.** Cannabis laws vary federally and from state to state.

4. **Answer: A.** True

5. **Answer:**

   B. Mexicans and/or Latinos

   C. Musicians

   D. Artists

   E. African Americans

   F. Veterans

   G. AIDS victims

   H. Cancer patients

   J. LBGTQ populations

6. **Answer: A.** Controlling immigrants, people of color, and vulnerable/marginal populations.

7. **Answer:**

Dennis Peron	"Prince of Pot"
Mary Lynn Mathre	"Mother of Cannabis Nursing"
Robert Randall	"Father of the Medical Marijuana Movement"
Raphael Mechoulam	"Grandfather of Cannabis Science"
Alice O'Leary-Randall	"First Lady of Medical Marijuana"
Harry Jacob Anslinger	"Commissioner of the FBN"

References

Alligood, M. R. (2013). *Nursing theory utilization and application.* Elsevier.

American Nurses Association. (2016). *Therapeutic use of marijuana and related cannabinoids: Position Statement.* NursingWorld.org. https://www.nursingworld.org/~49a8c8/globalassets/practiceandpolicy/ethics/therapeutic-use-of-marijuana-and-related-cannabinoids-position-statement.pdf

American Nurses Association. (2018). *Nursing scope and standards of practice* (3rd ed.). Author.

Backes, M. (2014). *Cannabis pharmacy: The practical guide to medical marijuana.* Black Dog & Leventhal Publisher.

Brand, E. J., & Zhao, Z. (2017). Cannabis in Chinese medicine: Are some traditional indications referenced in ancient literature related to cannabinoids? *Frontiers in Pharmacology, B3*(17), 108. https://doi.org/10.3389/fphar.2017.00108

Clark, C. S., Bernard, C., Quigley, N., Smith, K., Theisen, E., & Smith, D. (2019). *Scope and standards of practice for cannabis nurses.* American Cannabis Nurses Association. https://cannabisnurses.org/Scope-of-Practice-for-Cannabis-Nurses

Conley, K. (2017). Did aliens bring pot to Earth: National UFO day. *DOPE Magazine.* https://dopemagazine.com/aliens-bring-pot-earth/

Gaoni, Y., & Mechoulam, R. (1964). Isolation, structure, and partial synthesis of an active constituent of hashish. *Journal of the American Chemical Society, 86*(8), 1646–1647. https://doi.org/10.1021/ja01062a046

Grotenhermen, F., & Russo, E. (2012). *Cannabis and cannabinoids: Pharmacology, toxicology, and therapeutic potential.* Haworth Press, Inc.

Hand, A., Blake, A., Kerrigan, P., Phineas, S., & Friedberg, J. (2016). History of medical cannabis. *Journal of Pain Management, 9*(4), 387–394. https://medreleaf.com/app/uploads/2018/03/1.History-of-medical-cannabis.pdf

Holland, J. (2010). *The pot book: A complete guide to cannabis.* Park Street Press.

IFLScience. (2019). *Cannabis may have eased breast cancer symptoms of Siberian ice princess.* https://www.iflscience.com/health-and-medicine/cannabis-may-have-eased-breast-cancer-symptoms-siberian-ice-princess/

Konieczny, E., & Wilson, L. (2018). *Healing with CBD: How cannabidiol can transform your health without the high.* Ulysses Press.

Krumm, B. (2016). Cannabis for posttraumatic stress disorder: A neurobiological approach to treatment. *Nurse Practitioner, 41*(1), 50–54. https://doi.org/10.1097/01.NPR.0000434091.34348.3c

Lee, M. A. (2012). *Smoke signals.* Scribner.

Mathre, M. L. (1997). *Cannabis in medical practice: A legal, historical and pharmacological overview of the therapeutic use of marijuana* (1st ed.). McFarland & Company.

Mathre, M. L. (2017). *A historical, legal and evidence-based review of medical cannabis.* Presented at the National Council of State Boards of Nursing (NCSBN) 2017 Annual Institute of Regulatory Excellence Conference: Practice Breakdown, Discipline and Patient Safety, Clearwater Beach, FL. McFarland & Co., Inc.

National Council of States Boards of Nursing. (2018). THE NCSBN national nursing guidelines for medical marijuana. *Journal of Nursing Regulation, 9*(2), S5–S46. https://doi.org/10.1016/S2155-8256(18)30098-X

Nightingale, F. (1882, December 21). *Letter to Margaret Varney.* https://books.google.com/books?id=GAT1r2c_sIC&q=verney#v=snippet&q=verney&f=false

Ohio Plants Organization. (2019). *One-seeded dry fruits.* Ohio Plants. https://ohioplants.org/fruits-achene/

O'Leary-Randall, A. (2014). *Medical marijuana in America: Memoir of a pioneer.* Author.

Patients Out of Time. (2019). *About us: Mission statement.* https://www.medicalcannabis.com/about/

Ren, M., Zihua, T., Wu, X., Spengler, R., Jiang, H., Yang, Y., & Boivin, N. (2019). The origins of cannabis smoking: Chemical residue evidence from the first millennium BCE in the Pamirs. *Science Advances, 5*(6). https://advances.sciencemag.org/content/5/6/eaaw1391

Russo, E., Dreher, M., & Mathre, M. L. (2003). *Women and cannabis: Medicine, science, and sociology.* Hawthorne PR Inc.

Sloman, L. (1979). *Reefer madness: A history of marijuana.* St. Martin's Press.

Sloman, L. R. (1998). *Reefer madness: A history of marijuana.* Author.

Tikun Olam. (2019). *Medical cannabis. About us.* Retrieved from https://www.tikunolam.com/

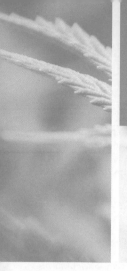

2

The Human Endocannabinoid System (ECS): Physiology

Denise A. Foster, PhD, MSN, RN, CNE

CONCEPTS AND CONSIDERATIONS

This chapter supports nursing knowledge of the endocannabinoid system (ECS) and its endogenous components, thereby fulfilling the call "to provide nurses with principles of safe and knowledgeable practice to promote patient safety when caring for patients using medical marijuana" (National Council of State Boards of Nursing [NCSBN], 2018, p. S23). The ECS is a very complex and large receptor system in the human body, and this chapter focuses on the intricate physiology of how this system functions to maintain homeostasis in the human body. In 2018, the NCSBN recommended that all nurses have an understanding of the ECS, cannabinoid receptors, cannabinoids (endo-, phyto-, and synthetic cannabinoids), and the interactions between them (NCSBN, 2018).

Learning Outcomes

Upon completion of this chapter, the learner will:

- Describe the components of the ECS.
- Explain the role of the ECS and endocannabinoids in maintaining homeostasis.
- Describe the entourage effect.
- Examine disease states associated with clinical endocannabinoid deficiency.

THE HUMAN ENDOCANNABINOID SYSTEM: A BRIEF OVERVIEW

The human ECS includes cannabinoid receptors, endocannabinoids, and enzymes that synthesize and degrade the endocannabinoids. Cannabinoid receptors are embedded in cell membranes throughout the body systems of all mammals (McPartland et al., 2001, 2006) and are responsible for promoting homeostasis and preventing disease and aging (McPartland et al., 2014; Paradisi et al., 2006). The ECS may also play an important role in the regulation of reactive oxygen species (ROS) by altering the expression and/or activity of enzymes responsible for the production of oxygen free radicals in the mitochondria of cells (Javed et al., 2016; Lipina & Hundal, 2016; Mukhopadhyay et al., 2010). Mitochondria are organelles found in large amounts in cells that are responsible for the biochemical processes of energy production and cellular respiration. The production of ROS in mammalian mitochondria has been linked to many disease processes (Birben et al., 2012; Murphy, 2009). The ECS is important in scavenging the human body for oxygen free radicals. Almost all disease processes occur simultaneously with inflammation, which occurs from the action of roaming oxygen free radicals. These free radicals cause damage as they tear through the body searching for other oxygen molecules with which to pair. Oxygen free radicals are a by-product of normal cellular processes in the body, such as elimination and nutrition. They are also formed from external sources, such as pollution, radiation, and pesticides (Birben et al., 2012). When oxygen free radicals overwhelm the body, they cause damage as they interact with cellular components such as cellular DNA or cell membranes. Oxidative stress formed by the production of ROS is thought to contribute to aging, cancer, inflammation associated with all diseases, neurologic disorders, and many other health disorders (Birben et al., 2012). The ECS has been found to protect neurons and cells against these free radicals. The concurrent role of the ECS as an immune function modulator is another way that it protects against oxidative stress as it works to suppress inflammation (Javed et al., 2016; Lipina & Hundal, 2016).

The human body creates its endocannabinoids from substances found within its cell membranes. The two principal endocannabinoids, arachidonoyl ethanolamine (AEA, or anandamide) and 2-arachidonoylglycerol (2-AG), are chemical messengers that activate receptors found on cellular membranes (Katona & Freund, 2008; Pertwee & Ross, 2002). These endocannabinoids are synthesized and degraded through multiple complex enzymatic pathways.

DISCOVERY OF THE ENDOCANNABINOID SYSTEM AND ENDOCANNABINOIDS

Discovery of the Phytocannabinoids

In 1932, British chemist Dr. Robert Sidney Cahn isolated the first known phytocannabinoid from hashish, a concentrated resinous extract of the *Cannabis sativa* plant. The pharmacologically inactive compound was named cannabinol (CBN) (Cahn, 1932). This was the first recognized scientific approach to understanding the molecular compounds contained within the cannabis plant. From this publication, other investigations followed, and in 1940, Jacob and Todd isolated another cannabis compound, cannabidiol (CBD), from Egyptian hashish (Jacob & Todd, 1940). Also in 1940, Adams et al. isolated CBD while working at the University of Illinois, which revealed this cannabis molecule is present in Minnesota wild hemp (Adams et al., 1940). This discovery led to the recognition that cannabis plant compounds are found in both forms of *C. sativa*, hemp and cannabis. These discoveries generated interest in possible other compounds found in the plants, and in 1942, Wollner et al. isolated the first known physiologically active cannabinoid, tetrahydrocannabinol (THC), from *C. sativa* resin while working in the U.S. Bureau of Narcotics Laboratory (Wollner et al., 1942). Their research was conducted using dogs, and although the physiologic actions of this compound were not fully described, researchers noted that the isolated

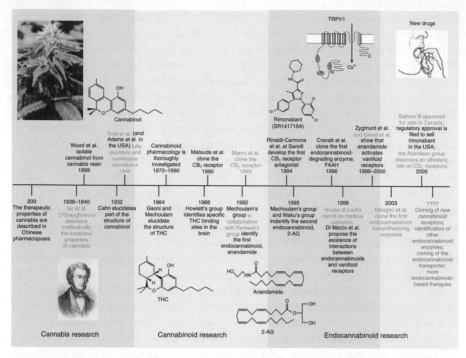

Figure 2.1: Major breakthroughs in the recent history of cannabis, cannabinoid, and endocannabinoid research. The use of cannabis as medicine stretches back to its use in the Far East. In the early part of the 19th century, cannabis was used regularly as medicine in many cultures. The discovery of the structures of cannabis compounds led to the discovery of the cannabinoid receptors, the endocannabinoids, and the synthesizing and degrading compounds that interact with them. Abbreviations: 2-AG, 2-arachidonoylglycerol; CB, cannabinoid; FAAH, fatty acid amide hydrolase; THC, tetrahydrocannabinol.

THC was "of high physiological potency" (Wollner et al., 1942, p. 29). Figure 2.1 illustrates a timeline of the breakthroughs in the recent history of cannabis, cannabinoids, and endocannabinoid research.

Throughout the 1940s and 1950s, pharmacologic studies were carried out involving THC, CBN, and CBD. Although the experiments involving separate phytocannabinoids helped to establish their effects on animal behavior, it was not until 1963 that Raphael Mechoulam and Yuval Shvo confirmed the chemical structure of CBD, which was isolated from hashish while working at the Weizmann Institute of Science in Israel (Mechoulam, 2016; Mechoulam & Shvo, 1963). Building on this knowledge, Gaoni and Mechoulam fully identified and synthesized the first pure form of the psychoactive constituent of *C. sativa*, which they named Δ^1-3,4-*trans*-THC (Gaoni & Mechoulam, 1964). This was the first time that THC was identified as the explicit mind-altering phytocannabinoid compound and duplicated in the laboratory setting. In 1967, Mechoulam and Gaoni further refined the compound's chemical structure to what is now recognized as Δ^9-THC, the psychoactive component of cannabis (Mechoulam & Gaoni, 1967).

For decades after the clarification of the structure and synthesis of THC, most of the scientific research focused on this one plant compound. Studies involving behavioral patterns associated with THC were conducted in numerous animal and human models around the world. For example, Paton and Pertwee (1973) examined the sedative and analgesic properties of THC and its metabolism in mammals in England, whereas Lemberger et al. (1970) administered intravenous THC to three human subjects to determine its pharmacokinetics at the National Institute of Mental Health. Although the mind-altering effects of THC were studied and classified, the physiologic mechanisms of its action remain poorly understood. The compounds found in the cannabis plant did not fit into any class of drug known at the time, and the cellular processes related to their activities remained vague. Additionally, the technology available to investigate the actions of cannabis and other drugs was not as advanced, and scientists lacked the equipment and methods to study these compounds and their effects on the human body.

Discovery of the Cannabinoid Receptors and Endocannabinoids

The knowledge that the chemical compounds found in cannabis affected physiologic and psychological functioning in both animals and humans suggested the presence of endogenous cannabinoid receptors in the body. The presence of endogenous cannabinoid receptors was confirmed in the early 1980s, when Allyn Howlett, working at Saint Louis University, produced evidence that the human body contained receptor sites that specifically interacted with the THC molecule. Howlett and her colleagues discovered that the psychotropic compounds found in cannabis were able to inhibit adenylate cyclase, an enzyme that regulates key activities in all cells, by acting through G-protein-coupled receptors (GPRs) found in cell membranes (Howlett, 1984; Howlett & Fleming, 1984; Howlett et al., 1986, 2002). The finding that GPRs were influenced by phytocannabinoids to inhibit an intracellular enzyme led to the discovery of the first cannabinoid receptor.

In 1988, William Devane and his team of investigators published their groundbreaking research on the discovery of the first known cannabinoid receptor, named cannabinoid receptor 1 (CB1R), found in the brains of rats. CB1R was found in abundance in the brain, especially in areas that are responsible for mental and physical processes (Devane et al., 1988, 1992). This discovery explained the physiologic effects of THC, including its effects on memory, cognition, motor coordination, movement, appetite, and mood. Working in Belgium and France, the human CB1R was cloned by Gérard, Mollereau, Vassart, and Parmentier, who verified the abundance of CB1R in the brain as well as in the testis, noting that the cloning of the CB1R "will be instrumental in the discovery of its endogenous ligand(s), promoting it from its role as a plant substance receptor to that of an important component of the neurotransmitter network" (Gérard et al., 1991, p. 133).

Because each GPR in the human body has an endogenous, or internal, molecule that binds with it, the search for CB1R endogenous ligands, or binding molecules, began swiftly. Devane and Mechoulam provided evidence that the human body produces its cannabinoid-like compound in 1992. Working in Israel, the first endogenous cannabinoid, AEA, was discovered. As the pharmacologist of the team, Devane was given the honor of naming the compound, and he chose the name "*anandamide*," which is derived from the Sanskrit word "*Ananda*," meaning "supreme joy" (Devane et al., 1992).

The period between 1980 and 2000 saw an escalation of cannabis-related research. Scientists and pharmaceutical companies around the world focused on either the physiologic effects of the cannabis plant or the endogenous cannabinoid systems found in all mammals (Institute of Medicine, 1999a). As studies indicated that THC could be useful in the treatment of pain, synthetic cannabinoid analogs of the compound were developed. In 1985, the U.S. Food and Drug Administration approved dronabinol, the first THC synthetic analog, for the treatment of chemotherapy-related nausea and vomiting and anorexia in acquired immunodeficiency syndrome (AIDS) patients (Institute of Medicine, 1999b).

Experimental models using both animals and humans further revealed the roles of CB1R concerning health and disease. In 1993, Munro et al. cloned what came to be known as cannabinoid receptor 2 (CB2R). Their findings distinguished CB2R from CB1R, as CB2R was found in macrophages in the spleen, suggesting that this receptor had "an immune-modulatory role in addition to its neuronal functions" (Munro et al., 1993, p. 65). This discovery further classified the cannabinoid receptors as either brain receptor (CB1R) or peripheral receptor (CB2R). The search for the endogenous ligand for CB2R began after this significant finding.

The year 1995 was busy in the field of cannabis science. Several breakthrough discoveries were made that year as scientists began to piece together the workings of phytocannabinoids, cannabinoid receptors, and the endogenous ligands that bind to them. While describing the pharmacokinetic and pharmacodynamic properties of anandamide, Di Marzo and Fontana (1995) suggested the term "endocannabinoid" to describe the endogenous cannabinoid receptors and their corresponding ligands, assigning it a similar name as the previously discovered morphine-like endorphin system.

The second endocannabinoid was discovered in 1995 by a team led once again by Mechoulam (Mechoulam et al., 1995). This new endogenous cannabinoid was isolated from canine gut and was the first to be found in peripheral tissue. The compound was named 2-AG for its chemical structure. During the same year, 2-AG was discovered in the brain and found to bind to CB1R at approximately a thousand times higher than that of anandamide, which confirmed the presence of this second endocannabinoid (Sugiura et al., 1995).

Discovery of Other Cannabinoid-Like Receptors and Endocannabinoid-Like Compounds

The discovery of the body's cannabinoid receptors and endocannabinoid ligands that bind to them led to other extensive breakthroughs involving the ECS. As researchers examined other endogenous substances that interacted with the CB1R and CB2R, additional endocannabinoid-like compounds were revealed. In 2001, 2-arachidonoyl glyceryl ether, or noladin ether (NE), was discovered. NE was found to interact with CB1R in brain tissue (Hanuš et al., 2001). A fourth compound, O-AEA, was discovered and given the name virodhamine for the Sanskrit word "opposition" because it displayed antagonistic activity at CB1R but agonistic activity at CB2R (Porter, 2002). Price et al. (2004) recognized that N-arachidonoyl dopamine (NADA) interacted with CB1R to decrease pain sensation, thus classifying this endogenous lipid as another endocannabinoid-like compound. Through the discovery that GPR18, an "orphan receptor," was an endocannabinoid receptor, N-arachidonoyl glycine (NaGly) was subsequently identified as its endogenous ligand (Kohno et al., 2006).

Other physiologic orphan receptors were investigated for their possible interactions with endogenous cannabinoids. In 2006, GPR119 was classified as a cannabinoid receptor when its interactions with oleoylethanolamide (OEA), another endocannabinoid-like compound, were found to influence food intake and glucose metabolism (see the section "Cannabinoid Receptors") (Godlewski et al., 2009; Overton et al., 2008). GPR55, another orphan receptor, was found to interact with anandamide,

2-AG, and virodhamine, as well as lysophosphatidylinositol (LPI), which was further identified as another endocannabinoid-like substance (Oka et al., 2007; Ryberg et al., 2007). Oleoyl serine (OS) was found to interact with cannabinoid receptors to regulate bone remodeling (Smoum et al., 2010), possibly through the activation of peripheral skeletal CB2R. Oleoyl glycine (OG) was discovered as another endocannabinoid-like compound that promotes adipogenesis through activation of CB1R (Wang et al., 2015).

To date, three GPRs that act as cannabinoid receptors have been identified (see the section below). GPR18 (Pertwee et al., 2010), GPR55 (Ryberg et al., 2007), and GPR119 (Overton et al., 2011) interact with endocannabinoid and endocannabinoid-like ligands to affect numerous physiologic processes. Other receptors that are not GPR have also been found to act within the ECS, including transient receptor potential vanilloid subtype 1 (TRPV1) receptor, serotonin 5-hydroxytryptamine (5-HT_3) receptor, and peroxisome proliferator–activated receptors (PPARs). As global interest in cannabinoid receptors and endocannabinoids continues to intensify, the identification of additional receptors and ligands will surely follow. Table 2.1 summarizes the cannabinoid receptors and their anatomic locations.

TABLE 2.1.	Cannabinoid receptors and their anatomic locations
Cannabinoid receptor	**Anatomic location**
Cannabinoid receptor 1 (CB1R)	Adipose tissue: Adipocytes Adrenal gland Blood vessels Bone Bone marrow Brain: Olfactory bulb, accumbens nucleus, hippocampus, basal ganglia, cerebellum, cerebral cortex, septum, amygdala, hypothalamus, pituitary gland, parts of the brain stem, astrocytes, microglial cells, striatum, globus pallidus, substantia nigra, dorsal horn Central nervous system: Dorsal horn of spinal cord Gastrointestinal (GI) tract Heart: Sympathetic nerve terminals of superior cervical ganglion Kidney Liver Lung Ovary Pancreas Peripheral nervous system Prostate Reproductive system: Uterus, testis, vas deferens Retina Skeletal muscle Spleen Thymus Tonsils Urinary bladder Uterus

(continued)

TABLE 2.1.	Cannabinoid receptors and their anatomic locations (*continued*)
Cannabinoid receptor	**Anatomic location**
Cannabinoid receptor 2 (CB2R)	Brain: Brain stem, microglia
	GI tract epithelial cells
	Immune: Tonsils, spleen, thymus, immune cells (B-cells, macrophages, natural killer cells, polymorphonuclear cells, T-cells)
	Osteoclasts/osteoblasts
	Retina
	Spleen
G-protein-coupled receptor 18 (GPR18)	Adipose tissue
	Appendix
	Brain: Cortex, thalamus, hypothalamus, cerebellum, brain stem
	Chondrocytes
	Colon
	Endometrium
	Kidney
	Lungs
	Lymph nodes
	Ovary
	Peripheral leukocytes: B-cells, T-cells
	Prostate
	Skin
	Small intestine
	Spleen
	Testis
	Thymus
	Uterus
G-protein-coupled receptor 55 (GPR55)	Adipose tissue: Subcutaneous, visceral
	Adrenal gland
	Bone
	Brain: Brain stem, hippocampus, hypothalamus, caudate putamen, cerebellum, frontal cortex, thalamus, pons, striatum
	Breast
	GI tract: Colon, ileum, jejunum, stomach
	Immune cells: Lymphocytes, macrophages, monocytes, neutrophils
	Kidney
	Liver
	Lung
	Pancreas: β-cells, islets of Langerhans
	Spleen
	Testis
	Urinary bladder
	Uterus
	Vascular endothelium
	Vascular smooth muscle

TABLE 2.1.	Cannabinoid receptors and their anatomic locations (*continued*)
Cannabinoid receptor	**Anatomic location**
G-protein-coupled receptor 119 (GPR119)	Intestines: Colon, ileum Pancreas: β-cells, islets of Langerhans Stomach
Transient receptor potential vanilloid 1 (TRPV1) receptor	Chondrocytes Brain neurons Cells: Epithelial, endothelial, smooth muscle, mast, dendritic, lymphocytes, keratinocytes, osteoclasts, hepatocytes, myotubes, fibroblasts, pancreatic β-cells
5-Hydroxytryptamine serotonin receptors (5-HT$_3$, serotonin receptors)	Central nervous system: Cortex, hippocampus, nucleus accumbens, substantia nigra, ventral tegmental area, brain stem Peripheral nervous system: Enteric nervous system of GI tract, smooth muscle of urinary tract
Peroxisome proliferator–activated receptors (PPAR)	PPARα: Colon, duodenum, heart, kidney, liver, macrophages, skeletal muscle, smooth muscle PPARδ: Abdominal adipose tissue, adrenal gland, brain, intestine, kidney, liver, lung, skeletal muscle, spleen PPARγ: Adipose tissue, colon, heart, kidney, liver, large and small intestines, macrophages, pancreas, spleen, skeletal muscle, smooth muscle

CANNABINOID RECEPTORS

The ECS is a lipid signaling system that evolved in humans and consists of the cannabinoid receptors, the endogenous ligands (endocannabinoids) that bind to them, and the enzymes that control their synthesis and degradation (Console-Bram et al., 2012; McPartland et al., 2006). Three forms of cannabinoid receptor agonists initiate a physiologic response when linked to the receptor: phytocannabinoids, which are compounds contained in the *C. sativa* plant, such as CBD, CBN, and THC; synthetic cannabinoids, such as dronabinol; and endocannabinoids, such as anandamide and 2-AG (Pertwee, 2005).

Cannabinoid receptors were named after their response to exogenously administered cannabinoid drugs, such as Δ^9-THC, and are part of the GPR family of proteins found on presynaptic nerve terminal cell membranes (McAllister & Glass, 2002). Both CB1R and CB2R transect, or cross through, the cell membrane seven times. Both cannabinoid receptors have been identified in many mammalian species, including humans, dogs, rats, pigs, fish, monkeys, and mice (Martin et al., 2000; McPartland et al., 2001, 2006). The main function of all cannabinoid receptors is to mediate inhibition of the release of neurotransmitters from presynaptic neurons, which have inhibitory or stimulatory effects on the postsynaptic neuron (Console-Bram et al., 2012; Katona & Freund, 2008). It is from this inhibition of neurotransmitter release that the ECS activates a wide variety of neurologic and immunologic processes that directly or indirectly influence physiologic actions in each major body system. The most well-researched cannabinoid receptors are CB1R and CB2R.

Cannabinoid Receptor 1

CB1Rs were previously thought to be confined to the brain. Although their highest concentration is in the brain, CB1Rs are also found in the peripheral nervous system and peripheral tissues, such as cardiovascular, gastrointestinal (GI), and reproductive tissues. CB1Rs are the most abundant GPRs in the brain and are highly expressed in areas of the brain and spinal cord associated with pain modulation (Calignano et al., 1998; Richardson et al., 1998). CB1Rs are also expressed in adipose tissue, bone, skeletal muscle, and the kidneys (Larrinaga et al., 2010; Tam, 2006). Activation of CB1R regulates fertility and influences oocyte maturation and embryonic development in the female reproductive system (Svizenska et al., 2008). Figure 2.2 illustrates the major locations and associated functions of CB1R in the human body.

CB1R is primarily located on cell membranes in the presynaptic neurons and their main function is to modulate neurologic function through the inhibition of neurotransmitter release (Katona & Freund, 2008). Repetitive activation of CB1R causes an increase in intracellular calcium (McAllister & Glass, 2002), which then leads to synthesis and mobilization of the endocannabinoid 2-AG. 2-AG then activates

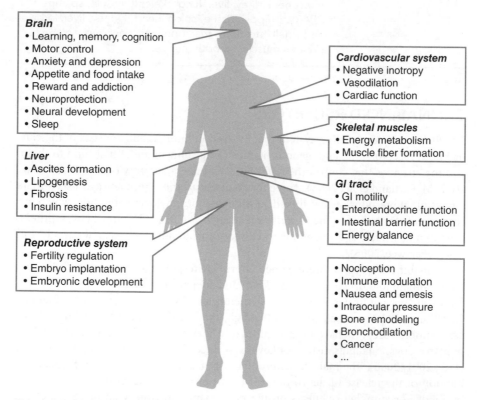

Brain
- Learning, memory, cognition
- Motor control
- Anxiety and depression
- Appetite and food intake
- Reward and addiction
- Neuroprotection
- Neural development
- Sleep

Liver
- Ascites formation
- Lipogenesis
- Fibrosis
- Insulin resistance

Reproductive system
- Fertility regulation
- Embryo implantation
- Embryonic development

Cardiovascular system
- Negative inotropy
- Vasodilation
- Cardiac function

Skeletal muscles
- Energy metabolism
- Muscle fiber formation

GI tract
- GI motility
- Enteroendocrine function
- Intestinal barrier function
- Energy balance

- Nociception
- Immune modulation
- Nausea and emesis
- Intraocular pressure
- Bone remodeling
- Bronchodilation
- Cancer
- ...

Figure 2.2: Major localization sites and associated functions of the cannabinoid receptor 1 (CB1R) in the human body. The majority of CB1R expressed in the human body are found in the brain, where they are involved in various neurologic activities. CB1R are expressed on the peripheral sites, although to a lesser extent, and participate in the regulation of local tissue functions. Abbreviation: GI, gastrointestinal.

postsynaptic potassium channels resulting in hyperpolarization and decreased neuronal excitability. Therefore, CB1R located on the presynaptic terminal reduces the neuronal firing of either excitatory or inhibitory neurotransmitters (Katona & Freund, 2008). CB1R in the brain is primarily expressed in gamma-aminobutyric acid (GABA)ergic and glutamatergic terminals, where inhibition of both excitatory (eg, glutamate) and inhibitory (eg, GABA) neurotransmitter release occurs (Andrzejewska et al., 2018; Katona & Freund, 2008). Figure 2.3 depicts the seven transmembrane structures of CB1R (Andrzejewska et al., 2018).

In the brain, CB1R stimulation is responsible for most of the mind-altering, psycho-impairing effects of THC found in cannabis. CB1R in the brain regulates appetite and food intake (Kirkham, 2009; Pagotto et al., 2006), learning and memory, anxiety and depression, neural development, and sleep (Zanettini et al., 2011; Zou & Kumar, 2018). In microglia cells of the brain and spinal cord, CB1R activation plays a critical role in the regulation of inflammatory cytokines in response to central nervous system (CNS) inflammation (Pertwee & Ross, 2002). Microglia are specialized nerve cells within the CNS that function as macrophages, the immune system's cellular scavengers, which search out and clear cellular debris and dead neurons from nervous tissue as well as destroy any foreign agents that may have penetrated the CNS. Other beneficial physiologic effects of CB1R activation include a reduction in intraocular pressure (IOP) (Laine et al., 2002), relief from muscle spasticity (Pertwee, 2005), decreased intestinal motility (Sharkey & Wiley, 2016), sedation (Pertwee, 2005), and a reduction in chemotherapy-induced nausea and vomiting (Parker et al.,

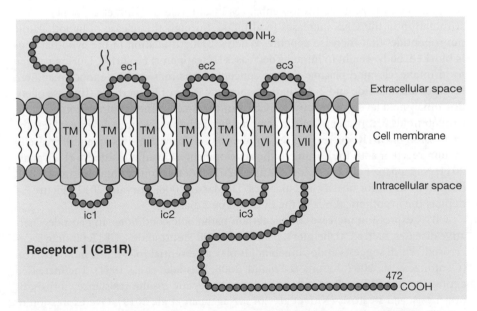

Figure 2.3: **Seven transmembrane construction of cannabinoid receptor 1 (CB1R).** The numbers at the beginning of the transmembrane chain (1) and end of the transmembrane chain (472) indicate the direction of numbers of amino acids along the chain. Terminal residues, amino (N-) and carboxy (C-), transmembrane domains (TM1-VII), intracellular (ic), and extracellular (ec) chain loops are also marked.

2010). A decrease in CB1R expression has been associated with aging in the human brain (Paradisi et al., 2006).

Cellular activity related to CB1R stimulation depends on the type of tissue or organ involved as well as the specific binding endogenous agonist. Activation of CB1R in the hypothalamus regulates energy homeostasis, increases food intake, and stimulates lipogenesis in peripheral tissues (Pagotto et al., 2006; Zou & Kumar, 2018). In the accumbens nucleus located in the midbrain, the dopaminergic reward pathway is activated by CB1R stimulation, triggering the impulse to eat, smoke tobacco, or use addictive drugs (Gardner, 2005).

In peripheral neurons, CB1R stimulation inhibits calcium channels (McAllister, 2002), which subsequently reduces neurotransmitter release from presynaptic neurons. CB1R stimulation also activates inwardly correcting potassium channels, balancing the intracellular/extracellular ratios of these important electrolytes, which then decreases neuronal excitability (Pertwee, 2005). In peripheral tissues and neurons, CB1R stimulation inhibits adenylate cyclase (McAllister & Glass, 2002). Adenylyl cyclase is the only enzyme used to synthesize cyclic adenosine monophosphate (cAMP). cAMP is a second intracellular messenger that regulates numerous essential physiologic processes, such as glucose and lipid metabolism, cell growth and differentiation, gene transformation, protein expression, and apoptosis, or programmed cell death (Yan et al., 2016). When CB1R is activated and adenylyl cyclase is inhibited, the production of cAMP is diminished, modifying these important physiologic functions (Bow & Rimoldi, 2016).

An important function of CB1R expression relates to its activity in the β-cells of the pancreas, where its activation enhances insulin release (Kim et al., 2011). CB1R stimulation in the CNS increases food intake through the release of hypothalamic neuropeptides that increase appetite. When CB1R stimulation in the hypothalamus is blocked, body weight in humans decreases (Nagappan et al., 2019). During normal food intake, elevated plasma glucose concentrations increase the endocannabinoid levels of anandamide and 2-AG in the pancreatic islets of Langerhans. This rise of endocannabinoid levels then activates CB1R in the β-cells. The accumulation of endocannabinoids within the β-cells in the presence of hyperglycemia downregulates the expression of CB1R, decreasing the number of CB1R, with a subsequent decrease in insulin receptor activity, leading to the development of insulin resistance (Kim et al., 2011; Nagappan et al., 2019; Zou & Kumar, 2018). Activation or antagonism of CB1R has implications for obesity and diabetes (Di Marzo, 2008; Horváth, 2012). Figure 2.4 depicts the hypothetical role of the ECS in type 2 diabetes.

CB1R expression increases under certain pathologic conditions. In neurodegenerative diseases, such as Alzheimer's, Parkinson's, and Huntington's, CB1R binding is decreased, which suggests endocannabinoids play an essential role in fine motor control (Centonze et al., 2007; Katona & Freund, 2008; Westlake et al., 1994). The increased expression of CB1R in liver cells contributes to hepatic insulin resistance, fibrosis, lipogenesis, and steatosis (Kim et al., 2011; Nagappan et al., 2019). Overexpression of CB1R and CB2R in the liver also results in hepatic vasodilation and hepatic inflammation, leading to cirrhosis and other liver pathologies (Xu et al., 2006). Overexpression of CB1R in adipose tissue can lead to obesity, dyslipidemia, and other metabolic complications, including insulin resistance (Di Marzo, 2008; Zou & Kumar, 2018).

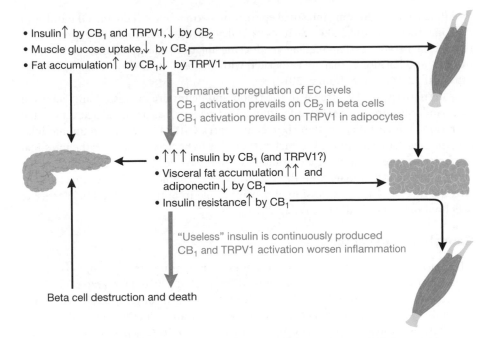

- Insulin↑ by CB_1 and TRPV1,↓ by CB_2
- Muscle glucose uptake,↓ by CB_1
- Fat accumulation↑ by CB_1,↓ by TRPV1

Permanent upregulation of EC levels
CB_1 activation prevails on CB_2 in beta cells
CB_1 activation prevails on TRPV1 in adipocytes

- ↑↑↑ insulin by CB_1 (and TRPV1?)
- Visceral fat accumulation ↑↑ and adiponectin↓ by CB_1
- Insulin resistance↑ by CB_1

"Useless" insulin is continuously produced
CB_1 and TRPV1 activation worsen inflammation

Beta cell destruction and death

Figure 2.4: **Hypothetical role of the endocannabinoid system in type 2 diabetes.** After a meal in a normal weight individual, endocannabinoid-induced CB1R and TRPV1 stimulatory actions on insulin release might be counteracted by CB2R, possibly as a result of high concentrations of 2-AG (most active on both CB1R and CB2R) over anandamide (most active on CB1R and TRPV1 receptor) levels. In hyperglycemia and obesity, both anandamide and 2-AG levels are increased in the pancreas, causing overstimulation of CB1R and TRPV1, and enhancing insulin release. At the same time, insulin sensitivity is decreased by elevated 2-AG levels in the skeletal muscle, whereas elevation of 2-AG in adipocytes causes activation of prolipogenetic CB1R versus antilipogenetic TRPV1 receptors, visceral fat accumulation, and reduced adiponectin production. These concurrent events cause more insulin resistance and hyperinsulinemia, thus leading to β-cell hypertrophy and damage, ultimately contributing to type 2 diabetes, possibly also through CB1R- and TRPV1-mediated proinflammatory actions. Abbreviations: 2-AG, 2-arachidonoylglycerol; CB1R, cannabinoid receptor 1; CB2R, cannabinoid receptor 2; TRPV1, transient receptor potential vanilloid subtype 1.

Cardiovascular expression of CB1R results in negative inotropy, weakening the force of contraction, and causes cardiovascular vasodilation, decreasing peripheral blood pressure. In pathologic cardiovascular conditions, CB1R is expressed in cardiac tissue, which promotes the progression of cardiovascular disease and dysfunction brought on by oxidative stress and fibrosis of cardiomyocytes, vascular endothelial cells, and smooth muscle cells (Horváth, 2012). In the skeleton, activation of CB1R modulates bone development by inhibiting the sympathetic neuronal release of norepinephrine, limiting bone formation (Bab & Zimmer, 2008; Tam, 2006). Expression of CB1R in skeletal muscle results in decreased energy metabolism by decreasing basal and insulin-mediated glucose uptake, promoting insulin resistance (Nagappan et al., 2019), and stimulates the formation of muscle fibers (Di Marzo, 2008). In the GI tract, CB1R activation alters GI motility by decreasing the secretion of gastric acids and fluids and modulating intestinal epithelium permeability, reducing GI motility of its contents (Izzo et al., 2001; Sharkey & Wiley, 2016). Overall, CB1R expression in the enteric nervous system regulates endocrine function, energy balance, neurotransmitters, and hormones that are associated with glucose intake (Di Marzo, 2008; Pagotto et al., 2006; Zou & Kumar, 2018).

Alternatively, CB1R present in the colon and ileum are expressed and activated by anandamide in the presence of pathologic states, such as paralytic ileus, intestinal secretion, and GI inflammation (Izzo et al., 2001). CB1Rs have an immunomodulatory/homeostatic role in the GI tract, responding to bacteria that enter the intestinal lumen to ensure an appropriate immune response to normal gut flora. During the acute phase of inflammatory GI disorders, such as irritable bowel syndrome (IBS) or Crohn's disease, CB2R expression also plays a role in anti-inflammation (Pacher & Mechoulam, 2011; Sharkey & Wiley, 2016).

Cannabinoid Receptor 2

CB2R is located in microglial cells, astrocytes, oligodendrocytes, spleen, tonsils, thymus, mast cells, blood cells, and neurons (Bisogno et al., 2016; Di Marzo et al., 1998; Svizenska et al., 2008). Like CB1R, CB2R also crosses through the cell membrane seven times. Figure 2.5 depicts the seven transmembrane structure of CB2R.

CB2R is expressed primarily by immune cells in the hematopoietic system, where it controls proliferation, differentiation, and survival of both neuronal and

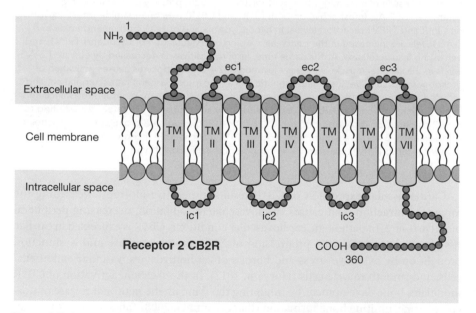

Figure 2.5: **Seven transmembrane construction of cannabinoid receptor 2 (CB2R).** The numbers at the beginning of the transmembrane chain (1) and end of the transmembrane chain (360) indicate the direction of numbers of amino acids along the chain. Terminal residues, amino (N-) and carboxy (C-), transmembrane domains (TM1-VII), intracellular (ic), and extracellular (ec) chain loops are also marked.

non-neuronal cells (Guzmán et al., 2001; Malfitano et al., 2014; Valk et al., 1997). The primary function of CB2R is to modulate chemical messengers (cytokines) from immune cells. During normal physiologic states, the human body does not express high densities of CB2R; it is only during the pathologic changes in organ systems that CB2R is significantly upregulated in affected cells and tissues (Pacher & Mechoulam, 2011; Roche & Finn, 2010).

The presence of disease in organ systems concurrently stimulates the elevation of endocannabinoid levels as part of the body's homeostatic inflammatory and immune response. During brain trauma, CB2R expression increases in astrocytes and microglial cells (Bisogno et al., 2016; Lu & Mackie, 2016; Witting et al., 2004). Neuronal damage stimulates increased CB2R expression in the CNS, which then provides a neuroprotective mechanism by reducing cell death as it blocks cell apoptosis (Bisogno et al., 2016; Guzmán et al., 2001; Viscomi et al., 2009). CB2R activation has been associated with neuronal homeostasis and survival (Javed et al., 2016).

Similar to CB1R activation, activation of CB2R also inhibits the production of adenylyl cyclase, which diminishes the production of cAMP (Bow & Rimoldi, 2016; Lutz, 2002). When endocannabinoids activate CB2R on immune B- and T-cells, adenylyl cyclase release is inhibited, which reduces the body's response to immune threats. During inflammation and tissue injury, endocannabinoid levels in the body rise. This elevation in endocannabinoid concentrations initiates CB2R upregulation and activation that suppress immune responses, which, in turn, decreases inflammation and associated tissue injury. This process of anti-inflammation subsequently reduces pain associated with tissue injury. CB2R activation can also suppress the antibody-mediated immune response, which demonstrates its ability to potentially moderate autoimmune diseases such as multiple sclerosis, systemic lupus erythematosus, and Crohn's disease (Basu & Dittel, 2011; Cabral & Griffin-Thomas, 2009; Leinwand et al., 2017; Navarini et al., 2018). Figure 2.6 displays CB2R expression and its known cellular functions.

CB2R is expressed on osteoblasts (bone-resorbing cells) and osteoclasts (bone-forming cells) (Pacher & Mechoulam, 2011; Whyte et al., 2009). Anandamide and 2-AG are present in bone in concentrations nearly as high as brain levels of these endocannabinoids (Zou & Kumar, 2018). When activated by endocannabinoids, CB2R limits bone resorption and enhances bone formation. This suggests CB2R agonism is a potential therapeutic target for anti-osteoporosis therapies (Bab & Zimmer, 2008; Malfitano et al., 2014).

When CB2R is expressed in cells and tissues, much of the subsequent physiologic activity is directed toward inhibition of inflammation and tissue injury. In cardiovascular diseases, such as heart failure, cardiomyopathy, myocardial infarction, and atherosclerosis, CB2R is expressed in the myocardium, cardiomyocytes, endothelial cells, and circulating immune cells to decrease inflammation, promote monocyte chemotaxis, and reduce endothelial activation and/or vascular smooth muscle proliferation (Pacher & Mechoulam, 2011).

In the presence of CNS disorders, such as stroke and spinal cord injury, CB2R activation in the brain, microglia, and circulating immune cells decreases endothelial activation and leukocyte infiltration, decreasing tissue injury (Bisogno et al., 2016; Malfitano et al., 2014; Pacher & Mechoulam, 2011). In GI disorders, such as IBS,

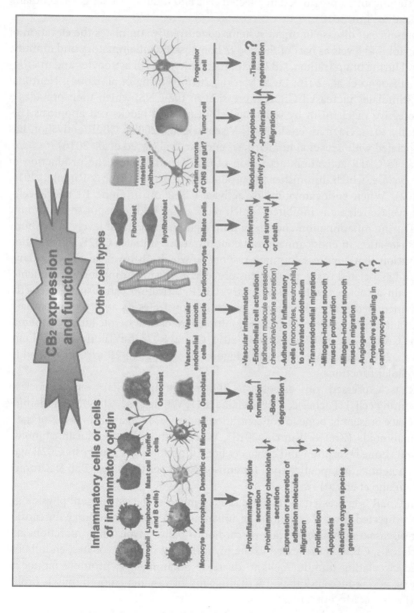

Figure 2.6: **Cannabinoid receptor 2 (CB2R) and its known cellular functions.** CB2R are the most abundantly expressed in cells of the immune system and cells of immune origin. In these cells, CB2R mostly mediate immunosuppressive effects. CB2R expression has been reported in activated/diseased other cell types. In various pathologic conditions, CB2R were reported to be markedly upregulated in most of the shown cell types and were found to play important roles in various cellular functions. Some of these effects are largely determined by the type of injury/inflammation and its stage.

colitis, and diverticulitis, epithelial cells sense inflammation in the gut, which activates CB2R expression. Thus, CB2R is upregulated in the presence of inflamed GI mucosa (Pacher & Mechoulam, 2011; Wright et al., 2005). The activation of CB2R decreases tissue inflammation and visceral sensitivity and promotes GI epithelial tissue healing (Wright et al., 2005). In pancreatitis, activation of CB2R has been shown to decrease inflammation (Nagarkatti et al., 2009), and activation during kidney nephropathy decreases cytokine signaling and chemotaxis, which subsequently decreases inflammatory cell infiltration and endothelial activation (Mukhopadhyay et al., 2010).

The expression of CB2R in microglia and damaged brain tissue has been shown to decrease inflammation by activating microglia, decreasing immune cell infiltration, and facilitating neuronal growth (Witting et al., 2004). CB2R activation in the presence of neurodegenerative and neuroinflammatory diseases such as multiple sclerosis, Alzheimer's disease, Parkinson's disease, Huntington's disease, and spinal cord injury has significant implications for treatment and restoration of damaged nerves and tissues (Centonze et al., 2007).

Disease states associated with tumor development in cancer are also affected by CB2R expression. In animal models of various tumor or cancer cells, CB2R expression decreases tumor growth through apoptosis, inhibiting angiogenesis, proliferation, and migration of tumor cells, which directly stops cancer cell growth by inducing programmed cell death, blocking vascular blood supply to the tissue, and preventing cancer cell metastasis to other tissues (Velasco et al., 2016). The endocannabinoids anandamide and 2-AG have also been shown to inhibit the proliferation of breast (De Petrocellis et al., 1998) and prostate cancer cells (Melck et al., 2000; Piñeiro et al., 2011).

Reproductive disease and dysfunction are also influenced by CB2R expression. In normal reproductive activity, CB2R expressed in testes, ovaries, and uterus induces spermatogenesis and affects embryo development (Battista et al., 2012). In endometriosis, CB2R expression attenuates the inflammation of uterine tissue and the proliferation of immune cells (Dmitrieva et al., 2010).

In some disease states, dysregulation of CB2R may enhance or even produce tissue damage. Numerous pathologic conditions are associated with dysfunctional CB2R expression, including diseases associated with the cardiovascular system, GI system, liver, kidney, lung, neurodegeneration (ie, Alzheimer's, Parkinson's, and Huntington's), psychiatric, skeletal, cancer, pain, reproduction, and skin (Pacher & Mechoulam, 2011). Figure 2.7 illustrates the disease states in which CB2R dysregulation plays a role in the development of the disease.

Putative Cannabinoid Receptors

As researchers began to understand the physiologic and pharmacologic effects of endocannabinoids and phytocannabinoids, additional targets for these ligands were theorized and eventually discovered. A group of GPRs, previously known as the orphan receptors, was found to be directly and indirectly activated by endocannabinoids and endocannabinoid-like ligands. The endogenous cannabinoids and related compounds bind to these receptors, and although they have not been formally classified as cannabinoid receptors, they nevertheless modulate physiologic processes when activated by their respective ligands.

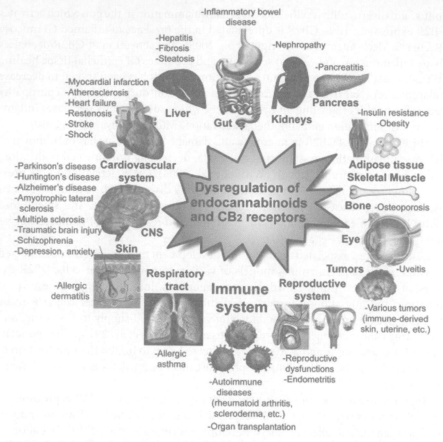

Figure 2.7: **Role of cannabinoid receptor 2 (CB2R) activation in various diseases affecting humans.** Selected disease conditions are shown in which dysregulation of CB2R is implicated in the pathophysiology. Conversely, in these conditions, pharmaceutical modulation of CB2R may represent a novel therapeutic strategy. Abbreviation: CNS, central nervous system.

G-protein-coupled receptor 18

GPR18 is expressed in the lymph nodes, leukocytes (including neutrophils, monocytes, macrophages, and B- and T-cells), spleen, and testes (Gantz et al., 1997; Kohno et al., 2006). When activated by the endogenous endocannabinoid-like ligand NaGly, GPR18 regulates the migration of leukocyte and microglial cells, which leads to apoptosis of inflammatory leukocytes, reducing local inflammation (Kohno et al., 2006; McHugh et al., 2010). GPR18 has been suggested to play a role in the modulation of acute and chronic pain (Guerrero-Alba et al., 2019). In mouse models of glaucoma, activation of GPR18 lowers IOP (Miller et al., 2018). GPR18 is expressed in chondrocytes within the cartilage of patients with osteoarthritis, suggesting that it plays a role in the development of pathologic musculoskeletal conditions (Dunn et al., 2016).

G-protein-coupled receptor 55

GPR55 is considered an atypical cannabinoid-like receptor (Kapur et al., 2009). Its expression plays a role in inflammatory pain and may also influence the development of cardiovascular diseases, osteoporosis, diabetes, and cancer (Piñeiro et al., 2011). GPR55 is expressed in brain regions that are associated with memory, learning, and motor function, such as the frontal cortex, cerebellum, striatum, hypothalamus, and brain stem (Nevalainen & Irving, 2010). In the peripheral tissues, GPR55 is found in the adrenal gland, testis, spleen, liver, lung, tonsils, breast, adipose tissue (including visceral and subcutaneous adipose tissues), uterus, urinary bladder, stomach, kidney, dorsal root ganglia neurons, and immune cells (lymphocytes, macrophages, monocytes, neutrophils) (Balenga et al., 2011; Yang et al., 2016). GPR55 is also found in vascular endothelium and smooth muscle (Bondarenko et al., 2011), and in GI tissues, including the jejunum, ileum, and colon (Godlewski et al., 2009).

Anandamide, 2-AG, O-AEA (also known as virodhamine), and palmitoylethanolamide (PEA) (see the section below) are agonists at GPR55 (Nevalainen & Irving, 2010; Reggio, 2010; Sharir et al., 2012). One of the endocannabinoid-like compounds, LPI, is considered the most potent endogenous ligand of GPR55 (Bełtowski, 2012; Bondarenko et al., 2011; Kargl et al., 2012; Reggio, 2010). GPR55 is expressed by osteoclasts, and when activated by LPI, osteoclast activity and survival is increased, suggesting it has therapeutic potential in the treatment of osteoporosis (Kargl et al., 2012). When expressed in mouse bone, GPR55 stimulates osteoclast function and reduces bone resorption (Whyte et al., 2009).

GPR55 controls the vascular tone and regulates immune cell function and cell migration through its activation by PEA (Ryberg et al., 2007). Intracellularly, GPR55 increases calcium concentrations, which activates signaling pathways that increase neuronal excitability (Lauckner et al., 2008). GPR55 may also play a role in obesity, as increased expression of this receptor in subcutaneous and visceral adipose tissues is found in obese subjects, including obese subjects with type 2 diabetes (Moreno-Navarrete et al., 2012). As LPI is considered the endogenous ligand for GPR55, circulating levels of this compound also increase in these patients, suggesting that the LPI/GPR55 system is positively correlated to obesity (Bełtowski, 2012; Moreno-Navarrete et al., 2012). Expression of GPR55 in visceral adipose tissue is positively associated with type 2 diabetes, as its activation may play an important role in the pathogenesis of visceral fat accumulation and insulin resistance (Moreno-Navarrete et al., 2012).

GPR55 and CB1R are highly expressed in similar levels of brain tissues, such as the striatum, hypothalamus, and brain stem (Kargl et al., 2012). GPR55 signaling is inhibited in the presence of CB1R activation, whereas CB1R signaling is enhanced in the presence of GPR55, suggesting that receptor "cross-talk" between the two receptors plays an important role in the development of cancer, bone formation, pain sensation, and inflammation (Godlewski et al., 2009; Guerrero-Alba et al., 2019; Kargl et al., 2012). In other pathologic conditions, GPR55 has been proposed to play a role in disorders that involve the GI tract, inflammatory and neuropathic pain, and diseases related to inappropriate innate and adaptive immune responses (Guerrero-Alba et al., 2019).

GPR55 also regulates CB2R responses in inflammatory cells and plays a significant role in inflammation, regulating ECS participation in the inflammatory process to maintain homeostasis (Yang et al., 2016). When LPI activates GPR55, neutrophil degranulation and ROS products are diminished, which creates a response that increases CB2R-mediated migration of 2-AG, thereby limiting tissue-injuring inflammatory responses while synergistically working with CB2R to recruit other inflammatory cells (Piñeiro et al., 2011). This "cross-talk" between GPR55 and CB2R is important for adjusting the homeostatic inflammatory and immune response that prevents excessive tissue injury.

G-protein-coupled receptor 119

GPR119 is expressed in pancreatic and intestinal cells, and it controls insulin release in response to glucose (Dhayal & Morgan, 2010; Godlewski et al., 2009). In the pancreas, GPR119 is restricted to the β-cells in the islets of Langerhans, and activation stimulates β-cell regeneration (Free et al., 2016). In the intestines, the ileum and colon express the highest densities of GPR119, where activation stimulates the secretion of gut hormones, such as glucagon-like peptide-1 (GLP-1) and glucose-dependent insulinotropic polypeptide (GIP), to enhance glucose secretion and improve hepatic glucose metabolism (Overton et al., 2008; Syed et al., 2012). Because of its location in these tissue cells, GPR119 is linked to the control of glucose homeostasis and obesity (Godlewski et al., 2009). In in vitro and animal models, GPR119 activation plays a role in the control of feeding and glucose homeostasis when activated by oleoyl ethanolamine (OEA) (Overton et al., 2006, 2008). Activation of this receptor improves glucose tolerance as it acts on β-cells to enhance insulin release (Syed et al., 2012). From these actions, GPR119 is proposed as a potential target for the treatment of type 2 diabetes and obesity (Dhayal & Morgan, 2010; Overton et al., 2008; Syed et al., 2012). Figure 2.8 describes the proposed mechanisms of GPR119 agonist action with glucose metabolism.

Non-CB1, Non-CB2 Receptors

In addition to the known CB1R, CB2R, and GPR, other types of receptors interact with endocannabinoids and endocannabinoid-like compounds. These include the TRPV1 receptor, serotonin (5-HT$_3$) receptor, and PPARs.

Transient receptor potential vanilloid 1 receptor

TRPV1 receptor is an ion-gated channel located in brain neurons and other cells, including epithelial, endothelial, smooth muscle, mast, lymphocytes, osteoclasts, and pancreatic β-cells. In the CNS, TRPV1 is expressed in the dopaminergic neurons of the midbrain (Romanovsky et al., 2009). TRPV1 is considered an inotropic cannabinoid receptor and is found together with CB1R in the brain, dorsal root ganglia, and spinal cord. It also occurs concurrently with CB2R in sensory neurons and osteoclasts. This colocalization between TRPV1, CB1R, and CB2R enhances intracellular "cross-talk" between the receptors, which amplifies endocannabinoid activity and has important physiologic consequences from each receptor's activation (Lutz, 2002; Pertwee et al., 2010; Smart et al., 2002). In animal models, TRPV1 activation on pancreatic islet β-cells modulates insulin secretion (Akiba et al., 2004). TRPV1

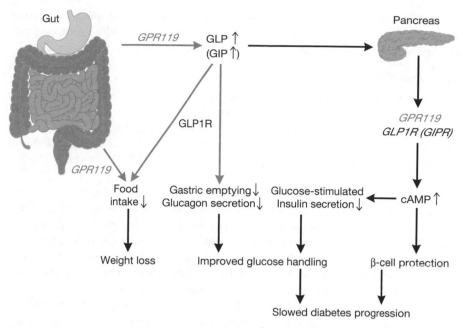

Figure 2.8: **Proposed mechanisms of GPR119 agonist action with glucose metabolism.**
The presence of GPR119 in the enteroendocrine cell lines suggests that intestinally expressed
receptors may also increase plasma glucagon-like peptide-1 (GLP-1) levels, thus decreasing
blood sugar levels in a glucose-dependent manner by enhancing the secretion of insulin.
GPR119 agonists might exert a twofold effect in lowering blood glucose, acting directly at
the pancreatic β-cell to promote glucose-stimulated insulin secretion (GSIS) and, indirectly,
via the enteroendocrine cells, by stimulating the release of the incretin hormones GLP-1
and glucose-dependent insulinotropic peptide (GIP), which are powerful antihyperglycemic
agents. GLP-1 also exerts its actions by suppressing meal-associated glucagon secretion and
regulating the delivery of food to the gut by reducing gastric motility involved in glucose
homeostasis via the modulation of incretin hormone release. Enteroendocrine cells are known
to secrete the incretin hormone GLP-1, and they respond to the signals controlling GLP-1
release. GPR119 agonists have been shown to elevate cyclic adenosine monophosphate
(cAMP) levels and stimulate GLP-1 secretion from enteroendocrine cells.

receptors and CB1R have opposite effects on calcium channel movement, indicating
that physiologic responses produced by TRPV1 receptor activation can be opposed
by the simultaneous activation of CB1R (Casarotto et al., 2012).

TRPV1 is activated by anandamide, thus anandamide is also referred to as an endovanilloid as well as an endocannabinoid (Pertwee & Ross, 2002; Smart et al., 2002).
TRPV1 is involved in the signaling processes of several physiologic stimuli, including
temperature, light, taste, and smell, and mechanical and osmotic stimuli, including
hypotonic cell swelling. TRPV1 is also involved in a number of physiologic functions, including autonomic thermoregulation, pain signaling, and synaptic plasticity
in the brain (Romanovsky et al., 2009). TRPV1 activated by anandamide produces
local vasodilation (Zygmunt et al., 1999), bronchoconstriction (Ross, 2003), and
anti-inflammation (Bisogno et al., 2001). Increased expression of TRPV1 has been
noted in pathologic conditions. TRPV1 is activated by noxious stimuli, such as heat,

protons, and other natural toxins (Brito et al., 2014). TRPV1 receptors are expressed in chondrocytes of patients with osteoarthritis, suggesting that TRPV1 receptors may be responsive to the therapeutic administration of cannabinoids (Dunn et al., 2016).

Serotonin 5-HT$_3$ receptor

The serotonin 5-HT$_3$ receptor (5-HT$_3$) is an ion-gated channel located in the enteric nervous system of the intestines that is activated by the endocannabinoid anandamide (Galligan, 2002; Haj-Dahmane & Shen, 2011; Pertwee et al., 2010; Rácz et al., 2008). Disturbances of 5-HT$_3$ may contribute to pathologies of the GI system, including diseases such as dyspepsia, gastroesophageal reflux disease (GERD), and IBS (Davies, 2011; Thompson & Lummis, 2006).

The serotonin receptor is found in the central and peripheral nervous systems, where it is stimulated by sympathetic, parasympathetic, and sensory activity. In the CNS, 5-HT$_3$ is located in areas that affect the vomiting reflex, pain processing, the reward system, cognition, depression, and anxiety, with the highest concentration found in brain stem areas involved in the vomiting reflex. In the peripheral nervous system, the serotonin receptor is found in neurons and immune cells (Haj-Dahmane & Shen, 2011; Thompson & Lummis, 2006; Walstab et al., 2010).

Functions of serotonin receptors in the GI tract include regulating gut motility and peristalsis (Browning & Travagli, 2014), while in the urinary tract smooth muscle, serotonin receptors regulate urinary bladder function (Ritter et al., 2017). Anandamide serves as a serotonin receptor antagonist, suppressing receptor activity, thus inhibiting nausea and anxiety (Parker et al., 2011) and decreasing pain associated with GI inflammation (Calignano et al., 1998; Davies, 2011; Haj-Dahmane & Shen, 2011; Sharkey & Wiley, 2016; Walker et al., 2002; Walstab et al., 2010).

Endocannabinoid signaling controls the function and expression of 5-HT$_3$ receptors in the CNS (Haj-Dahmane & Shen, 2011). Additionally, ECS signaling plays a critical role in the regulation of stress-related behaviors through the control of body temperature, feeding behavior, sleep and arousal, and emotional processes (Haj-Dahmane & Shen, 2011). The release of the 5-HT$_3$ neurotransmitter, serotonin, is involved in these physiologic processes. Anandamide blocks activation at the 5-HT$_3$ receptor (Davies, 2011), increasing 5-HT$_3$ receptor desensitization and modulating serotonin release. Serotonin release in the CNS is reduced when CB1R is activated by anandamide, resulting in reduced body temperature, decreased feeding behavior, and reduced stress response (Rácz et al., 2008).

Peroxisome proliferator–activated receptors

PPARs are lipid sensors that regulate lipid metabolism, the storage and catabolism of dietary fats, glucose homeostasis, hepatic enzyme expression, insulin sensitivity, and monitor for local changes in metabolism (Chinetti et al., 2000; Sun & Bennett, 2007; Willson et al., 2000). PPARs also regulate cellular differentiation, development, and inflammation (Le Menn & Neels, 2018; Müller et al., 2008). There are three PPAR isoforms: PPARα (alpha), PPARδ (delta), and PPARγ (gamma), and each is activated by a different ligand. Table 2.2 describes the anatomic location of these three receptors.

Activation of PPARα lowers cholesterol, prevents atherosclerosis, improves glucose tolerance and insulin resistance, lowers blood pressure, and inhibits inflammation

TABLE 2.2.	Location of PPAR isoforms
PPAR isoform	**Anatomic location**
PPARα	Brain (amygdala, prefrontal cortex, nucleus accumbens, ventral tegmental area), endothelial cells, heart, kidneys, liver, macrophages, skeletal muscle, smooth muscle (Chinetti et al., 2000; Pertwee et al., 2010; Peyrou et al., 2012; Tyagi et al., 2011; Warden et al., 2016)
PPARδ	Adipose tissue, brain (amygdala, prefrontal cortex, nucleus accumbens, ventral tegmental area), adrenal gland, heart, intestines, kidneys, liver, lung, skeletal muscle, spleen (Chinetti et al., 2000; Pertwee et al., 2010; Peyrou et al., 2012; Sun & Bennett, 2007; Warden et al., 2016)
PPARγ	Adipose tissue, brain (amygdala, prefrontal cortex, nucleus accumbens, ventral tegmental area), endothelial cells, heart, intestines, kidneys, liver, macrophages, mammary gland, skeletal muscle (Chinetti et al., 2000; Pertwee et al., 2010; Peyrou et al., 2012; Sun & Bennett, 2007; Tyagi et al., 2011; Warden et al., 2016)

PPAR, peroxisome proliferator–activated receptor.

(Chinetti et al., 2000; Willson et al., 2000). Anandamide weakly agonizes PPARα but strongly agonizes PPARγ, whereas 2-AG activates PPARγ (Pertwee et al., 2010). Through activation of PPARγ, anandamide stimulates adipocyte differentiation and inhibits the secretion of proinflammatory cytokines (O'Sullivan et al., 2005). 2-AG decreases the expression of proinflammatory cyclooxygenase 2 (COX2) enzymes through activation of PPARγ and inhibits amyloid formation found in Alzheimer's disease (O'Sullivan et al., 2005).

The endocannabinoid-like compounds OEA and PEA agonize PPARα (Lo Verme et al., 2005; Pertwee et al., 2010; Sun & Bennett, 2007). When OEA activates PPARα in animal models, lipolysis and fatty acid oxidation occur, which results in decreased liver and fat triacylglycerol concentrations with inhibition of food intake, subsequently reducing body weight (Guzmán et al., 2004). Significantly, synthetic PPARα agonists, such as the pharmaceutical fibrates (eg, gemfibrozil, fenofibrate), are currently prescribed for their lipid-lowering and anticholesterol effects (Pertwee et al., 2010; Sun & Bennett, 2007). OEA is 500 to 900 times more potent as PPARα in lowering cholesterol, with the added effect of reducing food intake, suggesting that a novel antiobesity drug designed to activate PPARα could have important therapeutic potential (Guzmán et al., 2004). Acting at brain PPARα, OEA reduces infarct size and brain edema after cerebral artery occlusion, which improves neurologic dysfunction after cerebrovascular injury (O'Sullivan et al., 2005).

Inflammatory responses to tissue injury are moderated through PPARα activation by endocannabinoid-like compounds. When PPARα is activated by PEA, inflammatory responses are inhibited by reducing COX and nitric oxide (NO) activity, which are major contributors to tissue inflammation (Costa et al., 2002; Lo Verme et al.,

2005). This reduction in inflammation thus decreases corresponding pain caused by inflammation, suggesting that alterations of endogenous PEA might be useful as anti-inflammatory treatments (Costa et al., 2002; Walker et al., 2002).

There are currently several pharmaceutical synthetic PPARγ agonist medications, including thiazolidinediones (TZDs), such as rosiglitazone and pioglitazone (Sun & Bennett, 2007). These pharmaceuticals have antidiabetic and insulin-sensitizing activities. Anandamide and 2-AG are endogenous PPARγ agonists that also mediate anti-inflammatory activity when this receptor is stimulated (Sun & Bennett, 2007). Activation of PPARγ by these endocannabinoid and endocannabinoid-like compounds suggests that they may play an important role in the development of obesity and type 2 diabetes.

ENDOCANNABINOIDS

Endocannabinoids are molecular derivatives of arachidonic acid (AA) that act as neuromodulators and immunomodulators (Alhouayek & Mucciolo, 2017; Di Marzo et al., 1998; Lutz, 2002). AA is an endogenous polyunsaturated omega-6 fatty acid that is present in the cell membrane of all body cells and is found in abundance in the brain, muscles, and liver. AA "is critically essential for the development and optimal performance of the nervous system, especially the brain and cognitive functions, the skeletal muscle, and immune systems. Additionally, [AA] promotes and regulates type 2 immune responses against intestinal and blood flukes" (Tallima & El Ridi, 2018, p. 38). Endocannabinoids are derived from fatty acid precursors that exist in cell membranes and include the classes of ethanol-amides, glycerols, and glycerol ethers (Reggio, 2010). Because of their lipophilic, or lipid-loving, structure, endocannabinoids bind to cannabinoid receptors (eg, CB1R and CB2R) and ion channels (eg, TRPV1) in tissues. More recently, endocannabinoid and endocannabinoid-like compounds have been found to interact with potassium channels, PPARs (eg, PPARα and PPARγ), and the serotonin 5-HT$_3$ receptor. Each endocannabinoid is a member of the lipid family of endogenous compounds. Two separate processes mediate the release of endocannabinoids from presynaptic neurons: neurotransmitter release from presynaptic neurons and neuronal depolarization. These two processes work simultaneously in a continual fashion (Lu & Mackie, 2016).

When the cellular membrane of cannabinoid receptors is depolarized, endocannabinoids are synthesized from phospholipid precursors that are already present in the membrane. Unlike other neurotransmitters that are stored in synaptic vessels, 2-AG is produced on demand in response to a rise in intracellular calcium levels in the postsynaptic neuron. When calcium levels rise in the postsynapse, 2-AG is released by both neuronal and non-neuronal cells (Kano, 2014; Reggio, 2010). Anandamide is stored in intracellular adiposomes, known as "lipid rafts" (Fowler, 2013; Oddi et al., 2008), which act as anandamide reservoirs and serve as "ferry lipids" to transport endocannabinoids between the plasma membrane and intracellular sites. Once released from the postsynaptic terminal, endocannabinoids travel backward across the synaptic cleft and work in reverse fashion at the presynaptic nerve terminal to modulate neurotransmitter release through cannabinoid receptors found on presynaptic neurons (see the section below) (Christie & Vaughan, 2001; Kreitzer & Regehr, 2001; Lu & Mackie, 2016).

Once an endocannabinoid binds to its corresponding receptor, an intracellular signal transduction pathway is activated, sending an extracellular signal through the receptor membrane to stimulate intracellular activities. Endocannabinoids act as both autocrine (ie, messaging the cell itself) and paracrine (ie, messaging nearby cells) messengers, which produce inhibitory effects on responses in both local and peripheral cells (Howlett et al., 2011). Endocannabinoids have been shown to inhibit acetylcholine, dopamine, GABA, glutamate, and norepinephrine release, supporting the physiologic effects that are associated with CB1R and CB2R activation (Di Marzo et al., 1998; Manzanares et al., 2006). The most well-researched endocannabinoids are AEA and 2-AG. Table 2.3 lists the proposed neuromodulatory actions of these two known endocannabinoids in the nervous system.

The two most thoroughly investigated concerning synthesis and degradation pathways are anandamide and 2-AG (Mechoulam & Ben-Shabat, 1999; Sugiura et al., 2002). Endocannabinoids are synthesized from physiologic compounds already found in cell membranes and are degraded intracellularly through hydrolysis via enzymatic activity. Once endocannabinoids are released from postsynaptic terminals and travel back across the synaptic cleft, they enter the presynaptic cell through a combination of simple diffusion and facilitated, carrier-mediated transport (Maccarrone, 2002; Rakhshan et al., 2000; Toczek & Malinowska, 2018). These distinct transport mechanisms are used by different cells, depending on the need for either cannabinoid receptor activation or endocannabinoid release, which represents the essential homeostatic-controlling properties of the ECS (Fowler, 2013).

Accepted Endocannabinoids

Arachidonoyl ethanolamide (or anandamide)

Anandamide (also known as AEA) was the first endogenous cannabinoid to be identified as the natural ligand for CB1R (Devane et al., 1992). It is a partial agonist at both CB1R and CB2R, with a slightly higher affinity for binding at CB1R. In addition to binding at CB1R and CB2R, anandamide also binds to other receptors, such as PPARα, PPARγ, and TRPV1. GPR55, GPR18, and GPR119 are also activated by anandamide. In the CNS, anandamide plays an important role in modulating pain (Calignano et al., 1998; Walker et al., 2002), learning, memory, and anxiety (Zanettini et al., 2011).

Anandamide is produced from phospholipid precursors in the postsynaptic lipid cell membrane and released into the synaptic cleft. Once it is taken up by cells through one of the receptors, anandamide moves to intracellular lipid adiposomes, or "lipid rafts" (Fowler, 2013; Maccarrone, 2017). Adiposomes act as shuttles for the rapid delivery of anandamide from the cell membrane to intracellular sites, where hydrolysis occurs (Oddi et al., 2008). Anandamide mediates tonic (ie, a slow, physiologic response) signaling at the presynaptic terminal, and in states of chronic neuronal inactivity, such as found in neurodegenerative disorders and trauma, anandamide uptake and degradation are increased, which then downregulates cannabinoid receptors, decreasing the number of available receptors for binding by endocannabinoids.

TABLE 2.3. Neuromodulatory actions of endocannabinoids in the nervous system

Brain or peripheral region	Neurotransmitter	Modulating activity	Possible CB1R containing cell target	Endocannabinoids	Possible effect
Hippocampus	Glutamate	Inhibition of release	Glutamatergic neurons	AEA 2-AG	Inhibition of long-term potentiation
	Acetylcholine	Inhibition of release	Cholinergic neurons	AEA 2-AG	Inhibition of learning and memory
Cerebellum	Glutamate	Inhibition of glutamate receptor activation of calcium channels	Glutamatergic neurons	AEA	Inhibition of motor coordination, neuroprotection
Cortex	Glutamate	Inhibition of glutamate receptor activation of calcium channels	Cortical layers	AEA 2-AG	Inhibition of memory and motor behavior, neuroprotection
Spinal cord	Glutamate	Inhibition of release/ glutamate receptor–mediated action	Dorsal horn neurons	2-AG	Spinal antinociception
Basal ganglia and substantia nigra	GABA	Inhibition of reuptake	GABAergic neurons	AEA	Inhibition of locomotor activity
	Dopamine	Inhibition of synthesis/ release/action	Dopaminergic neurons	AEA	Inhibition of locomotor activity
Sympathetic pre-junctional fibers	Norepinephrine	Inhibition of release	Renal endothelial cells	AEA	Hypotension
	Norepinephrine	Inhibition of release from postganglionic fibers	Superior cervical ganglion	AEA	Hypotension, bradycardia

2-AG, 2-arachidonoylglycerol; AEA, arachidonoyl ethanolamide, or anandamide; CB1R, cannabinoid receptor 1; GABA, gamma-aminobutyric acid. Adapted from Di Marzo, V., Melck, D., Bisogno, T., & De Petrocellis, L. (1998). Endocannabinoids: Endogenous cannabinoid receptor ligands with neuro-modulary action. *Trends in Neuroscience, 21*, 526. https://doi.org/10.1016/S0166-2236(98)01283-1

Downregulation of cannabinoid receptors subsequently decreases CB1R suppression of neurotransmitter inhibition (Di Marzo & De Petrocellis, 2012; Kim & Alger, 2010), reducing endocannabinoid tone (see the section below) and exacerbating the progression of neurodegeneration.

Structurally, anandamide is chemically similar to capsaicin and olvanil, which are noxious compounds found naturally in hot peppers. This chemical resemblance explains why anandamide acts as a full agonist at the TRPV1 receptor, classifying it as an endovanilloid compound as well (Smart et al., 2002). In healthy states of balanced homeostasis, the continuous elevation of anandamide concentrations produces a sustained agonist action without concurrent downregulation of CB1R (Di Marzo & De Petrocellis, 2012).

Anandamide has many physiologic functions. In the cardiovascular system, anandamide induces bradycardia and hypotension by inhibiting peripheral sympathetic nervous stimulation and norepinephrine release through activation of TRPV1 receptors, causing local vasodilation and decreasing systemic vascular resistance (Högestätt & Zygmunt, 2002). When CB1R in renal endothelial cells are activated by anandamide, norepinephrine release from renal sympathetic nerve stimulation is inhibited, producing renal vasodilation (Deutsch et al., 1997). Anandamide acts as a cardiovascular regulatory agent against atherosclerosis, ischemia reperfusion, and blood pressure regulation problems (Högestätt & Zygmunt, 2002; Pacher & Mechoulam, 2011). In the vascular circulation, anandamide stimulates platelet aggregation and platelet shape change (Braud et al., 2000; Maccarrone et al., 2001). In times of psychological stress, circulating anandamide concentrations have been shown to decrease (Dlugos et al., 2012). In pathologic conditions associated with excessive vasodilation, such as migraine, inflammation, and hemorrhagic and septic shock, anandamide levels in the blood are elevated (Bátkai & Pacher, 2009; Liu et al., 2006; Russo, 2008). More specifically, septic shock triggers macrophages to produce anandamide and 2-AG in platelets through CB1R activation, which then causes systemic vasodilation and subsequent hypotension (Liu et al., 2006; Maccarrone et al., 2001; Varga et al., 1998). The activation of these ECS mechanisms in the presence of both septic and hemorrhagic shock underscores its significance in cardiovascular pathophysiology.

Through activation at CB2R, anandamide enhances the response to human growth factor for hematopoietic cells, enlarging the populations of precursor blood cell lines in preparation for cell differentiation (Malfitano et al., 2014; Valk et al., 1997). Through activation of CB1R in the brain, specifically the forebrain and thalamus, anandamide decreases the firing of wake–active neurons, which increases the accumulation of adenosine (AD), a neuromodulating molecule believed to play a role in promoting sleep and suppressing arousal (Murillo-Rodriguez et al., 2003). This CB1R-AEA-AD mechanism then induces sleep, thus supporting the body's sleep homeostasis (Murillo-Rodriguez et al., 2003). Microglia extracellular vesicles have been found to carry anandamide on their surface, which stimulate CB1R throughout the CNS and inhibit either GABA (an inhibitory neurotransmitter) or glutamate (an excitatory neurotransmitter) release from presynaptic terminals (Gabrielli et al., 2015; Katona & Freund, 2008). Microglia cells produce and release endocannabinoids at a rate 20 times higher than neurons or astrocytes, suggesting that microglia play a possible role as the main source for modulating inflammatory responses after brain trauma or disease (Zou & Kumar, 2018).

Endocannabinoids regulate cell growth and differentiation, and anandamide facilitates control over the cell's choice between growth and death in both neuronal and immune cells (Eljaschewitsch et al., 2006). Anandamide activates several receptors to initiate programmed cell death. When CB1R, CB2R, and TRPV1 are activated by anandamide, apoptosis is initiated in neuronal and immune cells (Maccarrone et al., 2000; Zou & Kumar, 2018). The ECS's ability to modulate cell survival and death may be important as a novel therapy to treat cancer (Guzmán et al., 2001; Mukhopadhyay et al., 2010). Anandamide has been shown to inhibit breast (De Petrocellis et al., 1998) and prostate cancer (Melck et al., 2000) cell proliferation.

At low doses, anandamide increases food intake when CB1R is activated (Hao et al., 2000; Kirkham, 2009; Williams & Kirkham, 1999). It also reverses neurotransmitter changes caused by dietary restrictions, suggesting it as a potential treatment of cachexia that is associated with many wasting diseases such as cancer, anorexia nervosa, and AIDS (Hao et al., 2000). Anandamide has been reported to reduce neuronal injury in animal models of brain injury, resulting in smaller infarcts to brain tissue (Eljaschewitsch et al., 2006; van der Stelt et al., 2001).

Anandamide is a major pain modulator and works synergistically with PEA at two distinct receptors to inhibit the transmission of pain sensation. Through activation of CB1R, anandamide diminishes peripheral nervous signaling of pain, while at the same time PEA exerts its anti-inflammatory actions through local peripheral CB2R activation (Calignano et al., 1998; Clapper et al., 2010; Walker et al., 2002).

Anandamide synthesis and degradation

Most neurotransmitters are released from cells through intracellular vesicle mechanisms, which then travel through the cell's cytoplasm and then attach to the lipid cell membrane of the synapse in preparation for their release. Endocannabinoids are not stored or released from intracellular vesicles to the synapse (Pagotto et al., 2006) but are instead released through the process of either simple diffusion or through facilitated, carrier-mediated transport. Recent studies suggest that endocannabinoids are transported via a carrier-mediated system that facilitates the diffusion from one side of the lipid extracellular membrane to the intracellular membrane (Maccarrone, 2002; Nicolussi & Gertsch, 2015; Toczek & Malinowska, 2018). These dual mechanisms for transporting endocannabinoids across cell membranes support the rapid influx and outflow of molecules in a way that helps ensure the rapid handling of large localized endocannabinoid concentrations (Fowler, 2013). Figure 2.9 describes the proposed mechanism for anandamide transport through the cell membrane and within the cell.

In the CNS, astrocytes, oligodendrocytes, and microglial cells contain the biosynthetic mechanisms to produce anandamide and 2-AG; these specialized nerve cells also express both CB1R and CB2R (Di Marzo et al., 1998; Lu & Mackie, 2016). Activation of CB1R and CB2R by anandamide in astrocytes and microglial cells regulates inflammatory responses and produces neuroprotective effects (Bisogno et al., 2016; Di Marzo et al., 1998; Lu & Mackie, 2016; Viscomi et al., 2009). Anandamide synthesis is also triggered by increases in pre- and postsynaptic intracellular calcium and

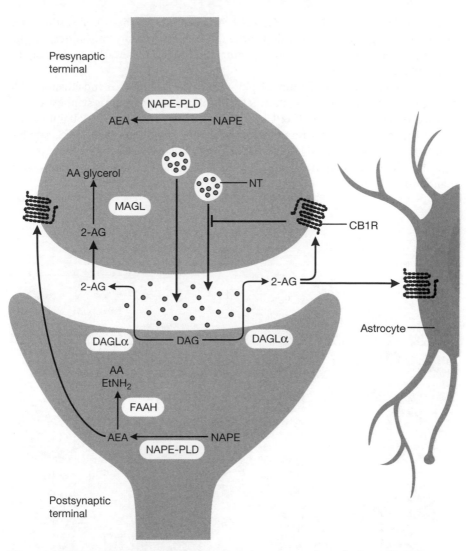

Figure 2.9: **Proposed mechanisms for anandamide transport through the cell membrane and within the cell.** Simple diffusion of anandamide through the cell membrane might be driven by fatty acid amide hydrolase (FAAH). Binding of anandamide to intracellular carrier proteins is also possible for transport across the cell membrane in a mechanism known as endocannabinoid membrane transporter (EMT). An additional proposed mechanism for anandamide uptake is where anandamide binds to a membrane carrier protein located within lipid rafts (adiposomes) and is subsequently introduced to the cell by endocytosis. Abbreviations: 2-AG, 2-arachidonoylglycerol; AA, arachidonic acid; AEA, anandamide; CB1R, cannabinoid receptor 1; DAG, diacylglycerol; DAGL-α, diacylglycerol lipase-α; EtNH$_2$, ethanolamine; FAAH, fatty acid amide hydrolase; MAG-L, monoacylglycerol lipase; NAPE, N-acyl-phosphatidyl ethanolamine; NAPE-PLD, NAPE phospholipase D; NT, neurotransmitter.

by activated GPR18, GPR55, and GPR119. Anandamide synthesis is also stimulated by the physiologic activation of dopamine (an inhibitory neurotransmitter) or glutamate (a major excitatory neurotransmitter) receptors (Lu & Mackie, 2016; Sugiura et al., 2002).

Anandamide is produced from the physiologic compounds AA and ethanolamide through an enzyme process (Deutsch & Chin, 1993). Anandamide is synthesized and released on demand (Deutsch & Chin, 1993; Di Marzo et al., 1996; Sugiura et al., 2002). This on-demand release of endocannabinoids is unique to the ECS, as other neurotransmitters are stored in presynaptic intracellular vesicles, where they are kept until they are released at the synapse. Figure 2.10 depicts the metabolic pathways of anandamide.

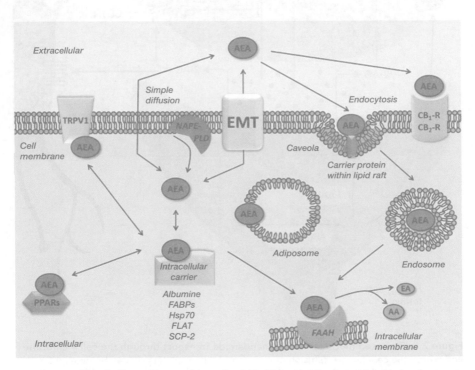

Figure 2.10: **Metabolic pathways of anandamide.** Biosynthesis of anandamide has been proposed to occur by several pathways. One simplified biosynthetic pathway is represented here. (1) The synthesis of anandamide begins when cell membrane phospholipid precursors PE and PC are released. (2) The enzyme NAT cleaves the two compounds into (3) the phospholipid NAPE. (4) NAPE is then cleaved by the enzyme NAPE-LPD, (5) producing anandamide and PA. (6) Degradation of anandamide occurs mainly through the enzyme FAAH. (7) FAAH cleaves anandamide into AA and ethanolamine. Abbreviations: AA, arachidonic acid; AEA, anandamide; CB1R, cannabinoid receptor 1; CB2R, cannabinoid receptor 2; EA, ethanolamine acid; EMT, endocannabinoid membrane transporter; FAAH, fatty acid amide hydrolase; NAPE, N-arachidonoyl phosphatidylethanolamine; NAPE-LPD, NAPE phospholipase D; NAT, N-acyltransferase; PA, phosphatidic acid; PC, phosphatidylcholine; PE, phosphatidyl ethanolamine; PPAR, peroxisome proliferator–activated receptor; TRPV1, transient receptor potential vanilloid subtype 1.

The synthesis pathway of anandamide begins when intracellular calcium rises and two cellular membrane precursors, phosphatidylethanolamine (PE) and phosphatidylcholine (PC), are cleaved by the enzyme N-acyltransferase (NAT). The product of this cleavage is N-arachidonoyl phosphatidylethanolamine (NAPE) (Alhouayek & Mucciolo, 2017; Liu et al., 2006; Maccarrone, 2017; Mechoulam & Ben-Shabat, 1999). After forming, NAPE is hydrolyzed by the enzyme phospholipase D (NAPE-PLD), producing anandamide and phosphatidic acid (PA). In animal models, anandamide is also produced outside the CNS in vascular endothelium and macrophages (Liu et al., 2006; Sugiura et al., 2002). An anandamide synthesis and signaling system is also present in renal endothelial cells, which causes arterial vasodilation and suppresses norepinephrine release from renal sympathetic nerves on arteries, reducing arterial resistance within the kidney (Deutsch et al., 1997; Pacher & Mechoulam, 2011).

Immediately after activating either CB1R or CB2R, anandamide is taken up by presynaptic cells through either simple diffusion or by a protein carrier–mediated transporter known as endocannabinoid membrane transporter (EMT) (Nicolussi & Gertsch, 2015; Toczek & Malinowska, 2018). This enables the lipophilic endocannabinoids to readily cross through the cell membrane. Both anandamide and 2-AG are transported across the cell membrane via EMT, and this mechanism has been proposed to be bidirectional (Chicca et al., 2012; Maccarrone, 2002; Toczek & Malinowska, 2018), indicating that the two endocannabinoids can move back and forth easily across cell membranes via a protein carrier–mediated transport, which supports their important role in regulating homeostasis. This transport of anandamide and 2-AG across the lipid membrane of cells via EMT occurs in both peripheral nervous system and CNS (Fowler, 2011; Nicolussi & Gertsch, 2015).

After entry into the cell, anandamide rapidly moves to adiposomes, which are organelles within cells that serve as intracellular lipid storage areas. Adiposomes, also known as "lipid rafts," are involved in endocytosis and trafficking of multiple signaling molecules within the cell (Maccarrone, 2017; Maccarrone et al., 2010; Toczek & Malinowska, 2018). Adiposomes isolate and metabolize anandamide via degradation pathways (Fowler, 2013). Adiposomes deliver anandamide from the plasma membrane to intracellular organelles in a rapid, efficient manner. Intracellular movement and storage of anandamide initiate its signaling, hydrolysis, and eventual degradation processes (Maccarrone, 2017). Once the intracellular activity of anandamide terminates, anandamide is inactivated by fatty acid amide hydrolase (FAAH), an essential cell membrane enzyme that is widely distributed in animal tissues (Ahn et al., 2009; Deutsch et al., 2001; Di Marzo et al., 1998; Zou & Kumar, 2018).

The catabolic enzymes responsible for the degradation of anandamide are also found in intracellular membranes. FAAH is the primary enzyme responsible for cleaving anandamide into AA and ethanolamine (Ahn et al., 2009), where AA is readily available to be reused as an endocannabinoid precursor. The accumulation of anandamide, as well as its by-products of catabolism (eg, AA and ethanolamine), correlates with the amount of enzymatic FAAH activity, which suggests that the breakdown of anandamide is also part of the driving force for its uptake (Deutsch et al., 2001; Sugiura et al., 2002). When FAAH is inhibited, the breakdown of anandamide is also inhibited, making more anandamide available for extracellular uptake. The development of FAAH antagonists, therefore, may have therapeutic potential for treating diseases such as chronic pain, depression, and anxiety (Ahn et al., 2009; Lever et al., 2009; Minkkilä et al., 2010; Walker et al., 2002). However, a French phase 1 clinical trial in 2016 by the Portuguese drug company Bial that tested an FAAH inhibitor proved to be dangerous to participants (one death and hospitalization of five others), as the FAAH inhibitor may have also targeted other enzymes that metabolize lipids and created damaging neurologic effects beyond inhibiting FAAH and extending the function of endocannabinoids.

2-Arachidonoylglycerol

2-AG is a full agonist at both CB1R and CB2R, where it binds strongly to both receptors with equal strength. 2-AG is considered the principal ligand for both cannabinoid receptors. In the brain, its levels are approximately 1,000 times higher than those of anandamide and thus it is considered the primary CB1R ligand of the brain and CNS (Zou & Kumar, 2018). In the brain, 2-AG only activates CB2R in response to brain injury or inflammation. 2-AG is also a full agonist at other endocannabinoid-like receptors, including TPRV1, PPARα, PPARγ, and GPR55. 2-AG has also been found to serve as a major source of AA for synthesizing prostaglandins, which are lipid compounds formed at sites of tissue damage or infection that control processes such as inflammation, blood flow, and the formation of blood clots (Baggelaar et al., 2018). Physiologic actions of 2-AG include modulating immune function, cell proliferation, neuroprotection and neuromodulation (Di Marzo et al., 1998), cardiovascular function, the inflammatory response, and embryo development (Zou & Kumar, 2018). Other physiologic processes modulated by 2-AG include food intake and energy metabolism (Jung et al., 2012), motor activity, learning and memory (Zanettini et al., 2011), pain sensation (Walker et al., 2002), regulation of body temperature, stress and anxiety, and addiction and reward behaviors (Baggelaar et al., 2018).

2-AG plays an important role in cardiovascular homeostasis and pathology as it regulates inflammation and thrombosis. Cardiovascular endothelial cells and platelets synthesize 2-AG. Cardiovascular endothelial cells function as a protective barrier and serve as a source for several vasoactive substances, and endothelial cell damage is associated with disorders that affect the cardiovascular system. 2-AG binds to the surface of platelets and leads to platelet activation, making this endocannabinoid an important contributor to the coagulation process and hemostasis (Keown et al., 2010; Maccarrone et al., 2001). The role of 2-AG in platelet function also mediates the aggregation of platelets via metabolism by the enzyme monoacylglycerol lipase (MAG-L) to generate AA, which is the substrate for the platelet activator thromboxane A_2. Thromboxane A_2 is a substance that stimulates the activation of new platelets and increases platelet aggregation to seal damaged tissue. This role as a platelet agonist to induce activation and aggregation suggests therapeutic potential for clinical applications of 2-AG cannabinoid receptor antagonists to inhibit platelet function, similar to pharmaceutical anticoagulants (Baldassarri et al., 2008; Brantl, Khandoga, & Siess, 2014; Cunha et al., 2011).

In times of psychological stress, 2-AG concentrations in the brain increase, which supports the role of 2-AG as an anxiolytic when it acts on CB1R in the CNS (Volkow et al., 2017). Dietary fasting also increases levels of 2-AG in the forebrain limbic area and hypothalamus, suggesting it as a possible treatment of metabolic disorders (Ginsberg & Woods, 2009).

Like anandamide, 2-AG inhibits the proliferation of breast (De Petrocellis et al., 1998) and prostate cancer cells (Melck et al., 2000). In the CNS, 2-AG modulates pain, memory, and anxiety (Zanettini et al., 2011). When GPR55 receptors found on neutrophils are activated by 2-AG, the migratory response of these granulocytes toward 2-AG is enhanced (Balenga et al., 2011). Through activation of CB2R in the periphery, 2-AG enhances chemotaxis in peripheral blood cells and modulates the migration of macrophages, monocytes, and T-cells, thereby helping to regulate inflammatory and immune responses (Chiurchiù, 2016). 2-AG, like anandamide, also promotes cardioprotection in regard to atherosclerosis, ischemic reperfusion, and regulation of blood pressure (Cunha et al., 2011).

During inflammatory reactions to brain injury, 2-AG has been shown to reduce the acute release of proinflammatory cytokines, which subsequently reduces the inflammatory response and limits damage to brain tissue. In animal models, levels of 2-AG increase sharply after closed head injury (CHI) (Mechoulam, 2002). When synthetic 2-AG was administered to mice after CHI, significant reductions of brain edema, better clinical recovery, reduced infarct volume, and reduced hippocampal cell death were noted. Continuous CB1R activation in the brain through increased 2-AG concentrations inhibits excitotoxicity, induces cerebral hypotension, reduces cerebral blood flow, and regulates microglial immune response to tissue trauma (Varga et al., 1998). This suggests 2-AG exerts a neuroprotective effect on brain tissues as it reduces excitatory glutamate release and diminishes excitotoxicity (Katona & Freund, 2008; Mechoulam, 2002; Piomelli et al., 2000). 2-AG also activates CB2R found on microglial cells in the brain and, when activated, inhibits the release of cytotoxic agents by invading immune cells after tissue injury. Microglial activation of CB2R does not occur under basal conditions, suggesting a protective role for endocannabinoids and cannabinoid receptors when exposed to damaging inflammatory stimuli (Zogopoulos et al., 2013).

2-AG has been investigated as a treatment for addiction and withdrawal from noxious substances, including nicotine, cocaine, and morphine. In animal models, 2-AG administration reduced the intensity of withdrawal signs in morphine-dependent mice and prevented naloxone-precipitated morphine withdrawal symptoms, including tremors, diarrhea, and weight loss (Yamaguchi et al., 2001). This suggests the augmentation of 2-AG as a potential treatment for addiction and withdrawal from opiates and other harmful drugs.

Increased levels of 2-AG have been shown to reduce clinical models of inflammatory pain. Neuropathic, peripheral inflammatory, GI, and chemotherapy-induced neuropathy were all shown to be effectively treated by either administration of 2-AG or preventing its degradation at CB1R (Pacher & Kunos, 2013). 2-AG has also been shown to affect IOP in a biphasic manner, with an initial increase followed by a reduction in IOP through the mediation of the ocular CB1R (Laine et al., 2002).

2-Arachidonoylglycerol synthesis and degradation

The synthesis of 2-AG begins in the lipid membrane of the cell wall located on postsynaptic neurons. Two synthesis pathways for 2-AG have been proposed and are often stimulated simultaneously (Baggelaar et al., 2018; Lu & Mackie, 2016). The first pathway produces the rapid formation of 2-AG and is dependent on the type of tissues and cells under various stimulus conditions, including increases in intracellular calcium (Baggelaar et al., 2018; Sugiura et al., 2002). In this synthesis process, phosphatidylinositol biphosphate (PIP2), a phospholipid found in neural cell membranes that plays a key role in intracellular signaling and modulation of receptor activation (Falkenburger et al., 2010; Traynor-Kaplan et al., 2017), is hydrolyzed by the enzyme phospholipase C (PL-C) into phosphatidylinositol (PL), which produces diacylglycerol (DAG). This is followed by the hydrolysis of DAG by the enzyme diacylglycerol lipase (DAG-L) to produce 2-AG. DAG-L has been found to regulate the majority of 2-AG production and it may contribute to the synaptic plasticity in the adult CNS (Lu & Mackie, 2016; Tanimura et al., 2010). DAG-L may also play an important role in the production of 2-AG during immune responses (Lu & Mackie, 2016).

A second 2-AG synthesis pathway begins at the same PL, but instead of being hydrolyzed by PL-C, it is broken down first into LPI by the enzyme phospholipase A (PL-A). After LPL is formed, it is hydrolyzed by PL-C into 2-AG. PL-C is a unique enzyme found in CNS neural synaptosomes, which are isolated synaptic terminals found on neurons (De Belleroche & Bradford, 1973; Sugiura et al., 2002; Weller, 2009). Synaptosomes contain high concentrations of glutamate and GABA and function as essential physiologic mechanisms to regulate the uptake, storage, and release of neurotransmitters (De Belleroche & Bradford, 1973; Sugiura et al., 2002; Weller, 2009). Figure 2.11 depicts the metabolic pathways of 2-AG.

Once synthesized and released, 2-AG travels backward across the synaptic cleft to bind with cannabinoid receptors located on presynaptic neurons (Alhouayek & Mucciolo, 2017). There, it physiologically activates the cannabinoid receptor, inhibiting neurotransmitter release in the presynaptic cell by inhibiting calcium channels while enhancing inward potassium channels in the cell membrane (Sugiura & Waku, 2000; Sugiura et al., 2002). After receptor activation, 2-AG enters the cell via EMT, where it is immediately inactivated by the enzyme MAG-L, an enzyme primarily found in the presynaptic membrane of neuronal axon terminals that readily interact with the presynaptic CB1R. MAG-L is considered the primary enzyme in the 2-AG degradation process, whereas FAAH has also been found to degrade 2-AG (Di Marzo & Maccarrone, 2008; Murataeva et al., 2014; Tsuboi et al., 2018). Although FAAH plays a minor role in the degradation of 2-AG (Bow & Rimoldi, 2016; Di Marzo et al., 1998; Lu & Mackie, 2016; Sugiura et al., 2002), it is not as central in the degradation process as compared to its significance in anandamide degradation. The rapid, immediate inactivation of 2-AG by two distinct degradation pathways prevents excess concentrations that may exert detrimental undesired physiologic effects. Upon hydrolysis by either MAG-L or FAAH, 2-AG degrades into AA and glycerol (Baggelaar et al., 2018; Sugiura et al., 2002).

Manipulating 2-AG synthesis and degradation pathways may provide a wide range of targeted therapeutic effects that are separate from its activities within the ECS (Minkkilä et al., 2010). For example, 2-AG found in the brain, liver, and lung, but not in the GI tract, heart, kidney, or spleen, is the major source of AA used for prostaglandin synthesis (Lu & Mackie, 2016). By potentially increasing the synthesis of 2-AG using AA, less of it would be available to produce an immune response to

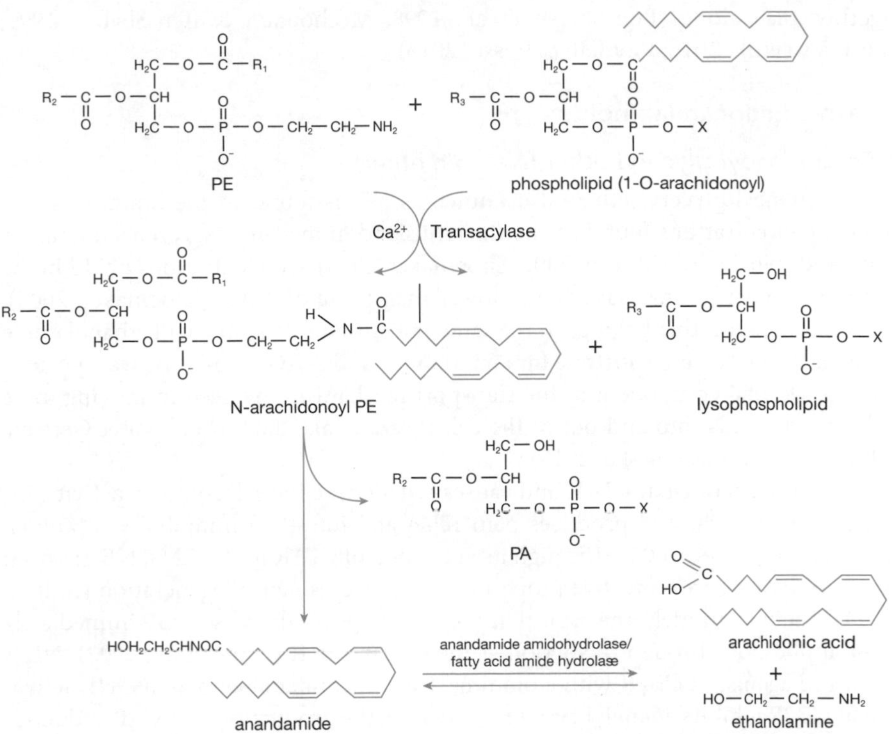

Figure 2.11: **Metabolic pathways of 2-arachidonoylglycerol (2-AG).** Two pathways have been proposed for the synthesis of 2-AG. A simplified overview of the two metabolic pathways is presented here. (1) PIP_2 is converted into PL by enzyme (2) PL-C, leading to (3) the production of DAG. (4) Hydrolysis of DAG by the enzyme DAG-L produces (5) 2-AG. Another synthesis pathway involves (2) conversion of PL by (6) enzyme PL-A, (7) producing LPL. (8) The enzyme PL-C then hydrolyzes LPL into (5) 2-AG. After entering the cell, 2-AG is immediately inactivated by the enzyme (9) MAG-L and produces (10) AA and glycerol. Abbreviations: 2-AG, 2-arachidonoylglycerol; AA, arachidonic acid; DAG, diacylglycerol; DAG-L, diacylglycerol lipase; LPL, lysophosphatidylinositol; MAG-L, monoacyl glycerol lipase; PIP_2, phosphatidylinositol biphosphate; PL, phosphatidylinositol; PL-A, phospholipase A; PL-C, phospholipase C.

injury, thus decreasing inflammation associated with high prostaglandin concentrations (Lu & Mackie, 2016; Minkkilä et al., 2010).

Endocannabinoid-modulating compounds

Two endocannabinoid-modulating compounds, 2-linoleoyl glycerol (2-LG) and 2-palmitoylglycerol (2-PG), enhance the neuroprotective activity of 2-AG (Murataeva et al., 2016) (see the section below). 2-LG and 2-PG are present in the brain but do not bind to either CB1R or CB2R; instead, these compounds enhance the activity of 2-AG by partially blocking its uptake and inhibiting 2-AG enzymatic hydrolysis. 2-LG and 2-PG also potentiate the binding of 2-AG to CB1R and CB2R. These combinations of 2-AG, 2-LG, and 2-PG work synergistically to support the "entourage effect" (see below), which may explain why endocannabinoids work more effectively together than alone (Ben-Shabat et al., 1998; Mechoulam & Ben-Shabat, 1999; Murataeva et al., 2016; Piomelli & Russo, 2016).

Putative Endocannabinoids

2-Arachidonoyl glyceryl ether (Noladin ether)

2-Arachidonoyl glyceryl ether, also known as NE, is found in the brain, with the highest concentrations found in the thalamus and hippocampus, cerebellum, brain stem, and spinal cord (Milton, 2002; Shoemaker, 2005). Concentrations of NE in the brain are similar to anandamide but lower than those of 2-AG (Shoemaker, 2005). NE is a compound that belongs in the same polyunsaturated fatty acid ethanolamide group as 2-AG. NE is a substrate for anandamide and 2-AG membrane transporters, making it a vital component of the transport mechanism involved in moving these endocannabinoids into and out of the cell (Fezza et al., 2002; Nicolussi & Gertsch, 2015; Toczek & Malinowska, 2018).

NE is a full agonist at CB1R and causes sedation, reduces locomotor activity, induces hypothermia, and produces pain relief and intestinal immobility in animal models (Shoemaker, 2005). Through its activation of CB1R in the CNS, NE has been shown to have neuroprotective properties and prevents neurodegeneration (Milton, 2002). In animal models, the topical use of NE in the eye decreases IOP immediately upon application through mediation at the ocular CB1R (Laine et al., 2002). NE is also a full agonist at CB2R with a binding strength comparable to 2-AG. NE activation at CB2R inhibits adenylyl cyclase, decreasing the production of cAMP and modifying important physiologic functions. Chronic activation of CB2R by NE causes receptor desensitization and downregulation (Fezza et al., 2002; Shoemaker, 2005).

O-arachidonoyl ethanolamine (virodhamine)

O-AEA, also known as virodhamine, is an atypical endocannabinoid-like compound in that in high concentrations, it acts as an antagonist against anandamide at CB1R, but acts as a full agonist at CB2R (Porter, 2002; Sharir et al., 2012). It is found in the brain in the hippocampus. Virodhamine is also present in peripheral tissues that express CB2R, such as the skin, spleen, kidney, and heart tissues, where it is found in higher concentrations than anandamide (Porter, 2002). It also interacts with cannabinoid receptors in the airway epithelium and on the pulmonary artery, suggesting that it controls pulmonary vascular tone under both physiologic and pathophysiologic conditions (Kozłowska et al., 2008). Virodhamine is a full agonist at GPR55, indicating that it plays an important role in inflammatory pain and cardiovascular diseases (Piñeiro et al., 2011). GPR55 is also found in brain regions associated with memory, learning, and motor function (Sharir et al., 2012). Virodhamine's name is derived from the Sanskrit word "*virodha*," which means opposition, because its chemical structure linkage of AA and ethanolamine is the exact opposite of the linkages found in anandamide (Porter, 2002).

Virodhamine diminishes anandamide-induced activation of CB1R in the CNS. Virodhamine blocks anandamide transport and produces hypothermia (Porter, 2002). Through an as-yet unknown vascular endothelial receptor, it modulates vasodilation in mesenteric arteries in the small intestines (Carnevale et al., 2018). Virodhamine interacts with both CB1R and CB2R in airway epithelial tissues to inhibit cAMP accumulation, which produces an anti-inflammatory effect in the airway by modifying cytokine release from the bronchial epithelium (Gkoumassi et al., 2007). Through activation of GPR55 on pulmonary vascular tissue, it relaxes the pulmonary artery, suggesting it may be an effective pharmacologic therapeutic for the treatment of pulmonary hypertension (Kozłowska et al., 2008).

It is proposed that virodhamine interacts with CB2R in cardiovascular tissues to regulate cardiovascular function and anti-inflammatory activity (Carnevale et al., 2018). Like anandamide (Braud et al., 2000), virodhamine stimulates platelet activation in blood and induces platelet shape change, secretion, and aggregation in the plasma (Brantl et al., 2014).

Another possible role for virodhamine is in the treatment of neurologic disorders caused by monoamine oxidate (MAO) dysregulation (Pandey et al., 2018). MAOs are important enzymes in brain development and function, and two subtypes, MAO-A and MAO-B, have been associated with psychological disorders. Nonselective MAO-A pharmaceutical inhibitors are widely used to treat depression, panic disorder, and anxiety, whereas selective MAO-B inhibitors are used to treat depression, attention deficit hyperactivity disorder (ADHD), Parkinson's, and Alzheimer's disease. Administration of selective MAO-B inhibitors leads to increases in phenylethylamine levels in the brain. Phenylethylamine is a compound that promotes dopamine-releasing activity, which stimulates the CNS, thus promoting positive effects on behavior and motor function. Virodhamine has been shown to inhibit MAO-B and thus it may have potential as a treatment for Parkinson's and Alzheimer's disease (Pandey et al., 2018).

N-arachidonoyl dopamine

NADA is an endogenous capsaicin-like compound found in CNS tissues, with the highest concentrations in the striatum, hippocampus, and cerebellum (Huang et al., 2002). It is also present in dorsal root ganglion. NADA is present in those brain areas that are associated with pain processing, and so it plays a role in pain modulation (Walker et al., 2002). NADA is an agonist at both CB1R and TRPV1, making it one of the dual endocannabinoids/endovanilloids, along with anandamide (Marinelli et al., 2007). NADA is considered the endogenous principal ligand for TRPV1 activation (Lawton et al., 2017). At both CB1R and TRPV1, NADA inhibits calcium channels, reducing the number of channels available to open during neuronal depolarization (Ross et al., 2009). NADA also inhibits FAAH, the enzyme responsible for the hydrolysis of both anandamide and 2-AG, thus inhibiting endocannabinoid inactivation. NADA itself is also degraded by FAAH (Bisogno et al., 2000).

When NADA activates CB1R, it produces analgesia, hypothermia, and catalepsy, which is a condition characterized by loss of sensation and consciousness accompanied by rigidity of the body (Manzanares et al., 2006). When NADA stimulates TRPV1, it causes hyperalgesia (pain) and contraction of smooth muscles (Marinelli et al., 2007). Like virodhamine, NADA causes vasodilation in the intestines in the small mesenteric arteries by acting on both CB1R and TRPV1 (Grabiec & Dehghani, 2017). The activity of NADA at both CB1R and TPRV1 aligns with its function as an excitatory glutamatergic modulator, through either increasing or decreasing transmission through CB1R and TRPV1 receptors, or by decreasing inhibitory GABA transmission through CB1R activation (Ryskamp et al., 2014). The pro- and antinociceptive effects of NADA also depend on which receptor is activated, as its contrasting action of hyperalgesia at TRPV1 receptors with simultaneous analgesia at CB1R demonstrates its complex function within the ECS (Marinelli et al., 2007). Modulation of either inhibitory GABA transmission or excitatory glutamate transmission is an important homeostatic mechanism in the CNS control of pain, temperature regulation, and GI function.

N-arachidonoyl glycine

NaGly is a by-product of the metabolism of anandamide. Its physiologic activities include antinociception, anti-inflammation, induction of apoptosis in proinflammatory macrophages, and reduction of cytokine production (Takenouchi et al., 2012). NaGly is proposed as the natural endogenous ligand for GPR18 (Kohno et al., 2006). NaGly is also degraded by FAAH to form AA and glycine.

In the periphery, NaGly induces proliferation of T-cells and causes insulin release in β-cells of the pancreas (Kohno et al., 2006). In the CNS, NaGly promotes proliferation and migration of microglia to support homeostatic maintenance and tissue repair (McHugh et al., 2010). When NaGly is released in the endometrium of the uterus and activates GPR18 receptors located there, it causes the migration of endometrial cells. This suggests it may have a potential role in the treatment of endometriosis, as GPR18 regulates the migration of leukocyte and microglial cells, which leads to apoptosis of inflammatory leukocytes and subsequently reducing local inflammation (McHugh et al., 2012).

Related Endogenous Fatty Acid Derivatives

Additional endogenous fatty acid derivatives regulate the activity of endocannabinoids and interact with cannabinoid and cannabinoid-like receptors. These fatty acid derivatives are a family of arachidonoyl amino acids that are especially important in the modulation of pain sensation. Although these endogenous substances do not directly interact with the cannabinoid or cannabinoid-like receptors, they potentiate the activity of endocannabinoids through inhibition of enzymes, prevention of endocannabinoid degradation, or improving the affinity for endocannabinoids to bind to the cannabinoid receptor.

N-acyl ethanolamides—oleoyl ethanolamide, palmitoylethanolamide, stearoyl ethanolamide

Fatty acid ethanolamides were discovered in the cerebrospinal fluid of sleep-deprived cats (Cravatt et al., 1995). Ethanolamides are lipids that have been investigated for their sleep-inducing properties in mammals, and although they do not interact with CB1R or CB2R, they have been associated with the indirect "entourage effect" associated with the synergism of endocannabinoids (see section below) (Murataeva et al., 2016; Piomelli & Russo, 2016; Ross, 2003). Three ethanolamides, OEA, PEA, and stearoyl ethanolamide (SEA), have important physiologic influence on the ECS.

Oleoyl Ethanolamide

OEA is a lipid that does not bind to either CB1R or CB2R. Instead, it is a full agonist at GPR55, GPR119, TRPV1, and PPARα (Brito et al., 2014; Syed et al., 2012). OEA is synthesized on demand in the small intestines, where its concentrations decrease during food starvation and increase upon refeeding (Overton et al., 2006). OEA inhibits the metabolism of other endocannabinoids and is inactive at CB1R and CB2R. Because of these supplemental physiologic actions within the ECS, OEA is considered one of the compounds that contribute to the "entourage effect" (see the section below) (Ho et al., 2008).

Through activation of PPARα, OEA regulates feeding behavior and energy homeostasis (Ezzili et al., 2010; Fu et al., 2003; Piomelli, 2013). OEA stimulation of intestinal PPARα reduces food intake and body weight gain by producing a feeling of satiety (or "fullness") and stimulating lipolysis. It also inhibits gastric emptying and intestinal motility, slowing down the upper GI transit of food (Fu et al., 2003; Guzmán et al., 2004). OEA regulates feeding behavior and motor activity through activation of TRPV1 (Ezzili et al., 2010; Syed et al., 2012) and increases fatty acid uptake by adipocytes through increased enzyme expression (Guzmán et al., 2004).

A significant physiologic action of OEA concerning the GI system is inhibition of the breakdown of anandamide. This action therefore potentially indirectly activates CB1R located in the enteric nervous system (Zou & Kumar, 2018). Anandamide also inhibits small intestine transit of food, which suggests a synergistic sensation of satiety when both OEA and anandamide are present (Fu et al., 2003). OEA also agonizes GPR119 found in the stomach and small intestines. GPR119 activation then stimulates the release of GLP-1, which is a hormone that inhibits intestinal transit of food (Overton et al., 2006).

Palmitoylethanolamide

PEA is found in the brain, liver, skeletal muscle, and small intestines (Ezzili et al., 2010) and is an endogenous ligand of PPARα (Verme et al., 2005). In animal models, PEA is produced by macrophages. PEA decreases inflammatory-related pain by inhibiting mast cell activation, thus reducing the inflammatory response (Ezzili et al., 2010; Gatti et al., 2012; Verme et al., 2005).

Although PEA lacks strong affinity for either CB1R or CB2R, it regulates the transmission of pain sensation and pain integration at CB2R (Calignano et al., 1998) and has been suggested as part of the endogenous group of compounds responsible for the "entourage effects" of cannabinoids (see section below) (Murataeva et al., 2016; Piomelli & Russo, 2016; Smart et al., 2002). PEA increases the physiologic activities of anandamide (Smart et al., 2002). Both anandamide and PEA activate peripheral CB1R and CB2R, producing antinociception by stimulating norepinephrine release (Romero et al., 2013). In addition to decreasing the peripheral response to pain, PEA has been shown to act synergistically with anandamide to enhance its antiproliferative effects of breast cancer cells by inhibiting the expression of FAAH (Di Marzo et al., 2001; Ross, 2003), further substantiating the "entourage effect" (see section below) in the presence of neoplastic activity.

PEA reduces allergic reactions, inhibits peripheral inflammation and mast cell de-generation, and exerts neuroprotective effects (Verme et al., 2005). PEA is a full agonist at GPR55 and PPARα (Kramar et al., 2017; O'Sullivan, 2016). In animal models, PEA exerts a hypophagic effect through activation of CB2R, which decreases appetite and potentially improves body weight (Onaivi et al., 2008). PEA has anti-inflammatory effects on adipocytes, which suggests it could be effective in the prevention of obe-sity-associated insulin resistance, which is one of the primary causes of metabolic syndrome (Hoareau et al., 2009). When PEA is found simultaneously with other en-docannabinoids, PEA interferes with their inactivation, which enhances the activities of other endogenous cannabinoids at cannabinoid and cannabinoid-like receptors (De Petrocellis et al., 2001).

Stearoyl Ethanolamide

SEA is another compound of the ethanolamide family found in tissues that also contain anandamide, including central neurons, brain, testes, basophils, and macro-phages (Maccarrone, 2002). PEA and SEA are the two most abundant N-acyl ethanol-amides found in tissues (Ezzili et al., 2010).

As another ethanolamide, SEA regulates appetite and food intake by producing satiety in the small intestine. SEA does not bind to either CB1R or CB2R (Ezzili et al., 2010), but studies are still investigating its specific receptor activity. SEA is considered an "endocannabinoid-like" compound that stimulates apoptosis in glioma cells and acts similarly to anandamide (Maccarrone, 2002). SEA theoretically binds to and is carried by new components of the ECS that are yet to be revealed (Maccarrone, 2002).

Endocannabinoid Modulators

Other endogenous lipid compounds influence endocannabinoid release and activity. These compounds do not directly interact with cannabinoid receptors but instead regulate the physiologic actions of other receptors and the binding of endocannabi-noids to both cannabinoid and noncannabinoid receptors. The actions of these en-docannabinoid modulators support the "entourage effect" (see the section below), which describes the synergism that endocannabinoids exhibit when working to-gether, rather than as isolated compounds (Piomelli & Russo, 2016).

2-Linoleoyl glycerol and 2-palmitoylglycerol

2-LG and 2-PG are two lipid monoacylglycerol compounds that have been isolated from the spleen, brain, and gut tissues. Neither of these lipid compounds interacts with CB1R or CB2R but instead significantly increases the binding power of 2-AG and its capacity to inhibit adenylyl cyclase, which then enhances the neuroprotective activity of 2-AG. Both 2-LG and 2-PG significantly increase the binding of 2-AG to both CB1R and CB2R, either separately or together (Ben-Shabat et al., 1998; Console-Bram et al., 2012).

The combination of 2-AG, 2-LG, and 2-PG is also more potent than 2-AG alone in the ability to inhibit adenylyl cyclase. Each of these compounds enhances 2-AG activity through inhibition of 2-AG inactivation, thus increasing the concentrations of 2-AG and the amount of time in which to bind to cannabinoid receptors. These mechanisms of cannabinoid receptor binding power significantly enhance the physiologic activity of 2-AG throughout the tissues. 2-LG and 2-PG also increase the behavioral effects produced by 2-AG (Ben-Shabat et al., 1998; Console-Bram et al., 2012).

Lysophosphatidylinositol

LPI is a phospholipid produced in endothelial cells that plays a key role in cellular signaling pathways. Several important physiologic functions of LPI include reproduction, angiogenesis, apoptosis, cell proliferation, inflammation, adipose tissue function, cardiovascular, lipid metabolism, glucose homeostasis, and autoimmune diseases (Bełtowski, 2012; Bondarenko et al., 2011; Yamashita et al., 2013). LPI is found abundantly in brain tissues and plays a neuroprotective role, preventing excitatory glutamate-induced hippocampal cell death and cerebral ischemia (Blondeau et al., 2002). LPI is considered to be the primary endogenous ligand of GPR55 (Bondarenko et al., 2011; Oka et al., 2007; Yamashita et al., 2013) and activates PPARγ to affect lipogenesis (Bełtowski, 2012).

When LPI activates GPR55, it synergistically increases the CB2R-mediated inflammatory migratory response to 2-AG and inhibits neutrophil degranulation and ROS production. The cross-talk that occurs between GPR55 and CB2R enables neutrophils to migrate toward sites of inflammation while preventing amplified tissue injury mediated by ROC production (Balenga et al., 2011).

Although the complete list of physiologic functions of LPI is still not well-defined, increased LPI levels have been linked to different forms of cancer. High levels of LPI and GPR55 expression were found in patients with breast, ovarian, and prostate cancer, suggesting it functions as an autocrine factor that regulates the growth, invasiveness, and proliferation of cancer cells (Piñeiro et al., 2011). LPI has been shown to stimulate cell proliferation in epithelial cells. When GPR55 receptors found on neutrophils are activated by LPI, the migratory response of neutrophils toward 2-AG is enhanced, increasing 2-AG's anti-inflammatory effects (Balenga et al., 2011).

LPI stimulation of GPR55 causes a rise in intracellular calcium concentrations and activation of inward potassium channels, much like the cellular activity of other endocannabinoids (Bondarenko et al., 2011). However, recent research indicates that LPI stimulation on endothelial cells also inhibits, as well as activates, potassium channels, which suggests that it may serve as a potent inter- and intracellular signaling molecule regulating potassium channels in the vasculature. This signaling of LPI to either stimulate or inhibit calcium channels within vascular endothelial cells may contribute to the homeostatic "fine-tuning" and control of adequate blood flow in various organs and tissues (Bondarenko et al., 2011). LPI also increases the number of resorbing human osteoclasts and increases the resorption area through GPR55 activation, suggesting that it could play a role in regulating bone loss. The agonist action of LPI at GPR55 in the skeletal system suggests it may have therapeutic potential to prevent bone remodeling and osteoporosis (Arifin & Falasca, 2016).

LPI influences the physiologic activity of adipose tissue. LPI levels have been shown to increase the adipose tissue of obese subjects and even more so in obese subjects with type 2 diabetes. GPR55 expression also increases in these individuals, indicating LPI activation of GPR55 positively correlates with fat percentage and

BMI; this physiologic mechanism is also gender specific, with higher levels found more in women than in men, suggesting that estrogen might also be important in the GPR55 signaling pathway (Moreno-Navarrete et al., 2012). The expression of GPR55 in visceral adipose tissue by LPI is positively associated with type 2 diabetes (Arifin & Falasca, 2016). Through PPARγ activation, LPI increases the expression of enzymes that promote lipogenesis, such as fatty acid synthesis, by inducing lipid storage and promoting adipocyte differentiation. The GPR55/LPI system is positively associated with obesity in humans, with women having a stronger correlation with weight, BMI, and body fat percentage. These differences in the distribution of fat between men and women seem to underscore the metabolic activity of GPR55/LPI (Moreno-Navarrete et al., 2012). Because of these physiologic activities, GPR55 agonists and antagonists may have potential therapeutic roles for the treatment of obesity and insulin sensitivity.

Through its action of increasing intracellular calcium in the pancreatic islets of Langerhans, LPI also stimulates insulin release via GPR55 receptors (Metz, 1986). GPR55 expression increases glucose tolerance and plasma insulin levels. This suggests that LPI may regulate body metabolism via pancreatic islet insulin stimulation (Arifin & Falasca, 2016; Metz, 1986). LPI also has a protective role in the brain, where it prevents excitatory glutamate-induced neuronal cell death and cerebral ischemia (Blondeau et al., 2002).

RETROGRADE TRANSMISSION

Endocannabinoids are released from the postsynaptic terminal after neuronal depolarization and act at the presynaptic terminal in a retrograde, or reverse, manner (Christie & Vaughan, 2001; Wilson & Nicoll, 2001). This type of reverse transmission—from postsynapse to presynapse—is unlike the action of classic neurotransmitters. Although both endocannabinoids 2-AG and anandamide are involved in retrograde signaling, 2-AG is considered the main endocannabinoid regulator of CNS retrograde signaling (Baggelaar et al., 2018). The mechanism by which endocannabinoids cross backward across the synaptic gap has become the most prominent example of retrograde signaling molecules in the CNS (Heifets & Castillo, 2009). Figure 2.12 depicts a scheme representing endocannabinoid retrograde signaling synaptic transmission.

The release of endocannabinoids from postsynaptic membranes causes the inhibition of two forms of synaptic regulation: depolarization-induced suppression of inhibition (DSI) and depolarization-induced suppression of excitation (DSE). DSI generates reduced GABA (an inhibitory neurotransmitter) release, whereas DSE generates reduced glutamate (an excitatory neurotransmitter) release. Figure 2.13 presents a simplified scheme of DSI/DSE.

The DSI/DSE synaptic regulatory processes are unique to the ECS function in the CNS (Lu & Mackie, 2016). DSI is triggered by postsynaptic depolarization and inhibits GABA neurotransmitter release by presynaptic neurons after CB1R activation, which then modifies neuronal plasticity. DSE is also triggered by postsynaptic depolarization and is mediated by the release of endocannabinoids and CB1R activation at the presynapse (Diana & Marty, 2004). DSE is proposed as a way for neurons to use their firing rate to regulate synaptic input (Kano et al., 2009), which emphasizes

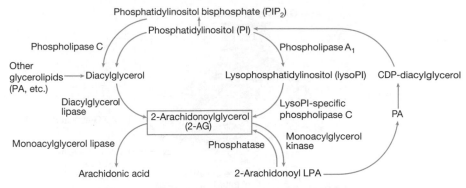

Figure 2.12: **Scheme representing endocannabinoid retrograde signaling.** Endocannabinoids are produced from postsynaptic terminals upon neuronal depolarization. 2-AG is biosynthesized from DAG by DAGL-α, and AEA is synthesized from NAPE by NAPE-PLD. Activated CB1R then inhibits NT release through the suppression of calcium influx. 2-AG in the synaptic cleft is taken up into the presynaptic terminals and degraded to AA and glycerol by MAG-L. FAAH is primarily found in postsynaptic terminals and is responsible for degrading anandamide to AA and EtNH$_2$. Thin arrows indicate enzymatic process; thick arrows indicate the direction of movement; blunted arrow indicates inhibition. Abbreviations: 2-AG, 2-arachidonoylglycerol; AA, arachidonic acid; AEA, anandamide; CB1R, cannabinoid receptor 1; DAG, diacylglycerol; DAGL-α, diacylglycerol lipase-α; EtNH$_2$, ethanolamine; FAAH, fatty acid amide hydrolase; MAG-L, monoacylglycerol lipase; NAPE, N-acyl-phosphatidyl ethanolamine; NAPE-PLD, NAPE phospholipase D; NT, neurotransmitter.

the significance of this process in maintaining homeostasis in the CNS. Kreitzer and Regehr (2001) note:

> DSE provides a feedback mechanism by which a postsynaptic cell can regulate the strength of excitatory inputs on a scale of tens of seconds ... by acting rapidly through a presynaptic mechanism, the postsynaptic cell does not simply scale its inputs but also changes short-term synaptic plasticity. Therefore, retrograde inhibition provides a means for altering both the strength and the properties of presynaptic inputs for tens of seconds during periods of high postsynaptic activity. (p. 726)

The mechanisms surrounding CNS neurotransmitter response to DSI/DSE are proposed as the primary cortical tissue process that is mediated by endocannabinoid activity, which may contribute to neuronal plasticity and synaptic strengthening in the CNS (Heifets & Castillo, 2009; Kreitzer & Regehr, 2001; Lovinger, 2008; Lu & Mackie, 2016; Pertwee & Ross, 2002). DSI may control the output of neuronal firing in the cerebral cortex, which then produces synchronized activity in larger groups of neurons that could influence cognitive processes. DSE may play a neuroprotective role in the CNS as it is triggered by postsynaptic endocannabinoid response during neuronal tissue injury, subsequently inhibiting the presynaptic release of neuronal-damaging excitatory glutamate (Diana & Marty, 2004).

The discovery of the DSI/DSE mechanisms, which affect only the presynaptic neuronal release of GABA or glutamate neurotransmitters, led to the recognition that endocannabinoids diffuse backward across the synaptic cleft once they are released from postsynaptic neurons to activate cannabinoid receptors found

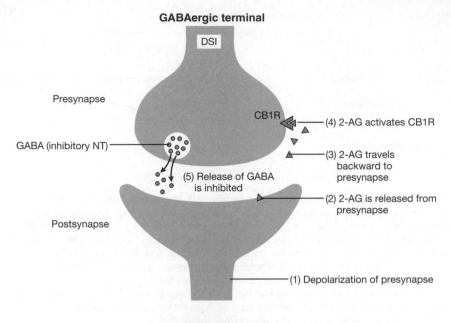

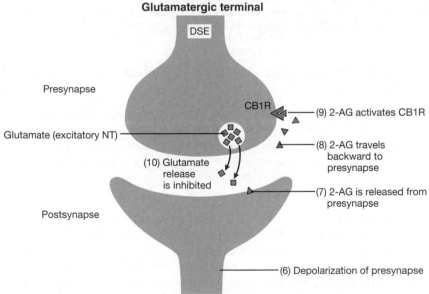

Figure 2.13: **Simplified scheme of depolarization-induced suppression of inhibition and depolarization-induced suppression of excitation (DSI/DSE).** (1) DSI is triggered by post-synaptic depolarization. (2) 2-AG is released from postsynapse and (3) travels backward across the synaptic cleft. (4) 2-AG activates CB1R and (5) inhibits GABA neurotransmitter release. (6) DSE is also triggered by postsynaptic depolarization. (7) 2-AG is released from postsynapse and (8) travels backward across the synaptic cleft. (9) 2-AG activates CB1R and (10) inhibits glutamate neurotransmitter release. Abbreviations: 2-AG, 2-arachidonoylglycerol; CB1R, cannabinoid 1 receptor; DSI, depolarization-induced suppression of inhibition; DSE, depolarization-induced suppression of excitation; GABA, gamma-aminobutyric acid; NT, neurotransmitter.

on presynaptic neurons, reducing either inhibitory or excitatory neurotransmitter release (Pertwee & Ross, 2002). No other neurotransmitter mechanism in the body works this way, as the predominant flow of neurotransmitters in the CNS is antegrade, with neurotransmitters moving from presynaptic neurons to activate postsynaptic receptors. This retrograde DSI/DSE is proposed to provide a self-regulating mechanism for the neuron to adjust its rate of firing to actively regulate neurotransmitter receptor expression (Heifets & Castillo, 2009; Lovinger, 2008; Lu & Mackie, 2016).

Activation of CB1R on the presynapse CB1R in the CNS results in reduced presynaptic neurotransmitter release (Bow & Rimoldi, 2016). Although the direction in which neurotransmitters are released from the presynaptic terminal remains constant (moving from pre- to postsynapse), the quantity of neurotransmitters released varies. Additionally, the length of time between CB1R activation and the release of neurotransmitters differs (Kano et al., 2009). Endocannabinoids can be released from presynaptic neurons in two distinct ways: either briefly in phases in an activity-dependent manner or continuously under homeostatic basal conditions. Once released from postsynaptic neurons to activate presynaptic CB1R, neurotransmitter release is suppressed either temporarily or persistently. These two types of endocannabinoid-mediated suppression of neurotransmitters are known as short-term and long-term depression of neurotransmitter release (Kano et al., 2009).

Short-term depression of neurotransmitter release has a rapid onset of less than 1 s, but it is a short-term event lasting seconds or sometimes minutes (Katona & Freund, 2008). Brief, short-term synaptic depression influences the local effects of neurotransmitter release, involving nearby tissues. During short-term depression, intracellular calcium concentrations in the presynapse are elevated by postsynaptic depolarization, which then stimulates the production of 2-AG in the postsynapse. 2-AG then travels from the postsynaptic neuron across the synaptic gap to activate CB1R on the presynaptic terminal. This activation of CB1R on presynaptic neurons causes inhibition of calcium influx into the cell, consequently inhibiting neurotransmitter release (Kano et al., 2009).

Long-term depression of neurotransmitter release requires a longer induction phase but its repression effects on presynaptic neurotransmitter inhibition can last for several hours (Katona & Freund, 2008). Long-term synaptic depression of neurotransmission release is exhibited only through CB1R activation (Kano, 2014). Although long-term depression of neurotransmitter release is generated in a similar manner as short-term depression, the mechanism for suppression of neurotransmitter release is through a different process: the decrease in the production of cAMP, which is the second intracellular messenger that triggers important physiologic changes at cellular level such as proliferation, differentiation, migration, survival, apoptosis, and depolarization (Nair et al., 2019). This depression of long-term neurotransmitter release can influence both local and remote tissue effects and has been implicated in learning and memory. Long-term synaptic depression of neurotransmitter release mediates a persistent change in the ability of neurons to generate synaptic plasticity, known as metaplasticity, suggesting that this basal long-term suppression of neurotransmitter release serves as a self-regulating mechanism for CB1R signaling in the brain (Di Marzo & De Petrocellis, 2012; Kano, 2014: Kano et al., 2009).

Long- and short-term synaptic depression of neurotransmitter release is associated with the homeostatic mechanism known as "endocannabinoid tone," or the overall rate of cannabinoid receptor activation and subsequent suppression of neurotransmitter inhibition (Howlett et al., 2011; Kim & Alger, 2010; Toczek & Malinowska, 2018). Fluctuations in endocannabinoid tone determine the extent and duration of endocannabinoid production through retrograde signaling. Modification of endocannabinoid tone, rather than directly targeting specific cannabinoid receptors (eg, via synthetic cannabinoids), has been suggested as a therapeutic approach with which to treat endocannabinoid-mediated disease states (Ahn et al., 2009; McPartland et al., 2014; Pertwee & Ross, 2002; Piomelli et al., 2000; Toczek & Malinowska, 2018). Additionally, different tissues may use only one or both forms of neurotransmission inhibition (short-term and/or long-term depression), depending on the location and need for DSI/DSE to maintain homeostasis or modulate disease states (Di Marzo & De Petrocellis, 2012).

The identification of short-term and long-term retrograde signaling in CB1R underscores the important role of this unique process as a presynaptic regulator of synaptic transmission. This action of short- or long-term neurotransmitter inhibition serves to control excessive presynaptic activity (Zou & Kumar, 2018). It is well known that increased concentrations of specific neurotransmitters, such as glutamate, can cause excitotoxicity and neuronal inflammation, which can lead to conditions such as cerebrovascular ischemia or seizures. In traumatic CNS disorders, such as CHI, 2-AG levels have been shown to increase sharply in animal models (Mechoulam, 2002). Administration of synthetic 2-AG to mice after CHI resulted in reduced brain edema, improved clinical recovery, reduced infarct volume, and reduced hippocampal cell death (Magid et al., 2019). 2-AG prevents the formation of tumor necrosis factor-α (TNF-α), a cytokine involved in the process of inflammation, and suppresses the formation of ROS, which are chemically reactive oxygen radicals that can damage cells; these inhibitory activities contribute to the neuroprotective properties of 2-AG (Panikashvili et al., 2001; Patel et al., 2018). Regulation of DSI/DSE patterns and timing of neuronal activity to affect specific neurons could play a role in the activation of cannabinoid receptors as well as the release of endocannabinoids to diminish the tissue-damaging effects of CHI (Lovinger, 2008). The effects associated with short- and long-term retrograde transmission and DSI/DSE offer a possible explanation as to why 2-AG can exert both neuroprotective and neuroregenerative effects both directly and remotely.

The unique processes of DSI/DSE and retrograde signaling in the ECS may have a critical role in some neurologic diseases, either as a contributing factor to the development of the disease or as a treatment for the impaired neuronal signaling pathways associated with the disease. Approaches to either antagonize or potentiate endocannabinoid signaling through blockage of endocannabinoid degradation may provide an effective treatment for neurologic disorders, such as depression, Alzheimer's disease, Huntington's disease, Parkinson's disease, and addiction behaviors (Centonze et al., 2007).

The ECS is remarkable in its ability to respond to both internal and external stimuli to support homeostasis. Depending on the input stimulus, the ECS can be up- or downregulated. When the ECS responds to either external or internal stimuli that call for more endocannabinoids to be produced, cannabinoid receptors increase expression on associated cells, upregulating their ability to bind to their respective ligands. Downregulation of cannabinoid receptors can also occur because of chronic exposure to cannabinoid receptor ligands (eg, endo- and phytocannabinoids), which subsequently reduces the number of available receptor binding sites. Long-term cannabis users downregulate their CB1R population, hence reducing psychoactivity and impairment associated with THC (McPartland et al., 2014).

Endocannabinoids vary greatly in their ability to activate cannabinoid receptors in a retrograde fashion, which then modulate inhibitory and excitatory neurotransmitter release from presynaptic neurons. This unique mechanism exemplifies the substantial role that the ECS plays in regulating neuronal synaptic function throughout the CNS.

CLINICAL ENDOCANNABINOID DEFICIENCY

First introduced in 2004, and then expounded and further explained in 2016, clinical endocannabinoid deficiency (CED) was proposed by the internationally renowned neurologist and psychopharmacologic/ethnobotanical researcher Dr. Ethan Russo as a possible causal explanation for a myriad of chronic pathophysiologic conditions. Russo's work in the field of cannabis botany and pharmacologic mechanisms of cannabis, as well as psychopharmacology, gave him extraordinary insight into the complex relationships between the chronic disease states of migraine, fibromyalgia, IBS, and other treatment-resistant conditions.

Pertwee (2006) noted that some physiologic disorders, such as pain, cancer, intestinal and cardiovascular diseases, multiple sclerosis, and traumatic head injury, along with psychological disorders, such as posttraumatic stress disorder (PTSD) and schizophrenia, involve fluctuations in tissue concentrations of endocannabinoids and cannabinoid receptor densities. Through upregulation of the ECS, expression of additional cannabinoid receptors, or increases in the concentrations of endocannabinoids, the severity of symptoms is reduced in these disease states, which slows the progression of the disease. Conversely, the upregulation of the ECS may result in other unwanted conditions, such as impaired fertility in women, obesity, cerebral injury in stroke, endotoxic shock, cystitis, ileitis, and paralytic ileus. One of the primary functions of the ECS is related to autoprotection by regulating homeostasis across several physiologic systems, and the recognition that pathologies can arise from either under- or overstimulation of endocannabinoid tone provides support for a plausible CED hypothesis (Pertwee, 2006).

Cannabinoid receptor density, or the number of cannabinoid receptors located within one distinct area, is greater in cells and tissues than in many other types of physiologic receptors (Russo, 2004). CED has been proposed as having two mechanisms: congenital or acquired. In congenital CED, there is an inherent deficiency within the ECS, in the number of receptors, a reduced binding capability of endocannabinoids, or a reduced concentration of endocannabinoids. For example, variations of CB1R and FAAH genes have been noted in patients with diarrhea-predominant and other forms of IBS (Sharkey & Wiley, 2016). Acquired CED occurs as a result of either injury or chronic disease that affects changes in endocannabinoid tone, such as desensitization of cannabinoid receptors (Russo, 2016). Multiple sclerosis is a likely example of acquired CED, where neurodegeneration occurs as a consequence of repeated axonal demyelination, which alters the excitotoxicity of neuronal channels (Correale et al., 2019). In either congenital or acquired CED conditions, the use of phytocannabinoids or synthetic cannabinoid receptor agonists has shown promise as a treatment, improving the symptoms and reducing the progression of these disease states (McPartland et al., 2014).

In the pathology of migraines, serotonin (5-HT$_3$) receptors play a prominent role in both etiology and treatment. In individuals who experience migraines, serum levels of both anandamide and 2-AG are significantly reduced. Anandamide is recognized as a partial CB1R agonist that reduces the release of serotonin from 5-HT$_3$ receptors. The activity of anandamide at CB1R and 5-HT$_3$ receptors provides support for its role in the endogenous therapeutic management of migraine. Migraine has also been linked to a genetic condition, but its pathology is similar to CHI, in that it is considered a condition of altered excitability in brain tissue (Goadsby et al., 2017). This suggests that the neuroprotective role of endocannabinoids also influences either the development or treatment of migraine symptoms. Alterations in either the ECS or endocannabinoid binding or concentrations may be a contributing factor in either congenital or acquired CED in migraine pathology (Russo, 2001, 2004, 2016). Figure 2.14 illustrates the common comorbidities that are observed in the disorders of migraine, fibromyalgia, and IBS that suggest the existence of CED.

Fibromyalgia is a condition in which central nervous sensitization increases over time, causing hyperalgesia and resulting in other comorbid conditions, such as sleep disturbances, dysfunction in the nerves that regulate involuntary body functions (dysautonomia), and depression (Russo, 2004, 2016). In individuals who experience fibromyalgia, low levels of anandamide in the cerebrospinal fluid suggest the lack of this endocannabinoid may be a factor in the development of the disorder. The ECS is an essential regulator of pain perception and pain thresholds, and hyperalgesia is associated with central endocannabinoid hypofunction in the spinal cord. The presence of endocannabinoids, such as anandamide and 2-AG, reduces associated hyperalgesia. Without a balanced endocannabinoid tone, chronic pain conditions develop. Anandamide activates CB1R in the CNS to reduce hyperalgesia as well as inflammation through its activity at peripheral CB2R and TRPV1 (Russo, 2016).

IBS is characterized as a condition that exhibits visceral hypersensitivity. The enteric nervous system expresses dense amounts of CB1R in both surface tissues and intestinal smooth muscle, and stimulation of this receptor in the gut depresses GI motility by inhibiting neurotransmitter release (Sharkey & Wiley, 2016). Chronic intestinal inflammation, therefore, causes upregulation and sensitization of cannabinoid receptors. Individuals experiencing IBS have been shown to have reduced levels of anandamide in GI tissues and an increase in TRPV1 (Russo, 2016). Anandamide, a partial agonist at CB1R, plays a role in decreasing pain associated with GI irritation. 2-AG, a full agonist at CB1R, has also been shown to modulate intestinal motility. As TRPV1 is also involved in IBS, increased concentrations of anandamide desensitize TRPV1 to painful stimuli and exert anti-inflammatory activities (Russo, 2016). The actions of anandamide at both CB1R and TRPV1 support the hypothesis for either congenital or acquired CED in the condition of IBS.

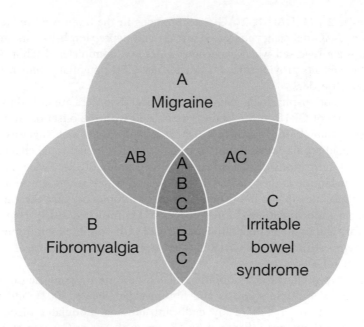

Figure 2.14: **Diagram depicting comorbidity of migraine, fibromyalgia, and IBS.** Chronic diseases such as migraine, fibromyalgia, and IBS share many common underlying pathologies that suggest the presence of clinical endocannabinoid deficiency. AB represents the number of migraine subjects (35.6%) who also fit the clinical criteria of fibromyalgia. BC represents the number of IBS subjects (31.6%) who were also diagnosed with fibromyalgia, which correlates to the number of fibromyalgia subjects (32%) who also fit the clinical criteria for IBS (Russo, 2004, 2016). AC represents the number of migraine subjects (24%) who also fit the clinical criteria for IBS (Tietjen et al., 2009). The overlap at the center of all three conditions illustrates the correlation of lifetime risk to develop another or all these chronic disease conditions simultaneously (Russo, 2004, 2016). Abbreviations: A, migraine; B, fibromyalgia; C, irritable bowel syndrome (IBS).

There are irrefutable similarities in the conditions of migraine, fibromyalgia, and IBS that offer clinical support for CED (see Figure 2.14). All three conditions share common characteristics, and Russo (2016) notes the similarities among the conditions:

- A state of hyperalgesia, or an abnormal increase in sensitivity to pain.
- Association with high levels of anxiety and depression.
- A lack of specific tissue pathology.
- Labeled as psychosomatic disorders or "wastebasket" diagnoses.
- Frequently present in the same individual simultaneously or at different points over time. (p. 155)

Although migraine, fibromyalgia, and IBS share these pathophysiologic properties, other disorders that are characterized by low pain thresholds and dysfunctions in digestion, mood, sleep, and neurologic function might also be explained by CED. In an animal model study that investigated the genetic deletion of the enzyme needed to synthesize 2-AG, DAG-L, 2-AG concentrations in the brain were reduced. This subsequent 2-AG deficiency increased anxiety and depression behaviors, and these behaviors were reversed when exogenous 2-AG was administered (Shonesy et al., 2014). These results provide further evidence that CED potentially influences mood and anxiety disorders.

Numerous other physiologic and psychological disorders are linked to ECS alterations. Loss of CB1R in the brain is associated with the onset of Huntington's disease symptoms before significant neuronal axon loss, which suggests that endocannabinoid regulation at these receptors is lost before neuronal changes cause the outward indications of this disease (Zou & Kumar, 2018). Twice the normal level of anandamide is seen in Parkinson's disease, which is thought to be a compensatory mechanism for the progressive loss of dopamine and the subsequent reduction in endocannabinoid tone (Toczek & Malinowska, 2018). Hyperrelease of excitatory glutamate in the brain is associated with Tourette's syndrome and epilepsy, whereas stimulation of CB1R in these areas reduces the release of glutamate (Piomelli et al., 2000).

Bladder hyperreflexia is a condition that is common among neurologic disorders, such as multiple sclerosis and fibromyalgia (Steers, 2002), and involves TRPV1. Activation of TRPV1 by endocannabinoids modulates bladder tone, decreasing spasticity and inflammation (Baker et al., 2003; Capasso et al., 2011; Toczek & Malinowska, 2018). Manipulation of the ECS to activate either TRPV1 or inhibit FAAH to increase endocannabinoid concentrations could also potentially restore endocannabinoid tone in CED disorders associated with bladder dysfunction (Bjorling & Wang, 2018).

Another disorder that is potentially linked to CED is infantile colic. Infantile colic has no apparent etiology and is associated with visceral sensitivity and general dysphoria. This disorder, which has furthermore been linked to migraines in children and adolescents aged 6 to 18 years (Romanello et al., 2013), is also resistant to traditional pharmaceutical intervention (Russo, 2004). Although there is currently a scarcity of studies that investigate the use of cannabinoids in pediatric populations, identification of the role of the ECS in this disorder could potentially explain an association to CED.

As the body strives to return to homeostasis, endocannabinoid levels may fall or rise. Individuals who suffer from PTSD have been shown to have significant reductions of anandamide and 2-AG in the brain (Papagianni & Stevenson, 2019; Shekhar & Thakur, 2018), whereas anandamide levels are higher in the cerebrospinal fluid of acute schizophrenics and individuals experiencing anorexia (Russo, 2016). Alterations in either cannabinoid receptor structure or expression have also been linked to anorexia and schizophrenia (Chase et al., 2016; Frieling et al., 2009; Gérard et al., 2011; Ishiguro et al., 2011; Perez et al., 2019), suggesting that although anandamide concentrations are excessive, activation of either CB1R or CB2R is dysfunctional in these psychological disorders. These alterations of endocannabinoids and cannabinoid receptors in the CNS support the presence of CED in individuals experiencing PTSD, anorexia, and schizophrenia.

The accumulating research regarding the complex relationships between the ECS, endocannabinoids, and exogenous sources of cannabinoids (ie, phyto- and synthetic cannabinoids) provides optimistic evidence that therapeutic adjustment of the ECS might reduce or even eliminate these chronic disease conditions. However, as deficits in these protective and homeostatic physiologic processes may be harmful, excesses may also be considered detrimental, as seen in upregulation of the ECS with accompanying rises in endocannabinoid levels that are associated with obesity and metabolic syndrome (Gatta-Cherifi & Cota, 2015; Hirsch & Tam, 2019). More scientific examination is needed to make the definitive case for CED, which should focus on whether a defective ECS or endocannabinoid activity underlies the pathology of disease states or whether these alterations are primary or secondary dysfunctions resulting from other causes.

 CASE STUDY
Interview with Dr. Ethan Russo
(Interview used with permission from Dr. Ethan Russo.)

Dr. Ethan Russo has been influential in the recognition and elucidation of CED. His work in associating the prospective mechanisms underlying chronic, misunderstood, and poorly treated disease states (ie, the "wastebasket" diseases of fibromyalgia, migraine, and irritable bowel disease) has been the focus of numerous investigations since his proposal that these disorders and others might be related to a deficiency of endocannabinoids or cannabinoid receptors. Dr. Russo provided some insight into the current state of CED research and the role of the cannabis nurse in helping to recognize its occurrence in the clinical patient.

Question 1: Where does current research stand concerning CED, as more chronic disorders are being linked to imbalances between endocannabinoids and endocannabinoid receptors?
Answer: Recent research supports the likelihood of autistic spectrum disorder as a CED disorder. Another study failed to show alterations in serum endocannabinoid levels in fibromyalgia, but this may or may not reflect what is going on in the brain.

Question 2: What other priorities in clinical research, besides the ones you mention, should be considered for CED?
Answer: I believe that CED should be considered in any disorder in a physiologic system for which we currently cannot discern the pathophysiology. Given that the ECS is everywhere, that covers a lot of territory.

Question 3: What can nurses do to assist patients in recognizing potential CED?
Answer: Nurses are the key communicators between patients and doctors and carry out an essential educational role. This is never as needed as in the case of the ECS and its pathology, wherein physicians lack the background to understand its implications.

Empirical Support for Clinical Endocannabinoid Deficiency

Empirical support for CED continues to accumulate. Experimental deletion of DAG-L, the enzyme required for the synthesis of 2-AG, was shown to decrease levels of 2-AG in the brain of mice (Shonesy et al., 2014). After reductions in 2-AG concentrations, the mice demonstrated anxiety-like behaviors and anhedonia, or the inability to feel pleasure. Restoration of 2-AG concentrations reversed anxiety and depression behaviors. In other studies, genetic deletion of CB1R produced anxiety behaviors in mice, generating chronic stress states (Shonesy et al., 2014). The deletion of DAG-L was repeated in another animal study that also investigated the effects of deletion on CB1R signaling and levels of anandamide (Jenniches et al., 2016). The increased anxiety- and stress-related behaviors noted after DAG-L deletion resembled those observed in animals lacking CB1R, and levels of anandamide were significantly decreased in brain areas associated with emotions and stress response. In one study, levels of 2-AG and anandamide were measured in individuals who were in close proximity to the World Trade Center at the time of the 9/11 attacks, and both 2-AG and anandamide levels were significantly reduced in individuals diagnosed with PTSD (Hill et al., 2013). These investigational models demonstrate the influence of CB1R and endocannabinoids in depression, stress, and anxiety behaviors.

Given that emotions are controlled by the amygdala in the brain's limbic system, the presence of CB1R in the amygdala and the knowledge that 2-AG is a full agonist at CB1R suggest that deficiencies in this brain endocannabinoid are linked to psychological states of anxiety and depression, which strengthen the argument that CED manifests from chronic alterations in either cannabinoid receptor densities or endocannabinoid concentrations. The concept of endocannabinoid tone, or the natural homeostatic balance of endocannabinoids and cannabinoid receptors, is also a significant concept that supports CED, as high doses of endocannabinoids induce anxiety-provoking effects, whereas low doses induce anxiety-relieving effects (Papagianni & Stevenson, 2019).

Complementary Modalities That Influence the Endocannabinoid System

McPartland et al. (2014) have suggested complementary modalities that can be utilized to enhance the ECS and support endocannabinoid tone by upregulating cannabinoid receptors, increasing endocannabinoid synthesis, or inhibiting endocannabinoid degradation. One of the first complementary modalities that serves to enhance endocannabinoid synthesis is the inclusion of polyunsaturated fats (PUFs) in the diet. The typical Western diet contains an overabundance of omega-6 PUF and a deficiency of omega-3 PUF; a proper balance in these two PUFs is essential to maintaining many cellular processes (Simopoulos, 2016). Endocannabinoids are synthesized from AA, which is an omega-6 PUF, and studies indicate that dietary inclusion of this substance increases serum levels of anandamide and 2-AG. Adequate levels of omega-3 PUF are also essential for proper endocannabinoid signaling. Dietary enhancement of omega-3 PUF produces a greater expression of CB1R and CB2R (McPartland et al., 2014).

Another dietary modification that enhances the ECS is the use of probiotics as a dietary supplement. Studies that investigated the use of probiotic compounds such as *Enterococcus faecium* and *Lactobacillus acidophilus* (Rousseaux et al., 2007) found increased expression of CB1R and CB2R in tissues, respectively. Administration of a probiotic to dogs diagnosed with GI motility disorders showed that CB1R and CB2R expression increased in colon epithelial tissue, which decreased signs of dysmotility (Rossi et al., 2020). It was hypothesized that probiotic administration modulated GI microbiota and epithelial cell receptor–mediated signaling in the intestinal mucosa, decreasing inflammation and preventing dysmotility.

Breastfeeding in newborns is also a beneficial method to enhance endocannabinoid tone. Human breast milk contains small amounts of anandamide and higher levels of 2-AG (Grant & Cahn, 2005). In animal studies, oral administration of anandamide, OEA, and 2-AG produced calming properties and enhanced infant suckling behavior (Crouzin et al., 2001; Fride et al., 2001). These ECS benefits support the rationale for breastfeeding in newborn infants.

Chronic stress reduces anandamide levels, whereas 2-AG levels either increase or decrease, depending on the nature of the stressor (Hill et al., 2010). Alternatively, relaxation and social play increase CB1R activation with enhanced anandamide levels in the brain (Trezza et al., 2012). The ECS is impaired in chronic stress, and stress management strategies that include regular interventions of yoga, meditation, mindfulness, deep breathing, and massage have been shown to upregulate the ECS while balancing endocannabinoid tone (McPartland et al., 2014).

Lifestyle modifications are also important in regulating the ECS. Numerous studies have indicated that diets rich in fats and sugars alter levels of anandamide, 2-AG, their metabolic enzymes (ie, DAG-L, MAG-L, and NAPE-PLD), and CB1R (Naughton et al., 2013). Upregulation of cannabinoid receptors driven by excessive levels of endocannabinoids is noted in obese disease states, and increased production of endocannabinoids is found in peripheral tissues such as visceral adipose tissue, liver, pancreas, and skeletal muscle (Côté et al., 2007). Decreased plasma anandamide and 2-AG levels were seen when obese individuals underwent programmed weight loss, with decreased 2-AG levels correlating with decreased visceral adipose tissue, triglycerides, and insulin resistance, with improved high-density lipoprotein-cholesterol levels (Di Marzo et al., 2009).

Exercise has also been shown to modulate the ECS. Anandamide levels significantly increased after ≥30 minutes of moderately intense running with subsequent increased cannabinoid receptor signaling (Sparling et al., 2003). Medium- to high-intensity voluntary exercise appears to increase endocannabinoid signaling through increased anandamide levels and CB1R expression. The "Runner's high" may be an endocannabinoid-rewarding response for intentional exercise (Raichlen et al., 2012).

CONCLUSIONS

The human ECS is likely the most important physiologic system in the body, regulating almost every organ system as it sustains a homeostatic balance between health and disease (Alger, 2013). The ECS is also responsible for prevention of disease, reduction of conditions associated with aging, and decreasing damage done by roaming oxygen free radicals (Javed et al., 2016; Lipina & Hundal, 2016; McPartland et al., 2014; Mukhopadhyay et al., 2010; Paradisi et al., 2006). The two principal endocannabinoids, anandamide and 2-AG, are synthesized in postsynaptic neurons using endogenous compounds found in the cell membrane. Once released from postsynaptic cells, endocannabinoids cross the synaptic cleft to activate presynaptic cannabinoid receptors, traveling backward in a retrograde fashion. Once the cannabinoid receptor has been activated, the endocannabinoids cross the cell membrane by either simple diffusion or facilitated carrier transport known as EMT and are degraded by intracellular enzymes into precursor molecules to be recycled again as endocannabinoids.

The significant discoveries of the cannabinoid and noncannabinoid receptors, endocannabinoids and endocannabinoid-like ligands, and the enzymes of synthesis and degradation have provided an extraordinary understanding of the multiple complex processes involved in homeostasis and disease states. The main function of CB1R is to mediate the release of neurotransmitters from presynaptic neurons, which modulates numerous physiologic processes that are responsible for health and disease. The main function of CB2R is to modulate cytokine release from immune cells. Although CB2R is found in lower densities than CB1R under basal conditions, their expression increases during pathologic states, supporting its role as a homeostatic regulator to help prevent tissue injury and disease progression.

The entourage effect is a phenomenon in which endocannabinoid activity is potentiated through a synergistic relationship with noncannabinoid compounds, such as OEA and 2-PG (PEA). Although entourage compounds do not directly interact with cannabinoid receptors, their presence enhances the activity of endocannabinoids at cannabinoid and cannabinoid-like receptors. Activation of cannabinoid and cannabinoid-like receptors causes numerous physiologic effects in almost every organ system; researchers around the world are currently performing rigorous investigations of the physiologic mechanisms underlying the effects of the ECS and its various components. Studies will continue to clarify the multifaceted roles of the ECS and the effects of alterations in endocannabinoid tone, and future discoveries will advance the knowledge of known and unknown ECS receptors, ligands, enzymes, and their effects on health and disease.

CED is proposed as an underlying pathophysiologic mechanism in which there are alterations in the ECS, through either acquired or congenital processes that decrease the number of cannabinoid receptors or decrease the activity or concentrations of endocannabinoids. These alterations cause an overall defect—either an intensification or a reduction—in endocannabinoid tone. Use of exogenous cannabinoids (eg, phyto- or synthetic cannabinoids) in disease states such as migraine, fibromyalgia, and IBS has been shown to improve the symptoms associated with these diseases by regulating endocannabinoid tone. However, humans are capable of modifying their endocannabinoid tone through a variety of holistic interventions that include diet, stress management, and lifestyle modifications. These interventions are similar to other recommendations that support reducing or altering disease states; perhaps the common denominator yet to be detected in all forms of identified diseases is an imbalance in endocannabinoid tone.

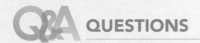 **QUESTIONS**

1. What are the primary functions of the ECS?
   A. Upregulate the immune system and prevent pain
   B. Inhibit cancer cells from forming and relaxing the body
   C. Regulate homeostasis and prevent disease and aging
   D. Implement retrograde signaling and endocannabinoid synthesis

2. Which term describes the potentiating effect of endocannabinoids?
   A. Cannabis effect
   B. Entourage effect
   C. Medical effect
   D. Phytocannabinoid production

3. What is the primary function of CB2R?
   A. Homeostasis of physiologic activities
   B. Modulate immune response
   C. Enhance CNS response
   D. Protection from external pathogens

4. How is anandamide transported to intracellular sites after it enters the cell?
   A. Through vesicular transport
   B. By facilitated diffusion
   C. Through enzymatic signaling
   D. By adiposomes

5. Why are endocannabinoids considered "retrograde messengers"?
   A. They are released and then act backward
   B. They are released and then create new endocannabinoids
   C. They are short-lived intracellular chemical signals
   D. They are released and then signal the cell to stop signaling

6. Where are endocannabinoids made?
   A. Postsynaptic neuron
   B. Presynaptic neuron
   C. Hippocampus
   D. Microglial cells

7. Which endocannabinoid modulator contributes to the entourage effect?
   A. Monoacylglycerol lipase (MAG-L)
   B. 2-Palmitoylglycerol (2-PG)
   C. 2-Arachidonoylglycerol (2-AG)
   D. Fatty acid amide hydrolase (FAAH)

8. Which is one way endocannabinoids are degraded?
   A. Excretion by the liver
   B. Exhaled as carbon dioxide
   C. Through intracellular enzyme activity
   D. Administration of cannabis antagonists

9. What is one proposed cause of CED?
   A. Overdose of synthetic cannabis
   B. Long-term use of phytocannabinoids
   C. Inadequate production of endocannabinoids
   D. Use of endocannabinoid antagonizing drugs

10. Which of these is one way to upregulate the ECS?
    A. Ride a bike
    B. Eat fast food
    C. Use alcohol in moderation
    D. Increase daily water intake

ANSWERS

1. **Answer: C.** The role of the ECS in homeostasis includes relaxation, eating, sleeping, forgetting, and protection. An altered balance in nervous, endocrine, cardiovascular, and immune systems characterizes aging and age-related disease change. By modifying endocannabinoid tone, the ECS can provide a protective role against disease and age-promoting physiologic processes.

2. **Answer: B.** Ben-Shabat and colleagues proposed the potentiating entourage effect of endocannabinoids in 1998. By that time, the two principal endocannabinoids, anandamide and 2-AG, had been identified, but additional endogenous compounds have subsequently been discovered to enhance their activities. Intense research into the complex relationships between endocannabinoids and cannabinoid receptors has led to the identification of a variety of physiologic mechanisms in which endocannabinoid activity is potentiated. Entourage effects occur because of the ability of entourage compounds to prevent the breakdown of endocannabinoids or by improving the affinity for them to bind to a cannabinoid receptor.

3. **Answer: B.** The primary function of CB2R is to modulate chemical messengers (cytokines) from immune cells. During normal physiologic states, the human body does not express CB2R; it is during the pathologic alterations of organ systems that CB2R is markedly upregulated in affected cells and tissues.

4. **Answer: D.** Once taken up by cells, anandamide moves to lipid adiposomes, or "lipid rafts." Adiposomes act as shuttles for the rapid delivery of anandamide from the cell membrane to intracellular sites, where hydrolysis occurs.

5. **Answer: A.** The endocannabinoids operate via retrograde signaling by moving backward across the synaptic cleft from the postsynapse to the presynapse.

6. **Answer: A.** Endocannabinoids are released from the postsynaptic terminal after neuronal depolarization and act at the presynaptic terminal in a retrograde, or reverse, manner.

7. **Answer: B.** 2-LG and 2-PG are two lipid monoacylglycerols that have been isolated from the spleen, brain, and gut tissues. Neither of these lipid compounds interacts with CB1R or CB2R but instead, significantly potentiate the binding of 2-AG and its capacity to inhibit adenylyl cyclase, which enhances the neuroprotective activity of 2-AG. Both 2-LG and 2-PG potentiated the binding of 2-AG to both CB1R and CB2R, either separately or together.

8. **Answer: C.** The two principal endocannabinoids, AEA (or anandamide) and 2-AG are synthesized and degraded through multiple complex enzymatic pathways.

9. **Answer: C.** Cannabinoid receptor density is found in greater quantities in cells and tissues than in many other types of physiologic receptors. CED has been proposed as having two mechanisms: congenital or acquired. In congenital CED, there is an inherent deficiency within the ECS, in the number of receptors, a reduced binding capability of endocannabinoids, or reduced concentrations of endocannabinoids.

10. **Answer: A.** The ECS is impaired in chronic stress, and stress management strategies that include regular interventions of yoga, meditation, mindfulness, deep breathing, and massage have been shown to upregulate the ECS while balancing endocannabinoid tone.

References

Adams, R., Hunt, M., & Clark, J. H. (1940). Structure of cannabidiol, a product isolated from the marihuana extract of Minnesota wild hemp. *Journal of the American Chemical Society, 62*(1), 196–200. https://doi.org/10.1021/ja01858a058

Ahn, K., Johnson, D. S., & Cravatt, B. F. (2009). Fatty acid amide hydrolase as a potential therapeutic target for the treatment of pain and CNS disorders. *Expert Opinion on Drug Discovery, 4*(7), 763–784. https://doi.org/10.1517/17460440903018857

Akiba, Y., Kato, S., Katsube, K., Nakamura, M., Takeuchi, K., Ishii, H., & Hibi, T. (2004). Transient receptor potential vanilloid subfamily 1 expressed in pancreatic islet β cells modulates insulin secretion in rats. *Biochemical and Biophysical Research Communications, 321*(1), 219–225. https://doi.org/10.1016/j.bbrc.2004.06.149

Alger, B. E. (2013). Getting high on the endocannabinoid system. *Cerebrum, 14.* https://www.ncbi.nlm.nih.gov/pmc/articles/PMC3997295/

Alhouayek, M., & Mucciolo, G. G. (2017). Pharmacological aspects of anandamide and 2-arachidonoylglycerol as bioactive lipids. In V. Preedy (Ed.), *Handbook of cannabis and related pathologies* (pp. 616–629). Academic Press.

Andrzejewska, A., Staszak, K., Kaczmarek-Ryś, M., Słomski, R., & Hryhorowicz, S. (2018). Understanding cannabinoid receptors: Structure and function. *Folia Biologica et Oecologica, 14*(1), 1–13. https://doi.org/10.1515/fobio-2017-0004

Arifin, S. A., & Falasca, M. (2016). Lysophosphatidylinositol signalling and metabolic diseases. *Metabolites, 6*(1), 1–11. https://doi.org/10.3390/metabo6010006

Bab, I., & Zimmer, A. (2008). Cannabinoid receptors and the regulation of bone mass. *British Journal of Pharmacology, 153*(2), 182–188. https://doi.org/10.1038/sj.bjp.0707593

Baggelaar, M. P., Maccarrone, M., & van der Stelt, M. (2018). 2-Arachidonoylglycerol: A signaling lipid with manifold actions in the brain. *Progress in Lipid Research, 71*, 1–17. https://doi.org/10.1016/j.plipres.2018.05.002

Baker, D., Pryce, G., Giovannoni, G., & Thompson, A. J. (2003). The therapeutic potential of cannabis. *Lancet Neurology, 2*(5), 291–298. https://doi.org/10.1016/S1474-4422(03)00381-8

Baldassarri, S., Bertoni, A., Bagarotti, A., Sarasso, C., Zanfa, M., Catani, M. V., Avigliano, L., Maccarrone, M., Torti, M., & Sinigaglia, F. (2008). The endocannabinoid 2-arachidonoylglycerol activates human platelets through non-CB1/CB2 receptors. *Journal of Thrombosis and Haemostasis, 6*(10), 1772–1779. https://doi.org/10.1111/j.1538-7836.2008.03093.x

Balenga, N. A. B., Aflaki, E., Kargl, J., Platzer, W., Schröder, R., Blättermann, S., Kostenis, E., Brown, A. J., Heinemann, A., & Waldhoer, M. (2011). GPR55 regulates cannabinoid 2 receptor-mediated responses in human neutrophils. *Cell Research, 21*(10), 1452–1469. https://doi.org/10.1038/cr.2011.60

Basu, S., & Dittel, B. N. (2011). Unraveling the complexities of cannabinoid receptor 2 (CB2) immune regulation in health and disease. *Immunologic Research, 51*(1), 26–38. https://doi.org/10.1007/s12026-011-8210-5

Bátkai, S., & Pacher, P. (2009). Endocannabinoids and cardiac contractile function: Pathophysiological implications. *Pharmacological Research: The Official Journal of the Italian Pharmacological Society, 60*(2), 99–106. https://doi.org/10.1016/j.phrs.2009.04.003

Battista, N., Meccariello, R., Cobellis, G., Fasano, S., Di Tommaso, M., Pirazzi, V., Konje, J. C., Pierantoni, R., & Maccarrone, M. (2012). The role of endocannabinoids in gonadal function and fertility along the evolutionary axis. *Molecular and Cellular Endocrinology, 355*(1), 1–14. https://doi.org/10.1016/j.mce.2012.01.014

Bełtowski, J. (2012). Lysophosphatidylinositol and the GPR55 receptor: A new regulatory system in the adipose tissue. *Clinical Lipidology, 7*(2), 135–139. https://doi.org/10.2217/clp.12.15

Ben-Shabat, S., Fride, E., Sheskin, T., Tamiri, T., Rhee, M.-H., Vogel, Z., Bisogno, T., De Petrocellis, L., Di Marzo, V., & Mechoulam, R. (1998). An entourage effect: Inactive endogenous fatty acid glycerol esters enhance 2-arachidonoylglycerol cannabinoid activity. *European Journal of Pharmacology, 353*(1), 23–31. https://doi.org/10.1016/S0014-2999(98)00392-6

Birben, E., Sahiner, U. M., Sackesen, C., Erzurum, S., & Kalayci, O. (2012). Oxidative stress and antioxidant defense. *World Allergy Organization Journal, 5*(1), 9–19. https://doi.org/10.1097/WOX.0b013e3182439613

Bisogno, T., Hanuš, L., De Petrocellis, L., Tchilibon, S., Ponde, D. E., Brandi, I., Moriello, A. S., Davis, J. B., Mechoulam, R., & Di Marzo, V. (2001). Molecular targets for cannabidiol and its synthetic analogues: Effect on vanilloid VR1 receptors and on the cellular uptake and enzymatic hydrolysis of anandamide. *British Journal of Pharmacology, 134*(4), 845–852. https://doi.org/10.1038/sj.bjp.0704327

Bisogno, T., Melck, D., Bobrov, M. Y., Gretskaya, N. M., Bezuglov, V. V., De Petrocellis, L., & Di Marzo, V. (2000). *N*-acyl-dopamines: Novel synthetic CB(1) cannabinoid-receptor ligands and inhibitors of anandamide inactivation with cannabimimetic activity *in vitro* and *in vivo. Biochemical Journal, 351*(Pt. 3), 817–824. https://www.ncbi.nlm.nih.gov/pmc/articles/PMC1221424/

Bisogno, T., Oddi, S., Piccoli, A., Fazio, D., & Maccarrone, M. (2016). Type-2 cannabinoid receptors in neurodegeneration. *Pharmacological Research, 111*, 721–730. https://doi.org/10.1016/j.phrs.2016.07.021

Bjorling, D. E., & Wang, Z. (2018). Potential of endocannabinoids to control bladder pain. *Frontiers in Systems Neuroscience, 12*, 17. https://doi.org/10.3389/fnsys.2018.00017

Blondeau, N., Lauritzen, I., Widmann, C., Lazdunski, M., & Heurteaux, C. (2002). A potent protective role of lysophospholipids against global cerebral ischemia and glutamate excitotoxicity in neuronal cultures. *Journal of Cerebral Blood Flow & Metabolism, 22*(7), 821–834. https://doi.org/10.1097/00004647-200207000-00007

Bondarenko, A. I., Malli, R., & Graier, W. F. (2011). The GPR55 agonist lysophosphatidylinositol acts as an intracellular messenger and bidirectionally modulates Ca2+-activated large-conductance K+ channels in endothelial cells. *Pflugers Archiv, 461*(1), 177–189. https://doi.org/10.1007/s00424-010-0898-x

Bow, E. W., & Rimoldi, J. M. (2016). The structure–function relationships of classical cannabinoids: CB1/CB2 modulation. *Perspectives in Medicinal Chemistry, 8*, 17–39. https://doi.org/10.4137/PMC.S32171

Brantl, S. A., Khandoga, A. L., & Siess, W. (2014). Mechanism of platelet activation induced by endocannabinoids in blood and plasma. *Platelets, 25*(3), 151–161. https://doi.org/10.3109/09537104.2013.803530

Braud, S., Bon, C., Touqui, L., & Mounier, C. (2000). Activation of rabbit blood platelets by anandamide through its cleavage into arachidonic acid. *FEBS Letters, 471*(1), 12–16. https://doi.org/10.1016/S0014-5793(00)01359-4

Brito, R., Sheth, S., Mukherjea, D., Rybak, L. P., & Ramkumar, V. (2014). TRPV1: A potential drug target for treating various diseases. *Cells, 3*(2), 517–545. https://doi.org/10.3390/cells3020517

Browning, K. N., & Travagli, R. A. (2014). Central nervous system control of gastrointestinal motility and secretion and modulation of gastrointestinal functions. *Comprehensive Physiology, 4*(4), 1339–1368. https://doi.org/10.1002/cphy.c130055

Cabral, G. A., & Griffin-Thomas, L. (2009). Emerging role of the CB2 cannabinoid receptor in immune regulation and therapeutic prospects. *Expert Reviews in Molecular Medicine, 11*, e3. https://doi.org/10.1017/S1462399409000957

Cahn, R. S. (1932). The constitution of cannabinol. *Journal of the Chemical Society*, 1342–1353.

Calignano, A., Rana, G. L., Giuffrida, A., & Piomelli, D. (1998). Control of pain initiation by endogenous cannabinoid. *Nature, 394*, 277–281. https://doi.org/10.1038/28393

Capasso, R., Aviello, G., Borrelli, F., Romano, B., Ferro, M., Castaldo, L., Montanaro, V., Altieri, V., & Izzo, A. A. (2011). Inhibitory effect of standardized *Cannabis sativa* extract and its ingredient cannabidiol on rat and human bladder contractility. *Urology, 77*(4), 1006.e9–1006.e15. https://doi.org/10.1016/j.urology.2010.12.006

Carnevale, L. N., Arango, A. S., Arnold, W. R., Tajkhorshid, E., & Das, A. (2018). Endocannabinoid virodhamine is an endogenous inhibitor of human cardiovascular CYP2J2 epoxygenase. *Biochemistry, 57*(46), 6489–6499. https://doi.org/10.1021/acs.biochem.8b00691

Casarotto, P. C., Terzian, A. L. B., Aguiar, D. C., Zangrossi, H., Guimarães, F. S., Wotjak, C. T., & Moreira, F. A. (2012). Opposing roles for cannabinoid receptor type-1 (CB1) and transient receptor potential vanilloid type-1 channel (TRPV1) on the modulation of panic-like responses in rats. *Neuropsychopharmacology, 37*(2), 478–486. https://doi.org/10.1038/npp.2011.207

Centonze, D., Finazzi-Agrò, A., Bernardi, G., & Maccarrone, M. (2007). The endocannabinoid system in targeting inflammatory neurodegenerative diseases. *Trends in Pharmacological Sciences, 28*(4), 180–187. https://doi.org/10.1016/j.tips.2007.02.004

Chase, K. A., Feiner, B., Rosen, C., Gavin, D. P., & Sharma, R. P. (2016). Characterization of peripheral cannabinoid receptor expression and clinical correlates in schizophrenia. *Psychiatry Research, 245*, 346–353. https://doi.org/10.1016/j.psychres.2016.08.055

Chicca, A., Marazzi, J., Nicolussi, S., & Gertsch, J. (2012). Evidence for bidirectional endocannabinoid transport across cell membranes. *Journal of Biological Chemistry, 287*(41), 34660–34682. https://doi.org/10.1074/jbc.M112.373241

Chinetti, G., Fruchart, J. C., & Staels, B. (2000). Peroxisome proliferator-activated receptors (PPARs): Nuclear receptors at the crossroads between lipid metabolism and inflammation. *Inflammation Research, 49*(10), 497–505. https://doi.org/10.1007/s000110050622

Chiurchiù, V. (2016). Endocannabinoids and Immunity. *Cannabis and Cannabinoid Research, 1*(1), 59–66. https://doi.org/10.1089/can.2016.0002

Christie, M. J., & Vaughan, C. W. (2001). Cannabinoids act backwards. *Nature, 410*(6828), 527–530. https://doi.org/10.1038/35069167

Clapper, J. R., Moreno-Sanz, G., Russo, R., Guijarro, A., Vacondio, F., Duranti, A., Tontini, A., Sanchini, S., Sciolino, N. R., Spradley, J. M., Hohmann, A., Calignano, A., Mor, M., Tarzia, G., & Piomelli, D. (2010). Anandamide suppresses pain initiation through a peripheral endocannabinoid mechanism. *Nature Neuroscience, 13*(10), 1265–1270. https://doi.org/10.1038/nn.2632

Console-Bram, L., Marcu, J., & Abood, M. E. (2012). Cannabinoid receptors: Nomenclature and pharmacological principles. *Progress in Neuro-Psychopharmacology & Biological Psychiatry, 38*(1), 4–15. https://doi.org/10.1016/j.pnpbp.2012.02.009

Correale, J., Marrodan, M., & Ysrraelit, M. C. (2019). Mechanisms of neurodegeneration and axonal dysfunction in progressive multiple sclerosis. *Biomedicines, 7*(1). https://doi.org/10.3390/biomedicines7010014

Costa, B., Conti, S., Giagnoni, G., & Colleoni, M. (2002). Therapeutic effect of the endogenous fatty acid amide, palmitoylethanolamide, in rat acute inflammation: Inhibition of nitric oxide and cyclo-oxygenase systems. *British Journal of Pharmacology, 137*(4), 413–420. https://doi.org/10.1038/sj.bjp.0704900

Côté, M., Matias, I., Lemieux, I., Petrosino, S., Alméras, N., Després, J.-P., & Di Marzo, V. (2007). Circulating endocannabinoid levels, abdominal adiposity and related cardiometabolic risk factors in obese men. *International Journal of Obesity, 31*(4), 692699. https://doi.org/10.1038/sj.ijo.0803539

Cravatt, B., Prospero-Garcia, O., Siuzdak, G., Gilula, N., Henriksen, S., Boger, D., & Lerner, R. (1995). Chemical characterization of a family of brain lipids that induce sleep. *Science, 268*(5216), 1506–1509. https://doi.org/10.1126/science.7770779

Crouzin, W. G., Berger, A., Di Marzo, V., Bisogno, T., de Petrocellis, L., Fride, E., & Mechoulam R. (2001). Lipids in neural function: Modulation of behavior by oral administration of endocannabinoids found in foods. *Nutrition and Brain, 5*, 169–184. https://doi.org/10.1159/000061850

Cunha, P., Romão, A. M., Mascarenhas-Melo, F., Teixeira, H. M., & Reis, F. (2011). Endocannabinoid system in cardiovascular disorders: New pharmacotherapeutic opportunities. *Journal of Pharmacy and Bioallied Sciences, 3*(3), 350–360. https://doi.org/10.4103/0975-7406.84435

Davies, P. A. (2011). Allosteric modulation of the 5-HT3 receptor. *Current Opinion in Pharmacology, 11*(1), 75–80. https://doi.org/10.1016/j.coph.2011.01.010

De Belleroche, J. S., & Bradford, H. F. (1973). The synaptosome: An isolated, working, neuronal compartment. *Progress in Neurobiology, 1*, 275–298. https://doi.org/10.1016/0301-0082(73)90015-4

De Petrocellis, L., Davis, J. B., & Di Marzo, V. (2001). Palmitoylethanolamide enhances anandamide stimulation of human vanilloid VR1 receptors. *FEBS Letters, 506*(3), 253–256. https://doi.org/10.1016/S0014-5793(01)02934-9

De Petrocellis, L., Melck, D., Palmisano, A., Bisogno, T., Laezza, C., Bifulco, M., & Di Marzo, V. (1998). The endogenous cannabinoid anandamide inhibits human breast cancer cell proliferation. *Proceedings of the National Academy of Sciences, 95*(14), 8375–8380. https://doi.org/10.1073/pnas.95.14.8375

Deutsch, D. G., & Chin, S. A. (1993). Enzymatic synthesis and degradation of anandamide, a cannabinoid receptor agonist. *Biochemical Pharmacology, 46*(5), 791–796. https://doi.org/10.1016/0006-2952(93)90486-G

Deutsch, D. G., Glaser, S. T., Howell, J. M., Kunz, J. S., Puffenbarger, R. A., Hillard, C. J., & Abumrad, N. (2001). The cellular uptake of anandamide is coupled to its breakdown by fatty-acid amide hydrolase. *Journal of Biological Chemistry, 276*(10), 6967–6973. https://doi.org/10.1074/jbc.M003161200

Deutsch, D. G., Goligorsky, M. S., Schmid, P. C., Krebsbach, R. J., Schmid, H. H., Das, S. K., Dey, S. K., Arreaza, G., Thorup, C., Stefano, G., & Moore, L. C. (1997). Production and physiological actions of anandamide in the vasculature of the rat kidney. *Journal of Clinical Investigation, 100*(6), 1538–1546. https://doi.org/10.1172/JCI119677

Devane, W., Hanus, L., Breuer, A., Pertwee, R., Stevenson, L., Griffin, G., Gibson, D., Mandelbaum, A., Etinger, A., & Mechoulam, R. (1992). Isolation and structure of a brain constituent that binds to the cannabinoid receptor. *Science, 258*(5090), 1946–1949. https://doi.org/10.1126/science.1470919

Devane, W. A., Dysart, F. A., & Johnson, M. R., Melvin, L. S., & Howlett, A. C. (1988). Determination and characterization of a cannabinoid receptor in rat brain. *Molecular Pharmaceutics, 34*, 605–613. https://pubmed.ncbi.nlm.nih.gov/2848184/

Dhayal, S., & Morgan, N. G. (2010). The significance of GPR119 agonists as a future treatment for type 2 diabetes. *Drug News & Perspectives, 23*(7), 418. https://doi.org/10.1358/dnp.2010.23.7.1468395

Diana, M. A., & Marty, A. (2004). Endocannabinoid-mediated short-term synaptic plasticity: Depolar-ization-induced suppression of inhibition (DSI) and depolarization-induced suppression of excitation (DSE). *British Journal of Pharmacology, 142*(1), 9–19. https://doi.org/10.1038/sj.bjp.0705726

Di Marzo, V. (2008). CB1 receptor antagonism: Biological basis for metabolic effects. *Drug Discovery Today, 13*(23–24), 1026–1041. https://doi.org/10.1016/j.drudis.2008.09.001

Di Marzo, V., Côté, M., Matias, I., Lemieux, I., Arsenault, B. J., Cartier, A., Piscitelli, F., Petrosino, S., Alméras, N., & Després, J.-P. (2009). Changes in plasma endocannabinoid levels in viscerally obese men following a 1 year lifestyle modification programme and waist circumference reduction: Asso-ciations with changes in metabolic risk factors. *Diabetologia, 52*(2), 213–217. https://doi.org/10.1007/s00125-008-1178-6

Di Marzo, V., & De Petrocellis, L. (2012). Why do cannabinoid receptors have more than one endogenous ligand? *Philosophical Transactions of the Royal Society B: Biological Sciences, 367*(1607), 3216–3228. https://doi.org/10.1098/rstb.2011.0382

Di Marzo, V., De Petrocellis, L., Sepe, N., & Buono, A. (1996). Biosynthesis of anandamide and related acyl-lethanolamides in mouse J774 macrophages and N18 neuroblastoma cells. *Biochemical Journal, 316*(Pt. 3), 977–984. https://doi.org/10.1042/bj3160977

Di Marzo, V., & Fontana, A. (1995). Anandamide, an endogenous cannabinomimetic eicosanoid: "Killing two birds with one stone." *Prostaglandins, Leukotrienes and Essential Fatty Acids, 53*(1), 1–11. https://doi.org/10.1016/0952-3278(95)90077-2

Di Marzo, V., & Maccarrone, M. (2008). FAAH and anandamide: Is 2-AG really the odd one out? *Trends in Pharmacological Sciences, 29*(5), 229–233. https://doi.org/10.1016/j.tips.2008.03.001

Di Marzo, V., Melck, D., Bisogno, T., & De Petrocellis, L. (1998). Endocannabinoids: Endogenous cannabi-noid receptor ligands with neuromodulatory action. *Trends in Neurosciences, 21*(12), 521–528. https://doi.org/10.1016/S0166-2236(98)01283-1

Di Marzo, V., Melck, D., Orlando, P., Bisogno, T., Zagoory, O., Bifulco, M., Vogel, Z., & De Petrocellis, L. (2001). Palmitoylethanolamide inhibits the expression of fatty acid amide hydrolase and enhances the anti-proliferative effect of anandamide in human breast cancer cells. *Biochemical Journal, 358*(1), 249–255. https://doi.org/10.1042/0264-6021:3580249

Dlugos, A., Childs, E., Stuhr, K. L., Hillard, C. J., & de Wit, H. (2012). Acute stress increases circulating anandamide and other N-acylethanolamines in healthy humans. *Neuropsychopharmacology, 37*(11), 2416–2427. https://doi.org/10.1038/npp.2012.100

Dmitrieva, N., Nagabukuro, H., Resuehr, D., Zhang, G., McAllister, S. L., McGinty, K. A., McGinty, K. A., Mackie, K., & Berkley, K. J. (2010). Endocannabinoid involvement in endometriosis. *Pain, 151*(3), 703–710. https://doi.org/10.1016/j.pain.2010.08.037

Dunn, S. L., Wilkinson, J. M., Crawford, A., Bunning, R. A. D., & Le Maitre, C. L. (2016). Expression of cannabinoid receptors in human osteoarthritic cartilage: Implications for future therapies. *Cannabis and Cannabinoid Research, 1*(1), 3–15. https://doi.org/10.1089/can.2015.0001

Eljaschewitsch, E., Witting, A., Mawrin, C., Lee, T., Schmidt, P. M., Wolf, S., Hoertnagl, H., Raine, C. S., Schneider-Stock, R., Nitsch, R., & Ullrich, O. (2006). The endocannabinoid anandamide protects neurons during CNS inflammation by induction of MKP-1 in microglial cells. *Neuron, 49*(1), 67–79. https://doi.org/10.1016/j.neuron.2005.11.027

Ezzili, C., Otrubova, K., & Boger, D. L. (2010). Fatty acid amide signaling molecules. *Bioorganic & Medici-nal Chemistry Letters, 20*(20), 5959–5968. https://doi.org/10.1016/j.bmcl.2010.08.048

Falkenburger, B. H., Jensen, J. B., Dickson, E. J., Suh, B.-C., & Hille, B. (2010). Phosphoinositides: Lipid regulators of membrane proteins. *Journal of Physiology, 588*(17), 3179–3185. https://doi.org/10.1113/jphysiol.2010.192153

Fezza, F., Bisogno, T., Minassi, A., Appendino, G., Mechoulam, R., & Di Marzo, V. (2002). Noladin ether, a putative novel endocannabinoid: Inactivation mechanisms and a sensitive method for its quantification in rat tissues. *FEBS Letters, 513*(2–3), 294–298. https://doi.org/10.1016/S0014-5793(02)02341-4

Fowler, C. J. (2013). Transport of endocannabinoids across the plasma membrane and within the cell. *FEBS Journal, 280*(9), 1895–1904. https://doi.org/10.1111/febs.12212

Free, A. C., Christopherson, J., Chen, Q., Gao, J., Liu, C., Naji, A., Rabinovitch, A., & Guo, Z. (2016). Activation of GPR119 stimulates human β-cell replication and neogenesis in humanized mice with functional human islets. *Journal of Diabetes Research, 2016*, 1620821. https://doi.org/10.1155/2016/1620821

Fride, E., Ginzburg, Y., Breuer, A., Bisogno, T., Di Marzo, V., & Mechoulam, R. (2001). Critical role of the endogenous cannabinoid system in mouse pup suckling and growth. *European Journal of Pharmacology, 419*(2–3), 207–214. https://doi.org/10.1016/S0014-2999(01)00953-0

Frieling, H., Albrecht, H., Jedtberg, S., Gozner, A., Lenz, B., Wilhelm, J., Hillemacher, T., de Zwaan, M., Kornhuber, J., & Bleich, S. (2009). Elevated cannabinoid 1 receptor mRNA is linked to eating disorder related behavior and attitudes in females with eating disorders. *Psychoneuroendocrinology, 34*(4), 620–624. https://doi.org/10.1016/j.psyneuen.2008.10.014

Fu, J., Gactani, S., Oveisi, F., Verme, J. L., Serrano, A., de Fonseca, F. R., Rosengarth, A., Luecke, H., Di Giacomo, B., Tarzia, G., & Piomelli, D. (2003). Oleoylethanolamide regulates feeding and body weight through activation of the nuclear receptor PPAR-α. *Nature, 425*, 90–93. https://doi.org/10.1038/nature01921

Gabrielli, M., Battista, N., Riganti, L., Prada, I., Antonucci, F., Cantone, L., Matteoli, M., Maccarrone, M., & Verderio, C. (2015). Active endocannabinoids are secreted on extracellular membrane vesicles. *EMBO Reports, 16*(2), 213–220. https://doi.org/10.15252/embr.201439668

Galligan, J. J. (2002). Ligand-gated ion channels in the enteric nervous system. *Neurogastroenterology & Motility, 14*(6), 611–623. https://doi.org/10.1046/j.1365-2982.2002.00363.x

Gantz, I., Muraoka, A., Yang, Y-K., Samuelson, L. C., Zimmerman, E. M., Cook, H., & Yamada, T. (1997). Cloning and chromosomal localization of a gene (GPR18) encoding a novel seven transmembrane receptor highly expressed in spleen and testis. *Genomics, 42*(3), 462–466. https://doi.org/10.1006/geno.1997.4752

Gaoni, Y., & Mechoulam, R. (1964). Isolation, structure, and partial synthesis of an active constituent of hashish. *Journal of the American Chemical Society, 86*(8), 1646–1647. https://doi.org/10.1021/ja01062a046

Gardner, E. (2005). Endocannabinoid signaling system and brain reward: Emphasis on dopamine. *Pharmacology Biochemistry and Behavior, 81*(2), 263–284. https://doi.org/10.1016/j.pbb.2005.01.032

Gatta-Cherifi, B., & Cota, D. (2015). Endocannabinoids and metabolic disorders. *Handbook of Experimental Pharmacology, 231*, 367–391. https://doi.org/10.1007/978-3-319-20825-1_13

Gatti, A., Lazzari, M., Gianfelice, V., Di Paolo, A., Sabato, E., & Sabato, A. F. (2012). Palmitoylethanolamide in the treatment of chronic pain caused by different etiopathogenesis. *Pain Medicine, 13*(9), 1121–1130. https://doi.org/10.1111/j.1526-4637.2012.01432.x

Gérard, C. M., Mollereau, C., Vassart, G., & Parmentier, M. (1991). Molecular cloning of a human cannabinoid receptor which is also expressed in testis. *Biochemical Journal, 279*(Pt. 1), 129–134. https://doi.org/10.1042/bj2790129

Gérard, N., Pieters, G., Goffin, K., Bormans, G., & Van Laere, K. (2011). Brain type 1 cannabinoid receptor availability in patients with anorexia and bulimia nervosa. *Biological Psychiatry, 70*(8), 777–784. https://doi.org/10.1016/j.biopsych.2011.05.010

Ginsberg, H. N., & Woods, S. C. (2009). The endocannabinoid system: Potential for reducing cardiometabolic risk. *Obesity, 17*(10), 1821–1829. https://doi.org/10.1038/oby.2009.107

Gkoumassi, E., Dekkers, B. G. J., Dröge, M. J., Elzinga, C. R. S., Schmidt, M., Meurs, H., Zaagsma, J., & Nelemans, S. A. (2007). Virodhamine and CP55,940 modulate cAMP production and IL-8 release in human bronchial epithelial cells. *British Journal of Pharmacology, 151*(7), 1041–1048. https://doi.org/10.1038/sj.bjp.0707320

Goadsby, P. J., Holland, P. R., Martins-Oliveira, M., Hoffmann, J., Schankin, C., & Akerman, S. (2017). Pathophysiology of migraine: A disorder of sensory processing. *Physiological Reviews, 97*(2), 553–622. https://doi.org/10.1152/physrev.00034.2015

Godlewski, G., Offertáler, L., Wagner, J. A., & Kunos, G. (2009). Receptors for acylethanolamides—GPR55 and GPR119. *Prostaglandins & Other Lipid Mediators, 89*(3–4), 105–111. https://doi.org/10.1016/j.prostaglandins.2009.07.001

Grabiec, U., & Dehghani, F. (2017). *N*-Arachidonoyl dopamine: A novel endocannabinoid and endovanilloid with widespread physiological and pharmacological activities. *Cannabis and Cannabinoid Research, 2*(1), 183–196. https://doi.org/10.1089/can.2017.0015

Grant, I., & Cahn, B. R. (2005). Cannabis and endocannabinoid modulators: Therapeutic promises and challenges. *Clinical Neuroscience Research, 5*(2–4), 185–199. https://doi.org/10.1016/j.cnr.2005.08.015

Guerrero-Alba, R., Barragán-Iglesias, P., González-Hernández, A., Valdez-Moráles, E. E., Granados-Soto, V., Condés-Lara, M., Rodríguez, M. G., & Marichal-Cancino, B. A. (2019). Some prospective alternatives for treating pain: The endocannabinoid system and its putative receptors GPR18 and GPR55. *Frontiers in Pharmacology, 9*, 1496. https://doi.org/10.3389/fphar.2018.01496

Guzmán, M., Lo Verme, J., Fu, J., Oveisi, F., Blázquez, C., & Piomelli, D. (2004). Oleoylethanolamide stimulates lipolysis by activating the nuclear receptor peroxisome proliferator-activated alpha (PPAR-alpha). *Journal of Biological Chemistry, 279*(2), 27849–27854. https://doi.org/10.1074/jbc.M404087200

Guzmán, M., Sánchez, C., & Galve-Roperh, I. (2001). Control of the cell survival/death decision by cannabinoids. *Journal of Molecular Medicine, 78*(11), 613–625. https://doi.org/10.1007/s001090000177

Haj-Dahmane, S., & Shen, R. Y. (2011). Modulation of the serotonin system by endocannabinoid signaling. *Neuropharmacology, 61*(3), 414–420. https://doi.org/10.1016/j.neuropharm.2011.02.016

Hanuš, L., Abu-Lafi, S., Fride, E., Breuer, A., Vogel, Z., Shalev, D. E., Kustanovich, I., & Mechoulam, R. (2001). 2-Arachidonoyl glyceryl ether, an endogenous agonist of the cannabinoid CB1 receptor. *Proceedings of the National Academy of Sciences, 98*(7), 3662–3665. https://doi.org/10.1073/pnas.061029898

Hao, S., Avraham, Y., Mechoulam, R., & Berry, E. M. (2000). Low dose anandamide affects food intake, cognitive function, neurotransmitter and corticosterone levels in diet-restricted mice. *European Journal of Pharmacology, 392*(3), 147–156. https://doi.org/10.1016/S0014-2999(00)00059-5

Heifets, B. D., & Castillo, P. E. (2009). Endocannabinoid signaling and long-term synaptic plasticity. *Annual Review of Physiology, 71*, 283–306. https://doi.org/10.1146/annurev.physiol.010908.163149

Hill, M. N., Bierer, L. M., Makotkine, I., Golier, J. A., Galea, S., McEwen, B. S., Hillard, C. J., & Yehuda, R. (2013). Reductions in circulating endocannabinoid levels in individuals with post-traumatic stress disorder following exposure to the World Trade Center attacks. *Psychoneuroendocrinology, 38*(12), 2952–2961. https://doi.org/10.1016/j.psyneuen.2013.08.004

Hill, M. N., Patel, S., Campolongo, P., Tasker, J. G., Wotjak, C. T., & Bains, J. S. (2010). Functional interactions between stress and the endocannabinoid system: from synaptic signaling to behavioral output. *The Journal of Neuroscience: the Official Journal of the Society for Neuroscience, 30*(45), 14980–14986. https://doi.org/10.1523/JNEUROSCI.4283-10.2010

Hirsch, S., & Tam, J. (2019). Cannabis: From a plant that modulates feeding behaviors toward developing selective inhibitors of the peripheral endocannabinoid system for the treatment of obesity and metabolic syndrome. *Toxins, 11*(5), 275. https://doi.org/10.3390/toxins11050275

Ho, W. S., Barrett, D., & Randall, M. (2008). "Entourage" effects of N-palmitoylethanolamide and N-oleoylethanolamide on vasorelaxation to anandamide occur through TRPV1 receptors. *British Journal of Pharmacology, 155*, 837–846. https://doi.org/10.1038/bjp.2008.324

Hoareau, L., Buyse, M., Festy, F., Ravanan, P., Gonthier, M-P., Matias, I., Petrosino, S., Tallet, F., d'Hellencourt, C. L., Cesari, M., Di Marzo, V., & Roche, R. (2009). Anti-inflammatory effect of palmitoylethanolamide on human adipocytes. *Obesity, 17*(3), 431–438. https://doi.org/10.1038/oby.2008.591

Högestätt, E. D., & Zygmunt, P. M. (2002). Cardiovascular pharmacology of anandamide. *Prostaglandins, Leukotrienes and Essential Fatty Acids, 66*(2–3), 343–351. https://doi.org/10.1054/plef.2001.0346

Horváth, B. (2012). The endocannabinoid system and plant-derived cannabinoids in diabetes and diabetic complications. *American Journal of Pathology, 180*(2), 432–442. https://doi.org/10.1016/ajpath.2011.11.003

Howlett, A. C. (1984). Inhibition of neuroblastoma adenylate cyclase by cannabinoid and nantradol compounds. *Life Sciences, 35*(17), 1803–1810. https://doi.org/10.1016/0024-3205(84)90278-9

Howlett, A. C., Barth, F., Bonner, T. I., Cabral., G., Casellas, P., Devane, W. A., Felder, C. C., Herkenham, M., Mackie, K., Martin, B. R., Mechoulam, R., & Pertwee, R. G. (2002). Classification of cannabinoid receptors. *Pharmacological Reviews, 54*(2), 161–202. https://doi.org/10.1124/pr.54.2.161

Howlett, A. C., & Fleming, R. M. (1984). Cannabinoid inhibition of adenylate cyclase: Biochemistry of the response in neuroblastoma cell membranes. *Molecular Pharmacology, 26*(3), 532–538. https://molpharm.aspetjournals.org/content/27/4/429

Howlett, A. C., Qualy, J. M., & Khachatrian, L. L. (1986). Involvement of Gi in the inhibition of adenylate cyclase by cannabimimetic drugs. *Molecular Pharmacology, 29*(3), 307–313. https://pubmed.ncbi.nlm .nih.gov/2869405/

Howlett, A. C., Reggio, P. H., Childers, S. R., Hampson, R. E., Ulloa, N. M., & Deutsch, D. G. (2011). Endocannabinoid tone versus constitutive activity of cannabinoid receptors. *British Journal of Pharmacology, 163*(7), 1329–1343. https://doi.org/10.1111/j.1476-5381.2011.01364.x

Huang, S. M., Bisogno, T., Trevisani, M., Al-Hayani, A., De Petrocellis, L., Fezza, F., Tognetto, M., Petros, T. J., Krey, J. F., Chu, C. J., Miller, J. D., Davies, S. N., Geppetti, P., Walker, J. M., & Di Marzo, V. (2002). An endogenous capsaicin-like substance with high potency at recombinant and native vanilloid VR1 receptors. *Proceedings of the National Academy of Sciences, 99*(12), 8400–8405. https://doi.org/10.1073/pnas.122196999

Institute of Medicine. (1999a). Cannabinoids and animal physiology. In J. E. Joy, S. J. Watson, and J. A. Benson (Eds.), *Marijuana and medicine: Assessing the science base* (pp. 33–82). National Academies Press.

Institute of Medicine. (1999b). Development of cannabinoid drugs. In J. E. Joy, S. J. Watson, & J. A. Benson (Eds.), *Marijuana and medicine: Assessing the science base* (pp. 193–213). National Academies Press.

Ishiguro, H., Onaivi, E. S., Horiuchi, Y., Imai, K., Komaki, G., Ishikawa, T., Suzuki, M., Watanabe, Y., Ando, T., Higuchi, S., & Arinami, T. (2011). Functional polymorphism in the GPR55 gene is associated with anorexia nervosa. *Synapse, 65*(2), 103–108. https://doi.org/10.1002/syn.20821

Izzo, A. A., Fezza, F., Capasso, R., Bisogno, T., Pinto, L., Iuvone, T., Esposito, G., Mascolo, N., Di Marzo, V., & Capasso, F. (2001). Cannabinoid CB1-receptor mediated regulation of gastrointestinal motility in mice in a model of intestinal inflammation. *British Journal of Pharmacology, 134*(3), 563–570. https://doi.org/10.1038/sj.bjp.0704293

Jacob, A., & Todd, A. R. (1940). Isolation of cannabidiol from Egyptian hashish: Observations on the structure of cannabinol. *Journal of the Chemical Society,* 649–653.

Javed, H., Azimullah, S., Haque, M. E., & Ojha, S. K. (2016). Cannabinoid type 2 (CB2) receptors activation protects against oxidative stress and neuroinflammation associated dopaminergic neurodegeneration in rotenone model of Parkinson's disease. *Frontiers in Neuroscience, 10,* 321. https://doi.org/10.3389/fnins.2016.00321

Jenniches, I., Ternes, S., Albayram, O., Otte, D. M., Bach, K., Bindila, L., Michel, K., Lutz, B., Bilkei-Gorzo, A., & Zimmer, A. (2016). Anxiety, stress, and fear response in mice with reduced endocannabinoid levels. *Biological Psychiatry, 79*(10), 858–868. https://doi.org/10.1016/j.biopsych.2015.03.033

Jung, K-M., Clapper, J. R., Fu, J., D'Agostino, G., Guijarro, A., Thongkham, D., Avanesian, A., Astarita, G., DiPatrizio, N. V., Frontini, A., Cinti, S., Diano, S., & Piomelli, D. (2012). 2-Arachidonoylglycerol signaling in forebrain regulates systemic energy metabolism. *Cell Metabolism, 15*(3), 299–310. https://doi.org/10.1016/j.cmet.2012.01.021

Kano, M. (2014). Control of synaptic function by endocannabinoid-mediated retrograde signaling. *Proceedings of the Japan Academy. Species B, Physical and Biological Sciences, 90*(7), 235–250. https://doi.org/10.2183/pjab.90.235

Kano, M., Ohno-Shosaku, T., Hashimotodani, Y., Uchigashima, M., & Watanabe, M. (2009). Endocannabinoid-mediated control of synaptic transmission. *Physiological Reviews, 89*(1), 309–380. https://doi.org/10.1152/physrev.00019.2008

Kapur, A., Zhao, P., Sharir, H., Bai, Y., Caron, M. G., Barak, L. S., & Abood, M. E. (2009). Atypical responsiveness of the orphan receptor GPR55 to cannabinoid ligands. *Journal of Biological Chemistry, 284*(43), 29817–29827. https://doi.org/10.1074/jbc.M109.050187

Kargl, J., Balenga, N., Parzmair, G. P., Brown, A. J., Heinemann, A., & Waldhoer, M. (2012). The cannabinoid receptor CB1 modulates the signaling properties of the lysophosphatidylinositol receptor GPR55. *Journal of Biological Chemistry, 287*(53), 44234–44248. https://doi.org/10.1074/jbc .M112.364109

Katona, I., & Freund, T. F. (2008). Endocannabinoid signaling as a synaptic circuit breaker in neurological disease. *Nature Medicine, 14*(9), 923930. https://doi.org/10.1038/nm.f.1869

Keown, O. P., Winterburn, T. J., Wainwright, C. L., Macrury, S. M., Neilson, I., Barrett, F., Leslie, S. J., & Megson, I. L. (2010). 2-Arachidonoylglycerol activates platelets via conversion to arachidonic acid and not by direct activation of cannabinoid receptors. *British Journal of Clinical Pharmacology, 70*(2), 180–188. https://doi.org/10.1111/j.1365-2125.2010.03697.x

Kim, J., & Alger, B. E. (2010). Reduction in endocannabinoid tone is a homeostatic mechanism for specific inhibitory synapses. *Nature Neuroscience, 13*(5), 592–600. https://doi.org/10.1038/nn.2517

Kim, W., Doyle, M. E., Liu, Z., Lao, Q., Shin, Y.-K., Carlson, O. D., Kim, H. S., Thomas, S., Napora, J. K., Lee, E. K., Moaddel, R., Wang, Y., Maudsley, S., Martin, B., Kulkarni, R. N., & Egan, J. M. (2011). Cannabinoids inhibit insulin receptor signaling in pancreatic β-cells. *Diabetes, 60*(4), 1198–1209. https://doi.org/10.2337/db10-1550

Kirkham, T. C. (2009). Cannabinoids and appetite: Food craving and food pleasure. *International Review of Psychiatry, 21*(2), 163–171. https://doi.org/10.1080/09540260902782810

Kohno, M., Hasegawa, H., Inoue, A., Muraoka, M., Miyazaki, T., Oka, K., & Yasukawa, M. (2006). Identification of N-arachidonoylglycine as the endogenous ligand for orphan G-protein-coupled receptor GPR18. *Biochemical and Biophysical Research Communications, 347*(3), 827–832. https://doi.org/10.1016/j.bbrc.2006.06.175

Kozłowska, H., Baranowska, M., Schlicker, E., Kozłowski, M., Laudański, J., & Malinowska, B. (2008). Virodhamine relaxes the human pulmonary artery through the endothelial cannabinoid receptor and indirectly through a COX product. *British Journal of Pharmacology, 155*(7), 1034–1042. https://doi.org/10.1038/bjp.2008.371

Kramar, C., Loureiro, M., Renard, J., & Laviolette, S. R. (2017). Palmitoylethanolamide modulates GPR55 receptor signaling in the ventral hippocampus to regulate mesolimbic dopamine activity, social interaction, and memory processing. *Cannabis and Cannabinoid Research, 2*(1), 8–20. https://doi.org/10.1089/can.2016.0030

Kreitzer, A. C., & Regehr, W. G. (2001). Retrograde inhibition of presynaptic calcium influx by endogenous cannabinoids at excitatory synapses onto Purkinje cells. *Neuron, 29*(3), 717–727. https://doi.org/10.1016/S0896-6273(01)00246-X

Laine, K., Järvinen, K., Mechoulam, R., Breuer, A., & Järvinen, T. (2002). Comparison of the enzymatic stability and intraocular pressure effects of 2-Arachidonoylglycerol and noladin ether, a novel putative endocannabinoid. *Investigative Ophthalmology & Visual Science, 43*(10), 3216–3122. https://iovs.arvojournals.org/article.aspx?articleid=2122899

Larrinaga, G., Varona, A., Pérez, I., Sanz, B., Ugalde, A., Cándenas, M. L., Pinto, F. M., Gil, J., & López, J. I. (2010.). Expression of cannabinoid receptors in human kidney. *Histology and Histopathology, 25*(9), 1133–1138. https://doi.org/10.14670/HH-25.1133

Lauckner, J. E., Jensen, J. B., Chen, H-Y., Lu, H-C., Hille, B., & Mackie, K. (2008). GPR55 is a cannabinoid receptor that increases intracellular calcium and inhibits M current. *Proceedings of the National Academy of Sciences, 105*(7), 2699–2704. https://doi.org/10.1073/pnas.0711278105

Lawton, S. K., Xu, F., Tran, A., Wong, E., Prakash, A., Schumacher, M., Hellman, J., & Wilhelmsen, K. (2017). N-Arachidonoyl dopamine modulates acute systemic inflammation via nonhematopoietic TRPV1. *Journal of Immunology, 199*(4), 1465–1475. https://doi.org/10.4049/jimmunol.1602151

Le Menn, G., & Neels, J. G. (2018). Regulation of immune cell function by PPARs and the connection with metabolic and neurodegenerative diseases. *International Journal of Molecular Sciences, 19*(6). https://doi.org/10.3390/ijms19061575

Leinwand, K. L., Jones, A. A., Huang, R. H., Jedlicka, P., Kao, D. J., de Zoeten, E. F., Ghosh, S., Moaddel, R., Wehkamp, J., Ostaff, M. J., Bader, J., Aherne, C. M., & Collins, C. B. (2017). Cannabinoid receptor-2 ameliorates inflammation in murine model of Crohn's disease. *Journal of Crohn's & Colitis, 11*(11), 1369–1380. https://doi.org/10.1093/ecco-jcc/jjx096

Lemberger, L., Silberstein, S. D., Axelrod, J., & Kopin, I. J. (1970). Marihuana: Studies on the disposition and metabolism of delta-9-tetrahydrocannabinol in man. *Science, 170*(3964), 1320–1322. https://doi.org/10.1126/science.170.3964.1320

Lever, I. J., Robinson, M., Cibelli, M., Paule, C., Santha, P., Yee, L., Hunt, S. P., Cravatt, B. F., Elphick, M. R., Nagy, I., & Rice, A. S. C. (2009). Localization of the endocannabinoid-degrading enzyme fatty acid amide hydrolase in rat dorsal root ganglion cells and its regulation after peripheral nerve injury. *Journal of Neuroscience, 29*(12), 3766–3780. https://doi.org/10.1523/jneurosci.4071-08.2009

Lipina, C., & Hundal, H. S. (2016). Modulation of cellular redox homeostasis by the endocannabinoid system. *Open Biology, 6*(4), 150276. https://doi.org/10.1098/rsob.150276

Liu, J., Wang, L., Harvey-White, J., Osei-Hyiaman, D., Razdan, R., Gong, Q., Chan, A. C., Zhou, Z., Huang, B. X., Kim, H.-Y., & Kunos, G. (2006). A biosynthetic pathway for anandamide. *Proceedings of the National Academy of Sciences, 103*(36), 13345–13350. https://doi.org/10.1073/pnas.0601832103

Lo Verme, J., Fu, J., Astarita, G. L. R., Russo, R., Calignano, A., & Piomelli, D. (2005). The nuclear receptor peroxisome proliferator-activated receptor mediates the anti-inflammatory actions of palmitoylethanolamide. *Molecular Pharmacology, 67*(1), 15–19. https://doi.org/10.1124/mol.104.006353

LoVerme, J., La Rana, G., Russo, R., Calignano, A., & Piomelli, D. (2005). The search for the palmitoylethanolamide receptor. *Life Sciences, 77*(14), 1685–1698. https://doi.org/10.1016/j.lfs.2005.05.012

Lovinger, D. M. (2008). Presynaptic modulation by endocannabinoids. *Handbook of Experimental Pharmacology, 184*, 435–477. https://doi.org/10.1007/978-3-540-74805-2_14

Lu, H. C., & Mackie, K. (2016). An introduction to the endogenous cannabinoid system. *Biological Psychiatry, 79*(7), 516–525. https://doi.org/10.1016/j.biopsych.2015.07.028

Lutz, B. (2002). Molecular biology of cannabinoid receptors. *Prostaglandins, Leukotrienes and Essential Fatty Acids, 66*(2–3), 123–142. https://doi.org/10.1054/plef.2001.0342

Maccarrone, M. (2002). Estrogen stimulates arachidonoylethanolamide release from human endothelial cells and platelet activation. *Blood, 100*(12), 4040–4048. https://doi.org/10.1182/blood-2002-05-1444

Maccarrone, M. (2017). Metabolism of the endocannabinoid anandamide: Open questions after 25 years. *Frontiers in Molecular Neuroscience, 10*. https://doi.org/10.3389/fnmol.2017.00166

Maccarrone, M., Bari, M., Menichelli, A., Giuliani, E., Del Principe, D., & Finazzi-Agrò, A. (2001). Human platelets bind and degrade 2-arachidonoylglycerol, which activates these cells through a cannabinoid receptor. *European Journal of Biochemistry, 268*(3), 819–825. https://doi.org/10.1046/j.1432-1327.2001.01942.x

Maccarrone, M., Dainese, E., & Oddi, S. (2010). Intracellular trafficking of anandamide: New concepts for signaling. *Trends in Biochemical Sciences, 35*(11), 601–608. https://doi.org/10.1016/j.tibs.2010.05.008

Maccarrone, M., Fiorucci, L., Erba, F., Bari, M., Finazzi-Agrò, A., & Ascoli, F. (2000). Human mast cells take up and hydrolyze anandamide under the control of 5-lipoxygenase and do not express cannabinoid receptors. *FEBS Letters, 468*(2–3), 176–180. https://doi.org/10.1016/s0014

Maccarrone, M., Lorenzon, T., Bari, M., Melino, G., & Finazzi-Agrò, A. (2000). Anandamide induces apoptosis in human cells via vanilloid receptors: Evidence for a protective role of cannabinoid receptors. *Journal of Biological Chemistry, 275*(41), 31938–31945. https://doi.org/10.1074/jbc.M005722200

Maccarrone, M., Pauselli, R., Di Rienzo, M., & Finazzi-Agrò, A. (2002). Binding, degradation and apoptotic activity of stearoylethanolamide in rat C6 glioma cells. *Biochemical Journal, 366*(Pt. 1), 137–144. https://doi.org/10.1042/BJ20020438

Magid, L., Heymann, S., Elgali, M., Avram, L., Cohen, Y., Liraz-Zaltsman, S., Mechoulam, R., & Shohami, E. (2019). Role of CB2 receptor in the recovery of mice after traumatic brain injury. *Journal of Neurotrauma, 36*(11), 1836–1846. https://doi.org/10.1089/neu.2018.6063

Malfitano, A. M., Basu, S., Maresz, K., Bifulco, M., & Dittel, B. N. (2014). What we know and do not know about the cannabinoid receptor 2 (CB2). *Seminars in Immunology, 26*(5), 369–379. https://doi.org/10.1016/j.smim.2014.04.002

Manzanares, J., Julian, M., & Carrascosa, A. (2006). Role of the cannabinoid system in pain control and therapeutic implications for the management of acute and chronic pain episodes. *Current Neuropharmacology, 4*(3), 239–257. https://doi.org/10.2174/157015906778019527

Marinelli, S., Di Marzo, V., Florenzano, F., Fezza, F., Viscomi, M. T., van der Stelt, M., Bernardi, G., Molinari, M., Maccarrone, M., & Mercuri, N. B. (2007). *N*-Arachidonoyl-dopamine tunes synaptic transmission onto dopaminergic neurons by activating both cannabinoid and vanilloid receptors. *Neuropsychopharmacology, 32*(2), 298–308. https://doi.org/10.1038/sj.npp.1301118

Martin, R. S., Luong, L. A., Welsh, N. J., Eglen, R. M., Martin, G. R., & MacLennan, S. J. (2000). Effects of cannabinoid receptor agonists on neuronally-evoked contractions of urinary bladder tissues isolated from rat, mouse, pig, dog, monkey and human. *British Journal of Pharmacology, 129*(8), 1707–1715. https://doi.org/10.1038/sj.bjp.0703229

McAllister, S. D., & Glass, M. (2002). CB1 and CB2 receptor-mediated signalling: A focus on endocannabinoids. *Prostaglandins, Leukotrienes and Essential Fatty Acids, 66*(2–3), 161–171. https://doi.org/10.1054/plef.2001.0344

McHugh, D., Hu, S. S., Rimmerman, N., Juknat, A., Vogel, Z., Walker, J. M., & Bradshaw, H. B. (2010). *N*-Arachidonoyl glycine, an abundant endogenous lipid, potently drives directed cellular migration through GPR18, the putative abnormal cannabidiol receptor. *BMC Neuroscience, 11*, 44. https://doi.org/10.1186/1471-2202-11-44

McHugh, D., Page, J., Dunn, E., & Bradshaw, H. B. (2012). Δ⁹-Tetrahydrocannabinol and *N*-arachidonoyl glycine are full agonists at GPR18 receptors and induce migration in human endometrial HEC-1B cells: Novel CB pharmacology at GPR18. *British Journal of Pharmacology, 165*(8), 2414–2424. https://doi.org/10.1111/j.1476-5381.2011.01497.x

McPartland, J., Di Marzo, V., De Petrocellis, L., Mercer, A., & Glass, M. (2001). Cannabinoid receptors are absent in insects. *Journal of Comparative Neurology, 436*(4), 423–429. https://doi.org/10.1002/cne.1078

McPartland, J. M., Guy, G. W., & Di Marzo, V. (2014). Care and feeding of the endocannabinoid system: A systematic review of potential clinical interventions that upregulate the endocannabinoid system. *PLoS One, 9*(3), e89566. https://doi.org/10.1371/journal.pone.0089566

McPartland, J. M., Matias, I., Di Marzo, V. & Glass, M. (2006). Evolutionary origins of the endocannabinoid system. *Gene, 370*, 64–74. https://doi.org/10.1016/j.gene.2005.11.004

Mechoulam, R. (2002). Discovery of endocannabinoids and some random thoughts on their possible roles in neuroprotection and aggression. *Prostaglandins, Leukotrienes and Essential Fatty Acids, 66*(2–3), 93–99. https://doi.org/10.1054/plef.2001.0340

Mechoulam, R. (2016). Cannabis—the Israeli perspective. *Journal of Basic and Clinical Physiology and Pharmacology, 27*(3), 181–187. https://doi.org/10.1515/jbcpp-2015-0091

Mechoulam, R., & Ben-Shabat, S. (1999). From gan-zi-gun-nu to anandamide and 2-arachidonoylglycerol: The ongoing story of cannabis. *Natural Product Reports, 16*(2), 131–143. https://doi.org/10.1039/A703973E

Mechoulam, R., Ben-Shabat, S., Hanuš, L., Ligumsky, M., Kaminski, N. E., Schatz, A. R., Goper, A., Almog, S., Martin, B. R., Compton, D. R., Pertwee, R. G., Griffin, G., Bayewitch, M., Barg, J., & Vogel, Z. (1995). Identification of an endogenous 2-monoglyceride, present in canine gut, that binds to cannabinoid receptors. *Biochemical Pharmacology, 50*(1), 83–90. https://doi.org/10.1016/0006-2952(95)00109-d

Mechoulam, R., & Gaoni, Y. (1967). The absolute configuration of Δ^1-tetrahydrocannabinol, the major active constituent of hashish. *Tetrahedron Letters, 8*, 1109–1111. https://doi.org/10.1016/S0040-4039(00)90646-4

Mechoulam, R., & Shvo, Y. (1963). The structure of cannabidiol. *Tetrahedron, 19*, 2073–2078. https://www.sciencedirect.com/science/article/abs/pii/004040206385022X

Melck, D., Petrocellis, L. D., Orlando, P., Bisogno, T., Laezza, C., Bifulco, M., & Di Marzo, V. (2000). Suppression of nerve growth factor Trk receptors and prolactin receptors by endocannabinoids leads to inhibition of human breast and prostate cancer cell proliferation. *Endocrinology, 141*(1), 118–126. https://doi.org/10.1210/endo.141.1.7239

Metz, S. A. (1986). Lysophosphatidylinositol, but not lysophosphatidic acid, stimulates insulin release. *Biochemical and Biophysical Research Communications, 138*(2), 720–727. https://doi.org/10.1016/S0006-291X(86)80556-3

Miller, S., Daily, L., Leishman, E., Bradshaw, H., & Straiker, A. (2018). Δ^9-Tetrahydrocannabinol and cannabidiol differentially regulate intraocular pressure. *Investigative Ophthalmology & Visual Science, 59*(15), 5904. https://doi.org/10.1167/iovs.18-24838

Milton, N. G. N. (2002). Anandamide and noladin ether prevent neurotoxicity of the human amyloid-beta peptide. *Neuroscience Letters, 332*(2), 127–130. https://doi.org/10.1016/s0304-3940(02)00936-9

Minkkilä, A., Saario, S. M., & Nevalainen, T. (2010). Discovery and development of endocannabinoid-hydrolyzing enzyme inhibitors. *Current Topics in Medicinal Chemistry, 10*(8), 828–858. https://doi.org/10.2174/156802610791164238

Moreno-Navarrete, J. M., Catalán, V., Whyte, L., Díaz-Arteaga, A., Vázquez-Martínez, R., Rotellar, F., Guzmán, R., Gómez-Ambrosi, J., Pulido, M. R., Russell, W. R., Imbernón, M., Ross, R. A., Malagón, M. M., Dieguez, C., Fernández-Real, J. M., Frühbeck, G., & Nogueiras, R. (2012). The L-α-lysophosphatidylinositol/GPR55 system and its potential role in human obesity. *Diabetes, 61*(2), 281–291. https://doi.org/10.2337/db11-0649

Mukhopadhyay, P., Rajesh, M., Pan, H., Patel, V., Mukhopadhyay, B., Bátkai, S., Gao, B., Haskó, G., & Pacher, P. (2010). Cannabinoid-2 receptor limits inflammation, oxidative/nitrosative stress and cell death in nephropathy. *Free Radical Biology & Medicine, 48*(3), 457–467. https://doi.org/10.1016/j.freeradbiomed.2009.11.022

Müller, R., Rieck, M., & Müller-Brüsselbach, S. (2008). Regulation of cell proliferation and differentiation by PPARβ/δ. *PPAR Research, 614852.* https://doi.org/10.1155/2008/614852

Munro, S., Thomas, K. L., & Abu-Shaar, M. (1993). Molecular characterization of a peripheral receptor for cannabinoids. *Nature, 365*(6441), 61–65. https://doi.org/10.1038/365061a0

Murataeva, N., Dhopeshwarkar, A., Yin, D., Mitjavila, J., Bradshaw, H., Straiker, A., & Mackie, K. (2016). Where's my entourage? The curious case of 2-oleoylglycerol, 2-linolenoylglycerol, and 2-palmitoylglycerol. *Pharmacological Research, 110*, 173–180. https://doi.org/10.1016/j.phrs.2016.04.015

Murataeva, N., Straiker, A., & Mackie, K. (2014). Parsing the players: 2-Arachidonoylglycerol synthesis and degradation in the CNS. *British Journal of Pharmacology, 171*(6), 1379–1391. https://doi.org/10.1111/bph.12411

Murillo-Rodriguez, E., Blanco-Centurion, C., Sanchez, C., Daniele, P., & Shiromani, P. J. (2003). Anandamide enhances extracellular levels of adenosine and induces sleep: An *in vivo* microdialysis study. *Sleep, 26*(8), 943–947. https://doi.org/10.1093/sleep/26.8.943

Murphy, M. P. (2009). How mitochondria produce reactive oxygen species. *Biochemical Journal, 417*(Pt. 1), 1–13. https://doi.org/10.1042/BJ20081386

Nagappan, A., Shin, J., & Jung, M. H. (2019). Role of cannabinoid receptor type 1 in insulin resistance and its biological implications. *International Journal of Molecular Sciences, 20*(9), 2109. https://doi.org/10.3390/ijms20092109

Nagarkatti, P., Pandey, R., Rieder, S. A., Hegde, V. L., & Nagarkatti, M. (2009). Cannabinoids as novel anti-inflammatory drugs. *Future Medicinal Chemistry, 1*(7), 1333–1349. https://doi.org/10.4155/fmc.09.93

Nair, A., Chauhan, P., Saha, B., & Kubatzky, K. F. (2019). Conceptual evolution of cell signaling. *International Journal of Molecular Sciences, 20*(13). https://doi.org/10.3390/ijms20133292

National Council of State Boards of Nursing. (2018). The NCSBN national nursing guidelines for medical marijuana. *Journal of Nursing Regulation, 9*(2), S5. https://doi.org/10.1016/S2155-256(18)30082-6

Naughton, S. S., Mathai, M. L., Hryciw, D. H., & McAinch, A. J. (2013). Fatty acid modulation of the endocannabinoid system and the effect on food intake and metabolism. *International Journal of Endocrinology, 361895*. https://doi.org/10.1155/2013/361895

Navarini, L., Bisogno, T., Mozetic, P., Piscitelli, F., Margiotta, D. P. E., Basta, F., Afeltra, A., & Maccarrone, M. (2018). Endocannabinoid system in systemic lupus erythematosus: First evidence for a deranged 2-arachidonoylglycerol metabolism. *International Journal of Biochemistry & Cell Biology, 99*, 161–168. https://doi.org/10.1016/j.biocel.2018.04.010

Nevalainen, T., & Irving, A. (2010). GPR55, a lysophosphatidylinositol receptor with cannabinoid sensitivity? *Current Topics in Medicinal Chemistry, 10*(8), 799–813. https://doi.org/10.2174/156802610791164229

Nicolussi, S., & Gertsch, J. (2015). Endocannabinoid transport revisited. *Vitamins & Hormones, 98*, 441–485. https://doi.org/10.1016/bs.vh.2014.12.011

Oddi, S., Fezza, F., Pasquariello, N., De Simone, C., Rapino, C., Dainese, E., Finazzi-Agrò, A., & Maccarrone, M. (2008). Evidence for the intracellular accumulation of anandamide in adiposomes. *Cellular and Molecular Life Sciences, 65*(5), 840–850. https://doi.org/10.1007/s00018-008-7494-7

Oka, S., Nakajima, K., Yamashita, A., Kishimoto, S., & Sugiura, T. (2007). Identification of GPR55 as a lysophosphatidylinositol receptor. *Biochemical and Biophysical Research Communications, 362*(4), 928–934. https://doi.org/10.1016/j.bbrc.2007.08.078

Onaivi, E. S., Carpio, O., Ishiguro, H., Schanz, N., Uhl, G. R., & Benno, R. (2008). Behavioral effects of CB2 cannabinoid receptor activation and its influence on food and alcohol consumption. *Annals of New York Academy of Sciences, 1129*, 426–433. https://doi.org/10.1196/annals.1432.035

O'Sullivan, S. E. (2016). An update on PPAR activation by cannabinoids. *British Journal of Pharmacology, 173*(12), 1899–1910. https://doi.org/10.1111/bph.13497

O'Sullivan, S. E., Tarling, E. J., Bennett, A. J., Kendall, D. A., & Randall, M. D. (2005). Novel time-dependent vascular actions of Delta9-tetrahydrocannabinol mediated by peroxisome proliferator-activated receptor gamma. *Biochemical and Biophysical Research Communications, 337*(3), 824–831. https://doi.org/10.1016/j.bbrc.2005.09.121

Overton, H. A., Babbs, A. J., Doel, S. M., Fyfe, M. C. T., Gardner, L. S., Griffin, G., Jackson, H. C., Procter, M. J., Rasamison, C. M., Tang-Christensen, M., Widdowson, P. S., Williams, G. M., & Reynet, C. (2006). Deorphanization of a G protein-coupled receptor for oleoylethanolamide and its use in the discovery of small-molecule hypophagic agents. *Cell Metabolism, 3*(3), 167–175. https://doi.org/10.1016/j.cmet.2006.02.004

Overton, H. A., Fyfe, M. C. T., & Reynet, C. (2008). GPR119, a novel G protein-coupled receptor target for the treatment of type 2 diabetes and obesity. *British Journal of Pharmacology, 153*(S1), S76–S81. https://doi.org/10.1038/sj.bjp.0707529

Pacher, P., & Kunos, G. (2013). Modulating the endocannabinoid system in human health and disease: Successes and failures. *FEBS Journal, 280*(9), 1918–1943. https://doi.org/10.1111/febs.12260

Pacher, P., & Mechoulam, R. (2011). Is lipid signaling through cannabinoid 2 receptors part of a protective system? *Progress in Lipid Research, 50*(2), 193–211. https://doi.org/10.1016/j.plipres.2011.01.001

Pagotto, U., Marsicano, G., Cota, D., Lutz, B., & Pasquali, R. (2006). The emerging role of the endocannabinoid system in endocrine regulation and energy balance. *Endocrine Reviews, 27*(1), 73–100. https://doi.org/10.1210/er.2005-0009

Pandey, P., Chaurasiya, N. D., Tekwani, B. L., & Doerksen, R. J. (2018). Interactions of endocannabinoid virodhamine and related analogs with human monoamine oxidase-A and -B. *Biochemical Pharmacology,* *155,* 8291. https://doi.org/10.1016/j.bcp.2018.06.024

Panikashvili, D., Simeonidou, C., Ben-Shabat, S., Hanuš, L., Breuer, A., Mechoulam, R., & Shohami, E. (2001). An endogenous cannabinoid (2-AG) is neuroprotective after brain injury. *Nature, 413*(6855), 527–531. https://doi.org/10.1038/35097089

Papagianni, E. P., & Stevenson, C. W. (2019). Cannabinoid regulation of fear and anxiety: An update. *Current Psychiatry Reports, 21*(6), 38. https://doi.org/10.1007/s11920-019-1026-z

Paradisi, A., Oddi, S., & Maccarrone, B. S. P. (2006). The endocannabinoid system in ageing: A new target for drug development. *Current Drug Targets, 7*(11), 1539–1552. https://doi.org/10.2174/1389450110607011539

Parker, L. A., Rock, E. M., & Limebeer, C. L. (2011). Regulation of nausea and vomiting by cannabinoids: Cannabinoids and nausea and vomiting. *British Journal of Pharmacology, 163*(7), 1411–1422. https://doi.org/10.1111/j.1476-5381.2010.01176.x

Patel, R., Rinker, L., Peng, J., & Chilian, W. M. (2018). Reactive oxygen species: The good and the bad. In C. Filip & E. Albu (Eds.), *Reactive oxygen species (ROS) in living cells.* IntechOpen.

Paton, W. D. M, & Pertwee, R. G. (1973). The actions of cannabis in man. In R. Mechoulam (Ed.), *Marijuana: Chemistry, pharmacology, metabolism and clinical effects* (pp. 288–334). Academic Press.

Perez, S. M., Donegan, J. J., Boley, A. M., Aguilar, D. D., Giuffrida, A., & Lodge, D. J. (2019). Ventral hippocampal overexpression of cannabinoid receptor interacting protein 1 (CNRIP1) produces a schizophrenia-like phenotype in the rat. *Schizophrenia Research, 206,* 263–270. https://doi.org/10.1016/j.schres.2018.11.006

Pertwee, R. G. (2005). Pharmacological actions of cannabinoids. In R. G. Pertwee (Ed.), *Cannabinoids* (pp. 1–51). Springer-Verlag.

Pertwee, R. G. (2006). Cannabinoid pharmacology: The first 66 years. *British Journal of Pharmacology, 147*(Suppl. 1), S163–S171. https://doi.org/10.1038/sj.bjp.0706406

Pertwee, R. G., Howlett, A. C., Abood, M. E., Alexander, S. P. H., Di Marzo, V., Elphick, M. R., Greasley, P. J., Hansen, H. S., Kunos, G., Mackie, K., Mechoulam, R., & Ross, R. A. (2010). Cannabinoid receptors and their ligands: Beyond CB1 and CB2. *Pharmacological Reviews, 62*(4), 588–631. https://doi.org/10.1124/pr.110.003004

Pertwee, R. G., & Ross, R. A. (2002). Cannabinoid receptors and their ligands. *Prostaglandins, Leukotrienes and Essential Fatty Acids, 66*(2–3), 101–121. https://doi.org/10.1054/plef.2001.0341

Peyrou, M., Ramadori, P., Bourgoin, L., & Foti, M. (2012). PPARs in liver diseases and cancer: Epigenetic regulation by microRNAs. *PPAR Research, 2012.* https://doi.org/10.1155/2012/757803

Piñeiro, R., Maffucci, T., & Falasca, M. (2011). The putative cannabinoid receptor GPR55 defines a novel autocrine loop in cancer cell proliferation. *Oncogene, 30*(2), 142–152. https://doi.org/10.1038/onc.2010.417

Piomelli, D. (2013). A fatty gut feeling. *Trends in Endocrinology and Metabolism, 24*(7), 332–341. https://doi.org/10.1016/j.tem.2013.03.001

Piomelli, D., Giuffrida, A., Calignano, A., & Rodriáguez de Fonseca, F. (2000). The endocannabinoid system as a target for therapeutic drugs. *Trends in Pharmacological Sciences, 21*(6), 218–224. https://doi.org/10.1016/S0165-6147(00)01482-6

Piomelli, D., & Russo, E. B. (2016). The *Cannabis sativa* versus *Cannabis indica* debate: An interview with Ethan Russo, MD. *Cannabis and Cannabinoid Research, 1*(1), 44–46. https://doi.org/10.1089/can.2015.29003.ebr

Porter, A. C. (2002). Characterization of a novel endocannabinoid, virodhamine, with antagonist activity at the CB1 receptor. *Journal of Pharmacology and Experimental Therapeutics, 301*(3), 1020–1024. https://doi.org/10.1124/jpet.301.3.1020

Price, T. J., Patwardhan, A., Akopian, A. N., Hargreaves, K. M., & Flores, C. M. (2004). Modulation of trigeminal sensory neuron activity by the dual cannabinoid-vanilloid agonists anandamide, *N*-arachidonoyl-dopamine and arachidonoyl-2-chloroethylamide. *British Journal of Pharmacology, 141*(7), 1118–1130. https://doi.org/10.1038/sj.bjp.0705711

Rácz, I., Bilkei-Gorzo, A., Markert, A., Stamer, F., Göthert, M., & Zimmer, A. (2008). Anandamide effects on 5-HT$_3$ receptors in vivo. *European Journal of Pharmacology, 596*(1–3), 98–101. https://doi.org/10.1016/j.ejphar.2008.08.012

Raichlen, D. A., Foster, A. D., Gerdeman, G. L., Seillier, A., & Giuffrida, A. (2012). Wired to run: Exercise-induced endocannabinoid signaling in humans and cursorial mammals with implications for the "runner's high." *Journal of Experimental Biology, 215*(8), 1331–1336. https://doi.org/10.1242/jeb.063677

Rakhshan, F., Day, T. A., Blakely, R. D., & Barker, E. L. (2000). Carrier-mediated uptake of the endogenous cannabinoid anandamide in RBL-2H3 cells. *Journal of Pharmacology and Experimental Therapeutics, 292*(3), 960–967.

Reggio, P. H. (2010). Endocannabinoid binding to the cannabinoid receptors: What is known and what remains unknown. *Current Medicinal Chemistry, 17*(14), 1468–1486. https://doi.org/10.2174/092986710790980005

Richardson, J. D., Aanonsen, L., & Hargreaves, K. M. (1998). Hypoactivity of the spinal cannabinoid system results in NMDA-dependent hyperalgesia. *Journal of Neuroscience, 18*(1), 451–457. https://doi.org/10.1523/jneurosci.18-01-00451.1998

Ritter, K. E., Wang, Z., Vezina, C. M., Bjorling, D. E., & Southard-Smith, E. M. (2017). Serotonin receptor 5-HT3A affects development of bladder innervation and urinary bladder function. *Frontiers in Neuroscience, 11*, 690. https://doi.org/10.3389/fnins.2017.00690

Roche, M., & Finn, D. P. (2010). Brain CB2 receptors: Implications for neuropsychiatric disorders. *Pharmaceuticals, 3*(8), 2517–2553. https://doi.org/10.3390/ph3082517

Romanello, S., Spiri, D., Marcuzzi, E., Zanin, A., Boizeau, P., Riviere, S., Vizeneux, A., Moretti, R., Carbajal, R., Mercier, J.-C., Wood, C., Zuccotti, G. V., Crichiutti, G., Alberti, C., & Titomanlio, L. (2013). Association between childhood migraine and history of infantile colic. *JAMA, 309*(15), 1607–1612. https://doi.org/10.1001/jama.2013.747

Romanovsky, A. A., Almeida, M. C., Garami, A., Steiner, A. A., Norman, M. H., Morrison, S. F., Nakamura, K., Burmeister, J. F., & Nucci, T. B. (2009). The transient receptor potential vanilloid-1 channel in thermoregulation: A thermosensor it is not. *Pharmacological Reviews, 61*(3), 228–261. https://doi.org/10.1124/pr.109.001263

Romero, T. R. L., Resende, L. C., Guzzo, L. S., & Duarte, I. D. G. (2013). CB1 and CB2 cannabinoid receptor agonists induce peripheral antinociception by activation of the endogenous noradrenergic system. *Anesthesia and Analgesia, 116*(2), 463–472. https://doi.org/10.1213/ANE.0b013e3182707859

Ross, H. R., Gilmore, A. J., & Connor, M. (2009). Inhibition of human recombinant T-type calcium channels by the endocannabinoid *N*-arachidonoyl dopamine: NADA inhibits T-type calcium channels. *British Journal of Pharmacology, 156*(5), 740–750. https://doi.org/10.1111/j.1476-5381.2008.00072.x

Ross, R. A. (2003). Anandamide and vanilloid TRPV1 receptors. *British Journal of Pharmacology, 140*(5), 790–801. https://doi.org/10.1038/sj.bjp.0705467

Rossi, G., Gioacchini, G., Pengo, G., Suchodolski, J. S., Jergens, A. E., Allenspach, K., Gavazza, A., Scarpona, S., Berardi, S., Galosi, L., Bassotti, G., & Cerquetella, M. (2020). Enterocolic increase of cannabinoid receptor type 1 and type 2 and clinical improvement after probiotic administration in dogs with chronic signs of colonic dysmotility without mucosal inflammatory changes. *Neurogastroenterology and Motility: the Official Journal of the European Gastrointestinal Motility Society, 32*(1), e13717. https://doi.org/10.1111/nmo.13717

Rousseaux, C., Thuru, X., Gelot, A., Barnich, N., Neut, C., Dubuquoy, L., Dubuquoy, C., Merour, E., Geboes, K., Chamaillard, M., Ouwehand, A., Leyer, G., Carcano, D., Colombel, J.-F., Ardid, D., & Desreumaux, P. (2007). *Lactobacillus acidophilus* modulates intestinal pain and induces opioid and cannabinoid receptors. *Nature Medicine, 13*(1), 35–37. https://doi.org/10.1038/nm1521

Russo, E. B. (2001). Hemp for headache: An in-depth historical and scientific review of cannabis in migraine treatment. *Journal of Cannabis Therapeutics, 1*(2), 21–92. https://doi.org/10.1300/J175v01n02_04

Russo, E. B. (2004). Clinical endocannabinoid deficiency (CECD): Can this concept explain therapeutic benefits of cannabis in migraine, fibromyalgia, irritable bowel syndrome and other treatment-resistant conditions? *Neuroendocrine Letters, 29*(2), 192–200. https://pubmed.ncbi.nlm.nih.gov/18404144/

Russo, E. B. (2008). Cannabinoids in the management of difficult to treat pain. *Therapeutics and Clinical Risk Management, 4*(1), 245–259. https://doi.org/10.2147/tcrm.s1928

Russo, E. B. (2016). Clinical endocannabinoid deficiency reconsidered: Current research supports the theory in migraine, fibromyalgia, irritable bowel, and other treatment-resistant syndromes. *Cannabis and Cannabinoid Research, 1*(1), 154–165. https://doi.org/10.1089/can.2016.0009

Ryberg, E., Larsson, N., Sjögren, S., Hjorth, S., Hermansson, N-O., Leonova, J., Elebring, T., Nilsson, K., Drmota, T., & Greasley, P. J. (2007). The orphan receptor GPR55 is a novel cannabinoid receptor. *British Journal of Pharmacology, 152*(7), 1092–1101. https://doi.org/10.1038/sj.bjp.0707460

Ryskamp, D. A., Redmon, S., Jo, A. O., & Križaj, D. (2014). TRPV1 and endocannabinoids: Emerging molecular signals that modulate mammalian vision. *Cells, 3*(3), 914–938. https://doi.org/10.3390/cells3030914

Sharir, H., Console-Bram, L., Mundy, C., Popoff, S. N., Kapur, A., & Abood, M. E. (2012). The endocannabinoids anandamide and virodhamine modulate the activity of the candidate cannabinoid receptor GPR55. *Journal of Neuroimmune Pharmacology, 7*(4), 856–865. https://doi.org/10.1007/s11481-012-9351-6

Sharkey, K. A., & Wiley, J. W. (2016). The role of the endocannabinoid system in the brain–gut axis. *Gastroenterology, 151*(2), 252–266. https://doi.org/10.1053/j.gastro.2016.04.015

Shekhar, A., & Thakur, G. A. (2018). Cannabinoid receptor 1 positive allosteric modulators for posttraumatic stress disorder. *Neuropsychopharmacology, 43*(1), 226–227. https://doi.org/10.1038/npp.2017.230

Shoemaker, J. L. (2005). The endocannabinoid noladin ether acts as a full agonist at human CB2 cannabinoid receptors. *Journal of Pharmacology and Experimental Therapeutics, 314*(2), 868–875. https://doi.org/10.1124/jpet.105.085282

Shonesy, B. C., Bluett, R. J., Ramikie, T. S., Báldi, R., Hermanson, D. J., Kingsley, P. J., Marnett, L. J., Winder, D. G., Colbran, R. J., & Patel, S. (2014). Genetic disruption of 2-arachidonoylglycerol synthesis reveals a key role for endocannabinoid signaling in anxiety modulation. *Cell Reports, 9*(5), 1644–1653. https://doi.org/10.1016/j.celrep.2014.11.001

Simopoulos, A. P. (2016). An increase in the omega-6/omega-3 fatty acid ratio increases the risk for obesity. *Nutrients, 8*(3), 128. https://doi.org/10.3390/nu8030128

Smart, D., Jonsson, K.-O., Vandevoorde, S., Lambert, D. M., & Fowler, C. J. (2002). "Entourage" effects of N-acyl ethanolamines at human vanilloid receptors: Comparison of effects upon anandamide-induced vanilloid receptor activation and upon anandamide metabolism. *British Journal of Pharmacology, 136*(3), 452–458. https://doi.org/10.1038/sj.bjp.0704732

Smoum, R., Bar, A., Tan, B., Milman, G., Attar-Namdar, M., Ofek, O., Stuart, J. M., Bajayo, A., Tam, J., Kram, V., O'Dell, D., Walker, M. J., Bradshaw, H. B., Bab, I., & Mechoulam, R. (2010). Oleoyl serine, an endogenous N-acyl amide, modulates bone remodeling and mass. *Proceedings of the National Academy of Sciences, 107*(41), 17710–17715. https://doi.org/10.1073/pnas.0912479107

Sparling, P. B., Giuffrida, A., Piomelli, D., Rosskopf, L., & Dietrich, A. (2003). Exercise activates the endocannabinoid system. *Neuroreport, 14*(17), 2209–2211. https://doi.org/10.1097/01.wnr.0000097048.56589.47

Steers, W. D. (2002). Pathophysiology of overactive bladder and urge urinary incontinence. *Reviews in Urology, 4*(Suppl. 4), S7–S18. https://www.ncbi.nlm.nih.gov/pmc/articles/PMC1476015/

Sugiura, T., Kobayashi, Y., Oka, S., & Waku, K. (2002). Biosynthesis and degradation of anandamide and 2-arachidonoylglycerol and their possible physiological significance. *Prostaglandins, Leukotrienes and Essential Fatty Acids, 66*(2–3), 173–192. https://doi.org/10.1054/plef.2001.0356

Sugiura, T., Kondo, S., Sukagawa, A., Nakane, S., Shinoda, A., Itoh, K., Yamashita, A., & Waku, K. (1995). 2-Arachidonoylgylcerol: A possible endogenous cannabinoid receptor ligand in brain. *Biochemical and Biophysical Research Communications, 215*(1), 89–97. https://doi.org/10.1006/bbrc.1995.2437

Sugiura, T., & Waku, K. (2000). 2-Arachidonoylglycerol and the cannabinoid receptors. *Chemistry and Physics of Lipids, 108*(1–2), 89–106. https://doi.org/10.1016/S0009-3084(00)00189-4

Sun, Y., & Bennett, A. (2007). Cannabinoids: A new group of agonists of PPARs. *PPAR Research, 2007*, 23515. https://doi.org/10.1155/2007/23513

Svizenska, I., Dubovy, P., & Sulcova, A. (2008). Cannabinoid receptors 1 and 2 (CB1 and CB2), their distribution, ligands and functional involvement in nervous system structures: A short review. *Pharmacology Biochemistry and Behavior, 90*(4), 501–511. https://doi.org/10.1016/j.pbb.2008.05.010

Syed, S. K., Bui, H. H., Beavers, L. S., Farb, T. B., Ficorilli, J., Chesterfield, A. K., Kuo, M. S., Bokvist, K., Barrett, D. G., & Efanov, A. M. (2012). Regulation of GPR119 receptor activity with endocannabinoid-like lipids. *American Journal of Physiology-Endocrinology and Metabolism, 303*(12), E1469–E1478. https://doi.org/10.1152/ajpendo.00269.2012

Takenouchi, R., Inoue, K., Kambe, Y., & Miyata, A. (2012). N-Arachidonoyl glycine induces macrophage apoptosis via GPR18. *Biochemical and Biophysical Research Communications, 418*(2), 366–371. https://doi.org/10.1016/j.bbrc.2012.01.027

Tallima, H., & El Ridi, R. (2018). Arachidonic acid: Physiological roles and potential health benefits—a review. *Journal of Advanced Research, 11*, 33–41. https://doi.org/10.1016/j.jare.2017.11.004

Tam, J. (2006). Involvement of neuronal cannabinoid receptor CB1 in regulation of bone mass and bone remodeling. *Molecular Pharmacology, 70*(3), 786–792. https://doi.org/10.1124/mol.106.026435

Tanimura, A., Yamazaki, M., Hashimotodani, Y., Uchigashima, M., Kawata, S., Abe, M., Kita, Y., Hashimoto, K., Shimizu, T., Watanabe, M., Sakimura, K., & Kano, M. (2010). The endocannabinoid 2-arachidonoylglycerol produced by diacylglycerol lipase α mediates retrograde suppression of synaptic transmission. *Neuron, 65*(3), 320–327. https://doi.org/10.1016/j.neuron.2010.01.021

Thompson, A. J., & Lummis, S. C. R. (2006). 5-HT$_3$ receptors. *Current Pharmaceutical Design, 12*(28), 3615–3630. https://www.ncbi.nlm.nih.gov/pmc/articles/PMC2664614/

Tietjen, G. E., Brandes, J. L., Peterlin, B. L., Eloff, A., Dafer, R. M., Stein, M. R., Drexler, E., Martin, V. T., Hutchinson, S., Aurora, S. K., Recober, A., Herial, N. A., Utley, C., White, L., & Khuder, S. A. (2009). Allodynia in migraine: Association with comorbid pain conditions. *Headache, 49*(9), 1333–1344. https://doi.org/10.1111/j.1526-4610.2009.01521.x

Toczek, M., & Malinowska, B. (2018). Enhanced endocannabinoid tone as a potential target of pharmacotherapy. *Life Sciences, 204*, 20–45. https://doi.org/10.1016/j.lfs.2018.04.054

Traynor-Kaplan, A., Kruse, M., Dickson, E. J., Dai, G., Vivas, O., Yu, H., Whittington, D., Hille, B. (2017). Fatty-acyl chain profiles of cellular phosphoinositides. *Biochimica et Biophysica Acta, 1862*(5), 513–522. https://doi.org/10.1016/j.bbalip.2017.02.002

Trezza, V., Damsteegt, R., Manduca, A., Petrosino, S., Van Kerkhof, L. W. M., Pasterkamp, R., Zhou, Y., Campolongo, P., Cuomo, V., Di Marzo, V., & Vanderschuren, L. J. M. J. (2012). Endocannabinoids in amygdala and nucleus accumbens mediate social play reward in adolescent rats. *Journal of Neuroscience, 32*(43), 14899–14908. https://doi.org/10.1523/jneurosci.0114-12.2012

Tsuboi, K., Uyama, T., Okamoto, Y., & Ueda, N. (2018). Endocannabinoids and related *N*-acylethanolamines: Biological activities and metabolism. *Inflammation and Regeneration, 38*, 28. https://doi.org/10.1186/s41232-018-0086-5

Tyagi, S., Gupta, P., Saini, A. S., Kaushal, C., & Sharma, S. (2011). The peroxisome proliferator-activated receptor: A family of nuclear receptors role in various diseases. *Journal of Advanced Pharmaceutical Technology & Research, 2*(4), 236–240. https://doi.org/10.4103/2231-4040.90879

Valk, P., Verbakel, S., Vankan, Y., Hol, S., Mancham, S., Ploemacher, R., & Mayen, A. (1997). Anandamide, a natural ligand for the peripheral cannabinoid receptor is a novel synergistic growth factor for hematopoietic cells. *Blood, 90*(4), 1448–1457. https://pubmed.ncbi.nlm.nih.gov/9269762/

van der Stelt, M., Veldhuis, W. B., Haaften, G. W. van, Fezza, F., Bisogno, T., Bär, P. R., Veldink, G. A., Vliegenthart, J. F. G., Di Marzo, V., & Nicolay, K. (2001). Exogenous anandamide protects rat brain against acute neuronal injury in vivo. *Journal of Neuroscience, 21*(22), 8765–8771. https://doi.org/10.1523/jneurosci.21-22-08765.2001

Varga, K., Wagner, J. A., Bridgen, D. T., & Kunos, G. (1998). Platelet- and macrophage-derived endogenous cannabinoids are involved in endotoxin-induced hypotension. *FASEB Journal, 12*(11), 1035–1044. https://doi.org/10.1096/fasebj.12.11.1035

Velasco, G., Sánchez, C., & Guzmán, M. (2016). Anticancer mechanisms of cannabinoids. *Current Oncology, 23*(Suppl. 2), S23–S32. https://doi.org/10.3747/co.23.3080

Viscomi, M. T., Oddi, S., Latini, L., Pasquariello, N., Florenzano, F., Bernardi, G., Molinari, M., & Maccarrone, M. (2009). Selective CB2 receptor agonism protects central neurons from remote axotomy-induced apoptosis through the PI3K/Akt pathway. *Journal of Neuroscience, 29*(14), 4564–4570. https://doi.org/10.1523/JNEUROSCI.0786-09.2009

Volkow, N. D., Hampson, A. J., & Baler, R. D. (2017). Don't worry, be happy: Endocannabinoids and cannabis at the intersection of stress and reward. *Annual Review of Pharmacology and Toxicology, 57*(1), 285–308. https://doi.org/10.1146/annurev-pharmtox-010716-104615

Walker, J. M., Krey, J. F., Chu, C. J., & Huang, S. M. (2002). Endocannabinoids and related fatty acid derivatives in pain modulation. *Chemistry and Physics of Lipids, 121*(1–2), 159–172. https://doi.org/10.1016/S0009-3084(02)00152-4

Walstab, J., Rappold, G., & Niesler, B. (2010). 5-HT$_3$ receptors: Role in disease and target of drugs. *Pharmacology & Therapeutics, 128*(1), 146–169. https://doi.org/10.1016/j.pharmthera.2010.07.001

Wang, S., Xu, Q., Shu, G., Wang, L., Gao, P., Xi, Q., Zhang, Y., Jiang, Q., & Zhu, X. (2015). *N*-Oleoyl glycine, a lipoamino acid, stimulates adipogenesis associated with activation of CB1 receptor and Akt signaling pathway in 3T3-L1 adipocyte. *Biochemical and Biophysical Research Communications, 466*(3), 438–443. https://doi.org/10.1016/j.bbrc.2015.09.046

Warden, A., Truitt, J., Merriman, M., Ponomareva, O., Jameson, K., Ferguson, L. B., Mayfield, R. D., & Harris, R. A. (2016). Localization of PPAR isotypes in the adult mouse and human brain. *Scientific Reports, 6*(1), 27618. https://doi.org/10.1038/srep27618

Weller, I. J. (2009). Synaptosomes. In L. R. Squire, F. E. Bloom, N. C. Spitzer, F. Gage, & T. Albright (Eds.), *Encyclopedia of neuroscience* (pp. 815–818). Academic Press. https://doi.org/10.1016/B978-008045046-9.02045-3

Westlake, T. M., Howlett, A. C., Bonner, T. I., Matsuda, L. A., & Herkenham, M. (1994). Cannabinoid receptor binding and messenger RNA expression in human brain: An *in vitro* receptor autoradiography and *in situ* hybridization histochemistry study of normal aged and Alzheimer's brains. *Neuroscience, 63*(3), 637–652. https://doi.org/10.1016/0306-4522(94)90511-8

Whyte, L. S., Ryberg, E., Sims, N. A., Ridge, S. A., Mackie, K., Greasley, P. J., Ross, R. A., & Rogers, M. J. (2009). The putative cannabinoid receptor GPR55 affects osteoclast function in vitro and bone mass in vivo. *Proceedings of the National Academy of Sciences, 106*(38), 16511–16516. https://doi.org/10.1073/pnas.0902743106

Williams, C. M., & Kirkham, T. C. (1999). Anandamide induces overeating: Mediation by central cannabinoid (CB1) receptors. *Psychopharmacology, 143*(3), 315–317. https://doi.org/10.1007/s002130050953

Willson, T. M., Brown, P. J., Sternbach, D. D., & Henke, B. R. (2000). The PPARs: From orphan receptors to drug discovery. *Journal of Medicinal Chemistry, 43*(4), 527–550. https://doi.org/10.1021/jm990554g

Wilson, R. I., & Nicoll, R. A. (2001). Endogenous cannabinoids mediate retrograde signalling at hippocampal synapses. *Nature, 410*(6828), 588–592. https://doi.org/10.1038/35069076

Witting, A., Walter, L., Wacker, J., Moller, T., & Stella, N. (2004). P2X7 receptors control 2-arachidonoylglycerol production by microglial cells. *Proceedings of the National Academy of Sciences, 101*(9), 3214–3219. https://doi.org/10.1073/pnas.0306707101

Wollner, H. J., Matchett, J. R., Levine, J., & Loewe, S. (1942). Isolation of a physiologically active tetrahydrocannabinol from cannabis sativa resin. *Journal of the American Chemical Society, 64*(1), 26–29. https://doi.org/10.1021/ja01253a008

Wright, K., Rooney, N., Feeney, M., Tate, J., Robertson, D., Welham, M., & Ward, S. (2005). Differential expression of cannabinoid receptors in the human colon: Cannabinoids promote epithelial wound healing. *Gastroenterology, 129*(2), 437–453. https://doi.org/10.1053/j.gastro.2005.05.026

Xu, X., Liu, Y., Huang, S., Liu, G., Xie, C., Zhou, J., Fan, W., Li, Q., Wang, Q., Zhong, D., & Miao, X. (2006). Overexpression of cannabinoid receptors CB1 and CB2 correlates with improved prognosis of patients with hepatocellular carcinoma. *Cancer Genetics and Cytogenetics, 171*(1), 31–38. https://doi.org/10.1016/j.cancergencyto.2006.06.014

Yamaguchi, T., Hagiwara, Y., Tanaka, H., Sugiura, T., Waku, K., Shoyama, Y., Watanabe, S., & Yamamoto, T. (2001). Endogenous cannabinoid, 2-arachidonoylglycerol, attenuates naloxone-precipitated withdrawal signs in morphine-dependent mice. *Brain Research, 909*, 121–126. https://doi.org/10.1016/S0006-8993(01)02655-5

Yamashita, A., Oka, S., Tanikawa, T., Hayashi, Y., Nemoto-Sasaki, Y., & Sugiura, T. (2013). The actions and metabolism of lysophosphatidylinositol, an endogenous agonist for GPR55. *Prostaglandins & Other Lipid Mediators, 107*, 103–116. https://doi.org/10.1016/j.prostaglandins.2013.05.004

Yan, K., Gao, L. N., Cui, Y. L., Zhang, Y., & Zhou, X. (2016). The cyclic AMP signaling pathway: Exploring targets for successful drug discovery. *Molecular Medicine Reports, 13*(5), 3715–3723. https://doi.org/10.3892/mmr.2016.5005

Yang, H., Zhou, J., & Lehmann, C. (2016). GPR55—a putative "type 3" cannabinoid receptor in inflammation. *Journal of Basic and Clinical Physiology and Pharmacology, 27*(3), 297–302. https://doi.org/10.1515/jbcpp-2015-0080

Zanettini, C., Panlilio, L. V., Aliczki, M., Goldberg, S. R., Haller, J., & Yasar, S. (2011). Effects of endocannabinoid system modulation on cognitive and emotional behavior. *Frontiers in Behavioral Neuroscience, 5.* https://doi.org/10.3389/fnbeh.2011.00057

Zogopoulos, P., Vasileiou, I., Patsouris, E., & Theocharis, S. (2013). The neuroprotective role of endocannabinoids against chemical-induced injury and other adverse effects: Endocannabinoids and neurotoxicity. *Journal of Applied Toxicology, 33*(4), 246–264. https://doi.org/10.1002/jat.2828

Zou, S., & Kumar, U. (2018). Cannabinoid receptors and the endocannabinoid system: Signaling and function in the central nervous system. *International Journal of Molecular Sciences, 19*(3), 833. https://doi.org/10.3390/ijms19030833

Zygmunt, P. M., Petersson, J., Andersson, D. A., Chuang, H., Sørgård, M., Di Marzo, V., Julius, D., & Högestätt, E. D. (1999). Vanilloid receptors on sensory nerves mediate the vasodilator action of anandamide. *Nature, 400*(6743), 452–457. https://doi.org/10.1038/22761

3

Cannabis Pharmacology: From the Whole Plant to Pharmaceutical Applications

Rachel A. Parmelee, MSN, RN, CRRN,
Carey S. Clark, PhD, RN, AHN-BC, RYT, FAAN, and
Deanna M. Sommers PhD, MSN, RN, CPNP-PC

CONCEPTS AND CONSIDERATIONS

Cannabis is a multifaceted plant, and how its therapeutic components interact with our endocannabinoid system (ECS) is essential for the cannabis care nurse to know. This chapter will focus on the fundamentals of cannabis pharmacokinetics and pharmacodynamics. The goal of this chapter is for the learner to have a foundational knowledge of how cannabis and cannabinoid medicines work to best support safe and effective use of cannabinoid therapeutics for cannabis care patients.

Learning Outcomes

Upon completion of this chapter, the learners will:

- Discuss the pharmacology, pharmacokinetics, and pharmacodynamics of cannabinoid medicines.
- Consider the entourage effect of whole-plant medicines versus isolates and synthetic plant medicines.
- Describe the adverse effects of cannabinoid medicines.
- Discern risks for cannabis substance use disorder.
- Consider safe and practical approaches to using cannabinoid medicines, including titration and dosing approaches.
- Gain awareness of drug-to-drug interactions.

DEFINITIONS

Cannabis: Dioecious, flowering herb *Cannabis sativa L.*, a genus of flowering plants in the family Cannabaceae, more commonly known as marijuana. Although the number of cannabis species of this plant is often debated, there are three commonly recognized species of cannabis, including *Cannabis sativa* (*C. sativa*), *Cannabis indica*

(*C. indica*), and *Cannabis ruderalis* (*C. ruderalis*). Scientists frequently debate how the plant evolved into three species, though it is likely related to various climate effects and human interventions.

Chemovars: This term (sometimes called chemotype) refers to the breakdown and categorization of a plant species as related to its chemical composition. A specific chemovar is identified with cannabis through its unique profile related to terpenes, cannabinoids, flavonoids, and the number of standard biomolecules. By examining these measurable chemical biomarkers, plants can be differentiated and the potential therapeutic effects discerned. Identifying the plant profile is a more precise approach to labeling that ensures consistency and replaces the need for inaccurate strain names.

Certificate of Analysis (COA): COA is a document that defines product specification through third-party accredited lab testing. COAs are used throughout the food, alcohol, and pharmaceutical industries. With cannabis, a COA should include cannabinoid and terpene profiles, along with evidence of testing for residues from solvents, pesticides, and heavy metals.

Delta-9-Tetrahydrocannabinol (THC): This is the psychoactive cannabinoid found in the cannabis plant. It is responsible for the euphoric feeling one experiences from cannabis ingestion and it is also related to many of the plant's side effects.

Endocannabinoids: Endogenous (naturally occurring) ligands that bind to cannabinoid receptors. The two best known and well-studied are anandamide (AEA) and 2-arachidonoylglycerol (2-AG), which are lipid-based, retrograde neurotransmitters.

Phytocannabinoids: Naturally occurring plant-based components that interact directly with the human ECS at the CB1, CB2, and other endocannabinoid receptor sites. They mimic the same action as naturally occurring human endocannabinoids. Cannabinoids have also been developed from synthesized chemicals/drugs.

Synthetic cannabinoids: Substances or chemical compounds created to mimic the effects of cannabis. "Spice" is an example of a synthetic cannabinoid, as is dronabinol, which is a synthetic form of THC.

Terpenes: Aromatic oils secreted from the same cannabis oil glands (trichomes) that produce cannabinoids. There are over 200 different terpenes produced by the cannabis plant (Russo, 2011).

Terpenoids (isoprenoids): A highly diverse class of natural products or a modified class of terpenes having different functional groups with an oxidized methyl group moved or removed at various positions. As the plant dries and cures, terpenes turn to terpenoids; however, they are often used interchangeably.

CANNABIS TAXONOMY

Although incessantly debated, how cannabis was historically categorized has become less relevant and, in some aspects, inaccurately defined. The methods used to identify cannabis and the plant's effects were thought to fall under three main species, which could also be combined to create hybrids:

- *Cannabis indica* grows rapidly, tends to be shorter (less than 6 feet tall), bushier, with more buds, and with darker green leaves. These chemovars tend to have more CBD and less THC.
- *Cannabis sativa* grows tall (12 feet), they have long leaves that may appear to be serrated, take longer to mature, and they may be a lighter green color. These plants tend to have higher ratios of THC and lower amounts of CBD.

- *Cannabis ruderalis* tends to be shorter (around 12 inches), stalky, and shaggier than the other species. It is quite rugged and is auto-flowering, which is what makes it attractive to cannabis breeders. Generally not used for medicinal needs, it does help to balance out chemotypes (formally known as strains) and shorten the period toward plant maturation.
- *Hybrids* tend to be either *sativa* dominant or *indica* dominant, depending on the breeding process. The appearance of these plants is related to how the parent plants are combined.

Historically, many believed that the two main types of cannabis plants had different effects on the body; *C. sativa* had energizing effects, creating a "head high," while also supporting creativity and focus, and *C. indica* had more sedating or calming effects with a full-body relaxation experience. Because of ongoing breeding and hybridization of cannabis plants, the two categories no longer relate to the effect of the plant. We also know now that terpenes play a much more significant role in how the person reacts to the specific plant chemovar (sometimes commonly called "strains" by laypeople and within the cannabis industry). The chemovars are better defined by assessing the plant's chemical profile, which is discussed later in this chapter.

CANNABIS PLANT: THERAPEUTIC COMPONENTS

The following section reviews the basics of the complex *C. sativa L.* (cannabis) whole-plant medicine. The cannabis plant produces well over 400 biochemicals, with at least 113 of these being cannabinoids that directly interact with the ECS. Terpenes are also explored as therapeutic components found in the cannabis plant.

Chemovars

Thousands of different cannabis chemovars (also known as chemotypes) define the unique profile and diversity of any given plant, with each one containing various concentrations of cannabinoids, flavonoids, and terpenes (MacCallum & Russo, 2018). The hybridization of cannabis plants has led to the development of many new chemical varieties with a wide range of effects. Some varieties are well established and maintain some consistency regardless of environmental factors, yet assigning a name to a chemical variation is an ongoing process. Given names (ie, Sour Diesel, Granddaddy Purple, MOB) do little to describe the effects of cannabis and confuse patients expecting predictability. The names of the cannabis flowers found in dispensaries serve to merely *identify* them, rather than truly *define* their pharmacologic properties. Hazekamp et al. (2016) called for cannabis plants that are being used for medical treatments to be fully mapped for their active components and for a "metabolomics" approach to be used, where terpenes and cannabinoids are mapped for each cannabis plant. Defining the plant's chemovar profile allows for a more accurate description of how the plant might interact with the ECS, versus limiting the plant's identification to the three categories of *indica*, *sativa*, or *ruderalis*.

In recent history, the vast majority of the chemovars in the United States were considered Type I cannabis (THC dominant; intoxicating). Nevertheless, as interest and the need for higher CBD ratios has grown, Type II (THC:CBD balanced ratios; less intoxicating) and Type III cannabis (CBD dominant: generally nonintoxicating; hemp) has allowed for improved therapeutic options aligning with patients' medical needs (MacCallum & Russo, 2018). Broadly classifying chemovars into these types, even without considering their specific terpene profiles, can assist with the selection and titrating; the knowledge of THC and CBD levels supports appropriate titration methods (as followed in this chapter).

Phytocannabinoids

Cannabis has over 400 chemical compounds, of which at least 100 are cannabinoids; the remaining compounds include terpenes, flavonoids, and fatty acids (Vadivelu et al., 2018). These active cannabinoid compounds are in the plant's trichomes, which are the sticky, resin glands found on the flower of the cannabis plant. Cannabinoids are a class of chemical compounds that act on the endocannabinoid receptors in our brains and elsewhere in the body and impact the physiologic functions of the ECS. There are endocannabinoids that our bodies make and exogenous phytocannabinoids that come from plant sources and synthetic cannabinoids. This section will cover some of the exogenous cannabinoids and their known effects. For more on how endogenous cannabinoids work in the body with the cannabinoid receptors found in the ECS, please see Chapter 2.

The two most well-known and highly studied phytocannabinoids are THC and CBD (see definitions). The cannabis plant does not directly manufacture these two cannabinoids. Instead, the cannabis plant makes chemicals that are the precursors to these cannabinoids: these precursors are called cannabinoid acids, which, when heated or given enough passage of time, will release different forms of the cannabinoids (Backes, 2017). All cannabinoids are contained within the trichomes of the raw cannabis flowers: these raw cannabinoids in the acidic form have a carboxylic acid group (COOH) attached to the benzene ring. The process of heating the plant to release different cannabinoids when the carboxyl group is removed is called decarboxylation. Additionally, as the raw cannabis plant is dried and cured over time, partial decarboxylation will occur. Vaporizing (at the right temperature) or smoking cannabis immediately decarboxylates cannabinoids, because of the high temperatures, allowing for more immediate absorption of the cannabinoids through inhalation; however, some valuable therapeutic chemical components such as terpenes may be lost in this process (Backes, 2017). Raw cannabis plant Δ^9-tetrahydrocannabinolic acid (THCA) is generally converted to THC and cannabidiolic acid (CBDA) into CBD through heating at 220 °F for 30 to 45 minutes. Terpenes may be better preserved by heating at lower temperatures for more extended periods.

The raw or acid forms of cannabinoids and the heated or decarboxylated forms of cannabinoids interact with the ECS, albeit in a different manner. For instance, when THCA is ingested, it is nonintoxicating, whereas THC is intoxicating. The challenge with using the acidic forms of cannabinoids is that they are not stable, and over time they degrade into their nonacidic forms (ie, CBDA becomes CBD) (see Tables 3.1 and 3.2).

The major phytocannabinoids

The following section provides readers with an overview of some of the many cannabinoids found in the cannabis plant and their reported therapeutic benefits. As the research in this area is continually emerging, the reader is encouraged to explore new findings related to each cannabinoid.

TABLE 3.1.	Fun fact about: decarboxylation

A simple way to decarboxylate raw cannabis is to preheat the oven to 235 °F (110 °C). Prepare the cured raw cannabis by placing it on a parchment paper–lined baking sheet or inside an oven bag (turkey bag). Larger cannabis buds may need to be broken up into smaller sizes so that the plant material will be thoroughly heated. Bake the cannabis for 40–60 min and remove it from the oven. Allow the cannabis to cool for 30 min. The majority of the THCA and CBDA should be converted to THC and CBD. Temperatures higher than 220° and approaching 300° can disrupt many terpene chemical structures and potentially leave behind aromas and flavors that are unfavorable, but also isolate specific cannabinoids for inhalation (Backes, 2017).

CBD, cannabidiol; CBDA, cannabidiolic acid; THC, delta-9-tetrahydrocannabinol; THCA, delta-9-tetrahydrocannabinolic acid.

Cannabigerol

Cannabigerol (CBG) was the first cannabis compound isolated from cannabis resin as a pure chemical substance (Elsohly & Slade, 2005). Cannabigerolic acid (CBGA) is considered the "mother" of all of the cannabinoids because, during photosynthesis, CBGA is converted into other cannabinoids. CBG, therefore, shows up as a minor cannabinoid in lab tests and the COAs of mature plants. CBG is nonintoxicating, neuroprotectant, antibacterial, a gamma-aminobutyric acid (GABA) reuptake inhibitor, and has been shown to boost the body's immune system (DePetrocellis et al., 2011).

Cannabichromene

Cannabichromene (CBC) is a nonintoxicating cannabinoid that targets TRPV1 (vanilloid) and TRPA1 (ankyrin) endocannabinoid receptors. Although it is a minor cannabinoid, it may come to play with the entourage effect and impact how other

TABLE 3.2.	A short history of cannabinoid discovery
Early 19th century	The first isolation of a phytocannabinoid (CBN).
1930s	Robert S. Cahn isolates and defines chemical structure of CBN.
1940	Roger Adams and Lord Todd et al. synthesize CBN in a lab in the United Kingdom. The team also isolated cannabidiol (CBD) during this time.
1942	Delta-9-tetrahydrocannabinol (THC) was first extracted from cannabis by H.J. Wollner, J. Matchett, J. Levine, and S. Loewe. Findings were published in the *Journal of the American Chemical Society*.
1963	Dr. Raphael Mechoulam isolates and reports the chemical structure of CBD.
1964	Mechoulam and colleagues isolate and define the chemical structure of THC.
1965	Mechoulam's laboratory synthesizes THC and CBD.

Pertwee, R. G. (2006). Cannabinoid pharmacology: The first 66 years. *British Journal of Pharmacology, 147*, S163–S171. https://doi.org/10.1038/sj.bjp.0706406

phytocannabinoids in cannabis interact with the ECS. CBC has been researched for its anticancer/antitumor neuroprotectant, pain alleviation, and anti-inflammatory effects (DePetocellis et al., 2011).

Cannabidiol

CBD is a well-known, popularly consumed, and highly researched cannabinoid, known for its antiepileptic, anti-inflammatory, antitumorigenic, immune-modulating, and mood-altering capacity. CBD is nonintoxicating and present in high percentages in the hemp plant, with many commercially available hemp-derived CBD products available. For more on CBD, please see Chapter 4.

Cannabidiolic Acid

CBDA interacts with the ECS by inhibiting cyclooxygenase-2 (COX2) enzymes responsible for inducing inflammation. Therefore, CBDA may act as a potent anti-inflammatory and reduce pain related to inflammation. CBDA interacts with serotonin signaling and may help with nausea and depression (Hen-Shoval et al., 2018).

Cannabinol

Cannabinol (CBN) is a cannabinoid that is a by-product of THCA degradation. Over time, as cannabis products are stored and age, the percentage of THCA decreases, and CBNA percentage increases. When the cannabis plant is heated, CBNA becomes CBN. CBN is a strong anti-inflammatory (DePetrocellis et al., 2011). CBN may also be mildly intoxicating, and although it has been reported to assist with sleep, this has not been a proven quality of this cannabinoid. CBN may help with appetite and stimulate bone growth (Farrimond et al., 2012).

Delta-9-Tetrahydrocannabinol

THC is the principal psychoactive and intoxicating component of the cannabis plant. THC helps to protect the plant against UV light, insect predators, and other environmental stressors. THC is known to help with pain, sleep, and nausea, and it is responsible for causing euphoria (DePetrocellis et al., 2011). It is generally the most abundant cannabinoid in the cannabis plant, though new chemovars with lower THC percentages are cultivated.

Δ^9-Tetrahydrocannabinolic Acid or 2-Carboxy-Tetrahydrocannabinolic Acid

THCA is an immunomodulator, antinausea, anti-inflammatory, neuroprotective, and antineoplastic cannabinoid. THCA begins as CBGA in the plant, and over time or with adequate heat, THCA degrades into THC (Moreno-Snaz, 2016).

Tetrahydrocannabivarin

Tetrahydrocannabivarin (THCV) does not begin as CBGA. Rather it stems from cannabigerovarin acid (CBGVA) converting to THCV. THCV is a minor cannabinoid

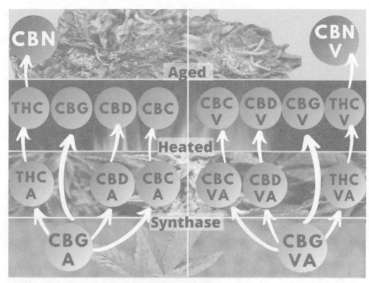

Figure 3.1: **Cannabinoids: chemical process.** (Based on Aryal, N., Orellana, D. F., & Bouie, J. (2019). Distribution of cannabinoid synthase genes in non-cannabis organisms. *Journal of Cannabis Research, 1*(8), 1–6. https://doi.org/10.1186/s42238-019-0008-7; Backes, M. (2017). *Cannabis pharmacy: The practical guide to medical marijuana.* Black Dog & Leventhal Publishers.)

found in some cannabis strains; it differs from THC because it has a three-carbon side chain rather than a five-carbon side chain. Longer carbon tails generally have higher affinity at CB1. In lower amounts, THCV may reduce the euphoria of THC by acting as a CB1 antagonist, whereas in higher amounts, it may indirectly cause the opposite. THCV may help treat obesity, type 2 diabetes, posttraumatic stress disorder (PTSD), and Parkinson's disease (García et al., 2011).

Figure 3.1 depicts how cannabinoids are derived from CBGA or CBGVA. Synthase occurs when an enzymatic reaction occurs. Once the acidic forms are heated or decarboxylated, they become the more commonly known neutral form of cannabinoids. When cannabis ages, the THC can convert to CBN.

Table 3.3 provides a summary of some commonly studied cannabinoids and their potential therapeutic effects.

Phytocannabinoids: personalized medicine

As we discover more about the individual cannabinoids found in cannabis and their healing properties, it may be possible for specialized chemovars to be grown to create greater percentages of specific cannabinoids. Additionally, specific beneficial cannabinoids may be isolated or synthesized and made available for patient use or to enhance specific products. For now, patients may be able to access the cannabis COA, a lab analysis of the plant contents generally provided by a third party, to determine the cannabinoid profile of a specific cannabis chemovar.

TABLE 3.3. A brief overview: cannabinoid benefits and health effects

Benefits	THC	THCA	THCV	CBN	CBD	CBDA	CBC	CBCA	CBG	CBGA	Health effects
Analgesic	X		X	X	X		X		X		Pain relief
Anti-inflammatory		X			X	X	X		X	X	Reduces inflammation
Anorectic			X								Suppresses appetite
Appetite stimulant	X										Stimulates appetite
Antiemetic	X	X			X						Reduces vomiting and nausea
Intestinal antiprokinetic					X						Reduces contractions of small intestine
Anxiolytic	X			X	X						Relieves anxiety
Antipsychotic					X						Tranquilizing/psychosis management
Antiepileptic	X		X		X						Reduces seizures and convulsions
Antispasmodic	X			X	X						Suppresses muscle spasms
Anti-insomnia				X							Aides sleep
Antidiabetic			X		X						Reduces blood sugar levels
Neuroprotective					X				X	X	Prevents nervous system degeneration
Antipsoriatic					X						Treats psoriasis
Anti-ischemic					X						Reduces risk of artery blockage
Antibacterial					X		X	X	X		Kills or slows bacterial growth
Antifungal								X	X		Treats fungal infection
Antiproliferative	X				X		X		X		Inhibits cell growth in tumors/cancer
Bone stimulant			X		X		X		X		Promotes bone growth

CBC, cannabichromene; CBCA, cannabichromenic acid; CBD, cannabidiol; CBDA, cannabidiolic acid; CBG, cannabigerol; CBGA, cannabigerolic acid; CBN, cannabinol; THC, delta-9-tetrahydrocannabinol; THCA, delta-9-tetrahydrocannabinolic acid; THCV, tetrahydrocannabivarin.
Adapted from Brenneisen, R. (2007). Chemistry and analysis of phytocannabinoids and other cannabis constituents. In M. A. ElSohly (Ed.), *Marijuana and the cannabinoids.* Humana Press.

The following is an example of a COA. Note that the cannabinoids, terpenes, and contaminants are addressed. A COA may help the patient determine if the medicine is safe (free from contaminants) and determine if it has the cannabinoids and terpenes that may be beneficial in addressing their needs. The cannabis care nurse can provide coaching and education on how to use a COA (see Certificate of Analysis).

Certificate of Analysis

		00000-00	GC/MS
		SAMPLE NO.	METHOD USED
J. Doe	Flower	Example	
CLIENT	SAMPLE TYPE	SAMPLE NAME	
2/26/20	3/2/20	1 gram	Lab Technician
DATE RECEIVED	DATE TESTED	SIZE OF SAMPLE	ANALYST SIGNATURE

Moisture Content: 8 %

Cannabinoid Profile	(% dry wt.)
THCa	21.8
Δ^9-THC	2.23
Δ^8-THC	0.00
CBDa	5.02
CBD	1.28
CBGa	0.14
CBG	0.03
CBC	0.00
CBN	0.00
THCv	0.00
Total THC:	21.34 %
Total CBD:	5.68 %

Terpene Profile	mg/kg
Mercene	2.18
Caryophyllene	1.23
Pinene	0.42
Limonene	0.28
Linalool	0.14
Humulene	0.03
Terpinene	0.00
Bisabolol	0.00

Purity	Pass/Fail
Water Activity	P
Pesticides	P
Microbials	P
Mycotoxins	P
Residual Solvents	P
Heavy Metals	P
Foreign Matter	P

Macro   Micro

Terpenes

Terpenes are the aromatic compounds in fruits, vegetables, trees, a few insects, and flowering plants, with over 50,000 terpenes found in nature and over 100 different terpenes identified in the cannabis plant. Terpenes are simple hydrocarbons, consisting of five-carbon isoprene units, which are assembled with many other isoprene units in thousands of different ways. Terpenes are responsible for the various fragrances and flavors of cannabis (cannabinoids are not fragrant) and may influence cannabis's effects. Terpenes perform an essential role by providing the plant with a natural protection or defense system from predatory insects, animals, bacteria, fungus, and other environmental stresses (Booth & Bohlmann, 2019). Although their fragrance acts as a repellent, terpenes attract bees to pollinate the cannabis flowers. Terpenes and cannabinoids are housed together in cannabis trichomes, the glandular and nonglandular "hairs" on the flower, bract, and leaves of the cannabis plant, which

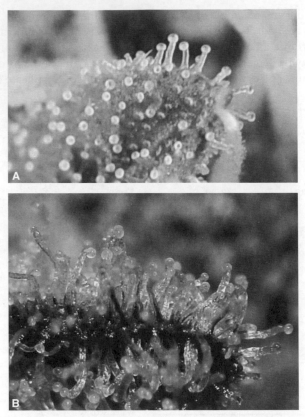

Figure 3.2: **Trichomes.** A. Multiple trichomes projecting from the cannabis flower.
B. The variations in the amount, stickiness, transparency, and slight color change depending on maturation and chemotype are illustrated. (Photo credit: Tim Hadley.)

have a sugary crystal–like appearance and sticky texture (Booth & Bohlmann, 2019) (see Figure 3.2). Although prevalent in any form of cannabis, high concentrations of terpenes can be found in unfertilized female cannabis flowers before senescence (the condition or process of deterioration with age) (Booth & Bohlmann, 2019).

Each cannabis chemovar has a unique terpene profile, which can be enhanced with light exposure during growth. Terpenes have a variety of characteristics, including flavor, smell, effects, and medicinal potential. The six prevalent fragrances and flavors are clove, lemon, pine, floral, pepper, and spicy wood. Terpenes are distinctly categorized: steam distilled, organic plant, synthetic, and cannabis derived. The most prevalent terpenes in cannabis are myrcene, with terpinolene, pinene, caryophyllene, and limonene also being predominantly found. Other commonly found terpenes in cannabis include linalool, terpinolene, ocimene, humulene, eudesmol, nerolidol, bisabolol, guaiol, terpineol, phellandrene, carene, pulegone, sabinene, and geraniol (Booth & Bohlmann, 2019) (see Table 3.4).

Chemical composition

Terpenes' and terpenoids' chemical structures contain an isoprene molecule (C_5H_8) as a repeating unit. Terpenes include carbon and hydrogen, and terpenoids' chemical composition includes carbon, hydrogen, and oxygen. The difference between

TABLE 3.4.	Fun facts about: terpenes

Terpenoids are biologically active and found in a variety of medicines, hormones, cosmetics, vitamins, etc. Terpenoids make up a large percentage of the essential oils found in cannabis plants, and there are over 100 different cannabis terpenoids, though only one terpenoid is unique to cannabis (monoterpenoid m-mentha-1,8(9)-dien-5-ol).

Turpentine is a fluid used as a solvent that is distilled from the resin of pine trees; it contains many terpenes, including pinene and terpinolene. Obviously, some terpenes are good for human health and others in certain combinations, like with this solvent, can be dangerous for one's health.

terpenes and terpenoids is that terpenes are hydrocarbons constructed from five-carbon isoprene units, which produce various molecular skeletons, and terpenoids have additional atoms that have been denatured or altered by oxidation. Denaturation occurs when cannabis flower has been dried, cured, or chemically modified: terpenes become terpenoids when cannabis is dried and cured, and terpene atoms are oxidized (Booth & Bohlmann, 2019). The cannabis terpene essential oil may be extracted from the plant material by steam distillation or vaporization (Booth & Bohlmann, 2019). Some terpenes vaporize at approximately the equivalent temperature as THC, though there is some volatility variance between terpenes, with their vaporization points tending to be higher (300 °F to 400 °F) compared to cannabinoids (Backes, 2017). High temperatures can jeopardize the terpene's integrity, and this is why high-temperature extraction can reduce the terpene content. After cannabinoid extraction, some processors may add terpenes back into their products for taste and smell, although it is unknown if this process has any medicinal value.

Modes of action

Until recently, it was hypothesized that terpenes could affect or influence the neuroreceptors by regulating the amount of THC that enters the brain through the blood–brain barrier, but no evidence exists that this is the case. Terpenes act on the receptors and neurotransmitters that are prone to combine or dissolve in lipids or fats (Booth & Bohlmann, 2019). Terpenes are lipophilic and hydrophobic. Some terpenes can act as serotonin uptake inhibitors and enhance norepinephrine activity, increase dopamine activity, and enhance GABA (Manayi et al., 2016). GABA's principal role is reducing neuronal excitability throughout the nervous system. Some terpenes may also influence the brain's neurotransmitters in different ways, including enhancing relaxation or altering mood or energy levels: relaxing or uplifting moods or energy levels (Booth & Bohlmann, 2019).

Prominent terpenes in cannabis

According to the United States Food and Drug Administration (USFDA, 2020), terpenes are food-safe additives. Terpene concentration changes as the cannabis plant dries (increased concentration) and then ages (decreased concentration). Soil, humidity, temperature, light, nutrition, and chemotype can affect the terpene composition.

Myrcene

Myrcene, a monoterpene, is the most abundant terpene in cannabis. Myrcene's aroma has been described as earthy, musky, and resembling cloves (Hartsel et al., 2016). It has been reported that myrcene acts as an analgesic, anti-inflammatory, antibacterial, antifungal, antioxidant, and neuroprotective; it has sedating and relaxing effects. Bay leaves, pine, juniper, citrus fruit, hops, eucalyptus, mango, and thyme also contain myrcene (Hartsel et al., 2016).

Limonene

Limonene is the second most common monoterpene found in cannabis. The aroma has hints of lemons, limes, and oranges (Hartsel et al., 2016). Limonene's medicinal value includes its actions as an antioxidant, anxiolytic, antibacterial, mood elevator, antifungal, antiacid (alleviates heartburn symptoms), and stress reducer. Citrus rind, pine, mint, rosemary, and juniper contain limonene (Hartsel et al., 2016).

Pinene

α- and β-Pinene, also monoterpenes, are the most abundant terpenes existing in nature. Pinene's aroma has been described as pine and fir trees. It has potential as an anti-inflammatory, bronchodilator, expectorant, antibiotic, analgesic, and anticonvulsant; pinenes may increase energy and alertness (Salehi et al., 2019). Pine trees, balsamic resin, rosemary, basil, and eucalyptus contain pinene (Hartsel et al., 2016).

β-Caryophyllene

β-Caryophyllene, the most common sesquiterpene, consists of three isoprene units and has a peppery, woody, and spicy aroma (Hartsel et al., 2016). β-Caryophyllene's pharmacologic medicinal value includes anti-inflammatory, antianxiety, mood elevation, anticancer, antibacterial, and analgesic effects (Hartsel et al., 2016). Cedarwood, black pepper, rosemary, cloves, basil, oregano, lavender, cinnamon, and hops contain β-caryophyllene. β-Caryophyllene is the only terpene that directly, although weakly, binds to the CB2 receptor (CB2 agonist), making it a cannabinoid and terpenoid (Gertsch et al., 2008). Because this terpene is found in many food sources, it may also be considered a dietary source of cannabinoids. This terpene is also the primary scent that police dogs are trained to detect and is often associated with chemovars that are high in THC (Mudge et al., 2019).

Humulene

Humulene is a sesquiterpene known as α-humulene and α-caryophyllene, an isomer of β-caryophyllene (Hartsel et al., 2016). Humulene's aroma is earthy, woodsy, and spicy. Humulene's pharmacologic medicinal value includes reports of anorectic, anti-inflammatory, antibacterial, antineoplastic, and analgesic effects. Clove, sage, ginseng, black pepper, and hops contain humulene (Hartsel et al., 2016).

Linalool

Linalool is a monoterpenoid, and its aroma resembles lavender with hints of spice (Hartsel et al., 2016). Reported benefits of linalool are anti-inflammatory, antianxiety, antidepressant, antiepileptic, immune booster, and calming-sedative effects. Cinnamon, lavender, mint, rosewood, and birch trees contain linalool (Hartsel et al., 2016).

Terpinolene

Terpinolene is a monoterpene. Terpinolene's aroma resembles piney and herbal fragrances with floral hints, and reported benefits include antianxiety, anticancer, sedation, and cognitive clarity effects (Hartsel et al., 2016). Allspice, juniper, rosemary, sage, and tea tree contain terpinolene, which are often found in soaps, perfumes, and insect repellent.

Camphene

Camphene's aroma bears a resemblance to damp woodlands, fir needles, and musky earth (Hartsel et al., 2016). Camphene's pharmacologic medicinal value has the potential of reducing cholesterol and triglycerides in the blood, further lowering the risk of cardiovascular diseases. Also, if camphene combines with vitamin C, it becomes a powerful antioxidant (Hartsel et al., 2016).

Terpineol

Terpineol has three closely related monoterpenes, α-terpineol, terpinen-4-ol, and 4-terpineol (Hartsel et al., 2016). Terpineol's floral aroma of lilacs and apple blossom with a hint of citrus aroma is beneficial for antibacterial, antioxidant, calming, and sedative effects (Hartsel et al., 2016). Pine trees, balsamic resin, rosemary, basil, and eucalyptus contain terpineol.

Less prominent terpenes in cannabis

- **α-bisabolol:** found in chamomile flower and candeia tree; antibacterial and analgesic
- **Borneol:** found in rosemary, mint, and camphor; insect repellent, anticancer
- **Carene:** found in rosemary, basil, bell peppers, cedar, and pine; analgesic, improves memory
- **Eucalyptol:** found in eucalyptus; analgesic, antibacterial, and antifungal
- **Geraniol:** found in lemons and tobacco; neuroprotectant and antioxidant
- **Guaiol:** found in guaiacum and cypress pine; antibacterial and antioxidant properties
- **Ocimene:** found in mint, mangoes, basil, and orchids; anti-inflammatory, antiviral, and antifungal
- **Nerolidol:** found in jasmine, ginger, and lavender; antifungal, antioxidant, antimicrobial, and anti-inflammatory agents
- **Phellandrene:** found in cinnamon, garlic, dill, ginger, parsley, turmeric, and eucalyptus oil; antifungal
- **Pulegone:** found in rosemary; sedative and antipyretic
- **Sabinene:** found in black pepper and basil; antioxidant and anti-inflammatory
- **Trans-nerolidol:** found in jasmine, lemongrass, and tea tree oil; antiparasitic, antioxidant, antifungal, anticancer, and antimicrobial
- **Valencene:** found in Valencia oranges; insect repellant

Benefiting from terpenes in cannabis

Terpenes are fragile structures that quickly degrade in the presence of high temperatures. Although not well studied, heating terpenes and cannabinoids below combustion lessens the toxic by-products and reduces the typical 30% to 50% loss from smoking (MacCallum & Russo, 2018). The lower temperatures used in vaporization help preserve more of the cannabis plant's therapeutic compounds and reduce the consumption of harmful by-products and pulmonary irritation that occurs if heated to combustion (MacCallum & Russo, 2018). Patients may opt to vaporize or smoke cannabis because it offers more immediate relief of symptoms, and the therapeutic components enter the bloodstream rapidly (see Table 3.5).

TABLE 3.5.	Terpenes common in cannabis		
Terpenes	**Aroma**	**Vaporizes**	**Commonly found in**
Myrcene	Cloves, earthy, herbal	334 °F (168 °C)	Bay leaves, mango, lemongrass, thyme, hops
Limonene	Citrus (lemon, lime, oranges)	350 °F (176 °C)	Fruit rinds, rosemary, pine, juniper, peppermint
Pinene	Pine, fir trees	313 °F (155 °C)	Pine needles, rosemary, basil, parsley, dill, pine trees, balsamic resin, eucalyptus
Caryophyllene	Pepper, spicy, woody, cloves	268 °F (130 °C)	Black pepper, cedarwood, rosemary, hops, cloves, cinnamon
Humulene	Woody, earthy, spicy	222 °F (106 °C)	Hops, coriander, cloves, sage, black pepper, basil
Linalool	Floral, lavender, spicy	388 °F (198 °C)	Cinnamon, mint, rosewood, birch trees, lavender
Terpinolene	Pine, floral, herbal	365 °F (185 °C)	Nutmeg, tea tree, conifers, apples, cumin, lilacs, allspice, juniper, rosemary, sage
Camphene	Damp woodlands, fir needles, musky, earth	318 °F (159 °C)	Turpentine, camphor oil, citronella oil, ginger oil
Terpineol	Floral, lilac, apple blossom, citrus	426.20 °F (219 °C)	Pine trees, balsamic resin, rosemary, basil, eucalyptus
Ocimene	Sweet, herbal, woody	122 °F (50 °C)	Mint, parsley, pepper, basil, mangoes, orchids, kumquats

Adapted from Backes, M. (2017). *Cannabis pharmacy: The practical guide to medical marijuana.* Black Dog & Leventhal Publishers; The Merck Index Online. (2020). *Version: 2020.0.26.0.* https://www.rsc.org/merck-index

However, in 2019, it was found that some contaminants (eg, vitamin E acetate) in cannabis-based oil cartridges designed for vaping were causing injury and death because of e-cigarette or vaping-associated lung injury (EVALI) (Centers for Disease Control and Prevention [CDC], 2020).

Flavonoids

Flavonoids are a group of naturally occurring substances with variable phenolic structures and are commonly found in fruits and vegetables, and some grains, bark, roots, stems, flowers, tea, and wine (Panche et al., 2016). Flavonoids are secondary polyphenolic metabolites that have a ketone group with a yellowish pigment, and they can be divided into four main groups, including flavonoids, isoflavonoids, neoflavonoids, and anthocyanins (referred to hereafter simply as flavonoids) (Foundacion Canna, 2020). Flavonoids in plants are not only responsible for the color and aroma of plants, but they also help to attract pollinators, protect from ultraviolet light, and act as antimicrobial agents. They support the overall growth and development of the plant, while also protecting the plant from stressors by enhancing frost hardiness, heat acclimatization, and drought resistance (Foundacion Canna, 2020; Panche et al.,

2016). They also act as the plant's cellular cycle regulator (Foundacion Canna, 2020). There are currently around 6,000 identified flavonoids that contribute to the color and pigment of fruits, herbs, vegetables, and medicinal plants (Panche et al., 2016).

Flavonoids are known to be anti-inflammatory, antioxidative, antimutagenic, and anticarcinogenic (*in vitro*) as they modulate key cellular enzymatic functions, being potent inhibitors of some enzymes such as xanthine oxidase, cyclooxygenase, lipoxygenase, and phosphoinositide 3-kinase (Panche et al., 2016). Some studies indicate that a diet rich in flavonoids may diminish cancer risks (Foundacion Canna, 2020).

Flavonoids are used widely in the nutraceutical, pharmaceutical, medicinal, and cosmetic industries. They are also found in the cannabis plant (leaves and flowers, primarily in the trichomes with the cannabinoids and terpenoids) but not in the cannabis roots or seeds (Foundacion Canna, 2020). They make up a very small percentage of the plant's total weight (around 1%). Flavonoids in cannabis include cannflavin A, cannflavin B, cannflavin C, vitexin, isovitexin, apigenin, kaempferol, quercetin, luteolin, and orientin (Foundacion Canna, 2020). Most flavonoids found in the cannabis plant are water soluble. Their potential healing properties are listed in Table 3.6,

TABLE 3.6.	Flavonoids and healing
Cannabis flavonoid(s)	**Potential healing properties**
Cannflavins A, B, C (Unique to the cannabis plant)	• Anti-inflammatory: inhibits the prostaglandin (PGE-2) inflammatory pathway • Shared mechanism with other terpenoids; work synergistically
Vitexin and isovitexin	• Inhibit thyroid peroxidase • May support healing from gout
Kaempferol	• Antidepressant • Possibly synergistic with cannabinoids to enhance antidepressive capacity • May reduce risks of cancer and heart disease
Apigenin	• Stimulates monoamine transporter • Acts as an anxiolytic and sedative on the gamma-aminobutyric acid (GABA) receptors • Synergistic effects with cannabinoids
Quercitin	• Antiviral effects: inhibits viral enzymes • Anti-inflammatory: inhibits production of prostaglandins • Inhibits monoamine oxidase enzyme (MAO) (metabolizes neurotransmitter and many pharmaceuticals: consider caution with drug interactions) • Synergistic with cannabinoids to decrease inflammation
Luteolin and orientin	• Antioxidant • Anti-inflammatory • Antibiotic • Anticancer (preclinical trials) • Synergistic with cannabinoids

Adapted from Foundacion Canna. (2020). *Flavonoids*. https://www.fundacion-canna.es/en/flavonoids

and it is clear that many of the cannabis plant flavonoids interact with cannabinoids and terpenes to create synergistic effects.

Flavonoids derived from the cannabis plant are still understudied. Of interest, one particular flavonoid found in cannabis, FBL-03G, was found in animal models to have efficacy with treating both local and metastatic pancreatic tumor progression. In a study by Moreau et al. (2019), FBL-03G delivered directly to the tumor, with and without radiotherapy, inhibited growth at the site of delivery and the distant untreated sites. As most people diagnosed with pancreatic cancer already have metastases, the concept of using cannabis-derived flavonoids to support oncology care and treatment is promising.

The Whole Cannabis Plant: Entourage Effect

The synergistic nature of cannabis offers a vast array of combinations that can be manipulated through hybridization to fit specific therapeutic needs. The theory of "entourage" or mechanisms in which phytochemical properties (cannabinoids, terpenes, and flavonoids) work together to achieve optimal expression is not a new concept. In 1998, Ben-Shabat and a team of researchers (including the esteemed Raphael Mechoulam) discovered how endogenous esters influenced endocannabinoid activity only in combination. It is important to highlight that, although some research indicates the entourage effect is likely, we have not yet determined how this complex process works from an accurate physiologic perspective.

Initially, researchers postulated that terpenes might have a direct effect on cannabinoid receptors. Whole-plant medicine may offer the benefits of other cannabinoids and terpenes that work in a multifaceted manner to provide therapeutic effects from layered angles, whereas isolates provide a single compound. Consequently, pharmaceutical synthetics mostly use cannabinoid isolates or synthetic versions requiring much higher doses to reach the therapeutic threshold, ultimately increasing the adverse side effects (Russo, 2019). For full-spectrum products, cannabinoids and terpenes from the natural plant are also included. Full-spectrum CBD-rich compounds often lack high amounts of THC to avoid the euphoric effects. Best practice is to check the COA or lab testing to verify what the product offers.

In a recent study, Namdar et al. (2019) used various extraction methods (hexane, ethanol, ethyl acetate, or a combination of these products) to determine other constituents in flower varieties of high THC versus high CBD chemovars. Once the cannabinoid and terpenoid profiles were determined, using various combinations together or individually, the researchers tested cell cytotoxicity for two prominent cancer cells (MDA-MB-231 breast cancer; HCT-116 colorectal cancer cells). The phytocannabinoid and terpene groups that showed the most efficacy for cell cytotoxicity were in combinations that mirrored those found in the plant naturally (Namdar et al., 2019), indicating that these work in unison to exert their effects.

The most recognized combination for cannabis is how the two main cannabinoids, CBD and THC, work in different ratios to create different effects (Russo, 2011). There are various levels of synergy between phytocannabinoids and non-phytocannabinoids (eg, terpenes) (Russo, 2011). Other combinations, including terpenes known to have specific effects, may also enhance the effects of cannabinoids, which are described in this chapter.

Finlay et al. (2020) studied terpenes' relationship with the CB1 and CB2 receptors and found that the terpenes did not appear to have any direct receptor action or other mechanisms of action (eg, terpenoid–endocannabinoid metabolism). For example, do some terpenes assist in inhibiting the metabolism of cannabinoids, or do they simply work as any other essential oil would and enhance the work of cannabinoids? These are not the only ways terpenes and cannabinoids could work in concert and we anticipate future research findings.

Other Plant Cannabinoids and Cannabimimetics

Although we often think of cannabis as the primary source of cannabinoids, other plants also produce cannabinoids or chemicals that interact with our ECS and may support homeostasis. Cannabimimetics are defined as phytochemicals and secondary metabolites that interact with the ECS (Kumar et al., 2019). Although this list is not exhaustive, it does point the reader toward other plants that may also support people in their efforts to supplement their diets with cannabinoids and support the health of the ECS. These plants should also likely be further researched for their healing properties in relationship to ECS tone (see Table 3.7).

TABLE 3.7.	Other cannabinoid plants and cannabimimetics
Plant(s)	**Endocannabinoid action and therapeutic benefits**
Acmella oleracea (electric daisy)	• Contains *N*-isobutyl amides, stimulates CB2 receptor • Herb from the Amazon • Used in managing dental pain; numbs area • Antifungal, antioxidant, anti-inflammatory
β-Caryophyllene-containing plants • Black peppercorn • *Cloves* • *Copaiba* • *Lemon balm* • *Hops* • *Rosemary*	• CB2 weak agonist • Supports immune system function, may decrease inflammation
Black truffles	• Creates anandamide, which may interact with the endocannabinoid system (ECS)
Carrots *Daucus carota*	• Contains falcarinol (carotatoxin), binds to CB1 as an inverse agonist • Acts as a pesticide/fungicide in the plant
Catechins • Tea: *Camellia sinensis* (black, green, yellow, white tea)	• Moderate CB1 binding affinity • Anti-inflammatory, neuroprotective
Chocolate	• Contains substances that inhibit FAAH enzyme, which breaks down anandamide. Therefore, anandamide functions for longer within the ECS.
Coffee	• Enhances the activation of CB1 receptors to both exo- and endocannabinoids • May counteract stress-related downregulation of CB1 receptors • Regular consumption
Diindolylmethane	Binds to CB2 receptors as a weak CBS partial agonist Anticarcinogenic Supplement and found in cruciferous vegetables: broccoli, cauliflower, brussels sprouts, cabbage, kale

(continued)

TABLE 3.7.	Other cannabinoid plants and cannabimimetics (*continued*)
Plant(s)	**Endocannabinoid action and therapeutic benefits**
Echinacea	Plant's alkamides interact with CB2 receptors Supports immune system health Decreases inflammation Helps fight infection May help with anxiety and depression
Helichrysum	Contains cannabinoids Primarily cannabigerol (CBG) South African plant Research around efficacy with skin conditions
Kava Kava	Kavalactone yangonin binds to CB1 receptor and acts as an agonist to CB2 receptor Sedative and anxiolytic properties
Kriya Hops	*Humulus kriya* contains high levels of CBD (18%) Terpenes: humulene and β-caryophyllene Hops are the closest botanical relative of cannabis
Liverwort (Perrottetinene)	Selectively binds to CB1 receptor agonist delta-9-tetrahydrocannabinol (THC) structural analog
Palmitoylethanolamide	Enhances ECS activity by inhibiting FAAH, it potentiates anandamide Used in European countries as a supplement

Adapted from Gertsch, J., Pertwee, R. G., & Di Marzo, V. (2010). Phytocannabinoids beyond the cannabis plant—do they exist? *British Journal of Pharmacology, 160*(3), 523–529. https://doi.org/10.1111/j.1476-5381.2010.00745.x; Russo, E. B. (2016). Beyond cannabis: Plants and the endocannabinoid system. *Trends in Pharmacological Science, 37*(7), 594–605. https://doi.org/10.1016/j.tips.2016.04.055; Wilcox. A. (2016). 6 plants that contain healing cannabinoids. https://herb.co/marijuana/news/plants-contain-healing-cannabinoids.

SYNTHETIC CANNABINOIDS

Synthetic cannabinoids are chemicals structurally manufactured to mimic the desired effects of naturally occurring cannabinoids. In the United States, the FDA approved synthetic cannabinoids such as dronabinol (Marinol/Syndros) and nabilone (Cesamet) for medical use. Reported adverse effects for synthetic cannabinoids include an elevated heart rate, postural hypotension, nausea and vomiting, psychiatric symptoms (mania, schizophrenia, impaired thinking, depression, and unusual thoughts or behaviors), potential habitual abuse, and inability to drive and operate machinery safely (Backes, 2017; Johnson, 2019).

Dronabinol (Marinol and Syndros)

Dronabinol (Marinol/Syndros) is a synthetic drug manufactured to mimic the cannabinoid THC and is in capsule form suspended in sesame oil. As a Schedule III drug, it is recognized by the Drug Enforcement Administration (DEA) to have a low to moderate potential for abuse. Therapeutic use includes appetite and weight stimulant associated with acquired immune deficiency syndrome (AIDS) and treatment of nausea and vomiting (antiemetic) often experienced during cancer therapy (Backes, 2017; Burchum & Rosenthal, 2019).

Dosing and titration of Marinol

Marinol is available in 2.5 mg, 5 mg, and 10 mg capsules for oral use (Burchum & Rosenthal, 2019; Johnson, 2019). Dosing and titration depend on the patient's condition. For adult anorexia associated with AIDS, the starting dose of Marinol is 2.5 mg an hour before lunch and 2.5 mg an hour before dinner to stimulate the appetite. According to provider recommendations, titration may occur to fit the needs of the patient, but not to exceed 20 mg total per day (RxList.com, 2020). The typical effective dose is 2.5 mg 1 hour before lunch and dinner, totaling 5 mg/day. If unpleasant reactions occur, the patient could attempt to build tolerance by taking a single dose of 2.5 mg in the evening for a few days.

Marinol may be titrated for chemotherapeutic regime reduction of adverse effects. For the diagnosis of *Nausea and Vomiting Associated with Cancer Chemotherapy in Adult Patients Who Failed Conventional Antiemetics*, the recommended dosage is calculated using the patient's body surface area (m^2), with Marinol 5 mg/m^2 PO administered 1 to 3 hours before the onset of chemotherapy administration. An additional 5 mg/m^2 PO of dronabinol may be administered every 2 to 4 hours after chemotherapy, for a maximum of four to six doses/day (RxList.com, 2020). For elderly patients, who are at higher risk for central nervous system (CNS) side effects, one dose of Marinol 2.5 mg/m^2 PO administered 1 to 3 hours before chemotherapy is advised (RxList.com, 2020). Titration of Marinol for chemotherapy can occur in 2.5 mg increments, with 15 mg/m^2 dose and a range of four to six doses/day. Titration of Marinol may change for specific populations and individual differences related to tolerance of side effects.

Dosing and titration of Syndros

Syndros comes in a liquid form, and packaging includes a 5 mg/mL calibrated syringe. Syndros may be taken orally or administered through an enteral feeding tube size 14 Fr or larger. Syndros should be ingested with a glass of water when administered orally or flushed with water after administration into an enteral feeding tube (RxList.com, 2020).

For *Anorexia Associated with Weight Loss in Adult Patients with AIDS*, the starting dose for Syndros is 2.1 mg PO BID, 1 hour before lunch and 1 hour before dinner. All CNS side effects and adverse reactions are related to THC content. If the patient is having concerning side effects such as feeling high, dizziness, confusion, or somnolence, they may move toward a single dose of 2.1 mg PO daily, before dinner *or* at bedtime. It may take several days for the tolerance to develop and side effects to diminish. The dosage may be gradually titrated up to 4.2 mg PO BID as related to the relief of symptoms. The maximum daily dosage of Syndros is 8.4 mg BID (RxList.com, 2020).

Syndros for *Nausea and Vomiting Associated with Cancer Chemotherapy in Adult Patients Who Failed Conventional Antiemetics* (chemotherapy patients) dosage is calculated based on body surface area (m^2). The starting dosage is 4.2 mg/m^2 PO, 1 to 3 hours before chemotherapy administration. This dose may be repeated every 2 to 4 hours after chemotherapy for a total of four to six doses/day. For the elderly, the starting dose may be reduced to 2.1 mg/m^2. Syndros should be administered on an empty stomach for the first dose of the day. After the titration schedule is determined, Syndros should be administered under the same mealtime conditions (RxList.com, 2020). Dosage for chemotherapy can be titrated in increments of 2.1 mg/m^2 for therapeutic effect, up to a maximum dose of 12.6 mg/m^2/dose, administered four to six times/day. Adverse reactions are dose related, and the risk for psychiatric side effects and symptoms escalates as dosing escalates (RxList.com, 2020).

Nabilone (Cesamet)

Cesamet is a Schedule II drug with therapeutic uses indicated for the treatment of nausea and vomiting (antiemetic) associated with cancer therapy when antiemetics have failed to provide relief (Backes, 2017; Burchum & Rosenthal, 2019). *Nabilone* is chemically similar to THC and has similar therapeutic effects.

Dosing and titration of Cesamet

Cesamet is available in 1.0 mg capsules for oral use. The recommended adult dose is 1 to 2 mg, twice a day, with the initial dose to be given 1 to 3 hours before chemotherapeutic agents are administered. Doses may be administered BID or TID, with a maximum dose of 2 mg, leading to a total of 6 mg each day (Johnson, 2019).

Standardized Cannabinoid Pharmacologic Preparations

The following section considers the few available standardized cannabinoid pharmaceutical preparations available as prescriptions for patients. These differ from the synthetic cannabinoids in that they are manufactured using components from the actual cannabis plant.

Nabiximols (Sativex)

Sativex is available in multiple countries, including Canada, New Zealand, and the United Kingdom. Sativex can provide relief for adults with spasticity related to multiple sclerosis (Backes, 2017). Sativex is a standardized herbal cannabinoid preparation, including THC, CBD, other minor cannabinoids, terpenes, and flavonoids. Sativex is an oral mucosal spray, absorbed in the lining of the mouth (sublingual route). The adverse effects and drug interactions are similar to synthetic cannabinoids (Backes, 2017; Johnson, 2019).

Dosing and titration of Sativex

Sativex is available as an oral mucosal spray: each single 100 mL spray contains 2.7 mg THC and 2.5 mg of CBD for a near THC:CBD ratio of 1:1. The recommended initial dose for adults is one spray once a day, then titrated per instructions (see Table 3.8).

Epidiolex

Epidiolex is an FDA-approved oral solution for people aged 2 years and older in the treatment of seizures associated with Lennox-Gastaut Syndrome (LGS) or Dravet Syndrome (DS). Greenwich Biosciences held the US drug/chemical patent since 2013, and the FDA approved Epidiolex as a prescription for those suffering from LGS in 2018 (Greenwich Biosciences, 2020).

Epidiolex is a CBD extraction from stabilized cannabis plants for consistency purposes. Adverse effects may include decreased appetite, diarrhea, rash, infections, elevated liver enzymes, sleepiness, weight loss, suicidal thoughts, hypersensitivity reaction, and possible withdrawal symptoms upon discontinuation (Backes, 2017; Greenwich Biosciences, 2020; Johnson, 2019).

Dosing and titration of Epidiolex

The oral solution concentration is 100 mg/mL. The recommended initial dose is 5 mg/kg daily, divided into two doses. After the first week, the dose may increase to

	Number of sprays in	Number of sprays in	Total number of
TABLE 3.8.	**Titration of sativex sprays**		
Day	the morning	the evening	sprays per day
1	0	1	1
2	0	1	1
3	0	2	2
4	0	2	2
5	1	2	3
6	1	3	4
7	1	4	5
8	2	4	6
9	2	5	7
10	3	5	8
11	3	6	9
12	4	6	10
13	4	7	11
14	5	7	12

Adapted from Datapharm. (2020). *Sativex oromucosal spray.* https://www.medicines.org.uk/emc/product/602

a maintenance dose of 10 mg/kg, orally twice a day, with a maximum maintenance dose of 20 mg/kg daily (Johnson, 2019). If a child weighs 45 lb, it is converted to 20.4 kg. The initial daily dose is 102 mg (5 mg × 20.41 kg). If we then divide the dose into two separate doses, each dose would be about 51 mg. In a solution of 100 mg/mL, the amount drawn into the oral syringe is 0.51 mL and is to be given twice daily; however, at the time of writing this, the instructions are to round up to 0.55 mL. Packaging typically includes two 5 mL syringes; for a more accurate dose, a 1 mL syringe may be requested from a pharmacist. Always check the latest drug insert before calculating dose. The solution is administered to the inside of the cheek by gently pressing the plunger (Greenwich Biosciences, 2020). Reductions or changes in other seizure medications should only be made with the guidance of the patient's physician.

Nonpharmaceutical Synthetic Cannabinoids: Global Recreational Drugs

All synthetic cannabinoids contain chemical compounds that attach to cannabinoid receptors. Unregulated synthetic cannabinoids are now illicitly manufactured and have become recognized as part of the recreational drug mainstream, which has become a global health issue (MacLaren, 2020). Many unregulated synthetic cannabinoids are illegal at the federal level, and others are illegal, depending on state and local laws (CDC, 2018). Manufacturing of the compounds may modify the chemical composition, resulting in new and, therefore, presumably legal, available synthetic cannabinoid compounds on the market (CDC, 2018).

Initially, the development of unregulated synthetic cannabinoid compounds served the structural and functional study of cannabinoid receptors, but in recent years they have emerged as drugs of abuse (CDC, 2020). Sales appeared first in European countries in 2005, and in 2008 for the United States (Gurney et al., 2014). In 2015, the United States DEA's National Forensic Laboratory Information System seized drugs from local, state, and federal forensic laboratories and identified 84 new synthetic cannabinoids (Gurney et al., 2014). All 50 states have reported adverse health effects in persons reporting the use of these unregulated synthetic cannabinoids (Gurney et al., 2014).

The adverse effects of unregulated synthetic cannabinoids include a range of symptoms including temporary changes in mental status, tingling, tremors, slurred speech, inability to concentrate, anxiety, anger, agitation, sleepiness, delirium, paranoia, suicidal thoughts, violent behavior, and psychosis. Other physical symptoms may include tachypnea, tachycardia, hypertension, severe nausea and vomiting, chest pain and heart attack, stroke, seizures, rhabdomyolysis, kidney failure, and death (Gurney et al., 2014). Various factors may impact the emergence and severity of these symptoms, such as time between synthetic cannabinoid use, symptom onset, the route of exposure (inhalation, ingestion), and the amount consumed (Gurney et al., 2014). Unregulated synthetic cannabinoids may be addictive. Chronic consumers have reported withdrawal symptoms, inclusive of headaches, nausea and vomiting, severe anxiety, sweating, and trouble sleeping (Gurney et al., 2014).

An unregulated synthetic cannabinoid, known as "spice," is used as an illicit or party-club drug. Spice street names include AK-47, K2, Mr. Happy, Scooby Snax, Kush, and Kronic. During the manufacturing process, acetones, other solvents, or mind-altering synthetic chemicals are used to transfer chemical compounds onto shredded plant-like material or a herbal mixture that provides an appearance similar to cannabis (Gurney et al., 2014). The difference between synthetic cannabinoids and phytocannabinoids is that synthetic cannabinoids have seven-carbon tails and are full agonists at CB1, which are more potent than phytocannabinoids (ie, THC has five-carbon tails). Other dangers occur by ingestion or exposure to chemicals that may be toxic or contaminated during the manufacturing process, and the transfer process to the plant material may lead to improper or uneven absorption of the synthetic cannabinoid (Gurney et al., 2014). These unregulated synthetic cannabinoids may be delivered in mega doses to the user as they smoke, vaporize, or ingest the spice (Gurney et al., 2014).

Clusters of illness related to unregulated synthetic cannabinoid use are typically identified through emergency department visits or calls to poison control centers, which receive thousands of reports of adverse health effects in persons using unregulated synthetic cannabinoids annually (Gurney et al., 2014). The American Association of Poison Control Centers received the highest number of calls at 7,794 in 2015, reporting adverse health effects in persons using synthetic cannabinoids; that number dropped to 1,163 in 2019 (American Association of Poison Control Centers, 2020). Unregulated synthetic cannabinoid use has similar patterns of other drug abuse and is not limited to a specific demographic population; that number dropped to 1,163 in 2019 (American Association of Poison Control Centers, 2020). A significant number of unregulated cannabinoid users are people aged 20 to 30 years, with higher use seen in males than females (CDC, 2018). Unregulated synthetic cannabinoid users are often polydrug users (CDC, 2018). However, many people may use unregulated synthetic cannabinoids in an attempt to avoid a positive drug screen from a condition of employment, in a substance abuse treatment program, or the criminal justice system (CDC, 2018).

Diagnosing synthetic cannabinoid–related illness without a history of exposure can be difficult for health care providers, which may require them to make a clinical diagnosis, without a toxicology result. A history of exposure to synthetic cannabinoids does not always indicate that the symptoms are related to synthetic cannabinoid exposure.

Diagnosing synthetic cannabinoid adverse side effects through laboratory results may be difficult for many reasons. Synthetic cannabinoids are not detectable with standard drug screening panels (CDC, 2018). Several commercial laboratories offer to test for synthetic cannabinoids in patients' urine samples (Redwood Toxicology Laboratory, 2012). However, the panels are often limited and may not detect all synthetic cannabinoids (CDC, 2018). Furthermore, the test results may not be available to the health care provider in a sufficient time frame to make a medical diagnosis. Lastly, patients with a history of mental illness or prior history of drug abuse are at higher risk of developing severe adverse side effects from synthetic cannabinoid use (CDC, 2018).

Treatment and education considerations

Synthetic cannabinoid adverse side effects have no specific antidote (CDC, 2018). Different synthetic cannabinoids are associated with different adverse health effects, including agitation and delirium, cardiac arrhythmias, seizures, and renal insufficiency (CDC, 2018). There are supportive treatments if a person demonstrates more severe adverse effects from cannabis or synthetic cannabinoids such as intravenous fluids, supplemental oxygen, airway protection, antiemetic medications, and intravenous benzodiazepines (CDC, 2018).

Nurses and health care providers need to educate the public on synthetic cannabinoids and their influence on health. Consumers should beware of purchasing products that claim to be "spice" or "mamba." Many have described spice as dried leaves with the appearance of oregano and other herbs colored light green to brown depending on what is used. The aroma is different compared to whole-plant cannabis (CDC, 2018). Additional information, guidance about the management of patients with possible synthetic cannabinoid–related illnesses, and common adverse side effects can be obtained from the local or national poison center (American Association of Poison Control Centers, 2017).

PHARMACOKINETICS

Pharmacokinetics is the branch of pharmacology that describes how the body manages drugs from entering to exiting the entire system. The route in which the substance enters the body determines the path it takes to reach the mechanism of action. Ingredient solubility, chemical properties, amount consumed, substance strength, and individual characteristics also play a major role in the effects felt. Each route has different aspects to consider in identifying the best approach for the patient. For example, when a drug enters the gastrointestinal system, typically via the oral route, most of the substance is taken to the liver through capillaries of the hepatic vein portal. During the metabolism phase, the liver breaks the drug down before it reaches the bloodstream, potentially affecting the absorption of the therapeutic components of cannabis: this is also known as the first-pass effect. Before one can fully understand how the various routes and forms of cannabis differ, one must understand how cannabis progresses through the four stages of pharmacokinetics: absorption, distribution, metabolism, and elimination.

Absorption

Absorption relies on the route of administration and the chemical properties of the substance, which translates as the "bioavailability." Bioavailability is the fraction of a drug that reaches the bloodstream and is highly dose and route dependent. Routes of administration for cannabis include inhalation, oral, sublingual, dermal, ophthalmic, and rectal. Intravenous is rarely used and is reserved for clinical situations or trials.

Routes of Administration

Patients have different preferences regarding how they use medicinal cannabis, but it is important to understand how their choice may impact their experience. The following details should be considered when choosing among the various routes of administration.

Inhalation:
> Rapid effects
> Simple to self-titrate
> Avoids first-pass effect

Smoking:
> No chemical processing
> Easier to access
> Combustion increases toxins
> Some cannabinoids and terpenes lost

Vaporization:
> May use whole plant cannabis or oil extractions
> Potential for chemical additives in extractions
> Adjust temperature to target effects
> Fewer toxins without combustion

Oral:
> First-pass effect
> Highly variable among patients
> Long-lasting
> Harder to titrate
> Delayed onset

Buccal/Sublingual:
> Highly vascularized
> Rapid onset
> Avoids first-pass effect (if absorbed correctly)
> Easy to titrate
> Difficult to do without swallowing

Dermal:
> Avoids first-pass effect
> Topicals applied directly to site
> Patches offer steady dose over time
> Absorption reliant on ingredients

Ophthalmic:
> Direct application
> Preparations only for eyes
> Relief is short-lived

Rectal:
  Difficult to absorb
  Highly vascularized
  Absorption depends on ingredients
  THC will cause euphoria if properly absorbed

Table 3.9 summarizes absorption, bioavailability, onset, and duration related to the specific administration route.

Distribution

Distribution occurs as the cannabinoids enter the bloodstream and travel to highly vascularized areas of the body (heart, brain, liver, and kidneys) and the less vascularized tissues (skin, muscles, and fat). Most cannabinoids attach to protein molecules (lipoproteins) and are metabolized by the liver before reaching the bloodstream (Grotenhermen, 2003). However, the remaining cannabinoids are smaller in size and exit capillary walls easier than if they were attached to protein molecules. Malnourished individuals have fewer proteins in circulation, which results in increased free (unattached to proteins) (Lilley et al., 2017) particles available to move beyond the bloodstream, possibly increasing the effects. Drug interactions may also occur as they compete for the same amount of proteins in the bloodstream, causing stronger or longer effects, or weaker or shorter effects of either substance. Once the cannabinoids leave the bloodstream, they will find their way to cell receptors.

TABLE 3.9.	Variability of cannabis effects: administration routes			
Method	**Absorption**	**Bioavailability**	**Onset**	**Duration**
Inhalation	Lung/capillaries	THC 25%–31% CBD 13%–19%	5–10 min	2–4 h
Oral	Gastrointestinal/ small intestine	6%–20%	1–3 h faster w/food	5–8 h
Sublingual	Oral mucosa/arterial	20%–30%	15–45 min	6–8 h
Topical	Skin/localized	Varies	30 min to 2 h	~1–8 h
Transdermal	Skin/capillaries	CBD and CBN 10× more than THC	20 min	<48 h
Suppository[a]	Rectal/vascular[a]	13%–40%[a]	10–45 min[a]	2–8 h[a]

[a]Hemisuccinate used for absorption.
CBD, cannabidiol; CBN, cannabinol; THC, delta-9-tetrahydrocannabinol.
Adapted from Knox, D. G. (2020). Clinical due diligence: Drug interactions with cannabis and cautions for practitioners: A clinician's perspective. *Townsend Letter, 438,* 62–65. https://www.townsendletter.com/article/438-townsend-table-of-contents-january-2020/; Lucas, C. J., Galettis, P., & Schneider, J. (2018). The pharmacokinetics and the pharmacodynamics of cannabinoids. *British Journal of Clinical Pharmacology, 84*(11), 2477–2482. https://doi.org/10.1111/bcp.13710; MacCallum, C. A., & Russo, E. B. (2018). Practical considerations in medical cannabis administration and dosing. *European Journal Internal Medicine, 49,* 12–19. https://doi.org/10.1016/j.ejim.2018.01.004; Mechoulam, R., Parker, L. A., & Gallily, R. (2002). Cannabidiol: An overview of some pharmacological aspects. *Journal of Clinical Pharmacology, 42*(S1), 11S–19S. https://doi.org/10.1002/j.1552-4604.2002.tb05998.x

Metabolism

Metabolism is when the body turns a substance into metabolites that are easier to excrete (biotransformation). More prominent with oral routes of the first-pass effect, the liver utilizes CYP450 enzymes to break down THC into 11-OH-THC, then 11-COOH-THC, a more water-soluble metabolite (Lucas et al., 2018). The 11-OH-THC metabolite is a stronger CB1 agonist than THC, resulting in a more intoxicating experience. Oral administration is more unpredictable than other routes because of this first-pass effect. Additionally, many drugs are also metabolized by the CYP450 group enzymes, which could alter the intended effects of those substances. These are described in the Drug–Drug Interactions section of this chapter.

Inhibitors and inducers

Enzyme inhibitors are substances that reduce the effectiveness of the enzyme. The drugs that are metabolized by the inhibited enzyme will increase in circulation, which can increase or lengthen the effects of the drug that is metabolized by the inhibited enzyme. Enzyme inducers behave by causing faster metabolism of the drug, thereby reducing or shortening the effects of the drug (Sinclair, 2016). Enzyme inhibitors and inducers are mostly responsible for the drug-to-drug interactions and thought to have a role in the entourage effect.

Elimination

Elimination is how the body rids itself of substances through the urinary and gastrointestinal systems. The time frame for eliminating cannabinoids is highly dependent on the previous three steps of pharmacokinetics. Absorption and how cannabinoids reach the bloodstream rely on mechanisms such as the first-pass effect and route of administration. Distribution depends on circulation, particle size, route, and dose. Metabolism is dependent on the structure and health of the digestive system; route, first-pass effect, and the amount of competing substances (ie, pharmaceuticals) determine the efficiency of turning substances into easier to eliminate metabolites. Elimination is highly variable to each situation, and reports reflect different measures. For regular or chronic cannabis users, THC metabolites accumulate in the lipid-based (fat) cells, which take longer for the body to eliminate. The wide range of findings for total elimination could be that a person's body fat has a significant effect on how cannabinoids are stored, yet research has not consistently included body fat as a variable of elimination (Millar et al., 2018).

Drug testing

Drug testing for cannabis remains a reality in many workplaces, despite the movement toward the end of the era of cannabis prohibition. The shift away from testing for a broad range of active and inactive metabolites in urine should be considered and based on science. The "behavior" of cannabis-related actions must be defined to reduce overarching speculations that cannabis use is the suspected cause of unsafe workplace practices. If an employee exhibits erratic behavior posing safety concerns in the workplace and this behavior is reasonably suspected to be related to cannabis use, then testing blood concentrations (>5 ng/mL) of THC would be more appropriate. Some tests have a 50 ng/mL cutoff, which determines cannabis use in the past few days, whereas others use 20 ng/mL, which may measure THC for 77 days postconsumption. Additionally, other chemical characteristics can prolong the

TABLE 3.10.	Fun facts about: workplace drug testing

Over time, many workplaces adopted similar testing approaches as the federal requirements out of concerns related to liability. As the cannabis prohibition era ends, we see a movement toward fewer requirements around mandatory drug testing. In 2020, Nevada became the first state to lawfully ban most employers from using preemployment drug screening tests that assess cannabis use. The ban does not apply to firefighters, emergency personnel, drivers, and those who could adversely affect others' safety. New York City amendments were made to its Human Rights Law effective in 2020 that prohibits employers, labor organizations, and employment agencies from requiring prospective employees to submit to cannabis/delta-9-tetrahydrocannabinol (THC) testing as a condition of employment. This also excludes safety or security-related positions, transportation workers, and caregivers. This law does not supersede federal government position requirements nor collective bargaining agreements.

elimination half-life of cannabinoids and extend the detection window beyond other substances (Kulig, 2017). As mentioned before, body fat should also be considered in drug-testing practices.

Determinants of metabolite detection:

Extended detection: higher doses, oral administration, chronic use, slow metabolism, higher body fat.

Range for positive result: 20 ng is detected longer than 100 ng, not representative of recent use, or intoxication.

Test sensitivity: Detection windows may not represent newer, more sensitive testing methods.

The 1988 Drug-free Workplace Act was intended for federal employees, or private businesses with at least $100,000 worth of federal contracts, to require workplace drug testing (Kulig, 2017). The cutoff for a positive screen was any cannabinoid metabolite higher than 50 ng/mL, followed by confirmation of a 15 ng/mL concentration of THCA, the nonintoxicating precursor for THC (Kulig, 2017). For employees with a prescription for Marinol, verification can be achieved by testing THCV, which is present in plant-based cannabis, not Marinol (Kulig, 2017) (see Table 3.10).

PHARMACODYNAMICS

Cannabis pharmacodynamics describes how cannabis affects or causes physiologic changes in the body, much of which mimics our natural ECS, as described in Chapter 2. Here are some key points to remember about cannabis and how it interacts with the ECS.

Ligands

Ligands, or in this case cannabinoids, bind to CB1 or CB2 receptors to exert actions within the cell. Actions within the cell then cause a cascade of effects inside and outside the cell through transporters (Klumpers & Thacker, 2019). An agonist is a ligand that perfectly fits in the receptor opening—filling the entire void and causing a strong positive or negative effect. A partial agonist is a shape that partially fills the void, but not quite all the way, causing a weak positive or negative effect. An antagonist is when

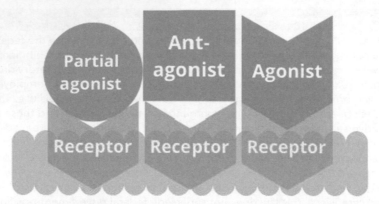

Figure 3.3: **Receptor site activity.**

the ligand blocks the receptor from all other shapes, preventing any effect even when the correct shape (ligand) is available. An allosteric modulator is when an enzyme interacts with another structure to change how the receptor and enzymes bind, causing stronger or weaker effects (see Chapter 2) (Figure 3.3).

Receptors

The two identified cannabinoid receptors are CB1 and CB2, although more novel receptors are likely to exist. Cannabinoids, much like our naturally occurring endogenous cannabinoids described in previous chapters (AEA; 2-AG), exert their action by connecting to CB1 and CB2 receptors, as described in Chapter 2.

CB1 receptors are more centrally located in the brain and spinal cord, although they are nearly nonexistent in the portion of the brain responsible for the cardiopulmonary functions of the body. The THC interaction with CB1 receptors is responsible for the intoxicating or euphoric effects of cannabis. CB2 receptors are more often peripherally located on immune cells. Cannabinoid and terpene combinations may enhance or dampen some effects of cannabis to provide better mechanisms of action to support homeostasis. This complex interaction of cannabis with the ECS is also known as the entourage effect (described earlier in this chapter).

A common misunderstanding is that THC is psychoactive, and CBD is not. Psychoactivity means being active within the CNS and often refers to changes in the way the brain functions by chemical mechanisms. CBD used for epilepsy is a perfect example of how CBD is thought to be psychoactive. Therefore, CBD is more accurately described as nonimpairing or nonintoxicating. Describing CBD as nonpsychoactive can be confusing for patients and others learning about cannabis-based medicines.

DOSING CONSIDERATIONS

One of the biggest challenges for practitioners when working with medical cannabis patients is supporting the proper dosing of cannabinoid medicines. Cannabis, particularly when accessed as whole-plant medicine, is self-titrating; therefore, doctors and advanced practice registered nurses (APRNs) generally refrain from writing precise dosing and chemovar recommendations, partly because of the lack of standardized

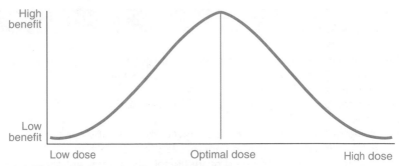

Figure 3.4: **The biphasic nature of cannabis medicine.**

production and distribution, with wide variations in potencies of the medicines as well. Some patients may need very little cannabis, and some may need substantial amounts of cannabis (Lee, 2019). As most medical doctors and APRNs have not been educated regarding medical cannabis, the issue becomes compounded by this lack of formal education around how to support patients in their ability to dose properly and to use cannabis safely and effectively, while also optimizing the results. However, there are several conventional approaches to supporting patients as they strive to find the right medicine, the right dose, the right route, and the right approaches.

Patients need to be aware that it is possible to get therapeutic effects from the medicine without getting "high," experiencing euphoria, or impairment because of the psychotropic effects. By starting low, going slow, and staying low with THC doses (MacCallum & Russo, 2018), the medical cannabis patient can alleviate symptoms, avoid the side and adverse effects, and optimize their use of medical cannabis.

Cannabis as a Biphasic Medicine

Cannabis medicine is biphasic in nature, which means that the medicine may have different effects at low versus high doses. For instance, a patient might feel relaxed and without anxiety when using a low dose of THC and experience anxiety and paranoia with higher doses of THC; higher doses of cannabis may create diminishing returns with escalating risks. In Figure 3.4, the reader can see that as cannabis and THC doses increase, there is a point of optimal beneficial effects, and yet, as doses increase beyond this "sweet spot," the benefits decline. With cannabis medicine, for many patients, less really is more.

Dosing and Titration of Cannabis: The MacCallum and Russo Approach

MacCallum and Russo (2018) stated that there is insufficient evidence to support medical cannabis patients starting their cannabinoid use with synthetic cannabinoids; if the patient can legally obtain cannabis in their state, they should start with a trial of whole-plant medicine. Tables 3.11 and 3.12 provide standardized ways that most medical cannabis patients can use to best support a safe and effective titration process.

The cannabis care nurse can share this published evidence-based approach to help coach and educate their patients toward success. Slow upward dosing also may allow

TABLE 3.11.	Titrating with inhaled cannabis

Inhalation:

- When available, patients should access cannabis flower tested for pesticides, molds, fungus, and heavy metals, with a certificate of analysis (COA) available.
- Start with one inhalation and wait 15 min.
- If needed, the patient may take one additional inhalation every 15–30 min, noting changes in symptoms.
- When symptom relief or palliation is achieved, the patient stops the inhalation process. The effects of inhalation generally last for several hours.
- The use of higher delta-9-tetrahydrocannabinol (THC)-dominant chemovars may allow for lower utilization of cannabis; however, patients should proceed with caution to avoid any unwanted effects of THC.
- The use of higher cannabidiol (CBD)-dominant chemovars may require the use of more cannabis to achieve symptom relief.

Adapted from MacCallum, C. A., & Russo, E. B. (2018). Practical considerations in medical cannabis administration and dosing. *European Journal Internal Medicine, 49*, 12–19. https://doi.org/10.1016/j.ejim.2018.01.004

for some tolerance for THC to develop, and by using CBD dominant chemovars, medical cannabis patients can get relief without the often undesired euphoria (MacCallum & Russo, 2018). Providers should educate patients on the risks and safety issues related to cannabis use, just as they would other psychotropic medications (MacCallum & Russo, 2018) (see Table 3.11).

For chronic conditions, longer-acting oral preparations are often the mainstay of treatment, with intermittent vaporization for acute exacerbations. Table 3.12 depicts

TABLE 3.12.	Titration of oral cannabis preparations

1. **Start with oral preparations, at bedtime.**
   Day 1–2: 1.25–2.5 mg THC
   Day 3–4: increase by 1.25–2.5 mg THC.
   Day 5–6: increase again by 1.25–2.5 mg THC every 2 days until symptom relief
   Side effects: reduce back to the best-tolerated dose.
2. **Add in daytime oral preparations if needed.**
   Daytime strategy, dose 2–3 times/day:
   Day 1–2: 2.5 mg THC once/day
   Day 3–4: 2.5 mg THC/BID
3. **Increase as tolerated.**
   Up to a max of 15 mg THC, divided BID or TID
   Doses: THC > 20–30 mg may increase adverse effects or cause tolerance with no increase in efficacy.
4. **Include CBD daily dose.**
   CBD: 5–20 mg, divided BID or TID

CBD, cannabidiol; THC, delta-9-tetrahydrocannabinol.
Adapted from MacCallum, C. A., & Russo, E. B. (2018). Practical considerations in medical cannabis administration and dosing. *European Journal Internal Medicine, 49*, 12–19. https://doi.org/10.1016/j.ejim.2018.01.004

a process that can help guide patients' self-titration with oral medications, such as tinctures and edibles.

In one study, most adult medical cannabis chronic pain patients used 1 to 3 g of *dried* herbal cannabis/day (please note this is flower weight, not dosage), with less than 5% of these patients using more than 5 g of *dried* herbal cannabis/day. Using this approach of 1 to 3 g of dried herbal cannabis/day, the group of 215 patients demonstrated that tolerance or the need for escalating doses of medical cannabis did not develop, and the dosing routines remained effective (Ware et al., 2015). MacCallum and Russo (2018) stated that the use of more than 5 g of *dried* herbal cannabis/day is likely unjustified except for primary cancer treatment.

A minimum of a 48-hour (or ideally longer) cannabis break or holiday can allow for a reset, and the patient may be able to experience symptom management using much lower doses. Taking regular cannabis holidays can also help support the patient in keeping cannabis doses low and allow for an opportunity to save on cannabis costs.

Backes (2017) suggested that for inhaling cannabis, the patient begins with just a match head size of cannabis, the typical amount to deliver one dose of cannabinoid medicine. According to Backes (2017), a cannabis cigarette, when smoked, will deliver about 27% of its THC content, whereas the use of a glass pipe leads to about 50% of THC being made available. In this way, delivery systems matter for patients who may be trying to optimize their use of cannabis as medicine and where finances are a concern, as cannabis is an expensive medicine that insurance typically does not cover. If a reliable lab has tested the cannabis, an inhaled dose may be calculated using the weight of the dose and the efficiency of the smoking method. For instance, one-thirtieth of a gram of dried herbal cannabis, having a THC percentage of 15%, would contain 5 mg of THC. If the patient uses a glass pipe, they expect to have about 2.5 mg of THC delivered, given the 50% efficiency. Cannabis should be inhaled and exhaled quickly, as holding the smoke in the lungs longer may do more damage and does not yield more THC absorption (Backes, 2017).

The formula for calculating THC dose in a sample of weighed dried herbal flower is:

- Convert grams (g) to milligrams (mg). Only use mg weight (1 g = 1,000 mg).
- Percentage of THC is used to calculate the approximate THC mg/weight of the flower.
- (X mg cannabis) × (% of THC) = mg THC in the flower by weight.

For patients making edibles, they are encouraged to use an online calculator to enter the weight of the cannabis used, the percentage of THC in the chemovar, and other variables associated with added ingredients, including the amount of alcohol or oil used within the infusion process.

Table 3.13 looks at more unscientific ways to estimate the THC dose or weight and commonly used weights for purchasing cannabis. Each state's medical cannabis law determines cannabis possession limits.

Figure 3.5 provides a visual representation of how dried cannabis flower appears in size. When considering calculating patient dose, or making edible preparations, actual weights of the cannabis should be obtained for accuracy.

TABLE 3.13.	Fun facts about: estimating cannabis doses		
Cannabis amount	**Looks like**	**Yields**	**Purpose of amount**
1 g *Commonly called a "G"*	The size of a large grape to the size of thumb, depending on density of the flower	1–3 cannabis cigarettes/"-joints"	Often used to "sample" personal effects of a particular cannabis chemovar
Eighth of an ounce *Commonly called "an eighth," "½ quarter," or a "slice"* = 3.5 g	The size of a walnut up to the size of a kiwi fruit depending on density of the flower	7, ½ g weight joints 14, ¼ g glass pipe "bowls"	Often affordable and convenient to purchase small amounts *Suitable for patients who use small amounts and can access flower regularly and with ease*
Quarter of an ounce *Commonly called a quarter, quad, or "Q"* = 7 g	Approximately the size of a small apple	14, ½ g weight joints 28, ¼ g glass pipe bowls	Useful for more frequent medicinal users or those who cannot access flower easily *Must be appropriately stored for longevity (low humidity, cool temperatures)*
Half of an ounce *Commonly called a half, or "half O"* =14 g	Approximately the size of a grapefruit or large orange	Yields many joints or bowls	This amount may be a good purchase for patients interested in cooking with cannabis, to making edible products
An ounce *Commonly called a "zip," "O," "Full O," or "Z"* = 28 g	Approximately the size of a coconut	May be used for cooking edibles	Most cost-effective way to purchase cannabis; must be stored properly

Adapted from Canuvo. (2020). THC dosage calculator. https://canuvo.org; Key to Cannabis. (2020). *What is an eighth, quarter, half or ounce of weed?* https://keytocannabis.com/what-is-an-eighth-quarter-half-or-ounce-of-weed-visual-guide/

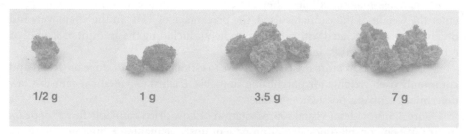

| 1/2 g | 1 g | 3.5 g | 7 g |

Figure 3.5: **Visual comparison of weights of dried herbal cannabis.** (Photo credit: Tim Hadley.)

Sulak Sensitization Process

On occasion, patients who find themselves using larger amounts of cannabis or those who have used cannabis from more of an adult use or "recreational" approach may find that they want to change their relationship with cannabis and find ways to have relief by using less medicine. Dr. Dustin Sulak has developed a cannabis sensitization protocol for such patients, which helps them lower their cannabis tolerance and optimize their cannabis use to the proper therapeutic dose. Keeping in mind the biphasic nature of cannabis as medicine and knowing that more cannabis does not mean greater therapeutic effect and may lead to diminishing returns, the program's goal is to help patients return to using cannabis in ways that optimize its interaction with the ECS. The full protocol with supportive worksheets and videos can be found here: https://healer.com/programs/sensitization-protocol/

Table 3.14 is a summary of the process.

TABLE 3.14.	Sulak cannabis sensitization protocol

Pre–Day 1: Track cannabis use and raise awareness of how much cannabis is being used. Review cannabis diary.

Day 1: Use cannabis as usual. At the end of the day, store away all cannabis products and associated ingestion tools (eg, vaporizers).

Day 2: Begin 48-h cannabis fast. Patients should be supported by eating endocannabinoid system (ECS)-enhancing foods, rest, voluntary exercise, and water.

Day 3: Goal to use a minimal amount of cannabis with the most therapeutic effect.
- Use intention and follow an inner inventory, where one walks through awareness of how the body feels, how the breath flows, and the mood (worksheet available online). Also, complete the inner inventory after cannabis is ingested.
- For inhalation: Take one inhalation and wait 5 min. Check inventory for any changes. Strive to feel the slightest of changes or enhancements. If no change at all is noted, have one more inhalation.
- For tinctures, take one administration at about ½ of the previously used dose. Wait 30 min and note any changes or enhancements in breath, body, and mood. Strive to feel the slightest of changes or enhancements. If no change at all is noted, have one more dose after the 30-min mark.
- Repeat up to 3 times/day.
- Continue to drink plenty of water, exercise, and eat ECS-enhancing diet.

Days 4–5: The goal remains the same, as does much of the process.
- Complete the inner inventory before and after use.
- Track progress.
- Go slow and wait the required time before repeating.
- Maximum use of 3 times/day.
- Continue to upregulate the ECS with water, exercise, ECS-enhancing diet.

Day 6: The goal is to find an optimal cannabis dose.
- Continue to use inventory and wait the recommended time between doses.
- Continue to upregulate the ECS with water, exercise, ECS-enhancing diet.
- The goal is to confirm the optimal dosage that relieves symptoms.
- Once an optimal dose is determined, cannabis can be used as needed without the waiting period between doses.

From Healer.com. (2015). *Cannabis sensitization 6 day protocol.* https://healer.com/programs/sensitization-protocol/

Successful Titration

For most patients using cannabis medicinally, the successful titration process means managing the euphoric effects. The sweet spot of dosing occurs when the dose is large enough to create therapeutic effects and small enough to avoid negative side effects. Although many people enjoy the euphoric feeling from cannabis, some do not, or they find it difficult to build tolerance for the THC effects. The person's sensitivity to THC is one of the main concerns when titrating cannabis.

Type I titration

Type I chemovars are THC dominant and may be quite intoxicating. Cautious titration with these chemovars is the best approach. Following the MacCallum and Russo (2018) protocol, the person must be careful to start low and go slow, as the small doses may also have greater effects at first, which may dissipate as the person develops tolerance and the biphasic effect happens. Less is more with this chemovar type, as the therapeutic range should remain around 15 mg of THC/day, divided into TID 5 mg dosing, with an equal balance of CBD (Lee, 2019).

Type II titration

When using chemovars with a more balanced THC:CBD ratio, the power of both cannabinoids can be maximized. CBD helps to decrease inflammation while also dampening the effects of THC. The CBD may also allow for lower THC doses to be used because of the therapeutic power of multiple cannabinoids working synergistically (Lee, 2019).

Type III titration

Type III cannabis is CBD dominant and generally is considered to be hemp plants. They will not have intoxicating effects. Whole-plant CBD will have different effects than CBD isolates, as isolates lack terpenes and the other cannabinoids that interact with the ECS. Full-spectrum CBD products tend to have a more significant therapeutic effect and window, whereas CBD isolates often require the patient to use more of the product and be more precise with dosing (Lee, 2019).

Selecting Chemovars

Chemovar selection for patients can be challenging. How does a patient find a chemovar to match their pharmacologic and healing needs? Ideally, this is where lab testing and the availability of cannabinoid and terpene profiles can help assist patients in determining what chemovar might best address their unique medical needs. Cultivar selection can be challenging, because factors from genetics to metabolism to THC tolerance can impact how the chemovar and the ECS interact, leading to different effects on each individual. Patients should, when possible, select products labeled with information around the cannabinoid and terpene profile. Ideally, a COA is available, which comes from third-party (lab) analysis and includes potency information (percentage of THC, THCa, CBD, CBDa), minor cannabinoids, terpene profiles, and also tests for pesticides, heavy metals, microbial (yeast and bacteria), and aflatoxins (indicates the presence of molds or fungi) (Project CBD, 2019).

With tinctures and edibles, patients look for labels that identify THC/CBD per serving and a definition of the serving size. Ideally, the patient can also select from stabilized varieties of cannabis where multiple lab analyses provide evidence that the cannabis product has consistently demonstrated the same chemical profile of active compounds; this occurs in some medical cannabis markets such as those in Germany and Canada. Unless a cannabis strain is stabilized and certified, the name or label is a poor indicator of the actual content and its potential effects (Weil, 2019).

Many patients will need to use a trial by error approach to select their medicine, including the following steps:

1. Patients should be supported or coached to review what the science says about their condition and specific combinations of THC, CBD, minor cannabinoids, and terpenes in relationship to palliating the symptoms of the condition.
2. Seek stabilized strains. These ideally come from a reputable cannabis distributor, which is also subject to regulations.
3. Consider what others have said or reported about the product and the producer. This sort of anecdotal information can be valuable but should not be the only consideration when selecting cannabis therapeutics.
4. Consult with a cannabis care nurse or other cannabis educator or coach if available for support with chemovar selection and titration process (Weil, 2019).

When selecting cannabis flower varieties or chemovars, one may also smell the plant. Although this seems to be reasonably nonscientific, we cannot underestimate the power of the terpenes' aromas and how they interact with our limbic system.

Pediatric Dosing

In the pediatric population, cannabis is most often used for seizure disorders, behavioral issues, perinatal brain injury, neuroblastoma, and as a palliative medication for oncologic treatments (Campbell et al., 2017). The American Academy of Pediatrics has recommended that the DEA move cannabis from a Schedule I drug to a Schedule II drug to be more easily researched. GW Pharma Ltd and Insys Development Company Inc have conducted clinical trials around using standardized cannabinoids to treat autism, DS, LGS, treatment-resistant epilepsy, pediatric schizophrenia, neonatal hypoxic–ischemic encephalopathy, infant spasm, fragile X syndrome, tuberous sclerosis complex, pediatric autoimmune neuropsychiatric disorders associated with streptococcal infections (PANDASs), cancer, and infantile spasms (Campbell et al., 2017; Goldstein, n.d.). The rationale for using medical cannabis with pediatric patients includes a favorable safety profile and tolerability, enhancement of quality of life and adherence with medical regimes, and support for palliation and compassionate care at end of life (Goldstein, n.d.).

It is suggested that for medically sensitive pediatric patients (as defined by currently using pharmaceuticals as part of the treatment plan with a diagnosed seizure disorder), CBD dosing would begin at 0.25 mg/lb/day in two to three divided doses (note that this dosing recommendation differs greatly from the Epidiolex dosing guidelines). **Caution: A knowledgeable health care provider should always be consulted prior to starting CBD with pediatric patients.**

The following formula would determine pediatric dosing for CBD for medically sensitive pediatric patients weighing less than 100 lb:

(weight in lb) × (mg/lb) = daily total mg

Daily total would then be divided equally between two and three administrations throughout the day.

For example, A patient weighing 50 lb

(50 lb) × (0.25 mg/lb) = 12.5 mg Daily Total

12.5 mg divided into two equal doses = 6.25 mg BID

For pediatric patients, sometimes THC and other cannabinoids may also prove beneficial for a given illness. All pediatric medicines should be lab-tested concentrates, with consistent profiles and sources (Goldstein, n.d.). Working with a physician or APRN specializing in cannabis care is the best way to ensure that the child and their family receive support and education around proper dosing and titration.

ADVERSE EFFECTS

One of the primary roles of cannabis care nurses is to ensure that patients can use medicinal cannabis safely and effectively. In turn, it may mean that nurses are aware of the contraindications, side effects, and adverse effects of cannabis. Although many people still believe that cannabis plants are completely safe, the reality is that cannabis is a potent medicine that can produce side effects (Backes, 2017). The THC intoxicating effects can be terrifying for the cannabis naive or novice user. A goal in cannabis care nursing is to support the patient in the safe, effective self-titration processes.

Common Adverse Effects

Cannabis's side effects are generally related to the THC-related euphoric effects, which is a reason to start low and go slow with dosing of THC. Combining CBD, limonene, and pinene with THC may help to mitigate some of the side effects (Backes, 2017). Mild and common side effects may include:

- Dry mouth and dry eyes (MacCallum & Russo, 2018). Staying hydrated and using moisturizing eye drops may help.
- Dizziness or light-headedness (Backes, 2017; MacCallum & Russo, 2018). Urge caution with movement and nighttime bathroom trips with the elderly or infirm.
- Coughing with inhaled products (Backes, 2017).
- Nausea (MacCallum & Russo, 2018).
- Mood changes: anxiety, euphoria, and/or cognitive effects.

More moderate and still common side effects, according to MacCallum and Russo (2018), include:

- Euphoria
- Blurred vision
- Headache

More severe and less frequent side effects or adverse effects:

- Tachycardia (MacCallum & Russo, 2018). With inhaled cannabis, this generally subsides quickly within 15 to 20 minutes, if other cardiac symptoms like chest pain accompany this, immediate emergency care should be sought (Backes, 2017).

- Orthostatic hypotension (MacCallum & Russo, 2018). Monitor blood pressure, caution upon standing by sitting first.
- Paranoia or psychosis (MacCallum & Russo, 2018). Discontinue use and seek appropriate care.
- Depression (MacCallum & Russo, 2018). Seek appropriate care.
- Cannabis hyperemesis syndrome (MacCallum & Russo, 2018). Discontinue use and seek appropriate care.

Overconsumption

If a person consumes too much cannabis, it will not be a fatal incident. Although the person may have seemingly severe symptoms that could develop into a sense of doom, no person has ever died from consuming too much cannabis (Backes, 2017). Overmedication or overconsumption usually occurs when cannabis is consumed by mouth or with edibles. Symptoms may include paranoia, anxiety, emotional distress, confusion, tachycardia, hallucinations, nausea, and vomiting (Backes, 2017).

If a child suffers from overconsumption, they should be brought to a hospital for treatment. Most adults can be managed at home with adequate hydration and rest. If the patient is able to eat, food may help support the person to feel grounded. They should be placed in a quiet environment with a trusted and supportive person to reassure them or hold their hand. They may alternately find a distracting activity like listening to music or watching a movie if it is helpful. In about 4 to 8 hours, the experience should dissipate (Backes, 2017). Although it has been said that CBD or chewing peppercorns may be helpful to dissipate the effects of THC, there are no data to prove this as a sufficient treatment for overconsumption.

Contraindications

There are some cases where cannabis is contraindicated or cautioned against, including:

- Pregnancy/lactation. Though cannabis has been used for centuries to support pregnant and lactating women, its use remains controversial, and we still lack strong studies demonstrating cannabis's efficacy with this population (MacCallum & Russo, 2018). Research for cannabis use during pregnancy and while breastfeeding has yielded inconsistent results thus far; attention to confounding factors such as tobacco or illicit drug use is also necessary to determine outcomes associated with cannabis use alone (Ryan et al., 2018). THC is, however, excreted in breast milk and can enter the placenta (Lucas et al., 2018). Thus, pregnant and breastfeeding women should avoid the ingestion of cannabis.
- Psychosis. Cannabis should also not be used during acute psychosis, though CBD preparations may be permissible (MacCallum & Russo, 2018). Use caution with schizophrenia, bipolar disease, and severe depression (Backes, 2017).
- Cardiac issues. Cannabis, particularly with high levels of THC or Type I cannabis, can cause tachycardia and hypotension; thus, it should be utilized with close monitoring and great caution in populations with unstable cardiac conditions like angina (MacCallum & Russo, 2018).
- Children and teens. The brain is still developing in these populations; thus, regular nonmedical use should be avoided; for medicinal purposes, risks and benefits must be weighed (MacCallum & Russo, 2018).

- Chronic obstructive pulmonary disease (COPD) and asthma. Avoid smoking (MacCallum & Russo, 2018).
- Substance use disorder. Although controversial, cannabis may be utilized as a harm reduction tool, and use should be weighed with risks and benefits (MacCallum & Russo, 2018).

Use caution with patients who have:

- Immune disorders. Patients undergoing medical treatments that compromise immune function should discuss cannabis use with the provider (Backes, 2017).
- Blood thinners. Closer monitoring of lab values may be called for and doses of medication adjusted accordingly (Backes, 2017).

CANNABIS USE DISORDER

"Cannabis abuse is considered to be an outdated term describing the continued use of cannabis despite impairment in psychological, physical, or social functioning" (Patel & Marwaha, 2019, p. 1). A better definition for people struggling with addiction issues related to cannabis is cannabis use disorder (CUD), and it is defined in the *Diagnostic and Statistical Manual of Mental Disorders (DSM)-V* by 11 patterns of pathology. Prolonged continuous use of cannabis can lead to anxiety and depressive moods. The *DSM-V* includes specific diagnostic criteria for cannabis intoxication, cannabis withdrawal, cannabis intoxication delirium, cannabis-induced psychotic disorder, cannabis-induced anxiety disorder, and cannabis-induced sleep disorder (Patel & Marwaha, 2019).

About 9% of the adult population who use cannabis may suffer from CUD, although the risk for CUD rises to 17% for adolescent cannabis users (Williams & Hill, 2019) (see Table 3.15).

TABLE 3.15.	Cannabis use disorder: *Diagnostic and Statistical Manual of Mental Disorders (DSM)-V* diagnostic criteria

A problematic pattern of cannabis use leading to clinically significant impairment or distress, as manifested by at least two of the following symptoms, occurring over a minimum of 12 mo:

1. Cannabis is often taken in more copious amounts or over a more extended period than was intended; difficulty containing use.
2. There is a persistent desire or unsuccessful effort to cut down or control cannabis use; failed attempts to discontinue or limit use.
3. A great deal of time is spent in activities necessary to obtain cannabis, use cannabis, or recover from cannabis's effects.
4. Craving, or a strong desire or urge to use cannabis. May include intrusive thoughts or images, or dreams about cannabis.
5. Recurrent cannabis use results in failure to fulfill role obligations at work, school, or home. Adverse consequences related to cannabis use.
6. Continued cannabis use, despite having persistent or recurrent social or interpersonal problems, caused or exacerbated by the effects of cannabis.
7. Important social, occupational, or recreational activities are given up or reduced because of cannabis use.

8. Recurrent cannabis use in situations in which it is physically hazardous or dangerous.
9. Cannabis use continues despite knowledge of having a persistent or recurrent physical or psychological problem that is likely to have been caused or exacerbated by cannabis (low motivation, chronic cough, anxiety).
10. Tolerance, as defined by either: (a) a need for markedly increased or progressively larger amounts of cannabis to achieve intoxication or desired effect or (b) a markedly diminished effect with continued use of the same amount of cannabis.
11. Withdrawal, as manifested by either (a) the characteristic withdrawal syndrome for cannabis or (b) cannabis or a similar substance is taken to relieve or avoid withdrawal symptoms.

Adapted from Patel, J., & Marwaha, R. (2019). *Cannabis use disorder*. StatPearls. https://www.ncbi.nlm.nih.gov/books/NBK538131/; American Psychological Association. (2013). *Diagnostic and statistical manual of mental disorders* (5th ed.). Author.

Risk factors for CUD may include family or personal history of chemical dependence, low socioeconomic status, cigarette smoking, traumatic childhood, sexual abuse, psychiatric issues (mood and personality disorders), antisocial behavior, impulsivity, early-onset anxiety disorders, other family members who smoke cannabis, and poor academic performance (Kosty et al., 2017; Patel & Marwaha, 2019; Williams & Hill, 2019). Interestingly, most CUD cases are associated with the onset of cannabis use in adolescence. This risk may continue to rise as they reach the 18- to 20-year-old range, then the CUD risk decreases. However, adolescents who continue to escalate use throughout their late 20s are the most at risk for CUD (Kosty et al., 2017). In one study, persistent CUD onset was generally well after high school, with later adolescence onset of use. The authors further noted that educational and occupational attainment might help to abate CUD (Kosty et al., 2017).

Treatment of CUD

Treatment begins with an assessment of use and a comprehensive psychiatric assessment (Williams & Hill, 2019). Williams and Hill suggested that using harm reduction techniques and gradually supporting the patient to lessen the use and move toward abstention may be more fruitful than going from a large amount of cannabis to no cannabis use. Outpatient treatment should address any ambivalence the patient feels toward being given the diagnosis; cognitive behavioral therapy, motivational interviewing, and psychosocial group approaches (Narcotics Anonymous) can prove helpful. Although many cannabis users may initially report using cannabis for comorbid issues such as insomnia or anxiety, cannabis use over time may worsen these symptoms because of rebound withdrawal (Williams & Hill, 2019).

There are currently no FDA-approved medical treatments for CUD. However, off-label use of some medications may be indicated; anticraving medications like naltrexone (50 mg daily), bupropion (150 to 450 mg daily), and the amino acid N-acetylcysteine (NAC) (1,200 mg twice daily) have all been explored as possible treatments for CUD (Williams & Hill, 2019). The person with CUD may find support from psychosocial groups such as Narcotics Anonymous or undertaking cognitive behavioral therapy. The person with CUD should also be worked up for other comorbidities such as anxiety disorder and treated appropriately.

DRUG–DRUG INTERACTIONS

Cannabis care nurses must be aware of drug–drug interactions between cannabis and both prescribed and over-the-counter medications to guide their patients toward using cannabis safely. Nurses should utilize resources that will enhance their coaching and educational efforts and help them support the patient when it becomes clear that drug–drug interactions could be impacting the patient's well-being. It is always important that the patient's primary and specialty health care providers are aware of the patient's choice to use cannabis for healing so that they can also ascertain any potential drug–drug interactions.

Cytochrome P450, Drug Metabolism, Cannabis, and CBD

Most cannabis drug–drug interactions are related to the various cannabinoid interactions with the liver's cytochrome P450 family of enzymes (Backes, 2017; Bornheim et al., 1993). CBD, although arguably one of the most commonly used cannabinoids, is the cannabinoid with the greatest interactions with the P450 enzymes, with potential interaction with approximately 60% of all medications (Backes, 2017). Serum levels of prescribed, over-the-counter, or supplement medications may increase with enzyme inhibitors or decrease with enzyme inducers (MacCallum & Russo, 2018). Additionally, the patient may experience the need for more or less cannabis based on the medications they are currently taking (see Tables 3.16 and 3.17).

Some years ago, it was discovered that grapefruit also interacts with the cytochrome P450 enzymes; therefore, any medication with a grapefruit ingestion warning may also be considered to have a CBD warning (Devitt-Lee, 2015). Additionally, the patient and provider should consider the potential for drug–drug interactions when high doses of CBD or CBD isolates are used are used in combination with drugs with a narrow therapeutic window or drugs that have serious and significant side-effect potential (Devitt-Lee, 2015).

TABLE 3.16.	Drug interference with oral cannabis: drugs that decrease effects of oral cannabis
Medication	**Purpose/treatment**
Amiodarone (Cordarone)	Arrhythmia management
Clarithromycin (Biaxin)	Antibiotic
Diltiazem (Tiazac, Cardizem, Dilacor)	High blood pressure/angina
Erythromycin (Roximycin, Ilosone, Acnasol)	Antibiotic
Fluconazole (Diflucan, Trican)	Antifungal
Isoniazid (Nydrazid, Rifamate)	Tuberculosis
Itraconazole (Sporanox)	Antifungal
Ketoconazole	Antifungal
Miconazole (Monistat)	Antifungal
Ritonavir (Norvir)	Human immunodeficiency virus protease inhibitor
Verapamil (Calan, Verelan, Isoptin)	Cardiac arrhythmias

Adapted from Backes, M. (2017). *Cannabis pharmacy: The practical guide to medical marijuana.* Black Dog & Leventhal Publishers.

TABLE 3.17.	Drug interference with oral cannabis: drugs that increase the effects of oral cannabis
Medication	**Purpose/treatment**
Carbamazepine (Tegretol, Equetro, Carbatrol)	Anticonvulsant
Phenobarbital	Sedative, anticonvulsant
Phenytoin (Dilantin)	Anticonvulsant
Primidone (Mylosine)	Anticonvulsant
Rifabutin (Mycobutin)	Mycobacterium avium complex (MAC) disease
Rifampicin (Rifampin, Rifadin, Rifater, Rimactane)	Antibiotic
St. John's Wort	Antidepressant (herbal)

Adapted from Backes, M. (2017). *Cannabis pharmacy: The practical guide to medical marijuana*. Black Dog & Leventhal Publishers.

MacCallum and Russo (2018) further stated that most medications could be used safely with cannabis. However, the most concerning drug interactions with cannabis are related to those drugs that are CNS depressants. Most current studies have not demonstrated toxicity or loss of effect of medications used while also consuming cannabis, except for clobazam with high-dose CBD, which requires a decrease in clobazam because of the production of a sedating metabolite (MacCallum & Russo, 2018). Benzodiazepines may also create an additive sedative effect with cannabis (Backes, 2017).

Websites to Check Drug–Drug Interactions

A website such as drugs.com can be used to look up drugs with major to moderate drug interactions with cannabinoids. At the time of this writing, drugs.com lists 24 significant drug interactions and 314 moderate interactions with cannabis (https://www.drugs.com/drug-interactions/cannabis-index.html). MacCallum and Russo noted that CNS depressants are the major class of drugs that interact with cannabis (2018). A reference list of drugs that interact with cannabis can be found on Drugs.com. Health care professionals should revisit resources as they may change over time. See Table 3.18 for the 23 drugs listed on the site as of September 2020.

TABLE 3.18.	Cannabis: major drug interactions	
Alfentanil		Morphine liposomal
Buprenorphine		Nalbuphine
Butorphanol		Oxycodone
Codeine		Oxymorphone
Dezocine		Pentazocine
Fentanyl		Propoxyphene
Hydrocodone		Remifentanil
Hydromorphone		Sodium oxybate
Levomethadyl acetate		Sufentanil
Levorphanol		Tapentadol
Meperidine		Tramadol
Morphine		

Cannabis may still be used safely with many of these drugs, including the opiate medications, but care should be taken to start low with THC doses and decrease other medications under the care of a prescribing health care provider.

Alcohol

Alcohol can increase the nervous system side effects of cannabis (Backes, 2017), including dizziness, drowsiness, and issues with concentrating, thinking, and judgment (Drugs.com, 2020). It is best to avoid the use of alcohol with cannabis, as both of these drugs exacerbate CNS effects.

Other Resources

- Chapter 7 of this textbook contains a table of some of the major drug interactions compiled by the author of that chapter.
- Project CBD website has many downloadable and updated readings regarding cannabinoid and drug interactions.
- Drugs.com allows the nurse to look up current cannabis and drug interactions.

CONCLUSION

This chapter provides a broad overview of the pharmacology of cannabis and implications for cannabis care nurses. This chapter also provides the cannabis care nurse with foundational information and begins to address the National Council of State Boards of Nursing (NCSBN [2018]) call for all nurses to understand cannabinoid pharmacology.

Although the nurse should work closely with the patient as a coach and educator to support them in the safe and effective titration and ongoing use of therapeutic cannabinoids, the nurse must understand their role and their scope and practice within their state. Working closely with patients to support their safe and effective use of cannabinoids is explored with more depth in the nurse's role chapter. Ideally, the nurse strives to coach the patient with their safe and effective use of cannabis by guiding them toward evidence-based best practices and navigating them toward the resources they might need to be successful.

Q&A QUESTIONS

1. Commonly prescribed drugs that can potentiate the effects of cannabis include:
   A. blood thinners
   B. antihypertensives
   C. narcotic pain relievers
   D. steroids

2. The most abundant terpene in the cannabis plant is:
   A. pinene
   B. myrcene
   C. terpinolene
   D. linalool

3. Most cannabis patients can adequately address their medicinal needs with how much *dried herbal cannabis plant*/day?
   A. 1–3 mg
   B. 3–5 g
   C. 1–3 g
   D. 5 g

4. When self-titrating cannabis for medicinal needs, in order to avoid adverse side effects, the patient should:
   A. be coached and educated around the self-titration process and the start low, go slow technique.
   B. use CBD to counteract THC effects.
   C. minimize all THC-containing products.
   D. be knowledgeable in all of the different available products to make the best choices.
   E. all of the above

5. According to MacCallum and Russo (2018), the maximum daily dosage for most patients using medical cannabis should be:
   A. 20–30 mg of THC divided into BID or TID dosing.
   B. 5–10 mg of THC divided into BID or TID dosing.
   C. 1–3 g THC divided into BID or TID dosing.
   D. 15 mg of THC divided into BID or TID dosing.

ANSWERS

1. Answer: C. narcotic pain relievers
2. Answer: B. myrcene
3. Answer: C. 1–3 g
4. Answer: E. all of the above
5. Answer: D. 15 mg of THC divided into BID or TID dosing.

References

American Association of Poison Control Centers. (2017). *Synthetic cannabinoids.* https://aapcc.org/track/synthetic-cannabinoids

American Association of Poison Control Centers. (2020). *Synthetic cannabinoid data: August 31, 2020.* https://piper.filecamp.com/uniq/oqxdcHUHKVLJNmZd.pdf

American Psychological Association. (2013). *Diagnostic and statistical manual of mental disorders* (5th ed). Author.

Aryal, N., Orellana, D. F., & Bouie, J. (2019). Distribution of cannabinoid synthase genes in non-cannabis organisms. *Journal of Cannabis Research, 1*(8), 1–6. https://doi.org/10.1186/s42238-019-0008-7

Backes, M. (2017). *Cannabis pharmacy: The practical guide to medical marijuana.* Black Dog & Leventhal Publishers.

Booth, J. K., & Bohlmann, J. (2019). Terpenes in cannabis sativa: From plant genome to humans. *Plant Science, 284,* 67–72. https://doi.org/10.1016/j.plantsci.2019.03.022

Bornheim, L. M., Everhart, E. T., Li, J., & Correia, M. A. (1993). Characterization of cannabidiol-mediated cytochrome P450 inactivation. *Biochemical Pharmacology, 45*(6), 1323–1331. https://doi.org/10.1016/0006-2952(93)90286-6

Brenneisen, R. (2007). Chemistry and analysis of phytocannabinoids and other cannabis constituents. In M. A. ElSohly (Ed.), *Marijuana and the cannabinoids.* Humana Press.

Burchum, J. R., & Rosenthal, L. D. (2019). *Lehne's pharmacology for nursing care.* Elsevier/Saunders.

Campbell, C. T., Phillips, M. S., & Manasco, K. (2017). Cannabinoids in pediatrics. *The Journal of Pediatric Pharmacology and Therapeutics, 22*(3), 176–185. https://doi.org/10.5863/1551-6776-22.3.176

Canuvo. (2020). *THC dosage calculator.* https://canuvo.org

Centers for Disease Control and Prevention. (2018, April 24). *Synthetic cannabinoids: A review for healthcare providers.* https://www.cdc.gov/nceh/hsb/chemicals/sc/healthcare.html

Centers for Disease Control and Prevention. (2020, February 28). *Outbreak of lung injury associated with the use of e-cigarette, or vaping, products.* https://www.cdc.gov/tobacco/basic_information/e-cigarettes/severe-lung-disease.html

Datapharm. (2020). *Sativex oromucosal spray.* Retrieved from https://www.medicines.org.uk/emc/product/602

DePetrocellis, L., Ligresti, A., Moriello, A. S., Allarà, M., Bisogno, T., Petrosino, S., Stott, C. G., & Di Marzo, V. (2011). Effects of cannabinoids and cannabinoid-enriched Cannabis extracts on TRP channels and endocannabinoid metabolic enzymes. *British Journal of Pharmacology, 163*(7), 1479–1494. https://doi.org/10.1111/j.1476-5381.2010.01166.x

Devitt-Lee, A. (2015). *CBD-drug interactions: Role of cytochrome P450.* https://www.projectcbd.org/medicine/cbd-drug-interactions/p450

Drugs.com. (2020). *Cannabis drug interactions.* https://www.drugs.com/drug-interactions/cannabis-index.html

Elsohly, M. A., & Slade, D. (2005). Chemical constituents of marijuana: The complex mixture of natural cannabinoids. *Life Sciences, 78*(5), 539–548. https://doi.org/10.1016/j.lfs.2005.09.011

Farrimond, J. A., Whalley, B. J., & Williams, C. M. (2012). Cannabinol and cannabidiol exert opposing effects on rat feeding patterns. *Psychopharmacology, 223*(1), 117–129. https://doi.org/10.1007/s00213-012-2697-x

Finlay, D. B., Sircombe, K. J., Nimick, M., Jones, C., & Glass, M. (2020). Terpenoids from cannabis do not mediate an entourage effect by acting at cannabinoid receptors. *Frontiers in Pharmacology, 11*(359), 1–9. https://doi.org/10.3389/fphar.2020.00359

Foundacion Canna. (2020). *Flavonoids.* https://www.fundacion-canna.es/en/flavonoids

García, C., Palomo-Garo, C., García-Arencibia, M., Ramos, J., Pertwee, R., & Fernández-Ruiz, J. (2011). Symptom-relieving and neuroprotective effects of the phytocannabinoid Δ^9-THCV in animal models of Parkinson's disease. *British Journal of Pharmacology, 163*(7), 1495–1506. https://doi.org/10.1111/j.1476-5381.2011.01278.x

Gertsch, J., Leonti, M., Raduner, S., Racz, I., Chen, J. Z., Xie, X. Q., Altmann, K. H., Karsak, M., & Zimmer, A. (2008). Beta-caryophyllene is a dietary cannabinoid. *Proceedings of the National Academy of Sciences of the United States of America, 105*(26), 9099–9104. https://doi.org/10.1073/pnas.0803601105

Gertsch, J., Pertwee, R. G., & Di Marzo, V. (2010). Phytocannabinoids beyond the cannabis plant—do they exist? *British Journal of Pharmacology, 160*(3), 523–529. https://doi.org/10.1111/j.1476-5381.2010.00745.x

Goldstein, B. (n.d.). *Medical cannabis: Practical treatment of pediatric patients for epilepsy, autism, cancer, and psychiatric disorders.* https://www.medicinalgenomics.com/wp-content/uploads/2016/05/Bonni-Goldstein-CannMed2016.pdf

Greenwich Biosciences. (2020). *Epidiolex.* https://www.epidiolex.com/about-epidiolex/story

Grotenhermen, F. (2003). Pharmacokinetics and pharmacodynamics of cannabinoids. *Clinical Pharmacokinetics, 42*(4), 327–360. https://doi.org/10.2165/00003088-200342040-00003

Gurney, S. M., Scott, K. S., Kacinko, S. L., Presley, B. C., & Logan, B. K. (2014). Pharmacology, toxicology, and adverse effects of synthetic cannabinoid drugs. *Forensic Science Review, 26*(1), 53–78.

Hartsel, J. A., Eades, J., Hickory, B., & Makriyannis, A. (2016). Cannabis sativa and hemp. In R. C. Gupta (Ed.), *Nutraceuticals: Efficacy, safety, and toxicity.* Elsevier.

Hazekamp, A., Tejalova, K., & Papadimitriou, S. (2016). Cannabis: From cultivar to chemovar II-A metabolomics approach to cannabis classification. *Cannabis and Cannabinoid Research, 1*(1), 1–14. https://doi.org/10.1089/can.2016.0017

Healer.com. (2015). *Cannabis sensitization 6 day protocol.* https://healer.com/programs/sensitization-protocol/

Hen-Shoval, D., Amar, S., Shbiro, L., Smoum, R., Haj, C. G., Mechoulam, R., Zalsman, G., Weller, A., & Shoval, G. (2018). Acute oral cannabidiolic acid methyl ester reduces depression-like behavior in two genetic animal models of depression. *Behavioural Brain Research, 351*, 1–3. https://doi.org/10.1016/j.bbr.2018.05.027

Johnson, S. (2019). *The endocannabinoid system and cannabis: The perfect partnership for self-regulation and healing.* Author.

Key to Cannabis. (2020). *What is an eighth, quarter, half or ounce of weed?* https://keytocannabis.com/what-is-an-eighth-quarter-half-or-ounce-of-weed-visual-guide/

Klumpers, L. E., & Thacker, D. L. (2019). A brief background on cannabis: From plant to medical indications. *Journal of AOAC International, 102*(2), 412–420. https://doi.org/10.5740/jaoacint.18-0208

Knox, D. G. (2020). Clinical due diligence: Drug interactions with cannabis and cautions for practitioners: A clinician's perspective. *Townsend Letter, 438*, 62–65. https://www.townsendletter.com/article/438-townsend-table-of-contents-january-2020/

Kosty, D. B., Seeley, J. R., Farmer, R. F., Stevens, J. J., & Lewinsohn, P. M. (2017). Trajectories of cannabis use disorder: Risk factors, clinical characteristics and outcomes. *Addiction, 112*(2), 279–287. https://doi.org/10.1111/add.13557

Kulig, K. (2017). Interpretation of workplace tests for cannabinoids. *Journal of Medical Toxicology, 13*(1), 106–110. https://doi.org/10.1007/s13181-016-0587-z

Kumar, A., Premoli, M., Aria, F., Bonini, S. A., Maccarinelli, G., Gianoncelli, A., Memo, M., & Mastinu, A. (2019). Cannabimimetic plants: Are they new cannabinoidergic modulators? *Planta, 249*(6), 1681–1694. https://doi.org/10.1007/s00425-019-03138-x

Lee, M. A. (2019). *CBD and cannabis dosage guide.* Project CBD interview with Dr. Sulak. https://healer.com/cbd-cannabis-dosage-guide-project-cbd-interview-with-dr-sulak/

Lilley, L. L., Rainforth-Collins, S., & Snyder, J. S. (2017). *Pharmacology and the nursing process* (8th ed.). Elsevier.

Lucas, C. J., Galettis, P., & Schneider, J. (2018). The pharmacokinetics and the pharmacodynamics of cannabinoids. *British Journal of Clinical Pharmacology, 84*(11), 2477–2482. https://doi.org/10.1111/bcp.13710

MacCallum, C. A., & Russo, E. B. (2018). Practical considerations in medical cannabis administration and dosing. *European Journal Internal Medicine, 49*, 12–19. https://doi.org/10.1016/j.ejim.2018.01.004

MacLaren, E. (2020). *The scary facts about designer drugs and legal highs.* https://drugabuse.com/the-scary-facts-about-designer-drugs-and-legal-highs/

Manayi, A., Nabavi, S. M., Daglia, M., & Jafari, S. (2016). Natural terpenoids as a promising source for modulation of GABAergic system and treatment of neurological diseases. *Pharmacological Reports, 68*(4), 671–679. https://doi.org/10.1016/j.pharep.2016.03.014

Mechoulam, R., Parker, L. A., & Gallily, R. (2002). Cannabidiol: An overview of some pharmacological aspects. *Journal of Clinical Pharmacology, 42*(S1), 11S--19S. https://doi.org/10.1002/j.1552-4604.2002.tb05998.x

Millar, S. A., Stone, N. L., Yates, A. S., & O'Sullivan, S. E. (2018). A systematic review on the pharmacokinetics of cannabidiol in humans. *Frontiers in Pharmacology, 9*(1365), 1–13. https://doi.org/10.3389/fphar.2018.01365

Moreau, M., Ibeh, U., Decosmo, K., Bih, N., Yasmin-Karim, S., Toyang, N., Lowe, H., & Ngwa, W. (2019). Flavonoid derivative of cannabis demonstrates therapeutic potential in preclinical models of metastatic pancreatic cancer. *Frontiers in Oncology, 9*(660), 1–8. https://doi.org/10.3389/fonc.2019.00660

Moreno-Snaz, G. (2016). Can you pass the acid test? Critical review and novel therapeutic perspectives of Δ^9-tetrahydrocannabinolic acid A. *Cannabis and Cannabinoid Research, 1*(1), 124–130. https://doi.org/10.1089/can.2016.0008

Mudge, E. M., Brown, P. N., & Murch, S. J. (2019). The terroir of cannabis: Terpene metabolomics as a tool to understand *Cannabis sativa* selections. *Planta Medica, 85*(9–10), 781–796. https://doi.org/10.1055/a-0915-2550

Namdar, D., Voet, H., Ajjampura, V., Nadarajan, S., Mayzlish-Gati, E., Mazuz, M., Shalev, N., & Koltai, H. (2019). Terpenoids and phytocannabinoids co-produced in cannabis sativa strains show specific interaction for cell cytotoxic activity. *Molecules, 24*(3031), 1–17. https://doi.org/10.3390/molecules24173031

National Council of State Boards of Nursing. (2018). The NCSBN national nursing guidelines for medical marijuana. *Journal of Nursing Regulation, 9*(2), S1–S60. https://www.ncsbn.org/The_NCSBN_National_Nursing_Guidelines_for_Medical_Marijuana_JNR_July_2018.pdf

Panche, A. N., Diwan, A. D., & Chandra, S. R. (2016). Flavonoids: An overview. *Journal of Nutritional Science, 5*, e47. https://doi.org/10.1017/jns.2016.41

Patel, J., & Marwaha, R. (2019). Cannabis use disorder. *StatPearls* [Internet]. https://www.ncbi.nlm.nih.gov/books/NBK538131/

Pertwee, R. G. (2006). Cannabinoid pharmacology: The first 66 years. *British Journal of Pharmacology, 147*, S163–S171. https://doi.org/10.1038/sj.bjp.0706406

Project CBD. (2019). *How do I choose a CBD product?* https://www.projectcbd.org/how-to/10-tips-for-buying-cbd

Redwood Toxicology Laboratory. (2012). *Synthetic cannabinoid testing—Urine.* https://www.redwoodtoxicology.com/docs/services/3370_sc_faq.pdf

Russo, E. B. (2011). Taming THC: Potential cannabis synergy and phytocannabinoid-terpenoid entourage effects. *British Journal of Pharmacology, 163*(7), 1344–1364. https://doi.org/10.1111/j.1476-5381.2011.01238.x

Russo, E. B. (2016). Beyond cannabis: Plants and the endocannabinoid system. *Trends in Pharmacological Science, 37*(7), 594–605. https://doi.org/10.1016/j.tips.2016.04.055

Russo, E. B. (2019). The case for the entourage effect and conventional breeding of clinical cannabis: No "strain," no gain. *Frontiers in Plant Science, 9*(1969), 1–8. https://doi.org/10.3389/fpls.2018.01969

RxList.com. (2020). *Marinol: Dronabinol capsules.* https://www.rxlist.com/marinol-drug.htm#description

Ryan, S. A., Ammerman, S. D., & O'Connor, M. E. (2018). Marijuana use during pregnancy and breastfeeding: Implications for neonatal and childhood outcomes. *Pediatrics, 143*(3), 1–15. https://doi.org/10.1542/peds.2018-1889

Salehi, B., Upadhyay, S., Erdogan Orhan, I., Jugran, A. K., Jayaweera, S. L. D., Dias, D. A., Sharopov, F., Taheri, Y., Martins, N., Baghalpour, N., Cho, W. C., & Sharifi-Rad, J. (2019). Therapeutic potential of α-and β-pinene: A miracle gift of nature. *Biomolecules, 9*(11), 738. https://doi.org/10.3390/biom9110738

Sinclair, J. (2016). An introduction to cannabis and the endocannabinoid system. *Australian Journal of Herbal Medicine, 28*(4), 107–117.

The Merck Index Online. (2020). *Version: 2020.0.26.0.* https://www.rsc.org/merck-index

United States Food and Drug Administration. (2020, March 11). *FDA regulation of cannabis and cannabis-derived products, including cannabidiol.* https://www.fda.gov/news-events/public-health-focus/fda-regulation-cannabis-and-cannabis-derived-products-including-cannabidiol-cbd

Vadivelu, N., Kai, A. M., Kodumudi, G., Sramcik, J., & Kaye, A. D. (2018). Medical marijuana: Current concepts, pharmacological actions of cannabinoid receptor mediated activation, and societal implications. *Current Pain and Headache Reports, 22*(3). https://doi.org/10.1007/s11916-018-0656-x

Ware, M. A., Wang, T., Shapiro, S., Collet, J. P., & Compass Team. (2015). Cannabis for management of pain: Assessment of safety study. *The Journal of Pain, 16*(12), 1233–1242. https://doi.org/10.1016/j.pain.2015.07.014

Weil, M. (2019). The different ways to choose a cannabis strain. *The Cannigma.* https://cannigma.com/treatment/how-to-choose-a-cannabis-strain-and-is-it-even-possible/

Wilcox. A. (2016). 6 plants that contain healing cannabinoids. https://herb.co/marijuana/news/plants-contain-healing-cannabinoids

Williams, A. R., & Hill, K. P. (2019). Cannabis and the current state of treatment for cannabis use disorder. *Focus, 17*(2), 98–103. https://doi.org/10.1176/appi.focus.20180038

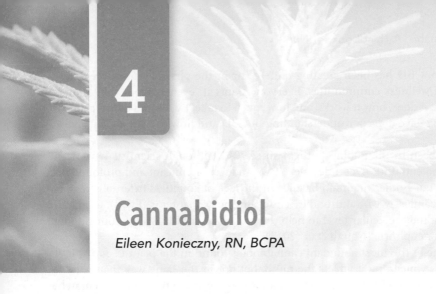

4

Cannabidiol

Eileen Konieczny, RN, BCPA

CONCEPTS AND CONSIDERATIONS

Cannabidiol or CBD has become a popularly used cannabinoid. You can find it online from hundreds of manufacturers, buy it from a dispensary, or see CBD gummies and tinctures displayed at the gas station check out. CBD interacts with many body systems, and nurses must be well educated to support patients' safe and effective use of this herbal medicine. This chapter provides readers with the information, science, and evidence that allow them to work effectively with patients using CBD.

Learning Outcomes

Upon completion of this chapter, the learners will:

- Understand the botany of, and differences between, industrial hemp and CBD-rich chemovars of *Cannabis sativa* L.
- Have a working knowledge of the current state of legalization of CBD in the United States.
- Have an understanding of CBD and the research associated with its use.
- Be able to identify the safety considerations for patient use of CBD.

CANNABIDIOL DEFINED

In the 2007 paper entitled "Cannabidiol—Recent Advances," Dr. Raphael Mechoulam and Professor Lionel Jacobson wrote, "CBD ... has been shown to produce a plethora of pharmacological effects, many of them associated with both central and peripheral actions.... The plethora of positive pharmacological effects observed with Cannabidiol makes this compound a highly attractive therapeutic entity in inflammation, diabetes, cancer, and affective or neurodegenerative diseases" (Mechoulam et al., 2007, p. 1678).

Since then, CBD has been creating quite a stir in the pharmaceutical, research, medical, and wellness communities. Everyone wants it, even without fully understanding what it does, how it works, and how much to take. By the end of this chapter, the reader will have a deeper understanding of CBD and how to help patients navigate its use.

CBD has been in the public spotlight since 2012, although scientists have been aware of its potential for over a decade. CBD produces significant and profound effects on how our bodies maintain balance in the face of countless external stressors by working seamlessly with our bodies' endocannabinoid systems (ECSs). Cannabinoids work at the molecular level to help the body heal, all the while producing no intoxication or euphoria (Naftali et al., 2013).

CBD is one of the most abundant cannabinoids found in the plant *C. sativa* L. It is psychoactive, meaning it affects the mind, but not in the same way that delta-9-tetrahydrocannabinol (THC) does. Dr. Ethan Russo suggested that "more accurately, CBD should be preferably labeled as 'non-intoxicating,' and lacking associated reinforcement, craving, compulsive use, etc., that would indicate a significant drug abuse liability" (Russo, 2017, p. 198).

CBD can be found in both cannabis and hemp plants. The genus *Cannabis* includes several closely related species. *C. sativa* L., known as industrial hemp, has many uses and generally contains less than 1% THC, whereas *C. indica* Lam., commonly known as "marijuana" or cannabis, averages between 13% and 30% THC (ElSohly et al., 2016).

C. sativa L. is an upright herb and one of humanity's oldest domesticated crops. All species of cannabis, regardless of whether it is a cannabis plant or a hemp plant, have the same structural features: stems, stalks, roots, flowers, and leaves. Female plants develop flowers. The flower is where the majority of the cannabinoids are developed. These flowers get very sticky, becoming covered with resinous glandular trichomes. These trichomes contain over 100 different compounds within them, which are designed to protect from grazing and insect predators as well as the ultraviolet (UV) rays from the sun.

Today, the classification of cannabis as either "marijuana" or hemp is based on a threshold concentration of THC. Although a level of 1% THC is considered a minimum value to elicit an intoxicating effect, current laws in the United States, Canada, and several other jurisdictions use 0.3% THC as the arbitrary threshold point at which cannabinoid content is used to distinguish cannabis strains of hemp from "marijuana" (Cherney & Small, 2016).

Throughout this chapter, the following definitions are used:

- CBD-rich plants, heavy with resinous flowers whose THC content is less than 0.3%, are **medicinal hemp.**
- Plants high in fiber or seed content with few flowers are **industrial hemp** or fiber-type.
- Plants heavy with resinous flowers whose THC content is greater than 0.3% are **cannabis** or THC-rich plants.

Industrial hemp, grown for fiber or seed, typically contains a much higher cannabidiolic acid (CBDA) to delta-9-tetracannabidiolic acid (THCA) ratio than do drug types of cannabis (the acid forms are the precursors to CBD and THC, respectively;

the acid forms of these cannabinoids are found in the plant before heating or processing). There are a large number of applications for this type of plant, from car parts to cooking oils, and clothing to body creams. Industrial hemp plants are genetically predisposed to grow tall and lanky with small flowers—using much of their energy for developing fibers or seed. The lack of flowers makes fiber types of hemp a less desirable crop for medicinal applications.

Medicinal hemp plants, on the other hand, are designed for phytochemical production. They grow short and bushy, with branches laden with flowers and, therefore, an abundance of therapeutic compounds. The cannabis industry has been busy developing new genetics of CBD-rich cultivars by cross-breeding medicinal strains of cannabis with industrial hemp plants to develop medicinal hemp strains with a THC content less than 0.3%.

Although it was discovered in 1940, we still have so much to learn about CBD. Since the beginning of cannabis research, THC has been the compound researchers have looked at the most. To better understand some of the regulations around CBD today, we need to take a look at how we got here.

A Brief Chronological Timeline

1940: In the laboratories of Roger Adams in the United States, CBD was separated as an isolated chemical compound from the cannabis plant probably in combination with CBDA (THC was not isolated until 1942). Adams was a prominent organic chemist at the University of Illinois, spending many years researching the chemical makeup of cannabis. Unfortunately, when they discovered CBD, they did not know what they had.

1946: Dr. Walter S. Loewe began trials on rabbits and mice using cannabinoids THC, CBD, and cannabinol (CBN). His research showed that THC caused catalepsy in mice, and CBD produced no observable changes. Findings in rabbits showed that THC caused a "central excitant action" in rabbits, whereas CBD did not.

1963: Dr. Raphael Mechoulam from the Hebrew University of Jerusalem identified the structure and stereochemistry of CBD.

The majority of research from the mid-1960s through the early 1970s focused on understanding the psychotropic properties of THC, with little emphasis placed on other cannabinoids (Figure 4.1).

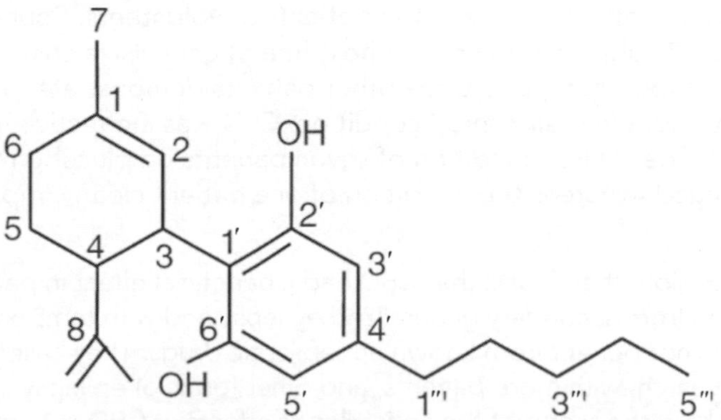

Figure 4.1: **Cannabidiol.**

1970: The Comprehensive Drug Abuse Prevention and Control Act of 1970, Pub.L. 91-513, 84 Stat. 1236, is signed into law. The Controlled Substances Act (CSA), Title II of the Comprehensive Drug Abuse Prevention and Control Act of 1970 is enacted, placing cannabis and all its cannabinoids within Schedule I, meaning they have no currently accepted medical use and have a high potential for abuse.

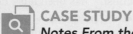 **CASE STUDY**
Notes From the Field

Ignored Research—1980 (Cunha et al., 1980)
    Dr. Mechoulam has said many times how disappointed he was that the results of this early research went unnoticed. As far back as the 1980s, it was understood that CBD had antiepileptic properties.

Phase 1 of the study
For 30 days, 16 healthy human volunteers, divided equally, were given either 3 mg/kg of CBD of placebo in a double-blind setting. Each week, each group underwent neurologic and physical examinations, blood and urine analysis, and ECG and EEG were also performed.

Phase 2 of the study
Fifteen patients with a diagnosis of secondary generalized epilepsy with temporal focus were randomly divided into two groups. This study was double blinded, and each group was given either 200 to 300 mg of CBD daily or placebo for as long as 4.5 months. At 15- or 30-day intervals, each group underwent neurologic and physical examinations, blood and urine analysis, and ECG and EEG. Patients remained on their prescribed antiepileptic medications even though they were not effective in controlling their disease.

Results
CBD was tolerated very well, and there were no signs of toxicity or serious side effects in any of the patients or volunteers. Four of the eight CBD subjects remained almost free of convulsive crises through-out the experiment, and three other patients demonstrated partial improvement in their clinical condition. CBD was ineffective in one patient. The clinical condition of seven patients on placebo remained unchanged, whereas the condition of one patient clearly improved.

Conclusion
In conclusion, they found that CBD had a beneficial effect in patients suffering from secondary generalized epilepsy and with temporal focus, who did not benefit from known antiepileptic drugs. They called for further research, with more patients, and other forms of epilepsy as needed to establish the scope of the antiepileptic effects of CBD in humans.

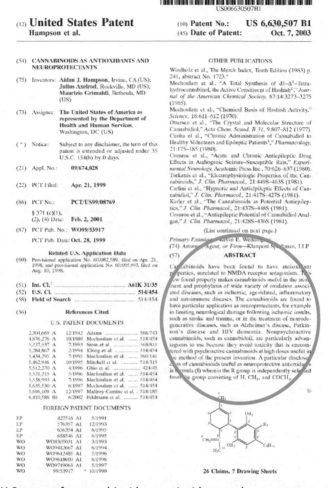

Figure 4.2: **U.S. patent for cannabinoids as antioxidants and neuroprotectants.**

1980: Dr. Mechoulam, in concert with a team from the Sao Paulo Medicine Faculty of Santa Casa, published the results of a phase 1 trial associated with CBD and epilepsy.

The year 1996 was the first in the United States where a state instituted its policy on the medical use of cannabis. California's Prop 15 allowed patients, with a doctor's recommendation, access to medical cannabis. Since that time, states began enacting their regulations, all with varying qualifying conditions and rules that govern the industry responsible for medicine.

2003: In October, the U.S. government patents cannabinoids for their antioxidant and neuroprotective qualities under Patent No.: US 6,630,507 B1 (Figure 4.2).

2013: GW Pharmaceuticals, a biopharmaceutical company focused on discovering, developing, and commercializing novel therapeutics from its proprietary cannabinoid product platform, begins phase 1 trials of a CBD-based epilepsy drug.

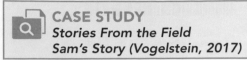

CASE STUDY
Stories From the Field
Sam's Story (Vogelstein, 2017)

Sam Vogelstein
Diagnosis: Hard-to-treat variant of epilepsy
Characteristics: Seizures; 5- to 20-second events where he would partially lose consciousness, eyes glaze over, jaw slackening, up to 100 events in a day
State of Residence: California
Story: Sam Vogelstein was diagnosed with a hard-to-treat variant of epilepsy when he was 4 years old. His parents Fred Vogelstein and Evelyn Nussenbaum tried multiple treatments and pharmaceuticals to help. They had also read anecdotal reports and literature on CBD's ability to treat seizures.

At the end of a long road of unsuccessful treatments, Evelyn learned that a nurse practitioner in one of their doctors' offices was starting a cannabis collective—outside of work—to help some of the physician's sickest children. Besides having a medical degree, the nurse was a herbalist. She had heard that cannabis—if made into oil-based tinctures, taken by the drop instead of smoked—could help people with intractable seizures. Evelyn liked the fact that the nurse sent her a 1980s paper from *The Journal of Clinical Pharmacology* on cannabinoids as potential antiepileptics. And she liked that the nurse assured her that the cannabis being used would not get anyone stoned. It would be high in CBD and low in THC.

They joined the collective.

Sam experienced success, but it was limited. His results varied from batch to batch.

These challenges surrounding reliable products sent Sam's parents looking for alternatives. Evelyn had read a study that had mentioned a British pharmaceutical company, GW Pharmaceuticals. At that time (2012), GW was one of only a handful of companies in the world doing legal, drug-company quality research on cannabis. Nussenbaum reached out to Geoffrey Guy, one of the company's cofounders.

She spent 4 months managing physicians and executives in two continents, navigating the intricate road of advocating for her son. One of the positive developments they learned is that the United Kingdom did not have the same regulatory oversights as did the United States. There, physicians can get promising medications for their patients directly from the manufacturer to be used under their direct responsibility; it was known as administering on a named patient basis.

Traveling to the United Kingdom, Sam became the very first person to take the drug that is now known as Epidiolex. Within days of using the medication, Sam's seizures virtually disappeared.

Today, Sam is seizure-free on a combination of Epidiolex and Depakote.

Speaking in front of a U.S. Food and Drug Administration (FDA) panel that was hearing testimony on whether to approve Epidiolex in April 2018, Sam said, "Now I can understand what goes on at school, and I can have adventures that never would have been possible before. I just went to South Africa for two weeks without my parents on a school trip. I had a bar mitzvah 18 months ago; I wouldn't have been able to do any of that if I hadn't tried this medication. It changed my life."

CASE STUDY
Stories From the Field
A Mother's Account

(Used with permission from Maa, E., Figi, P. (2014). *The case for medical marijuana in epilepsy. Epilepsia.* John Wiley and Sons.)
Charlotte Figi
Diagnosis: SCN1A, confirmed Dravet syndrome
Characteristics: Seizures, self-injury, violence, reluctance to make eye contact, autistic-like behavior
State of Residence: Colorado

A Mother's Account: Paige Figi

I had heard of a California parent successfully treating an epileptic child's seizure with cannabis, and because we live in Colorado, another state with legalized medical marijuana, I got busy doing research. I spoke with parents, doctors, scientists, chemists, marijuana activists, growers, medical marijuana patients, lawyers, and dispensary owners. The literature was confusing, with some papers suggesting that marijuana appeared to help seizures, and other papers suggesting that seizures got worse. What began to emerge, however, was interest in a less talked about component of marijuana, a phytocannabinoid called cannabidiol, or CBD.

It appeared to have no psychotropic properties, and the animal studies suggested that it might be very effective against seizures. Unfortunately, most people in the marijuana industry, as well as physicians, initially discouraged me from pursuing cannabis therapy, feeling that Charlotte was too much of a liability because she would be the youngest medical marijuana patient in the state at 5 years old.

Eventually, I found Joel Stanley, who, along with his brother, had dedicated themselves to breeding a rare, high-CBD strain of cannabis. After getting the green light from our team of epileptologists, pediatricians, and the reluctant state of Colorado, I started Charlotte on low doses of a sublingual preparation of the plant extract. I treated as I would with any antiepileptic drug (AED), starting low and slowly increasing the extract dose, keeping the THC content sufficiently low to avoid psychotropic effects. For the first time since her seizures started, Charlotte experienced 7 consecutive days without a single seizure!

With a baseline frequency of 300+ convulsions (generalized tonic-clonic [GTC]) per week, by month 3 of high-concentration CBD extract, Charlotte had a greater than 90% reduction in GTC seizures and had been weaned from her other AEDs. Now at 20 months after starting what the Stanley Brothers would eventually dub "Charlotte's web" (CW), Charlotte has only two to three nocturnal GTC seizures per month, is feeding and drinking orally and on her own, sleeps soundly through the night, and her autistic behaviors (self-injury, aggressiveness, self-stimulating behavior, poor eye contact, and poor social interaction) have improved. She has had only one episode of autonomic dysfunction associated with Dravet syndrome in the same time period. She is finally walking and talking again.

At first, it was too good to be true, but her control was so much better that we began to wean her off clobazam, which was the only medication she was taking at the time we started CW. By the end of the first month, she was entirely off clobazam and had only had three GTC seizures.

Several months later, we still could not believe that CW was working so well and started to slowly back down on the dose. When we reached 2 mg of CBD/lb per day (from her steady dose of 4 mg CBD/lb per day), Charlotte's seizures started coming back and when she was completely off the CW, her seizures returned to 5 to 10 GTC seizures per day for 3 days, at which time we restarted CW. To see whether the seizures would recur without CW, we have done this two other times and have had the same results each time.

On the basis of Charlotte's success, the Stanley Brothers created a nonprofit organization to address the needs of other patients with catastrophic epilepsy syndromes by helping them gain access to consistent, high-quality, laboratory-tested, high-CBD-content cannabis. They have successfully treated hundreds of patients. Families are moving from across the country and internationally to Colorado for treatment with CW.

2013: Sanjay Gupta's *Weed* documentary airs. Sanjay Gupta is an American neurosurgeon and an assistant professor of neurosurgery at Emory University School of Medicine and associate chief of the neurosurgery service at Grady Memorial Hospital in Atlanta, Georgia. He created a documentary to show why he "changed his mind on weed." The *Weed* documentary highlights the amazing story of Charlotte Figi, one of the youngest patients on medical cannabis in the country. After the documentary aired, parents across the country began advocating for access to medical cannabis in their states. Many families migrated to Colorado, to have access to CBD tinctures and oils because their states did not allow access to medical cannabis.

2014: GW Pharmaceutical gets investigational new drug (IND) designation from the FDA for approval of phase 2/3 trials for Epidiolex.

The United States saw a plethora of low-THC, high-CBD medical cannabis legislation across the country. Starting with Utah, other states such as Alabama, Kentucky, Wisconsin, Mississippi, Tennessee, Iowa, South Carolina, Florida, North Carolina, and Missouri all allowed access to state-regulated medicines high in CBD for patients with qualifying conditions. Qualifying conditions varied from state to state, but all had one common thread—epilepsy.

The 2014 Farm Bill U.S. Code § 5940 *Legitimacy of industrial hemp research* allowed for state-sponsored agricultural pilot programs that were partnered with institutions of higher education and state departments of agriculture to grow or cultivate industrial hemp and determine the economic viability of the domestic production and sale of industrial hemp.

2015: The U.S. Drug Enforcement Administration (DEA) eases regulatory requirements for those conducting FDA-approved clinical trials on CBD (DEA, 2015).

2016: GW Pharmaceuticals completes three positive phase 3 trials for Epidiolex.

The DEA established a new drug code for "Marijuana Extract," broadly defining the term as an "extract containing one or more cannabinoids that are derived from any plant of the genus *Cannabis*, other than the separate resin (whether crude or purified) obtained from the plant." CBD, regardless of its source, falls within this definition.

2017: The World Health Organization (WHO) officially recommended that CBD not be internationally scheduled as a controlled substance.

GW Pharmaceuticals' New Drug Application for Epidiolex is accepted.

2018: On June 25, GW Pharmaceuticals' Epidiolex received marketing authorization as an orphan drug by the FDA. It is now a Schedule V medication available by prescription. Epidiolex is a pharmaceutical formulation of highly purified, cannabis-derived CBD for the treatment of seizures associated with Lennox-Gastaut syndrome (LGS) and Dravet syndrome in patients 2 years of age or older.

On December 20, The Agricultural Improvement Act of 2018 Pub L. 115-334 (2018 Farm Bill) was signed into law, authorizing the production of hemp and removing hemp and hemp seeds from the DEA's schedule of controlled substances.

2019: The FDA held a public hearing on May 31, 2019, to hear from stakeholders regarding the soon-to-be-established guidelines on hemp products.

THERAPEUTIC BENEFIT

We are still uncovering the benefits and value of CBD as a medicinal tool. As of June 2019, a search in the U.S. National Library of Medicine, clinicaltrials.gov website, noted 191 studies on CBD associated with 309 different conditions ranging from acute graft-versus-host disease (aGVHD) to demyelinating disease. Being nonintoxicating, CBD is in great demand on several levels. Through new studies on the science of the entourage effect coupled with countless patient stories, it has been shown that CBD often works better with THC, even if it is only a minimal effect (Birdsall et al., 2016; McAllister et al., 2015; Ward et al., 2014).

THC and CBD share a special symbiotic relationship. They both offer potent anti-inflammatory and analgesic (pain-relieving) effects, but they do so through different mechanisms in the body and brain. CBD also famously mitigates some of the euphoric effects of THC, and with medicines containing high ratios of CBD:THC, the euphoria can be virtually nonexistent. CBD also prolongs the therapeutic effects of THC by delaying its breakdown by the body. This means a more robust overall effect.

SOURCE MATERIAL

The molecular structure of CBD is the same regardless of its source, cannabis or hemp. Understanding the botany of the plant, in regard to cannabinoid production, will help nurses ultimately to best understand issues with patients accessing quality legal CBD products. Both plants, although part of the same family, are genetically distinct in their ability to produce CBD.

Botany

Both cannabis and hemp are members of the same species, *C. sativa* L., which is one of humanity's oldest domesticated crops. Throughout history, cultivation and production of this plant have created a wide range of end products: foods, fabrics, paper, and other manufactured goods. Over thousands of years of genetic selection for function, coupled with varying growing environments, two distinct cultivars have emerged.

Let us take a look at the plant. *C. sativa* plants, regardless of whether it is a fiber or seed plant (hemp) or a medicinal plant (cannabis), all have the same structural features: stems and stalks, roots, flowers, and leaves (Figure 4.3).

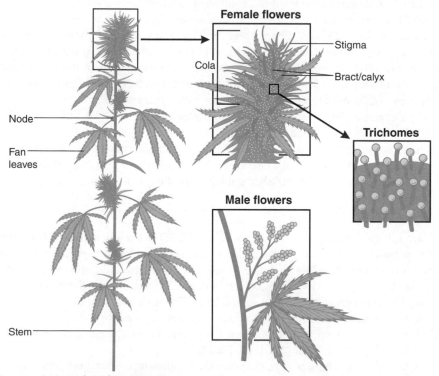

Figure 4.3: **Cannabis plant anatomy.**

TABLE 4.1.	Plant composition
Parts of the plant	**Percentage of cannabinoids**
Fan leaves	0.05%
Unfertilized flowers	Up to 30%
Capitate glandular trichomes	Up to 60%
Fertilized flowers	Up to 13%
Roots	0%
Stem and stalk	0.2%
Seed	0% + 35% essential fatty acids

Used with permission from Russo, E. B., & Marcu, J. (2017). Cannabis pharmacology: The usual suspects and a few promising leads. In D. Kendall and S. P. H. Alexander (Eds), *Cannabinoid pharmacology* (Vol. 80). Elsevier.

Cannabis is a tall, upright annual herb. The plant is generally dioecious, meaning seed stock can produce plants that are either male or female, whereas hemp varieties cultivated for fiber have been specifically bred to be hermaphrodite (monoecious). Industrial hemp plants are tall, sturdy plants grown for their fibrous stalk, seeds, and oil. Medicinal plants grow shorter and bushier, with multiple branches and flowers.

The leaves and flowers of *C. sativa* are covered, as is the entire plant, with tiny sticky hairs. These hairs, as with the hairs on so many other plant species, are almost microscopic spikes that develop on the plant's skin. The technical term for plant hairs is "trichomes." Trichomes are living cells that run the gamut in how they look and feel, getting classified as either "simple" or glandular.

The trichomes found on Cannabis are glandular trichomes. Within these trichomes, the biologically active compounds called phytochemicals—flavonoids, terpenoids, phenolic compounds, and cannabinoids—are found. This makes the female flower the most important plant part to those using it for medicinal and recreational purposes.

As the plant grows and develops, the chemical composition of the trichomes changes dramatically. The "chemical cocktail" found within the trichomes of each strain has a therapeutic effect that is unique to that plant. Both cannabis and hemp plants develop these trichomes; however, industrial hemp contains fewer and smaller flowers.

That said, CBD is the most abundant cannabinoid found in industrial hemp, but in amounts at or about 3.5% by dry weight. CBD-rich cannabis plants can have amounts as high as 20% CBD by dry weight, making this a more robust source for CBD medicines and wellness products.

Both hemp and cannabis products can be "full spectrum," meaning they contain CBD and THC in addition to the many other natural phytochemicals present in the plant. Hemp-derived extracts, by law, contain minimal amounts of THC (<0.3% by dry weight) (Table 4.1).

Utility

Industrial hemp has been used worldwide to produce a variety of industrial and consumer products. Industrial hemp is an excellent source of fiber and oilseed that is grown in more than 30 nations.

Cultivated industrial hemp plants usually consist of a spindly main stalk covered with leaves. Considered a low-maintenance crop, hemp plants typically reach between 6 and 15 feet in height. Depending on the purpose, variety, and climatic conditions, the period between planting and harvesting ranges from 70 to 140 days. One acre of hemp can yield an average of 700 pounds of grain, which in turn can be pressed into about 22 gallons of oil and 530 pounds of meal. The same acre will also produce an average of 5,300 pounds of straw, which can be transformed into approximately 1,300 pounds of fiber.

Industrial hemp may be an excellent rotation crop for traditional crops because it suppresses weeds and decreases outbreaks of insect and disease problems. Hemp may also rebuild and condition soils by replacing organic matter and providing aeration through its extensive root system. (Quote used with permission. © 2020 Agricultural Marketing Resource Center (AgMRC). www.agmrc.org.)

As with other plants, all cultivars of *C. sativa* take in nutrients and water from the soil. Cannabis is also a known bioremediatory, meaning it can remove pollution from its environment. This is a favorable characteristic, providing farmers with a rotational crop capable of pulling chemicals, pesticides, and heavy metals out of their soil. However, this is a positive only when these plants are not destined for human consumption because these toxins can remain in the plant if there is too much for the plant to digest, a process called "bioaccumulation." These toxins are held in their leaves, stems, stalks, roots, and flowers. When these plants are harvested and processed for consumption, these contaminants can be extremely hazardous to one's health, even at low levels (Potter, 2009).

One of the limiting factors of using industrial hemp for CBD-based products is that the bioaccumulation effects during extraction are compounded: It takes a lot of industrial hemp to get a little bit of CBD. This means that all things being equal, there would be comparatively more toxins in a hemp-derived CBD product than in a cannabis one. Without uniform regulations for heavy metal testing, consumers may be consuming products containing cadmium, lead, arsenic, or mercury—all of which pose serious health risks.

Best practices to ensure the quality of cannabis and/or hemp products should include testing for pesticides, heavy metals, mycotoxins, and microbes. "All these contaminants require monitoring because they can be introduced to cannabis products in the growth and/or processing stages of the plant, and consumers may be exposed to them. The toxicological effects of pesticides, heavy metals, mycotoxins, and pathogenic microbes are well-documented in the literature, including their carcinogenicity, neurotoxicity, and teratogenicity. Exposure to these contaminants through the consumption of cannabis products may lead to short- and long-term adverse health effects." (Used with permission from Craven, C. B., Wawryk, N., Jiang, P., Liu, Z., & Li, X.-F. (2019). Pesticides and trace elements in cannabis: Analytical and environmental challenges and opportunities. Journal of Environmental Sciences, 85, 82–93. Elsevier.)

Cannabis or hemp seeds are possibly the single most nutritionally complete food on earth and reportedly harbor powerful anti-inflammatory effects. Pollinated female flowers develop copious numbers of seeds. These have been collected by man over several millennia for their great nutritional value. They contain 35% protein as the digestible edestin and all of the essential amino acids. The seeds also contain 35% oil, rich in essential fatty acids in what is considered the ideal nutritional 3:1 ω-6:ω-3 ratio:75% linoleic acid (LA, ω-6), 25% linolenic acid (LNA, ω-3), and 9% γ-linolenic acid (GLA, ω-6) (Russo & Marcu, 2017).

The U.S. Department of Agriculture (USDA) has yet to promulgate federal regulations or approve state regulations relating to the cultivation and processing of hemp, and the FDA has not yet provided a clear path forward for the introduction of CBD and CBD-containing products into the marketplace. To ensure efficacy and consumer safety, a strong regulatory regime around hemp-derived CBD products would feature many of the same characteristics found in state-regulated cannabis or medical program, such as seed-to-sale track and trace functions, security requirements, product safety protocols, staff training, adverse event reporting, and recall procedures. Mandated laboratory testing would provide consumers in all states proof that their product is safe, reliable, and consistent.

CASE STUDY
Notes From the Field 2017/2018

Acute Poisoning From Synthetic Cannabinoid Sold as CBD
State of Residence: Utah
Story: On December 8, 2017, the Utah Poison Control Center (UPCC) notified the Utah Department of Health (UDOH) of reports of emergency department visits associated with reported exposure to products labeled as CBD. Five patients experienced adverse reactions, including altered mental status, seizures, confusion, loss of consciousness, and hallucinations. These reactions were inconsistent with known CBD effects, which prompted concern for potential adulteration.

State and federal health and law enforcement officials established a task force on December 11 to investigate cases and identify the source product. By the end of January 2018, there were 52 identified cases. Nine product samples (including one unopened product purchased by investigators from a store and a brand reported by a patient) were found to contain a synthetic cannabinoid, 4-cyano CUMYL-BUTINACA (4-CCB), but no CBD. Eight of the tested products were branded as "Yolo CBD oil" and indicated no information about the manufacturer or ingredients. Blood samples from four of five persons were positive for 4-CCB.

Press releases were distributed to media outlets dated December 19 to 21, 2017, with a warning regarding the dangers of using the counterfeit product; information with a description of the product and associated symptoms was disseminated to healthcare providers and law enforcement agencies. Hospitals and law enforcement agencies or persons experiencing CBD-associated reactions were asked to report any CBD-associated cases to the UPCC. Concomitantly, public health investigators searched UPCC's database and Utah's Syndromic Surveillance System as part of CDC's National Syndromic Surveillance Program for CBD-related events. UDOH interviewed patients over telephone, using a survey adapted from a synthetic cannabinoid investigation. The number of reported cases peaked during this outreach and dropped shortly thereafter. Thirty-four suspected cases were reclassified as confirmed if the person reported use of a Yolo product or laboratory testing found 4-CCB. Approximately one-quarter of persons were aged younger than 18 years, nearly three-fourths had vaped the CBD product, and approximately 60% were seen at an emergency department (Horth et al., 2018).

🔍 CASE STUDY
Notes From the Field 2018

8-Year-Old Boy
Diagnosis: Seizure disorder, not Dravet or LGS
Medication: Zonisamide (only antiepileptic medicines)
Characteristics: Seizure; 5- to 20-second events where he would partially lose consciousness, eyes would glaze over, jaw slackening, up to 100 events in a day
State of Residence: Washington State
State of Treatment: Oregon
Story: Parents discussed with their neurologist a trial of CBD oil. Although the parents lived in a state with retail, legal cannabis, and CBD products, they decided to purchase their CBD oil from what they believed to be a reputable online distributor from Colorado. After 9 days of seizure-free activity on the CBD oil, the boy was brought to the emergency room (ER) for evaluation, where within 24 hours he had 14 tonic-clonic episodes and intermittent agitation, delirium, depressed mental status, tachycardia, and mydriasis. The CBD oil was discontinued, with the physician sending off the remaining oil for testing. The patient was given midazolam in the ER for a tonic-clonic episode. Neurology was consulted, and the patient was given clorazepate and fosphenytoin for seizure control. Workup included magnetic resonance imaging (MRI) of the brain, electroencephalogram (EEG) monitoring, and lumbar puncture (LP). Within 2 days, the boy was baseline and discharged.

Analysis of the patient's CBD oil confirmed that it contained both CBD and AB-FUBINACA, a synthetic cannabinoid consistent with the boy's symptoms. Although the physician will not conclusively say that the contaminated oil caused the boy's symptoms, the symptoms that he exhibited are consistent with the drug's known effects.

The case study was published in the medical journal *Clinical Toxicology*. The physician declines to name the specific brand of CBD oil, but plans to enter it into the FDA Medwatch database (Rianprakaisang et al., 2019).

LEGAL ISSUES

Before the signing of the Agriculture Improvement Act of 2018 ("The 2018 Farm Bill"), on December 20, 2018, CBD, regardless of its source (cannabis or hemp), was held in Schedule I of the CSA. Language within this legislation effectively removed the CBD compound *procured from hemp* from the CSA, and federally recognized hemp as an agricultural commodity. It also made hemp production unlawful if done without a USDA license issued under a USDA plan or in a state without a USDA-approved industrial hemp production plan (National Institute of Food and Agriculture, 2019).

The following section sifts through the legal morass surrounding CBD, beginning with the international stage and moving toward implications for state and local restrictions.

International to Local Issues

International schedules encompass two treaties: the United Nations Single Convention on Narcotic Drugs (1961) and the United Nations Convention on Psychotropic Substances (1971). These two treaties provide the legal basis for the international prevention of drug abuse, together with the United National Convention Against the Illicit Traffic in Narcotic Drugs and Psychotropic Substances (1988) (WHO, 2017).

Since the signing of the Single Convention on Narcotic Drugs of 1961, all cannabinoids have been held within Schedule IV and Schedule I, concurrently. The Single Convention is the foundation for global drug control, guiding the production and supply of drugs, specifically narcotic drugs and other drugs with similar effects for medical treatment and research. The schedule includes:

Schedule I: Drugs liable to significant abuse and to produce ill effects, but have potential therapeutic uses (ie, cocaine, heroin, cannabis, morphine, fentanyl)

Schedule II: Drugs with somewhat lower abuse liability (ie, codeine, dextropropoxyphene)

Schedule III: Exempt preparations of drugs in Schedules I or II—specifically listed formulations (ie, codeine preparations when compounded with one or more ingredients and containing not more than 100 mg of the drug per dosage unit)

Schedule IV: Drugs in Schedule I that are particularly liable to abuse and to produce ill effects. Such liability is not offset by substantial therapeutic advantages (ie, cannabis, etorphine, heroin, and fentanyl analogs—only salts covered) (Lande, 1962).

The Commission on Narcotic Drugs and the WHO have the power to add, remove, and transfer drugs between the treaty's four schedules of a controlled substance. In November 2017, The WHO Expert Committee on Drug Dependence met in Geneva for its 40th meeting; on the agenda was a *"Critical Review of Cannabidiol."* The recommendation coming from that meeting was: "…that a footnote be added to Schedule I of the 1961 Single Convention on Narcotic Drugs to read: *Preparations containing predominantly cannabidiol and not more than 0.2 percent of delta-9-tetrahydrocannabinol are not under international control*" (WHO, 2017). They did this to remove CBD from the schedules. CBD would be unshackled from the strict international controls "of cannabis," inclusive of production and supply (WHO, 2017).

The WHO summary of cannabidiol:

> Cannabidiol (CBD) is one of the naturally occurring cannabinoids found in cannabis plants. It is a 21-carbon terpenophenolic compound which is formed following decarboxylation from a cannabidiolic acid precursor, although it can also be produced synthetically.
>
> CBD can be converted to tetrahydrocannabinol (THC) under experimental conditions; however, this does not appear to occur to any significant effect in patients undergoing CBD treatment.
>
> In experimental models of abuse liability, CBD appears to have little effect on conditioned place preference or intracranial self-stimulation. In an animal drug discrimination model, CBD failed to substitute for THC. In humans, CBD exhibits no effects indicative of any abuse or dependence potential.
>
> CBD has been demonstrated as an effective treatment of epilepsy in several clinical trials, with one pure CBD product (Epidiolex) currently in Phase III trials. There is also preliminary evidence that CBD may be a useful treatment for many other medical conditions.
>
> There is unsanctioned medical use of CBD-based products with oils, supplements, gums, and high-concentration extracts available online for the treatment of many ailments.
>
> CBD is generally well tolerated with a good safety profile. Reported adverse effects may be as a result of drug-drug interactions between CBD and patients' existing medications.
>
> Several countries have modified their national controls to accommodate CBD as a medicinal product.
>
> To date, there is no evidence of recreational use of CBD or any public health-related problems associated with the use of pure CBD. (WHO, 2017)

In the United States, all cannabinoids have been held within Schedule I since the schedule's inception in 1970. Schedule I drugs of the CSA are deemed to:

- Have a high potential for abuse.
- Have no currently accepted medical treatment use in the United States.
- Have a lack of accepted safety for use under medical supervision (DEA, 1970).

This is where CBD was scheduled, until the passing of the 2018 Farm Bill.

Historically, cannabis laws across the United States have been created by states exercising their rights and liberties observed under the Tenth Amendment, which declares, "the powers not delegated to the United States by the Constitution, nor prohibited by it to the States, are reserved to the States respectively, or to the people." California was the first state to flex its muscles when it came to the medical use of cannabis, passing legislation for medicinal use in 1996. As of this writing, there are 33 states with comprehensive medical cannabis legislation, with 11 states that have passed adult-use regulations. In addition, 12 states do not have a medical cannabis program, but allow for low-THC hemp-derived CBD products (Hanson, Karmen, & Garcia, 2019) including:

- Alabama
- Georgia
- Indiana
- Kentucky
- Mississippi
- North Carolina
- South Carolina
- Tennessee
- Texas
- Virginia
- Wisconsin
- Wyoming

This leaves patients across the country with varying degrees of access and product quality.

Living in 1 of the 11 adult-use states allows anyone older than age 21 access to a state-regulated dispensary, where they can purchase a variety of products with a multitude of cannabinoid ratios of CBD:THC. Living in a state with a medical cannabis program, access is limited to medical patients with a qualifying condition. Medical conditions that are covered vary from state to state, and proof-of-patient certification or a medicinal cannabis recommendation is required to enter a dispensary.

Most states with comprehensive cannabis and/or medical cannabis regulation require seed-to-sale tracking and product testing, adding a layer of oversight with product labeling, testing, and compliance.

In states with CBD-only laws, access to CBD is limited. Some states have allowed for interstate productions of products high in CBD, whereas others permit qualified patients to possess CBD products. Public approval of medical cannabis has remained above 77% since 2011, hitting 91% in January 2018. A 2017 survey of medical patient reports seems to be satisfied with the treatment they experience, with 72% reporting that they would be highly likely to recommend medical cannabis to friends or family for treatment (Statista, 2016).

With the production and acceptance of cannabis booming, the therapeutic benefits of CBD are increasingly being recognized. With that, we are seeing a tidal wave of CBD-infused products popping up everywhere: oils, creams, beverages, and even pet food. A handful of coffee shops in New York were adding a few drops of hemp-based CBD into the coffee served, for an extra $3.00 (Hemponair, 2019).

HEMP: CULTIVATION AND REGULATIONS

Understanding hemp cultivation and regulations across the globe will help one to understand the type and quality of imported products into the United States.

China appears to have had the longest continuous history of hemp cultivation (over 6,000 years). Since the 1990s, the cultivation of hemp restarted in Great Britain, then spread to the Netherlands, Germany, and throughout Europe (MIT, 2000). The European Union's regulations require the use of certified seeds of specified hemp varieties whose THC content does not exceed 0.2% (Food Safety—European Commission, 2019).

The gradual relaxation of regulations around the cultivation, processing, and production of hemp products coupled with the growing interest in CBD are contributing to the resurgence of hemp across the globe. The United States, in 2018, joined the ranks of the top six countries growing hemp:

#6—North Korea

Since the beginning of both North and South Korea's written history, traditional weavers turned hemp fiber into a fabric known as "sambe." North Korea continues to use hemp and even cultivates it on an industrial level. At least 47,000 m² of land is dedicated to hemp textiles in Pyongyang alone.

#5—Chile

Rules and regulations surrounding cannabis in Chile are quite strange. It is illegal to consume cannabis in public and forbidden to grow the plant on an industrial level. Yet, because there are no laws against private consumption and cultivation, many Chilenos take advantage of this. Within the Quillota Valley specifically, records of hemp cultivation go as far back as the year 1545. It has been used for many reasons, primarily for shipping and army support. However, some sources claim its main use is for seed oil production.

#4—France

France produced more than double the amount of hemp for the past few decades in comparison to all other European countries. The plant has mainly been used industrially for animal bedding, nautical applications, and textiles. As of 2017, France grew over 43,000 acres of hemp.

#3—The United States

With 78,176 total acres grown in up to 23 states, the country saw a massive expansion of industrial hemp cultivation. Right now, the vast majority of hemp in the United States is grown for CBD. Other forms of hemp, used in textiles, fabric, or hempcrete, are often imported.

#2—Canada

Health Canada, the federal agency in charge of distributing hemp licenses, reported that Canadian farmers saw an 80% increase in hemp production between 2016 and 2017, growing from 75,000 acres to 140,000. Harvest takes place primarily in three providences—Saskatchewan (56,000 acres), Alberta (45,000 acres), and Manitoba (30,000 acres). Most of this cultivation focuses on extracted seeds for hemp oils, hemp protein powders, and hulled hemp seeds (similar food to sunflower seeds).

#1—China

For some time, China has grown nearly 70% of the world's hemp. The earliest records of Chinese hemp use date as far back as the year 300 BCE. The main use for the plant, as with other countries on this list, was for fiber or survival food. In fact, after World War II, hemp saved many people from starving in areas of Northern China.

Not only did the Chinese government never place a ban on the plant but they also supported industrial growth, allowing hemp to prosper to an estimated 200,000 to 250,000 acres (James, 2019).

In 2009, a new hemp fiber processing plant was built in Dai Autonomous Prefecture in southern Yunnan. The factory, owned by China Hemp Industrial Holding Investment Co Ltd., has an annual capacity of 2,000 tonnes.

The United States remains the largest global importer of hemp products, which includes textiles from China, food and seed from Canada, and industrials from Europe (Hempbizjournal, 2017).

2014 Farm Bill Section 7606

In January of 2014, the American Farm Bureau Federation took a stance against the controlled substance classification of hemp, and a total of 10 states—California, Colorado, Kentucky, Maine, Montana, North Dakota, Oregon, Vermont, Washington, and West Virginia—had previously passed laws allowing hemp production.

Then, on February 7, 2014, President Obama signed the Farm Bill into law. Section 7606, Legitimacy of Industrial Hemp Research, defined industrial hemp as distinct from marijuana and allowed for state departments of agriculture or universities to grow and produce hemp as part of research or pilot programs.

Specifically, the law allowed universities and state departments of agriculture to grow or cultivate industrial hemp if:

1. "the industrial hemp is grown or cultivated for purposes of research conducted under an agricultural pilot program or other agricultural or academic research; and
2. the growing or cultivating of industrial hemp is allowed under the laws of the state in which such institution of higher education or state department of agriculture is located, and such research occurs." (USDA, 2019)

At least 41 states have enacted legislation to establish industrial hemp cultivation and production programs (NCSL, 2019).

The 2018 Farm Bill

On December 20, 2018, the Agriculture Improvement Act of 2018 (2018 Farm Bill) was signed into law.

> *This law changed certain federal guidelines and authorities relating to the production and marketing of hemp, defined as cannabis (Cannabis sativa L.), and derivatives of cannabis with extremely low (less than 0.3% on a dry weight basis) concentrations of the psychoactive compound delta-9-tetrahydrocannabinol (THC). It also removed hemp from the Controlled Substances Act, which means that it will no longer be an illegal substance under federal law.*
>
> *States and Tribes may impose additional restrictions or requirements on hemp production and the sale of hemp products, but they cannot interfere with the interstate transport of hemp or hemp products. Cannabidiol (CBD) derived from hemp is still undergoing evaluations for use as a food additive, and a determination has not yet been made relative to its use in products intended for consumption. There has been a small number of states, Maine, Massachusetts, NY, that have implemented regulations that prohibiting the sale of food and beverages infused with CBD. The FDA has indicated that hulled hemp seeds, hemp seed protein, and hemp seed oil*

are Generally Recognized as Safe (GRAS). The use of these hemp or hemp-derived products in food is legal (Gottlieb, 2018).

The Agricultural Marketing Service (AMS) was designated as the lead USDA agency to administer the new USDA Hemp Production Program. Under this bill, hemp cultivation in the United States will require licensing, either through the USDA or in accordance with a state plan developed by a state department of agriculture and approved by the USDA. At the time of this writing, the AMS is in the process of working toward developing regulations to implement the 2018 Farm Bill provisions. Until the final rule is implemented, all rules and restrictions must be followed per Section 7606 of the 2014 Farm Bill.

Food and Drug Administration

The FDA is a federal agency of the United States Department of Health and Human Services, one of the United States' federal executive departments. The FDA is empowered by the United States Congress to enforce the Federal Food, Drug, and Cosmetic Act (FD&C Act), which serves as the primary focus for the agency.

FDA recognizes the potential opportunities that cannabis or cannabis-derived compounds may offer and acknowledges the significant interest in these possibilities. However, FDA is aware that some companies are marketing products containing cannabis and cannabis-derived compounds in ways that violate the Federal Food, Drug and Cosmetic Act (FD&C Act) and that may put the health and safety of consumers at risk. The agency is committed to protecting public health while also taking steps to improve the efficiency of regulatory pathways for the lawful marketing of appropriate cannabis and cannabis-derived products (FDA, 2019).

Because CBD is an active ingredient in Epidiolex, an FDA-approved drug that was subject to substantial clinical investigations, hemp manufacturers cannot lawfully market food and dietary supplements containing CBD.

Epidiolex became the first FDA-approved drug that contains a purified extract from cannabis in June of 2018. It is a Schedule V medication available by prescription. Epidiolex is a pharmaceutical formulation of highly-purified, cannabis-derived cannabidiol for the treatment of seizures associated with Lennox-Gastaut Syndrome and Dravet syndrome in patients 2 years of age or older. This is GW Pharmaceutical's second plant-derived cannabinoid prescription drug. Their first cannabis-derived drug is Sativex (nabiximols), which is approved for the treatment of spasticity due to multiple sclerosis in numerous countries outside the United States. GW is in the process of working with the FDA to identify the optimal path to NDA submission for Sativex in the U.S. (GW Pharmaceuticals, 2019).

Another role of the FDA is to identify and take action against companies that are illegally selling unapproved CBD products that include claims to prevent, diagnose, treat, or cure serious diseases and target vulnerable populations. Part of this activity involves the FDA testing the chemical content of cannabinoid compounds in some of the products, and many were found to not contain the levels of CBD they claimed to contain. Since 2015, the agency has sent out dozens of warning letters to certain companies across the country, informing the companies that it has reviewed their websites and concluded that the companies have made unsubstantiated advertising claims, offered products that are unapproved, and misbranded new drugs sold in violation of the FD&C Act. A list of warning letters and associated companies/products can be found on their website.

According to estimates from the Brightfield Group, a leading predictive analytics and market research firm for the legal CBD and cannabis industries, CBD sales are expected to soar from $591 million globally in 2018 to $22 billion worldwide by 2022. Recently, nine major retailers across the United States are selling CBD-based products.

According to the FDA FAQ page, their position on cannabis and cannabis-derived ingredients in cosmetics is that:

> *A cosmetic is defined in 201(i) as "(1) articles intended to be rubbed, poured, sprinkled, or sprayed on, introduced into, or otherwise applied to the human body or any part thereof for cleansing, beautifying, promoting attractiveness, or altering the appearance, and (2) articles intended for use as a component of any such articles; except that such term shall not include soap."*
>
> *Under the FD&C Act, cosmetic products and ingredients are not subject to pre-market approval by FDA, except for most color additives. Certain cosmetic ingredients are prohibited or restricted by regulation, but currently, that is not the case for any cannabis or cannabis-derived ingredients. Ingredients not specifically addressed by regulation must nonetheless comply with all applicable requirements, and no ingredient—including cannabis or cannabis-derived ingredient—can be used in a cosmetic if it causes the product to be adulterated or misbranded in any way. A cosmetic generally is adulterated if it bears or contains any poisonous or deleterious substance which may render it injurious to users under the conditions of use prescribed in the labeling, or under such conditions of use as are customary or usual (section 601(a) of the FD&C Act [21 U.S.C. § 361(a)]).*
>
> *If a product is intended to affect the structure or function of the body, or to diagnose, cure, mitigate, treat or prevent disease, it is a drug, or possibly both a cosmetic and a drug, even if it affects the appearance. (See Question #3 for more information about drugs.)*
>
> *FDA can take action if it has information that an ingredient or cosmetic product is unsafe to consumers. Consumers can report adverse events associated with cosmetic products via the FDA's MedWatch reporting system, either online or by phone at 1-800-FDA-1088, or by contacting your nearest FDA district office consumer complaint coordinator (Figure 4.4).*

In March of 2019, CVS Health began to carry CBD topicals at roughly 800 of its stores spanning eight states. Walgreens Boots Alliance carries CBD-containing topicals in nearly 1,500 of its U.S. locations. Rite Aid plans to carry CBD products in two states (Washington and Oregon) (Duprey, 2019). Ulta Beauty is carrying five skin care products from Cannuka that blend CBD with manuka, a type of honey that is sourced from bees that pollinate Manuka trees. Ulta is currently able to sell these CBD skin care products in all but three states (Nebraska, South Dakota, and Idaho) where CBD laws remain very strict. GNC recently began selling a variety of CBD-infused topical creams of varying strengths (Williams, 2019). Designer Brands and Simon Property Group, the largest mall operator in America, have an agreement with Green Growth Brands to sell their CBD-infused products, creams, and balms.

CURALEAF, INC MARCS-CMS 579389 – JUL 22, 2019

fda.gov/inspections-compliance-enforcement–and–criminal–investigation/
warning-letters/curaleaf-inc-579289-07222019

Delivery method:

Via Overnight Delivery

Product:

Animal & Veterinary

Drugs

Recipient:

Joseph Lusardi

President

Curaleaf, Inc

301 Edgewater Place Suite 405 Wakefield, MA 01880 United States

Issuing Office:

Center for Drug Evaluation and Research

10903 New Hampshire Avenue, Silver Spring, MD 20993 United States

WARNING LETTER

VIA OVERNIGHT DELIEVERY

RETURN RECEIPT REQUESTED

July 22, 2019

Joseph Lusardi, President

Curaleaf, Inc.

301 Edgewater Place

Suite 405

Wakefield, MA 01880

RE: 579289

Dear Joseph Lusardi:

This letter is to advice you that the U.S. Food and Drug Administration (FDA) reviewed your website at the Internet address https://curaleafhemp.com_in April and June 2019 and has determined that you take orders there for the products "CBD Lotion," "CBD Pain – Relief Patch," "CBD Tincture" (5 versions), "CBD Disposable Vape Pen" (5 versions) and "Bido CBD for Pets" (3 versions), all of which you promote as products containing cannabidiol (CBD). *1* We have also reviewed your social media websites at and https://twitter.com/curaleafhemp; these websites direct consumers to you websites, https://curaleafhemp.com, to purchase your products. FDA has determined that your "CBD Lotion," "CBD Pain – Relief," "CBD Tincture," and "CBD Disposable Vape Pen" products are unapproved new drugs sold in violation of sections 505(a) and 301(d) of the Federal Food, Drug, and Cosmetic Act (the FD&C Act), 21 U.S.C 355(a) and 331(d). Furthermore, these products are misbranded drugs under section 502 (f) (1) of the FD&C Act, 21 U.S.C. 352 (f) (1). FDA has also determined that your "Bido CBD for Pets" products are unapproved new animal drugs that are unsafe under section 512 (a) of the FD&C Act, 21 U.S.C 360 b(a), and adulterated under section 501 (a)(5) of the FD&C Act, 21 U.S.C. 351 (a)(5). As explained further below, introducing or delivering these products for introduction into interstate commerce for such uses violates the FD&C Act. You can find the FD&C Act and FDA regulation through links on FDA's home page at www.fda.gov.

Figure 4.4: **FDA letter.** (www.fda.gov).

UNAPPROVED NEW AND MISBRANDED HUMAN DRUG PRODUCTS

Based on our review of your website, your "CBD Lotion," "CBD Pain-Relief Patch," "CBD Tincture," "CBD Disposable Vape Pen" products are drugs under section 201 (g)(1) of the FD&C Act, 21 U.S.C. 321 (g)(1), because they are intended for use in the diagnosis, cure, mitigation, treatment, or prevention of disease and/or intended to affect the structure or any function of the body.

Examples of claims observed on your website and social media accounts in April 2019 that establish the intended use of your products as drugs include, but may not be limited to, the following:

On your product webpage for CBD Disposable Vape Pen (Relieve):

- "[F]or chronic pain."

On your product webpage for CBD Tincture (Relieve):

- "[S]oothing tincture for chronic pain."

Additional claims observed on your website in June 2019 include, but are not limited to, the following:

On your Webpage titled "Can CBD Oil Used for ADHD?"

- "CBD oil becoming a popular, all-natural source of relief used to address the symptoms if many common conditions, such as chronic pain, anxiety…ADHD"
- "The benefits of CBD oil for ADHD… it's not usual for people with ADHD to feel anxious and on the edge. CBD is known for its anti-anxiety properties that can promote relaxation and stress relief. It can also help to restore focus and ability to concentrate on specific tasks, as well as reduce impulsivity."

On your webpage titled "How to Use CBD Oil for Anxiety"

- "CBD can successfully reduce anxiety symptoms, both alone and in conjunction with other treatments."
- "CBD oil can be used in variety of ways to help with chronic anxiety."

On your webpage titled "CBD Benefits Top 5 Research-Backed Benefits of CBD"

- "CBD has also been shown to be effective in treating Parkinson's disease."
- "CBD has been linked to the effective treatment of Alzheimer's disease…."
- "CBD is being adopted more and more as a natural alternative to pharmaceutical-grade treatments for depression and anxiety."
- "CBD can also be used in conjunction with opioid medications, and a number of studies have demonstrated that CBD can in fact reduce the severity of opioid-related withdrawal and lessen the buildup of tolerance."
- "CBD has been demonstrated to have properties that counteract the growth of spread of cancer."
- "CBD was effective in killing human breast cancer cells."
- "Heart disease is one of the leading causes of death in the United States each year, and CBD does a number of things to deter it. The two most important of these are the ability to lower blood pressure, and the ability to promote good cholesterol and lower bad cholesterol."

On your webpage titled "Hemp Oil vs. CBD Oil: Everything You Need to Know"

- "CBD… can be used to help manage a wide range of health conditions, such as…Anxiety and depression… Chronic or arthritic pain…"

Figure 4.4: (*continued*)

CANNABIDIOL INDICATIONS

Scientists continue to research focused on understanding the therapeutic effect of CBD. CBD has demonstrated anti-inflammatory, analgesic, antianxiety, and antitumor properties, among others (Mechoulam et al., 2007). Yet the mechanism of action remains unclear, regardless of all the attention it has gotten from the research community.

According to Morales et al. (2017), we do know that CBD:

• Lacks affinity for cannabinoid 1 (CB1) and cannabinoid 2 (CB2) receptors.
• With *in vitro* studies, there are weak antagonistic effects at CB1 and CB2.
• Is a negative allosteric modulator of delta-9-THC- and 2-AG.
• Inhibits cellular uptake of the endogenous CB1 ligand, anandamide, affecting endocannabinoid tone.
• Acts as an antagonist at the G protein–coupled receptor 55 (GPR55), preventing GTPγ S binding and Rho activation.
• Was inactive in Ca^{2+} mobilization assays and β-arrestin recruitment.
• Is antagonist of the putative cannabinoid receptor GPR18.
• Acts as a full 5HT1A agonist, a 5HT2A weak partial agonist and a noncompetitive antagonist of 5HT3A (serotonin receptors).
• Activates the A1A adenosine receptors.

As of July 31, 2019, www.clinicaltrials.gov lists 119 clinical trials examining CBD as an intervention for a variety of conditions. Of those 119 clinical trials, 27 are actively recruiting patients. The conditions and areas being researched are as follows:

1. CBD pharmacokinetics
2. Autism spectrum disorder
3. Post-traumatic stress disorder (PTSD)
4. Rett syndrome
5. Anxiety
6. Substance use disorder
7. Cocaine dependence
8. Withdrawal from addictive substances
9. Chronic pain
10. Pharmacokinetics, bioavailability
11. Epileptic encephalopathy
12. Parkinson's disease (PD)
13. Prader-Willi syndrome
14. Childhood absence epilepsy
15. Chronic pain, widespread
16. Prevention of aGVHD
17. Epilepsy
18. Fragile X syndrome
19. Drug-resistant epilepsy
20. Essential tremor
21. Schizophrenia
22. Atopic dermatitis
23. Psoriatic arthritis
24. Hand osteoarthritis
25. Pain
26. Drug abuse

The following sections highlight the health concerns, symptoms, and conditions that currently have the most evidence backing up the use of cannabis-derived CBD medicines.

Table 4.2 provides an overview of diseases for which CBD may have therapeutic benefits (Pisanti et al., 2017).

TABLE 4.2.	CBD and therapeutic effects
Disease	**Effects**
Alzheimer's disease	Anti-inflammatory, antioxidant, antiapoptotic *in vitro* and *in vivo* models of A-β-evoked neuroinflammatory and neurodegenerative responses
Parkinson's disease	Attenuation of the dopaminergic impairment *in vivo*; neuroprotection; improvement of psychiatric rating and reduction of agitation, nightmare, and aggressive behavior in patients
Multiple sclerosis	Improved signs of experimental autoimmune encephalomyelitis (EAE) in mice, anti-inflammatory and immunomodulatory properties
Huntington's disease	Neuroprotective and antioxidant in mice transgenic models; no significant clinically important differences in patients
Hypoxia-ischemia injury	Short-term neuroprotective effects; inhibition of excitotoxicity, oxidative stress, and inflammation *in vitro* and in rodent models
Pain	Analgesic effect in patients with neuropathic pain resistant to other treatments
Psychosis	Attenuation of the behavioral and glial changes in animal models of schizophrenia; antipsychotic properties on ketamine-induced symptoms
Anxiety	Reduction of muscular tension, restlessness, fatigue, problems in concentration, improvement of social interactions in rodent models of anxiety and stress; reduced social anxiety in patients
Depression	Antidepressant effect in genetic rodent model of depression
Cancer	Antiproliferative and anti-invasive actions in a large range of cancer types; induction of autophagy-mediated cancer cell death; chemopreventive effects
Nausea	Suppression of nausea and conditioned gaping in rats
Inflammatory diseases	Anti-inflammatory properties in several *in vitro* and *in vivo* models; inhibition of inflammatory cytokines and pathways
Rheumatoid arthritis	Inhibition of TNF-α in an animal model
Infection	Activity against methicillin-resistant *Staphylococcus aureus*
Inflammatory bowel and Crohn's diseases	Inhibition of macrophage recruitment and TNF-α secretion *in vivo* and *ex vivo*; reduction in disease activity index in patients with Crohn's disease
Cardiovascular diseases	Reduced infarct size through antioxidant and anti-inflammatory properties *in vitro* and *in vivo*
Diabetic complications	Attenuation of fibrosis and myocardial dysfunction

CBD, cannabidiol; TNF-α, tumor necrosis factor-alfa.
Used with permission from Pisanti, S., Malfitano, A. M., Ciaglia, E., Lamberti, A., Ranieri, R., Cuomo, G., Abate, M., Giorgio, F., Proto, M. C., Donatella, F., Laezza, C., & Bifulco, M. (2017). Cannabidiol: State of the art and new challenges for therapeutic applications. *Pharmacology & Therapeutics, 175*, 133–150. Elsevier.

Anxiety

Numerous animal studies and mounting patient evidence supports that CBD has powerful antianxiety properties. CBD works with the 5HT1A serotonin receptor and acts similarly as prescription serotonin reuptake inhibitors (SSRIs) such as Prozac and Zoloft to increase the availability of serotonin in the brain, which can reduce anxiety and boost moods. In one animal study (Linge et al., 2016), Spanish researchers found that CBD may affect serotonin levels in the brain faster than do SSRIs.

In another animal study, the researchers found that consistent use of CBD may help the hippocampus regenerate neurons (Campos et al., 2013); in fact, research shows that both SSRIs and CBD may promote neurogenesis. This is important because this evidence suggests that severely impaired neurogenesis may influence suicidal behavior.

In one human study, Brazilian researchers did a small double-blind study of patients suffering from generalized social anxiety (Crippa et al., 2011). After consuming CBD, the participants reported a significant decrease in anxiety. Researchers validated the patient reports by doing brain scans, and the scans showed cerebral blood flow patterns consistent with an antianxiety effect. In another small study, researchers had patients suffering from social anxiety disorder perform a simulated public speaking test (Bergamaschi et al., 2011). Participants reported significantly less anxiety, and these findings were supported by anxiety indicators such as heart rate and blood pressure.

Arthritis

A 2014 review of preclinical research showed that the ECS is an important therapeutic target for osteoarthritis pain (La Porta et al., 2014). The fact that cannabinoid receptors are located all over the body, along with the physiologic role of the ECS in the regulation of pain, inflammation, and even joint function, are the main ways that CBD can help treat arthritis-related pain.

 CASE STUDY
Notes From the Field

73-Year-Old Female
Diagnosis: Chronic knee pain r/t osteoarthritis with a history of chronic obstructive pulmonary disease (COPD)
State of Residence: California
Story: Living in an assisted living community. The patient wanted to try to alleviate chronic pain. Cannabis naive.
Treatment Plan: Included a topical and tincture. The tincture is a wellness formula (1 mL of which equals 3 mg THCa, 3 mg CBD, 3 mg CBDa and 1 mg THC) @ 10 mg 2× daily; reduced pain only slightly. Topical was only minimally effective. However, her COPD symptoms improved markedly, noting a decrease in shortness of breath and increased energy.

A 2016 study that used a transdermal CBD gel in arthritic mice confirmed CBD's common use for pain relief and reduced inflammation (Hammel et al., 2016). Another study in mice showed that oral and injected CBD helped prevent the joint damage associated with arthritis (Malfait et al., 2000).

Autoimmune Disease

There are more than 80 different types of autoimmune diseases, and they can affect almost any part of the body. Treatment depends on the disease, but in most cases, one important goal is to reduce inflammation, making CBD a great therapeutic candidate.

CBD is effective in treating disorders affecting the overactivation of immune response and its associated oxidative stress (Booz, 2011). CB1 and CB2 receptors are present in the immune system, although CB2 receptors are more abundant. CBD stimulates these receptors to support the regulation of the immune response.

A review by Parcher, Batkai, and Kunos (2006) supported research findings that cannabinoids are regulators of the immune system, and additional research (Cabral & Marciano-Cabral, 2005) further suggested that they work to suppress the immune response, which is helpful in many autoimmune diseases. Cannabinoids can also downregulate the production of inflammatory proteins called cytokines (Nagarkatti et al., 2009). Additional research found that CBD specifically caused levels of proinflammatory cytokines to decrease, whereas levels of anti-inflammatory proteins increased (Weiss et al., 2008).

Diabetes

Israeli doctor Raphael Mechoulam led the research that demonstrated CBD can be useful in treating diabetes by stabilizing blood sugars, reducing inflammation in nerves, and reducing the pain associated with neuropathy (Weiss et al., 2008). It can also act as a vasodilator that keeps blood vessels open and improves circulation. CBD can also decrease the arterial inflammation that is common in diabetes, and CBD does not just block the onset of diabetes but the development of it as well.

Cancer

Although cannabis is known for treating symptoms related to cancer and its treatments—such as nausea and vomiting, appetite stimulation, pain relief, and insomnia—there is mounting evidence that CBD can play a role in treating cancer as well.

Initial research with CBD shows promising results for various forms of cancer such as bladder, brain, breast, colon, endocrine, leukemia, lung, and skin cancers. Although better quality research is needed, Massi et al. (2013) concluded that cannabinoids work to reduce tumor size, interfere with cancer cell migration, adhesion, invasion, and metastasization. A 2015 review of studies using animal models demonstrated how CBD inhibits the progression of many types of cancer including glioblastoma (GBM) and breast, lung, prostate, and colon cancer (McAllister et al., 2015). CBD specifically has been shown to stop the proliferation of new cancer cells (Massi et al., 2013). CBD can also prevent angiogenesis, an important mechanism by which cancer promotes the formation of new arteries and veins to provide it with oxygen and nutrients (Solinas et al., 2012). A recent study found that CBD could also increase the efficacy of antitumor drugs (Fraguas-Sánchez et al., 2016).

Concussion, Brain/Spinal Injury

A 2003 trial used an equal combination of THC and CBD to treat symptoms arising from a variety of different brain and spinal cord injuries and found it effective in treating pain, muscle spasms, and improving bladder control (Wade et al., 2003). In 2012, a study showed that CBD could be useful in the treatment of spinal cord lesions (Kwiatkoski et al., 2012) and CBD has also been shown to be useful in treating neonatal brain injury.

Depression

CBD can help treat depression through its influence on the 5HT1A serotonin receptors. CBD acts to naturally increase the amount of serotonin available to the body, like common SSRIs that are often prescribed for depression. In 2006 researchers concluded that the ECS could provide a novel way to treat depression (Hill et al., 2006), whereas in 2016 CBD was recognized as a fast-acting antidepressant drug (Linge et al., 2016).

Inflammatory Bowel Conditions

Inflammatory bowel diseases, such as Crohn's, and syndromes such as inflammatory bowel syndrome (IBS), cause inflammation of the inner lining of the colon. Luckily, cannabinoid receptors are abundant, particularly CB2, in the gut. There have been several studies over the past decade or so showing a strong link between the ECS and the gastrointestinal (GI) system. Specifically, CBD works to inhibit the enzyme that breaks down anandamide (the fatty acid amide hydrolase [FAAH] enzyme) and this study showed that CBD might suppress colitis by reducing the activation of T cells and inflammatory response in the colon (Sharman et al., 2017). CBD has also been shown to reduce hypermotility (abnormally high activity) in the guts of mice (Capasso et al., 2008).

In one study (Jamontt et al., 2010), colitis was induced in rodents, and the results showed that THC was somewhat effective on its own, whereas CBD was not. A lower dose of THC combined with CBD proved the most effective. The combination of THC and CBD also improved colonic muscle movement. Another animal study (De Filippis et al., 2011) showed that administering CBD *after* inflammation was induced reduced the inflammation, whereas administering it *before* the inflammation was induced prevented it from happening at all.

Migraines

Migraines may be triggered by a variety of factors, such as hormonal changes, foods, food additives, drinks such as coffee and alcohol, stress and changes in sleep habits, for example. To be diagnosed with migraine, one must have had five or more unprovoked headaches, each lasting 4 to 72 hours, with a severity that restricts or prohibits daily routines, and is accompanied by nausea and/or light sensitivity (American Migraine Foundation, 2019).

In a recent study in human patients, results showed that THC and CBD in combination was an effective form of pain relief in high dosages (200 mg total) (Baron et al., 2018). In the second phase of this study, some patients were prescribed 25 mg of amitriptyline, an antidepressant commonly used for migraines, or 200 mg of the THC/CBD combination. After 3 months of use, it was shown that the THC/CBD medicine was most effective in treating acute pain during an attack, as opposed to decreasing the frequency or duration of attacks.

Multiple Sclerosis

Multiple sclerosis (MS) is an inflammatory and autoimmune disease with unclear causes and is characterized by the breakdown of fat-based myelin sheets in the brain and spinal cord, which leads to a degeneration of the nerve fibers. The most commonly associated symptoms of MS are muscle spasms, numbness, weakness, and slurred speech. Acute pain and chronic pain are also common symptoms.

Cannabis-based medicine, Sativex, is a 1:1 CBD:THC plant-based mouth spray developed by GW Pharmaceuticals. It is available in 30 countries around the world and is currently awaiting FDA approval for use in the United States. Each oral spray delivers 2.7 mg of THC and 2.5 mg of CBD.

There is not a lot of research looking at CBD's specific effects on MS in isolation. However, one study with mice showed promising results for CBD's ability to treat and possibly reverse some of the degenerative effects of MS in the brain and spine (Giacoppo et al., 2017). That said, there have been several studies supporting the use of a THC:CBD combination for spasticity and pain. It seems that the best dosage varies drastically from patient to patient, and that finding the best personal dose for MS symptoms requires some trial and error.

A cross-cultural study looking at American and Israeli patients showed that both groups suffered from high levels of stress, and experienced difficulty coping, along with feelings of hopelessness (Mei-Tal et al., 1970). Later studies revealed that stress seems to be involved in the onset, exacerbation, and relapse of MS (Ackerman et al., 2002).

Nausea/Vomiting

There have been many studies showing cannabis' efficacy in alleviating nausea and vomiting, many of these studies focusing on chemotherapy patients. This is one of the most commonly accepted medical uses of cannabis.

Less research has been done looking at CBD specifically, although a few animal studies show promising results. Because CBD works indirectly with the serotonin 5HT1A receptor, preliminary research (Rock et al., 2012) suggested it can be used to treat nausea and vomiting. CBD also acts as a reuptake inhibitor for our body's own cannabinoid, anandamide. A review of animal studies confirmed that CBD could be effective in treating several different types of induced vomiting, but not vomiting due to motion sickness (Parker et al., 2011).

CASE STUDY
Notes From the Field 2016

A 58-Year-Old Female
Diagnosis: MS in 1992 at the age of 31
Alternative Treatment: Acupuncture, chiropractic care, physical therapy, occupational therapy, gym, massage, meditation, consult with registered dietitian, supplements, essential oils, aromatherapy, homeopathy, energy healing work, and trigger point injections
State of Residence: New York
Story: Near-death accident in 1992 led to the diagnosis of MS. The neurologist at the University of Florida predicted she would be wheelchair-bound within 4 years. Donna chose a holistic approach to her diagnosis, refusing standards of care that included pharmaceutical intervention. This led to multiple physicians firing her as a patient.

Donna was able to walk again with the help of chiropractic adjustments, acupuncture, diet, and homeopathic interventions. She continues to work with a chiropractor, but unfortunately is unable to afford acupuncture. Donna has become very intuitive with her body, diagnosis, and symptoms; learning through experience what works to keep her functional with a good quality of life.

Is it all perfect? No, it is not. There are days where she has lost the function of her hands. Her speech, cognitive thinking, and vision become impaired. Painful spasms and muscle cramps can bring her to the point of screaming; dealing with fatigue seems to be the issue that consistently affects her quality of life. Donna has found that doing yoga daily helps her push through the fatigue most days. Life is a constant struggle.

In 2013, Donna describes hitting a wall. Depression set in, on top of everything else and no matter what she tried, nothing was helping. This was the first time she considered trying pharmaceutical intervention.

It was a mutual friend who introduced Donna to me due to my expertise in cannabis therapeutics. Cannabis was something Donna had used in her youth, but it was not something she enjoyed. I provided Donna with basic information on the ECS and how cannabis works as a medicine, the various delivery methods, the different components of the plant. Donna stated, "It has opened doors to a better life."

Donna began using THC-dominant products, which helped her battle the exacerbated symptoms and depression. Supply, trial, and error experimenting with new products helped break down the wall, to where her life is manageable and functional. Before starting cannabis therapy, Donna would sometimes need to wear adult incontinence underwear because of bladder control issues; these symptoms have disappeared *completely with the use of CBD and THC together.*

Donna uses multiple products, multiple times a day to maintain her quality of life.

She is using a full-spectrum hemp oil extract that helps her with depression. If she runs out of the product, within 4 days her depression returns. After consistent use over the course of a month, her body will remind her if she misses a dose. She uses this product three times daily, with some days where she uses an additional dose.

She also uses a hemp extract supplement that is enriched with clove, black pepper, hops, and rosemary that gives her an overall feeling of strength and well-being. She uses this product twice daily.

If she finds herself crashing, a tincture of CBDA helps decrease its severity.

A full-spectrum phytocannabinoid topical helps ease tight and painful muscles.

Throughout the day she uses inhaled cannabis at a 1:1 CBD:THC ratio, which allows her full function of her body.

She has experienced times when her MS begins to take over, leaving her bedridden, unable to afford the medicines that she needs to function. She feels that without cannabis, she would not have the quality of life or the function she currently experiences. She feels cannabis is a safe treatment option and she feels very confident in using it and attributes her health and well-being, in part, to its use.

Parkinson's Disease

CBD and cannabis therapies have shown great promise in treating the symptoms of PD and might also stop or greatly decrease the underlying nerve damage. Long-term daily use of CBD can have therapeutic effects on preventing the onset, halting the progression, and alleviating the symptoms associated with PD.

A study of 22 human patients showed a great improvement in symptoms such as rigidity, tremors, and slowness of movement, with improvements in sleep and pain reported as well (Lotan et al., 2014). There is also preliminary evidence that CBD can

 CASE STUDY
Notes From the Field 2016

73-Year-Old Male
Diagnosis: PD and dementia
State of Residence: California
Story: The patient is a retired pediatrician, living in an assisted living community. He began exhibiting aggressive behavior. Frequently walked into other residents' rooms. His wife was called nearly every night to come to the facility to calm him down.

The patient is cannabis naive. Consulted with a nurse practitioner with experience in cannabis medicine. Treatment plan—2.5 mg CBD + 2.5 mg THC 3× daily. After 3 nights, the wife was no longer called to come to the facility to help calm him. The patient was eventually weaned from Seroquel.

delay the progression of PD because of its potent neuroprotective, anti-inflammatory, and antioxidant properties. More and Choi (2015) concluded that CBD could help recover memory deficits induced by brain iron accumulation, which is a feature of several neurologic diseases. Another study showed measurable improvement in the quality of life and general well-being scores in patients with PD after only 1 week of treatment with CBD (Chagas et al., 2014).

Pain

CBD is effective for most forms of chronic pain, and for many forms of acute or short-term pain as well. Many studies have shown the ECS's role in the processing of pain signals.

CBD does not directly stimulate the CB1 receptors that are involved in pain perception (THC does), but it does have potent anti-inflammatory benefits, making it a great candidate for treating many types of pain. It can be used to reduce inflammation at the site of injury (eg, a sprained ankle) or can be used for chronic pain caused by pinched, irritated, or injured nerves.

A study looking into the use of CBD in combination with morphine and independently of it found that CBD could be combined with morphine in the treatment of acute pain conditions (Neelakantan et al., 2015). The results suggested that distinct mechanisms of action underlie the interactions between CBD and morphine in the three different behavioral assays and that the choice of appropriate combination therapies for the treatment of acute pain conditions may depend on the underlying pain type and stimulus. In addition, another study concluded that CBD has clinical value as a way to limit the rewarding effects of opioids, noting that CBD inhibits the rewarding effects of morphine, partially blocking the opioid's ability to produce pleasure and cause dependency (Katsidoni et al., 2013). In animal tests, CBD also reduced the animal's desire to seek heroin when responding to different cues.

One review assessed how well CBD works to relieve chronic pain (Russo, 2008). The review looked at studies conducted between the late 1980s and 2007. On the basis of these reviews, researchers concluded that CBD was effective in overall pain management without adverse side effects. They also noted that CBD was beneficial in treating insomnia related to chronic pain.

Several studies show that CBD can effectively decrease the prescribed dose of opioids for pain management, which is terrific news considering that so many people experience negative side effects or develop addictions to these medications. CBD can also lessen the symptoms of withdrawal from opioids (Russo & Hohmann, 2013).

Anecdotally, many patients report that a combination of THC and CBD proved to be most effective in treating pain.

Post-Traumatic Stress Disorder

Not only does CBD have wonderful antianxiety effects that are very important for patients suffering from PTSD but research also suggests that CBD might have an important role in storing traumatic memories through the "extinction process." The extinction process is the brain's way of diminishing the impact of traumatic memories;

	CASE STUDY
Q	*Notes From the Field*

46-Year-Old Female

Diagnosis: Acute colitis secondary to pseudomembranous *Clostridium difficile colitis*, polymyalgia rheumatica, malnutrition, pain, suicidal ideations, migraines, depression, insomnia, and failure to thrive

Medications: Polypharmacy, approximately more than five medications including different combinations of antibiotics, opioids, steroids, nonsteroidal anti-inflammatories, benzodiazepines, SSRIs, tricyclic antidepressants, neuroleptics, β-blockers, supplements, probiotics, and lidocaine patches and creams

Alternative Treatment: Acupuncture, chiropractic care, physical therapy, occupational therapy, gym, massage, meditation, consult with registered dietitian, supplements, essential oils, aromatherapy, homeopathy, energy healing work, and trigger point injections

Characteristics: Pain resulting in PTSD, debilitating depression, anxiety, insomnia, panic disorder, and agoraphobia

State of Residence: Massachusetts

State of Treatment: Massachusetts

Story: Healthy single mother of three working full time as a registered nurse (RN) in the Boston Hospitals. Specialty in holistic nursing with a focus on diet, nutrition, energy healing, and mind-body connection. Contracted pseudomembranous *C. difficile* colitis while working, resulting in disability

Started with flulike symptoms; fevers, sweats, chills, and irregular bowel patterns alternating between diarrhea and constipation. Progressing to severe urgency, cramping, and constipation, causing severe pain. Computed tomography (CT) scan revealed megacolon. Hospitalized in critical condition for pseudomembranous *C. difficile* colitis, requiring multiple antibiotics and stabilization secondary to malnutrition.

Once discharged, condition did not improve. Pain after eating, suffering from regular and unpredictable bouts of painful diarrhea. Abdominal distension. Prescribed opioids, steroids, and antibiotics.

Tried to return to work with exacerbation of symptoms. Patient experienced malnourishment, and failure to thrive. At this time, the autoimmune disorder, polymyalgia rheumatic, was diagnosed, causing muscle pain and stiffness, especially in the shoulders. Pain would be so severe that patient would vomit, exacerbating the ongoing cycle of malnutrition and pain.

Prescribed over 15 medications including different combinations of antibiotics, opioids, steroids, nonsteroidal anti-inflammatories, benzodiazepines, SSRIs, tricyclic antidepressants, neuroleptics, β-blockers, supplements, probiotics, lidocaine patches, and creams.

Traditional and complementary holistic healing including acupuncture, chiropractic care, physical therapy, occupational therapy, gym, massage, meditation, consult with registered dietitian, supplements, essential oils, aromatherapy, homeopathy, energy healing work, and trigger point injections.

Began experiencing horrible bouts of debilitating depression, anxiety, insomnia, panic disorder, and agoraphobia. Panic, anxiety, post-traumatic stress, insomnia, and pain were experienced daily, causing the patient to feel isolated, disconnected from family and community; began to experience the dissonance of wanting to live and die at the same time.

Exhausted conventional and holistic therapies. When introduced to cannabis, the patient stated, "two puffs of the cannabis joint and I felt the pain slowly dissolve away into background noise."

Her condition greatly improved, felt connected to family and community again.

Patient self-diagnosed clinical endocannabinoid deficiency. Over 2 years, the patient experimented with various ratios of THC and CBD to determine "sweet spot," the limits of intoxication to remain functional. Access was limited to start with. Lower doses of CBD isolate helped offset some of the negative side effects associated with THC.

Higher doses of CBD isolate did not help as much as the broad-spectrum and full-spectrum CBD products. CBD dosage was dependent on THC sensitivity. The use of broad-spectrum and full-spectrum CBD medicines and the other cannabinoids, specifically CBG, CBN, CBC, and terpene profiles rich in the terpene β-caryophyllene, helped lower the amount of THC needed to control pain.

The care plan included a combination of cannabis medicines, with CBD-rich profiles as a staple.

and for sufferers of PTSD, there is a failure in this process. Because traumatic memories do not fade in the same way for PTSD sufferers, these memories often produce symptoms such as nightmares, anxiety, flashbacks, and depression.

CBD injections are effective in reducing "freezing behavior" (a common fear response in animals of prey, think of a deer in the headlights) in rats that had been exposed to strong fear-based conditioning (Song et al., 2016). The rats given CBD were significantly less likely to be fearful when exposed to the same conditions at a later date, suggesting that CBD can be effective in hindering the development of fear around traumatic memories. Evidence also shows reduced levels of circulating endocannabinoids in patients with PTSD.

Seizure Disorders

CBD has gained much of its notoriety because of the almost miraculous results it has produced for many sufferers of epilepsy and other seizure disorders, especially in children.

Studies showed that CBD-rich oils had impressive impacts on reducing the frequency of seizures. A study in Colorado of 11 patients found that all of the participants reported a reduced frequency in seizures, with 73% reporting a near-complete to complete reduction (Reddy & Golub, 2016). A 2015 survey of 117 parents by pediatric neurologists at the UCLA Medical Center showed that 85% of parents reported a significant decrease in seizure frequency and 14% reported that their children were seizure-free with use of CBD (Hussain et al., 2015).

Because there is a risk of interaction with AEDs, patients should consult with their doctors before beginning treatment with CBD.

Sleep Disorders

The role of the ECS in sleep is clear: As the master regulator of our most basic human functions, the ECS has a direct impact on sleep. Our own endocannabinoids, anandamide and 2-AG, fluctuate with our natural circadian rhythms. Anandamide levels in the brain are higher at night, where it works with oleamide and adenosine to generate sleep. 2-AG levels in the brain are higher during the day, and they seem to promote wakefulness.

Cannabis's ability to help with sleep has been known and appreciated for hundreds of years, but CBD has impacts on sleep that we are only beginning to understand scientifically. Because of its biphasic properties, CBD has been reported to have both sedative and alerting effects in different people and at different doses. Low-moderate doses of CBD tend to create an alerting effect and might be helpful for narcoleptics or people suffering from excessive sleepiness during the day. In one insomnia study, high doses (160 mg) of CBD were shown to improve the length and quality of sleep (Carlini & Cunha, 1981).

Several terpenes found most potently in cannabis-derived products, and to some extent in hemp-CBD products, can also work both on their own and with cannabinoids to help promote sleep: Terpinolene, linalool, and myrcene all work as sedatives.

RESEARCH AND THE FUTURE OF CANNABIDIOL

The following section reviews where we are headed with future research endeavors related to CBD. Although CBD remains challenging to study, there is hope that as the prohibition era ends, we can move toward more high-quality studies.

Addiction

CBD is showing interesting potential in the realm of addiction. It has been shown to protect nerve cells from alcohol-induced neurodegeneration (neurodegeneration being a major consequence of alcoholism) and liver damage in animal studies. Another animal study shows that CBD can inhibit drug-seeking behaviors common in addiction.

Human clinical trials show that it can be very effective when it comes to quitting smoking, with the total number of cigarettes smoked per day decreasing by up to 40% when participants were given a CBD inhaler to use when they got cravings. Several states have also approved medical cannabis as a way to alleviate the symptoms of opioid withdrawal.

Attention Deficit Disorder/Attention Deficit Hyperactivity Disorder

Although limited data addresses CBD specifically, there has been some evidence of cannabis-based therapies helping attention deficit disorder/attention deficit hyperactivity disorder (ADD/ADHD) in human case studies. CBD's antianxiety effects could conceivably be helpful to patients, and CBD would also be great for treating side effects such as insomnia and nausea that are often caused by prescription drugs (Deiana & Zamberletti, 2018; Poleg et al., 2018).

Alzheimer's Disease

Evidence is mounting for CBD's efficacy in treating Alzheimer's disease (AD) (Hughes & Herron, 2019; Sharman et al., 2019). A connection between the ECS and AD has was historically investigated, and in more recent years CBD has been looked at specifically. Its neuroprotective, antioxidant, and anti-inflammatory benefits make it a natural fit for AD and other neurodegenerative diseases.

A 2006 study showed how CBD inhibits hyperphosphorylation of tau protein in A-beta-stimulated PC12 neuronal cells, which is one of the greatest hallmarks with AD. These results provide new molecular insight regarding the neuroprotective effect of CBD and suggest its potential role in the pharmacologic management of AD, especially considering its low toxicity in humans (Esposito et al., 2006). A recent review of preclinical research concludes that CBD can reduce the overall damage to the central nervous system (reactive gliosis) and curb the neuroinflammatory response. CBD has been shown to protect against memory loss and even help restore memory. CBD also promotes neurogenesis. New research is looking at how CBD can help treat and even reverse symptoms of dementia associated with AD and other neurodegenerative diseases.

Amyotrophic Lateral Sclerosis

Research around CBD and amyotrophic lateral sclerosis (ALS) is still in its infancy, although it is known that conventional therapies for ALS work by suppressing oxidative stress and inflammation while providing neuroprotection. CBD offers all these benefits, and it might be useful in prolonging the survival of neuronal cells and preventing the progression of the disease. In addition, CBD may help with other ALS symptoms through the promotion of bronchodilation and muscle relaxation as well as improving sleep.

A recent review concluded that the ECS seems to be involved in the pathology of ALS (Giacoppo & Mazzon, 2016). They believe there is great potential for cannabis as a treatment for both symptoms of and the disease itself, although more human clinical trials are needed.

Asthma

The use of cannabis to treat asthma is not entirely new, and the bronchodialating abilities of THC have been investigated. Because CBD is also a great bronchodilator, initial animal studies showed that it can be very effective in treating asthma and other issues caused by lung damage (Vuolo et al., 2015).

Autism

Although anecdotal evidence mounts for cannabis's efficacy in helping children on the spectrum, the evidence is still lacking. Initial research has shown that alterations in endocannabinoid signaling may contribute to autism (Foldy et al., 2013) and the CB2 receptor seems to play an important role (Siniscalco et al., 2013). An animal study showed that blocking the enzyme that breaks down anandamide improved antisocial behaviors (Doenni et al., 2016). CBD blocks that same FAAH enzyme, meaning it could help treat or manage symptoms of autism. Compelling anecdotal evidence suggests that cannabis can help reduce self-harming behaviors common in children on the spectrum, and CBD has been shown to help previously nonverbal patients speak their first words.

Schizophrenia

There is a growing body of preclinical and anecdotal evidence supporting the antipsychotic potential of CBD, which is great news because the side effects of antipsychotic pharmaceuticals are often severe and unpleasant. It also means that CBD might be useful in treating other psychiatric disorders such as bipolar disorder.

Although results are still preliminary and mostly at the preclinical level, research looking at schizophrenia and CBD has been largely positive. A systematic review of all CBD and schizophrenia studies was done by Iseger and Bossong (2015). They concluded:

> *"The first small-scale clinical studies with CBD treatment of patients with psychotic symptoms further confirm the potential of CBD as an effective, safe and well-tolerated antipsychotic compound, although large randomized clinical trials will be needed before this novel therapy can be introduced into clinical practice."*

Skin Conditions

The skin has a large number of CB1 and CB2 receptors. For this reason, cannabinoids can be quite useful in the treatment of skin conditions. CBD, in particular, has shown promise on several fronts.

CBD might be useful for acne because it increases the levels of anandamide, which, in turn, turns down the activity of our oil glands. CBD also acts on its own to curb oil glands (Olah et al., 2014). CBD's anti-inflammatory and antibacterial properties may be useful for acne sufferers as well.

For psoriasis, CBD seems to stop the overproduction of keratinocyte cells, the skin cells involved in producing the itchy, flaky layers of skin commonly associated with psoriasis (Wilkinson & Williamson, 2007).

SIDE EFFECTS

In 2017, the WHO conducted an extensive study on CBD and its effects on humans. They concluded "that naturally occurring CBD is generally well tolerated with a good safety profile in humans and animals, and is not associated with any negative public health effects. Reported adverse effects may be as a result of drug-drug interactions between CBD and patients' existing medications. To date, there is no evidence of recreational use of CBD or any public health-related problems associated with the use of pure CBD."

CBD has few dose-limiting side effects. In practice, dizziness, lightheadedness, increased heart rate, jitteriness, drowsiness, and diarrhea have all been noted, with less common side effects of irritability, decreased appetite, palpitations, and increased seizures also reported.

Several scientific reviews on CBD suggest that controlled CBD administration is safe and nontoxic in animals and humans with high doses up to 1,500 mg/day of CBD being well tolerated (in humans). These reviews conclude that CBD does not induce changes in food intake or affect physiologic parameters such as heart rate, body temperature, or blood pressure. CBD alone also does not produce significant psychoactivity, nor does it affect GI transit and psychomotor or psychological function (Bergamaschi et al., 2011; FDA, 2019).

Epidiolex research found that central nervous system adverse reactions have been reported in at least 10% of patients receiving CBD in phase 3 trials of CBD. Side effects included somnolence, fatigue, malaise, asthenia, insomnia, sleep disorders, poor-quality sleep, decreased appetite, diarrhea, rash, and elevated liver enzymes (FDA, 2019).

A 1986 study that focused on dystonia reported side effects of dry mouth, a small drop in blood pressure, lightheadedness, and sedation (Consroe et al., 1986). Research conducted in association with schizophrenia and psychosis suggested that CBD has a better safety profile compared to a commonly used medication, amisulpride, which could improve acute compliance and long-term treatment adherence (Iseger & Bossong, 2015).

The potential toxic effects of CBD have been extensively reviewed. The following are some noted relevant findings from *in vitro* and animal studies:

- CBD affects the growth of tumoral cell lines, but does not affect most nontumor cells. However, a proapoptotic effect has been observed in lymphocytes.
- CBD has no effect on embryonic development (limited research).
- Evidence related to potential hormonal changes is mixed, with some evidence of possible effects and other studies suggesting no effect, depending on the method used and the particular hormone.
- CBD has no effect on a wide range of physiologic and biochemical parameters or significant effects on animal behavior unless extremely high doses are administered (eg, in excess of 150 mg/kg intravenous [IV] as an acute dose or in excess of 30 mg/kg orally daily for 90 days in monkeys).
- Effects on the immune system are unclear; there is evidence of immune suppression at higher concentrations, but immune stimulation may occur at lower concentrations.
- There is potential for CBD to be associated with drug interactions through inhibition of some cytochrome P450 enzymes, but it is not yet clear whether these effects occur at physiologic concentrations (Figure 4.5).

Summary of AEs.

	Treatment group						
	Placebo (N = 37)	Alprazolam (N = 40)	Dronabinol 10 mg (N = 39)	Dronabinol 30 mg (N = 40)	CBD 750 mg (N = 38)	CBD 1500 mg (N = 39)	CBD 4500 mg (N = 40)
Any AE, n (%)	16 (43.2)	40 (100)	28 (71.8)	39 (97.5)	18 (47.4)	25 (64.1)	26 (65.0)
Somnolence, n (%)	8 (21.6)	35 (87.5)	14 (35.9)	22 (55.0)	9 (23.7)	12 (30.8)	12 (30.0)
Diarrhea, n (%)	0	0	2 (5.1)	0	1 (2.6)	4 (10.3)	8 (20.0)
Headache, n (%)	3 (8.1)	2 (5.0)	5 (12.8)	4 (10.0)	5 (13.2)	8 (20.5)	4 (10.0)
Abdominal pain, n (%)	0	0	2 (5.1)	1 (2.5)	0	1 (2.6)	4 (10.0)
Nausea, n (%)	4 (10.8)	1 (2.5)	7 (17.9)	7 (17.5)	2 (5.3)	4 (10.3)	3 (7.5)
Euphoric mood, n (%)	0	3 (7.5)	12 (30.8)	25 (62.5)	2 (5.3)	2 (5.1)	3 (7.5)
Fatigue, n (%)	2 (5.4)	7 (17.5)	3 (7.7)	5 (12.5)	2 (5.3)	2 (5.1)	2 (5.0)
Abdominal discomfort, n (%)	1 (2.7)	0	0	0	1 (2.6)	1 (2.6)	2 (5.0)
Feeling of relaxation, n (%)	1 (2.7)	5 (12.5)	0	2 (5.0)	0	1 (2.6)	2 (5.0)
Feeling abnormal, n (%)	1 (2.7)	1 (2.5)	1 (2.6)	2 (5.0)	0	0	2 (5.0)
Feeling cold, n (%)	0	0	0	0	0	0	2 (5.0)
Dry mouth, n (%)	0	0	3 (7.7)	8 (20.0)	1 (2.6)	1 (2.6)	1 (2.5)
Dizziness, n (%)	0	0	2 (5.1)	3 (7.5)	0	0	1 (2.5)
Sinus tachycardia, n (%)	0	4 (10.0)	4 (10.3)	10 (25.0)	0	2 (5.1)	0
Electrocardiogram T wave inversion, n (%)	0	2 (5.0)	1 (2.6)	1 (2.5)	0	0	0

AE, adverse event; CBD, cannabidiol.

Figure 4.5: **Summary of AEs.** Adverse effects were noted from a trial assessing abuse potential of CBD, using a range of doses up to a supratherapeutic dose of 4,500 mg in a highly sensitive population of recreational polydrug users. (Used with permission from Schoedel, K. A., Szeto, I., Setnik, B., Sellers, E. M., Levy-Cooperman, N., Mills, C., Tilden, E., & Sommerville, K. (2018). Abuse potential assessment of cannabidiol (CBD) in recreational polydrug users: A randomized, double-blind, controlled trial. *Epilepsy & Behavior, 88*, 162–171. Elsevier.)

INTERACTIONS

Orally ingested CBD is metabolized in the liver with a half-life of 18 to 32 hours. Although CBD has a good safety profile and is generally well tolerated, there is the potential for CBD to interact negatively with other medications. The number of people experiencing adverse reactions with polypharmacy is on the rise.

With the research completed by GW Pharmaceuticals for their cannabinoid-based drugs, we have a better understanding of potential drug interactions; however, these doses are not typical of what most people consume. Research has not been completed to indicate at what dose many of these interactions start to become a concern.

There are three main places in the body where CBD drug interactions may take place:

Intestine: Any drug taken orally is absorbed through the intestinal tract. The main cells of the intestines express both drug transporters and drug-metabolizing enzymes. A drug interaction here may decrease or increase bioavailability (the extent to which a drug is absorbed).

Liver: The liver is the main organ responsible for drug metabolism, and it also expresses drug transporters that can pump drugs or metabolites into the bile. Drug interactions in the liver may decrease or increase drug elimination. It can also impact bioavailability because blood from the intestines goes to the liver before heading to the rest of the body.

Brain: The blood-brain barrier expresses drug transporters that can control how much a drug penetrates the brain.

In preclinical studies, CBD is potentially able to influence the body's CYP enzymes through multiple methods, including the following:

Competitive inhibition: A chemical may bind to a CYP but not react with it, with the effect being blocking the other drug from entering the active site of the enzyme, where the metabolic reaction would ordinarily occur.

Allosteric modulation: A chemical may change how well a second molecule fits into or interacts with the enzyme, thereby either enhancing or decreasing the enzyme's binding affinity with the pharmaceutical ligand.

Heteroactivation: Certain CYP enzymes, such as CYP3A4, may not metabolize a drug normally; however, a second chemical may change the shape of CYP3A4 so that it can now metabolize a drug that it normally would not. This is a more extreme case of allosteric modulation.

Enzyme disintegration: Some drugs may cause the essential components of a CYP enzyme to dissociate, thereby potentially rendering the enzyme nonfunctional.

Altered gene expression: A compound may potentially impact the gene encoding a CYP enzyme, thereby increasing or decreasing the total amount of the enzyme in the cell (DeVitt-Lee, 2019).

CYP1A2

CYP1A2 clinically relevant substrates: *clozapine, cyclobenzaprine, duloxetine, fluvoxamine, haloperidol, imipramine, mexiletine, nabumetone, naproxen, olanzapine, riluzole, tacrine, theophylline, tizanidine, triamterene, zileuton, zolmitriptan* (Flock-hart Table, 2019).

According to a 2010 study, both THC and CBD inhibit CYP1A2a, although the potency is low and probably not clinically relevant at typical doses (Yamaori et al., 2010). The Epidiolex drug label indicates that at high doses, CBD has the potential to both induce and inhibit CYP1A2.

CYP2C9

CYP2C9 clinically relevant substrates: *diclofenac, ibuprofen, naproxen, piroxi-cam, tolbutamide, glipizide, glyburide, losartan, irbesartan, celecoxib, fluvastatin, phenytoin, rosiglitazone, torsemide, valproic acid, warfarin, zafirlukast* (Flockhart Table, 2019).

There is limited clinical evidence that CBD can inhibit CYP2C9 in humans at low doses (Yamaori et al., 2010), but higher doses are more likely to be clinically rele-vant. According to the Epidiolex drug label, inhibition of this enzyme is considered a risk. In addition, at doses of 5+ mg/kg/day, CBD appeared to rapidly increase war-farin levels, requiring a 27% decrease in warfarin dose to maintain therapeutic range (Grayson et al., 2018).

CYP2C19

CYP2C19 clinically relevant substrates: *esomeprazole, lansoprazole, omeprazole, pan-toprazole, diazepam, phenytoin, phenobarbitone, amitriptyline, carisoprodol, citalo-pram, clomipramine, clopidogrel, cyclophosphamide, imipramine, labetalol, proguanil, voriconazole* (Flockhart Table, 2019).

Caution should be applied when combining high-dose CBD with CYP2C19 sub-strates, because a dose adjustment is likely to be needed. High-dose CBD may act as a moderate to strong inhibitor, potentially causing two- to fivefold increases in expo-sure to sensitive substrates. There is not enough clinical data to characterize at exactly what dose CBD starts to become a concern.

CYP3A4/5

CYP3A clinically relevant substrates: *clarithromycin, erythromycin, telithromycin, quinidine, alprazolam, diazepam, midazolam, triazolam, cyclosporine, tacrolimus, sirolimus, indinavir, ritonavir, saquinavir, nevirapine, cisapride, astemizole, chlor-pheniramine, amlodipine, diltiazem, felodipine, nifedipine, nisoldipine, nitrendipine, verapamil, atorvastatin, lovastatin, simvastatin, sildenafil, tadalafil, vardenafil, al-fentanil, aripiprazole, boceprevir, buspirone, carbamazepine, Gleevec, haloperidol, pimozide, quinine, tamoxifen, telaprevir, trazodone, and vincristine* (Flockhart Table, 2019).

Research has indicated that CBD can weakly inhibit the activity of CYP3A4 and CYP3A5 *in vitro* (Yamaori et al., 2011), but further study indicated that CBD (50 to 100 mg/day oral) did not have a clear effect on levels of the CYP3A substrate tacroli-mus (Cuñetti et al., 2018).

> ### 🔍 CASE STUDY
> ### *Notes from the Field*
>
> Case Report: Warfarin
> A 44-year-old Caucasian male with Marfan syndrome, had a mechanical mitral valve replacement, was on warfarin therapy, and had post-stroke epilepsy. The patient was enrolled in the University of Alabama at Birmingham (UAB) open-label program for compassionate use of CBD for the management of treatment-resistant epilepsy. The patient's seizures began at age 27 concurrent with the diagnosis of stroke during the postoperative period after cardiac surgery. Despite initial control of seizures on monotherapy, seizures returned in 2011, prompting adjustment of antiseizure medications and eventual consideration of epilepsy surgery (Grayson et al., 2018).
>
> Following video EEG monitoring, the patient was determined to be a poor surgical candidate because of nonlocalized seizure onset. In addition, the need for anticoagulation due to the mechanical valve issue limited more invasive testing for localization of seizure focus and posed a challenge for the completion of any surgical resection. He was subsequently referred to the UAB CBD program.
>
> At the time of study enrolment, the patient was taking lamotrigine 400 mg and levetiracetam 1,500 mg, both bid. He was also taking warfarin 7.5 mg daily with a goal of international normalized ratio (INR) of 2 to 3. Before study entry, INR had been stable for 6 months, with levels ranging from 2.0 to 2.6. At the initial study visit, the patient's baseline INR was obtained and he was placed on the starting dose of CBD at 5 mg/kg/day divided twice daily. Per study protocol, CBD dose was increased in 5 mg/kg/day increments every 2 weeks.
>
> With uptitration of CBD oil as per protocol, a nonlinear increase in the INR was noted. Warfarin dosage adjustments were made by the primary care physician in an effort to maintain an INR within his therapeutic range while remaining on CBD treatment. Eventually, the patient's warfarin dose had been reduced by approximately 30%. The patient was followed up clinically without bleeding complications, but this points toward the need for close monitoring of INR when patients on warfarin use large doses of CBD.

OTHER CLINICAL EXAMPLES

A small number of clinical trials have specifically evaluated the risks of cannabinoid-drug interactions with opiates, antiepileptic drugs, and antiretroviral therapies. Although cannabinoids only had a slight impact on drug metabolism in most of these studies, the results were deemed clinically significant with respect to some antiepileptic drugs.

Several interactions have been noted between a formulation of pure cannabidiol, Epidiolex, and antiepileptic drugs, as described earlier. This may be, in part, because very high doses have been used in many of the Epidiolex trials. It is also likely due to simultaneous interactions with three sets of CYP enzymes: CYP3A4 in the intestines, CYP3A4 in the liver, and CYP2C19 in the liver. In 2015, researchers at Massachusetts General Hospital described a significant interaction with clobazam, a benzodiazepine. CYP3A4 metabolizes clobazam to an active metabolite, N-desmethylclobazam (nCLB), and CYP2C19 further breaks down nCLB. CBD increased nCLB concentrations by 500%, possibly by activating CYP3A4 activity while simultaneously inhibiting CYP2C19. But these authors concluded that "CBD is a safe and effective treatment of refractory epilepsy in patients on clobazam treatment," although "monitoring of clobazam and nCLB levels is necessary."

Another study on the interaction between Epidiolex and antiepileptic drugs noted that CBD caused statistically significant changes in the concentration of several antiepileptic drugs: clobazam, rufinamide, topiramate, zonisamide, and eslicarbazepine. Clobazam was the only drug whose concentration moved outside of the therapeutic window (roughly the range of concentrations where the effectiveness of the drug outweighs its side effects or toxicity). In particular, nCLB levels rose by about 100%, so the dose of clobazam had to be decreased.

Patients taking CBD with valproate had abnormal liver function, as previously discussed. Adults had slightly different drug interactions than did children.

Action

Sometimes a blood test may be necessary to see how the concentration of a drug changes—and if a change of dosage is required—when a patient begins taking CBD. This might be the case with chemotherapy, for example, because oncologists often utilize the maximum nonlethal dose to kill cancer cells. If CBD delays the metabolism of a chemotherapy agent, this could result in dangerous levels of a highly toxic drug.

Preclinical research indicates that administering CBD and/or THC in conjunction with first-line chemotherapy drugs could potentiate the latter, thereby reducing the dosage of chemotherapy necessary to treat the cancer. If this indeed translates to human experience, it would be a huge benefit.

Likewise, supplementing an opioid-based pain management regimen with cannabis could result in lower doses of opioids required for adequate pain relief. Lower doses of opioids will reduce the number of overdose deaths.

There is much more we need to learn about cannabinoid-drug interactions to avoid adverse reactions and harness potential synergies. But this uncertainty is not an excuse for medicine to continue to reject cannabinoid therapies—many pharmaceuticals are incompletely understood.

BIOAVAILABILITY, PRODUCTS, DOSING

The following section discusses the bioavailability of CBD, types of products, and dosing issues.

BioAvailability

Even with CBD's safety record and nonimpairing properties, best practice dictates that the smallest amount of medicine to elicit a satisfactory effect is appropriate. Each product has a different mechanism of action, with varying levels of bioavailability. Just as with high-THC cannabis products, inhalation, topical, and ingestible CBD have their unique onset of effect.

According to the WHO's prereview report from 2017:

> Oral delivery of an oil-based capsule formulation of CBD has been assessed in humans. Probably due to its poor aqueous solubility, the absorption of CBD from the gastrointestinal tract is erratic, and the resulting pharmacokinetic profile is variable. Bioavailability from oral delivery was estimated to be 6% due to significant first-pass metabolism.
>
> In healthy male volunteers, the mean ±SD whole blood levels of CBD at 1, 2 and 3 hours after administration of 600 mg oral CBD were reported to be 0.36 (0.64) ng/mL, 1.62 (2.98) ng/mL and 3.4 (6.42) ng/mL, respectively.
>
> Aerosolized CBD has been reported to yield rapid peak plasma concentrations in 5–10 minutes and higher bioavailability than oral administration. CBD is rapidly distributed into the tissues with a high volume of distribution of ~32 L/kg.
>
> Like THC, CBD may preferentially accumulate in adipose tissues due to its high lipophilicity. CBD is extensively metabolized in the liver. The primary route is hydroxylation to 7-OH-CBD which is then metabolized further resulting in several metabolites that are excreted in feces and urine.

In 2012, it was discovered that CBDA, the precursor of CBD, enhances the bioavailability of CBD by a factor of 2 (Eichler et al., 2012). A 2013 study noted that the bioavailability of THC via oral mucosal spray was greater than was CBD at single and multiple doses (Stott et al., 2013). A 2018 review article looked at pharmacokinetics in humans and reported that, "the half-life of cannabidiol was reported between 1.4 and 10.9 h after oromucosal spray, 2–5 days after chronic oral administration, 24 h after I.V., and 31 h after smoking. Bioavailability following smoking was 31%, however, no other studies attempted to report the absolute bioavailability of CBD following other routes in humans, despite I.V. formulations being available" (Millar et al., 2018).

Bell-Shaped Curve

Isolated CBD is the compound used in pharmaceutical research because it is CBD in its purest form. Product manufacturers also use isolates in product development because it is free of THC, odor, and taste.

If your patient is using a product manufactured using isolates, finding the therapeutic window may involve larger amounts of the product versus a full-spectrum or whole plant product. This is due to the limited dose range noted from isolates. According to research, using isolated CBD produces a very narrow window of efficacy, with no benefits noted at low or high doses.

Products

CBD comes in a wide range of product formulations, sizes, potency, and brands. What is available to patients depends on the laws within their state. Once the FDA develops regulations in association with the 2018 Farm Bill, hemp cultivation, production, manufacturing, and sales of nationwide hemp products will become legal.

There are two types of extraction methods used to remove the beneficial compounds from the cannabis plant, ethanol, and supercritical carbon dioxide. Each method produces a distinct end product.

In 1854, the U.S. Pharmacopeia recommended ethanol-based tinctures of "Indian hemp" to treat numerous ailments. Today, the FDA classifies ethanol as "generally regarded as safe: or GRAS," meaning that it is safe for human consumption. High-grade grain alcohol can be used to create high-quality cannabis oil that can be used in many products. One drawback of ethanol extraction is that it pulls in chlorophyll, which makes the extract dark green with a grassy bitter taste, making the final product less appealing to patients and consumers.

Supercritical carbon dioxide extraction uses carbon dioxide under high pressure and extremely low temperatures to isolate, preserve, and maintain the purity of the medicinal oil. This process requires expensive equipment and a steep operational learning curve. However, when done well, the end product is safe, potent, and free of chlorophyll. Once the plant material is processed and turned into an extract, that extract can be further processed to remove impurities that affect potency, flavor, and stability.

Let us take a closer look at some of the products and terminology available in the market today. At the time of this writing, CBD products are unregulated unless they are developed by a 2014 Farm Bill–compliant producer or within a state with cannabis/medical cannabis regulations.

Terminology

Full spectrum	Full-spectrum CBD products contain the widest range of cannabinoids, terpenes, and other plant compounds; they also contain essential vitamins, minerals, fatty acids, protein, chlorophyll, flavonoids, and fiber.
Broad spectrum	Broad-spectrum products contain an array of cannabinoids and terpenes, without the THC. These products go through additional processing to try to isolate and remove as much THC as possible while maintaining the other cannabinoids and terpenes.
Distillate	The distillate is a highly refined cannabis extract with the chlorophyll removed. It is often derived from high-CBD hemp flower and hemp biomass; typically, it contains around 80% CBD, with the balance including minor cannabinoids, terpenes, and other plant oils and extracts.
Isolate	Isolates contain nothing but CBD. Products labeled as isolates are generally highlighted as being 99+% "pure CBD." Epidiolex, which is an FDA-approved pharmaceutical available by prescription, was developed using isolated CBD.
Nanoemulsion	Nanoemulsions are solutions containing evenly distributed microscopic, insoluble particles within a mixture of water, oil, and other substances that reduce surface tension and stabilize the mixture. Researchers use nanoemulsions to increase the oral bioavailability of other drugs that have similar characteristics to CBD.

CBD, cannabidiol; FDA, U.S. Food and Drug Administration; THC, tetrahydrocannabinol. Adapted from Nakano, Y., Tajima, M., Sugiyama, E., Sato, V. H., & Sato, H. (2019). Development of a novel nanoemulsion formulation to improve intestinal absorption of cannabidiol. *Medical Cannabis and Cannabinoids, 2*, 35–42.

Types of Products

Ingestible	Inhalation	Topical
Tincture	Vape liquid	Creams
Capsules	Flower	Salves
Soft gels		Muscle rubs
Gummies		Cosmetics
Beverages		Toiletries
Water-soluble powders		

Tinctures

Tinctures are one of the easiest and most popular ways to consume CBD. Tinctures generally contain CBD diluted in food-grade oil (such as hemp oil, olive oil, or coconut oil). The tincture is sometimes flavored. Tinctures can be made using full-spectrum, broad-spectrum, and isolate or nanoemulsified CBD oil.

Tinctures made using full-spectrum oil often have a strong taste and the most abundant amount of plant compounds. Tinctures typically contain 1% to 10% CBD by weight (10 mg to 100 mg/mL) and often come in 30 mL (1 fl oz) containers. Tinctures are easy to administer a precise dose of CBD in a convenient and discrete format. Tinctures are normally taken sublingually: The liquid is held for 30 to 60 seconds under the tongue, and then swallowed. This likely allows some oral mucosal absorption, with the balance ingested.

Oral Spray

Oral spray delivers a metered dose of CBD into the mouth/cheek, allowing for mucosal absorption and accurate dosing. Oral sprays can be made using full-spectrum, broad-spectrum, isolate or nanoemulsified CBD oil, a diluent such as a food-grade oil, alcohol and/or vegetable glycerin, flavoring and other ingredients to improve flavor, mouthfeel, and absorption. Oral sprays have the added benefit of a metered dose.

Capsules

Capsules are hard capsules composed of two pieces that are joined together. Capsules come in a range of sizes, with typical dosages of 10, 25, 50, and 100 mg. Capsules generally contain powders of isolate and can be opened to apply the contents to food or consume orally.

Soft Gels

Soft gels, also known as gelatin capsules, contain full-spectrum, broad-spectrum, and isolated or nanoemulsified CBD oil along with a diluent such as food-grade oil. Soft gels deliver a precisely measured dose of CBD and are one of the simplest and most popular ways to take CBD oil. Soft gels are a great option for people who do not like taking oral liquids or who do not like the flavor or texture of tinctures. Soft gels may be made with gelatin (animal derived) or from vegan alternatives.

Gummies

Gummies are a popular way to consume CBD. Gummies combine a precise dose of broad-spectrum or isolated CBD oil with a small, tasty gummy candy. Gummies may be made with animal gelatin or a vegan alternative and may be sweetened with sugar or an alternative natural or artificial sweetener. Gummies typically contain doses of CBD such as 5, 10, or 25 mg.

Vape Liquid

Vape liquid or vape juice is a popular method to consume CBD. Most vape CBD products available (outside of adult-use legal or medical cannabis programs) contain small amounts of CBD oil diluted in an e-liquid containing a VG (vegetable glycerin), and/or PG (polyethylene glycol), or similar diluents. These products are usually called CBD e-liquids or CBD vape juice. The content of these products is normally low, typically similar to or less than a CBD tincture—that is: 1% to 5% or even less. PG and polyethylene glycol (PEG) are common thinning agents added to vape concentrates (particularly in hemp-derived products) that can be carcinogenic when heated and should be completely avoided. In the summer of 2019, after several deaths from vaping due to lung damage, the need for better testing and regulation of vaporized oils became apparent.

Flower

The cannabis/hemp flower contains all the beneficial compounds of the plant: cannabinoids, terpenoids, and flavonoids. Smoking remains the most popular way of consuming cannabis, and with the rise in popularity of CBD, cultivators have been busy growing and cross-breeding strains that are high in CBD and people are beginning to smoke nonindustrial grade hemp flower. Research supports that cannabis smoke is healthier than cigarette smoke is, but smoke is still smoke. Because smoking leads to irritation and inflammation in the lungs, it is not a preferable option for many patients, especially if they are already dealing with a compromised immune system or inflammatory conditions. In addition, the strong odor of cannabis smoke makes this the least discreet of the delivery methods available.

Herbal vaporizers function by heating the dry plant material to the point where the active ingredients are released without burning the material, meaning no smoke and almost none of the smoke's associated toxins. Instead, one inhales a vapor full of activated cannabinoids, which may (depending on temperature) produce a thick cloud of visible vapor.

Water-Soluble Powders and Liquids

Water-soluble powders contain isolated or nanoemulsified CBD and other agents that convert it to a powder, which allows the CBD to mix with water. In this form, CBD can readily be added to many different foods and liquids to allow highly versatile and convenient dosing. Because this product is more water-soluble than oils, it is thought to be more rapidly absorbed and it has greater bioavailability.

Powders and liquids can either come premixed or with a tablet or sachet, which is added before drinking. It should be noted that CBD may separate, so liquids should be shaken before drinking. UV light and other factors like heat may inactivate CBD, so CBD water and beverages may not be stable in storage.

Creams and Lotions

Creams are a topical product used to treat skin conditions such as acne or dermatitis. They are generally made using CBD isolate in modest amounts (1% to 2%). Lotions are similar to creams but lighter, and often have lower levels of CBD.

Salves and Rubs

Salves are another type of topical product applied locally to treat the skin, muscle aches, and pain. Salves can be a balm or an ointment. They are made with oils and waxes to create a semisolid material. Salves often contain other herbal ingredients or beeswax to give them a distinctive scent and a semisolid form.

Rubs contain CBD oil plus a liniment or rubbing alcohol and are used before, during, or after exercise or injury to promote recovery. Muscle rubs often contain menthol, camphor, or other ingredients that provide additional therapeutic benefits.

Cosmetics and Toiletries

Cosmetics are also becoming increasingly popular for infusion of CBD. From sunscreen to lip balm, CBD can provide local benefits in some cases, but it is often used as a novelty ingredient that is unlikely to provide therapeutic benefit.

Toiletries include products such as bath bombs, soaps, body washes, shaving creams, and other products. Bath bombs would provide the most benefits because of the absorption of CBD by the skin, but, generally, many of these products will have very low bioavailability and the CBD generally serves as a novelty ingredient.

Dosing

Currently, there is one FDA-approved marketed pure CBD medicinal product, Epidiolex. The manufacturer's website has a dosing tool to help practitioners determine a starting dose. This can be found at https://www.epidiolexhcp.com/. Because Epidiolex is the only medication on the market with dosing instructions, it should benefit the nurse to understand what this dosing might look like for the patient. Keep in mind that Epidiolex is an approved drug for patients with LGS or Dravet syndrome.

Week 1: Start Epidiolex with 5 mg/kg/day (2.5 mg/kg twice daily).
Week 2: Dosage can increase to a recommended maintenance dosage of 10 mg/kg/day (5 mg/kg twice daily).
If tolerated and required: Increase in weekly increments of 5 mg/kg/day (2.5 mg/kg twice daily) up to 20 mg/kg/day.
Additional dosing considerations
- For patients in whom a more rapid titration from 10 to 20 mg/kg/day is warranted, the dosage may be increased no more frequently than every other day.
- Administration of the 20 mg/kg/day dosage resulted in somewhat greater reductions in seizure rates than the recommended maintenance dosage of 10 mg/kg/day, but with an increase in adverse reactions.

Dosing Considerations
Epidiolex causes dose-related elevations of liver transaminases. Because of the risk of hepatocellular injury, obtain serum transaminases (alanine aminotransferase [ALT] and aspartate transaminase [AST]) and total bilirubin

levels in all patients before starting treatment with Epidiolex and periodically thereafter; https://www.epidiolexhcp.com/dosing-and-calculator

In clinical trials and research studies, CBD is generally administered orally as either a capsule or dissolved in an oil solution (eg, olive or sesame oil). It can also be administered through sublingual or intranasal routes. A wide range of oral doses has been reported in the literature, with most ranging from 100 to 800 mg/day (Fasinu et al., 2016).

Titration of Medication

Titration is a method used to determine the dose of medicine that reduces the greatest number of symptoms while avoiding as many side effects as possible. The process is very individualized and can occur quickly or slowly. Cannabis and CBD products are self-titrated medicines, meaning that the patient determines what dose best addresses their needs. Educating patients on this process is paramount to successful cannabinoid therapy, as health conditions are fluid, and dosing changes over time. The RN can provide the patient with information, coaching, and education to support their journey through the titration process, but, in general, RNs are not licensed to offer patients specific dosing guidelines, other than sharing the evidence-based approaches to dosing.

Providing step-specific instructions is important to determine the effectiveness of a product. If titrating a particular product over a period of weeks does not work to reduce a patient's symptoms, then suggesting a different product may be necessary. I have personally worked with several patients who had product-specific results with CBD products. I always recommend patients utilize one product for several weeks before throwing in the towel on CBD. Often switching from an isolate to a full-spectrum product is all that is necessary, while other times, changing the source from CBD-rich cannabis to hemp works.

There are normally two points that measure a therapeutic window or "sweet spot"; the lowest dose that begins to reduce symptoms and the high dose, where there is no further improvement in symptoms. More does not always equal better, it only equals additional expense.

Although the patient is titrating the dose, keeping a diary will help determine whether or not the medication is helping to alleviate symptoms as well as to what degree they experience side effects. Journaling (keeping a diary) is an important tool that can be used to help patients individualize their treatment. Sometimes improvements go unnoticed. I have had several patients notice the product they were using worked, only after they stopped using it. As patients' conditions improve, oftentimes, symptoms change, so having a therapeutic range of medicine helps patients maintain optimal health.

Titrating to an Ideal Level

Start with a low dose. If the product is a hemp-derived product with negligible THC or a CBD-rich cannabis product with a ratio of 20:1 or higher, this starting dose could be as little as 5 mg/day. For patients using a product that contains THC, they should use milligrams of THC to determine dosing, because THC will have more dose-limiting side effects.

As long as the product is reducing symptoms with few or no side effects, the patient may be educated to gradually adjust (titrate) the dose upward, using small incremental doses (5 to 10 mg). This gradual increase usually occurs every 3 to 4 days or weekly. Once there is no further improvement in symptoms, the dosage increases stop. This dose is the high end of the therapeutic dose or "sweet spot". Patients may now have a deep understanding of their therapeutic window and adjust their doses accordingly, with a good understanding of effect.

Depending on the condition and symptoms, dividing the dose may be appropriate. Patients who experience symptoms throughout the day, such as spasticity, may choose to divide their dose in half or thirds and medicate hour of sleep bid or tid. However, patients with sleep issues may choose to take just one dose at half-strength (HS).

CONCLUSION

Consumer interest in CBD continues to grow as our understanding of what it can do increases. "One in seven Americans say they personally use cannabidiol- (CBD-) based products, which have proliferated since last year's passage of a federal law legalizing this hemp form of cannabis. Younger Americans and those in the Western U.S. are most likely to report using these products, which are widely touted for their therapeutic benefits without any psychoactive effects because they contain a low level of THC. Twenty percent of adults younger than 30 say they use CBD, but usage and familiarity decrease progressively in older age groups. Just 8% of those aged 65 and older say they use CBD, and 49% are not familiar with it. CBD users in the U.S. cite relief from pain (40%), anxiety (20%), insomnia (11%) and arthritis (8%) as the top reasons for use" (Gallup, 2019).

The "FDA recognizes the potential opportunities that cannabis or cannabis-derived compounds may offer and acknowledges the significant interest in these possibilities, however, FDA is aware that some companies are marketing products containing cannabis and cannabis-derived compounds in ways that violate the Federal Food, Drug and Cosmetic Act (FD&C Act) and that may put the health and safety of consumers at risk" (FDA, 2019).

The 2018 Farm Bill will, in time, provide regulations that will provide transparency and quality control behind hemp-derived CBD products. Low-quality manufacturers will be pushed out of the market, and companies will learn how to increase their quality, decrease their prices, and still turn a profit. But until then, patients and consumers must do their product vetting.

Americans for Safe Access (Patient Guide to CBD, 2019) suggested the following:

- Consumers must pay close attention to how products are packaged, labeled, and stored to ensure product safety and efficacy.
- It is important that consumers closely read product labels, which should include all of the following:
  - Name and place of business of the manufacturer or distributor
  - Identity of the product
  - Cannabinoid content
  - Net quantity of contents in terms of weight, numerical count, or other appropriate measures

- A batch, lot, or control number
- Production date or expiration date (products susceptible to spoilage must bear a "use by" date and/or a "freeze by" date)
- Instructions for use
- Dosing guidance
- Appropriate warnings for use, including any individuals for whom the product is contraindicated, as appropriate
- Instructions for appropriate storage
- Edible products should be labeled with content and nutrition information, including the following:

  - Cannabinoid content
  - Total calories and fat calories (when >5 calories per serving)
  - Total fat, saturated fat, and transfat (when >0.5 g per serving)
  - Cholesterol (when >2 mg per serving)
  - Sodium (when >5 mg per serving)
  - Total carbohydrates (when >1 g per serving)
  - Dietary fiber (when >1 g per serving)
  - Sugars (when >1 g per serving)
  - Protein (when >1 g per serving)
  - Vitamin A, vitamin C, calcium, and iron (when present at >2% of the recommended daily intake)

Although this chapter attempted to provide an accurate portrayal of the current state of science, regulation, and laws regarding CBD, there are still many moving and evolving parts in this field. Between the continuous search for the mechanism of action around CBD and how it interacts with our bodies, to its symbiotic relationship with the other cannabinoids, CBD certainly has earned an important position helping consumers and patients alike influence their health and well-being in a nonintoxicating, positive manner.

Q&A QUESTIONS

1. The safest source of CBD comes from what?
   A. *C. sativa* L. (industrial hemp)
   B. Yeast
   C. *C. indica* L. (cannabis)

2. The 2018 Farm Bill removed CBD from the CSA as long as the compound is:
   A. Manufactured by a pharmaceutical company.
   B. Procured from hemp.
   C. Isolated from all other compounds found in cannabis.
   D. Is grown in a field.

3. An RN can provide patients with what?
   A. Coaching, education, and information
   B. Coaching, dosing guidelines, education, and information
   C. Coaching, diagnosing, and dosing guidelines
   D. Coaching, dosing, and edibles

4. The therapeutic window is:
   A. The lowest dose that reduces symptoms and the highest dose where there is not further improvement in symptom.
   B. The time when a treatment begins to start to take effect and the time the treatment begins to stop working.
   C. The start of a new medication and the first sign of a reduction in symptom.

5. CBD isolate:
   A. Is the purest form of the compound.
   B. Works better than whole plant formulations.
   C. Can be used in small amounts to reduce symptoms.

ANSWERS

1. **Answer: C.** *C. indica* L. (cannabis)
2. **Answer: B.** Procured from hemp
3. **Answer: A.** Coaching, education, and information
4. **Answer: A.** The lowest dose that reduces symptoms and the highest dose where there is not further improvement in symptoms
5. **Answer: A.** Is the purest form of the compound

References

Ackerman, K. D., Heyman, R., Rabin, B. S., Anderson, B. P., Houck, P. R., Frank, E., & Baum, A. (2002). Stressful life events precede exacerbations of multiple sclerosis. *Psychosomatic Medicine, 64*(6), 916–920. https://doi.org/10.1097/00006842-200211000-00009

American Migraine Foundation. (2019). *What is migraine?* https://americanmigrainefoundation.org/resource-library/migraine-chronification/

Americans for Safe Access. (2019). *Patient's guide to CBD.* https://www.safeaccessnow.org/patientscbd

Baron, E. P., Lucas, P., Eades, J., & Hogue, O. (2018). Patterns of medicinal cannabis use, strain analysis, and substitution effect among patients with migraine, headache, arthritis, and chronic pain in a medicinal cannabis cohort. *The Journal of Headache and Pain, 19*(1), 37. https://doi.org/10.1186/s10194-018-0862-2

Bergamaschi, M. M., Queiroz, R. H. C., Chagas, M. H. N., De Oliveira, D. C. G., De Martinis, B. S., Kapczinski, F., Quevedo, J., Roesler, R., Schröder, N., Nardi, A. E., Martín-Santos, R., Hallak, J. E. C., Zuardi, A. W., & Crippa, J. A. S. (2011). Cannabidiol reduces the anxiety induced by simulated public speaking in treatment-naive social phobia patients. *Neuropsychopharmacology, 36*(6), 1219. https://doi.org/10.1038/npp.2011.6

Bergamaschi, M. M., Queiroz, R. H. C., Zuardi, A. W., & Crippa, J. A. S. (2011). Safety and side effects of cannabidiol, a *Cannabis sativa* constituent. *Current Drug Safety, 6*(4), 237–249. https://doi.org/10.2174/157488611798280924

Birdsall, S. M., Birdsall, T. C., & Tims, L. A. (2016). The use of medical marijuana in cancer. *Current Oncology Reports, 18*(7), 40. https://doi.org/10.1007/s11912-016-0530-0

Booz, G. W. (2011). Cannabidiol as an emergent therapeutic strategy for lessening the impact of inflammation on oxidative stress. *Free Radical Biology and Medicine, 51*(5), 1054–1061. https://doi.org/10.1016/j.freeradbiomed.2011.01.007

Brenan, M. (2019). *14% of Americans say they use CBD products.* https://news.gallup.com/poll/263147/americans-say-cbd-products.aspx

Cabral, G. A., & Marciano-Cabral, F. (2005). Cannabinoid receptors in microglia of the central nervous system: Immune functional relevance. *Journal of Leukocyte Biology, 78*(6), 1192–1197. https://doi.org/10.1189/jlb.0405216

Campos, A. C., Fogaca, M. V., Aguiar, D. C., & Guimaraes, F. S. (2013). Animal models of anxiety disorders and stress. *Brazilian Journal of Psychiatry, 35*, S101–S111. https://doi.org/10.1590/1516-4446-2013-1139

Capasso, R., Borrelli, F., Aviello, G., Romano, B., Scalisi, C., Capasso, F., & Izzo, A. A. (2008). Cannabidiol, extracted from *Cannabis sativa*, selectively inhibits inflammatory hypermotility in mice. *British Journal of Pharmacology, 154*(5), 1001–1008. https://doi.org/10.1038/bjp.2008.177

Carlini, E. A., & Cunha, J. M. (1981). Hypnotic and antiepileptic effects of cannabidiol. *The Journal of Clinical Pharmacology, 21*(S1), 417S–427S. https://doi.org/10.1002/j.1552-4604.1981.tb02622.x

Chagas, M. H. N., Zuardi, A. W., Tumas, V., Pena-Pereira, M. A., Sobreira, E. T., Bergamaschi, M. M., dos Santos, A. C., Teixeira, A. L., Hallak, J. E. C., & Crippa, J. A. S. (2014). Effects of cannabidiol in the treatment of patients with Parkinson's disease: An exploratory double-blind trial. *Journal of Psychopharmacology, 28*(11), 1088–1098. https://doi.org/10.1177/0269881114550355

Cherney, J., & Small, E. (2016). Industrial hemp in North America: Production, politics and potential. *Agronomy, 6*(4), 58. https://doi.org/10.3390/agronomy6040058

Consroe, P., Sandyk, R., & Snider, S. R. (1986). Open label evaluation of cannabidiol in dystonic movement disorders. *International Journal of Neuroscience, 30*(4), 277–282. https://doi.org/10.3109/00207458608985678

Craven, C. B., Wawryk, N., Jiang, P., Liu, Z., & Li, X. F. (2019). Pesticides and trace elements in cannabis: Analytical and environmental challenges and opportunities. *Journal of Environmental Sciences, 85*, 82–93. https://doi.org/10.1016/j.jes.2019.04.028

Crippa, J. A., Derrenusson, G. N., Ferrari, T. B., Wichert-Ana, L., Duran, F. L. S., Martin-Santos, R., Simões, M. V., Bhattacharyya, S., Fusar-Poli, P., Atakan, Z., Santos Filho, A., Freitas-Ferrari, M. C., McGuire, P. K., Zuardi, A. W., Busatto, G. F., & Hallak, J. E. (2011). Neural basis of anxolytic effects of cannabidiol (CBD) in generalized social anxiety disorder: A preliminary report. *Journal of Psychopharmacology, 25*(1), 121–130. https://doi.org/10.1177/0269881110379283

Cuñetti, L., Manzo, L., Peyraube, R., Arnaiz, J., Curi, L., & Orihuela, S. (2018). Chronic pain treatment with cannabidiol in kidney transplant patients in Uruguay. *Transplantation Proceedings, 50*(2), 461–464. https://doi.org/10.1016/j.transproceed.2017.12.042

Cunha, J. M., Carlini, E. A., Pereira, A. E., Ramos, O. L., Pimentel, C., Gagliardi, R., Sanvito, W. L., Lander, N., & Mechoulam, R. (1980). Chronic administration of cannabidiol to healthy volunteers and epileptic patients. *Pharmacology, 21*(3), 175–185. https://doi.org/10.1159/000137430

De Filippis, D., Esposito, G., Cirillo, C., Cipriano, M., De Winter, B. Y., Scuderi, C., Sarnelli, G., Cuomo, R., Steardo, L., De Man, J. G., & Iuvone, T. (2011). Cannabidiol reduces intestinal inflammation through the control of neuroimmune axis. *PLoS One, 6*(12), e28159. https://doi.org/10.1371/journal.pone.0028159

DEA. (1970). *US Department of Justice. "Title 21 United States Code (USC) Controlled Substances Act." Title 21 United States Code (USC) Controlled Substances Act - Section 801–971,* 1970. www.deadiversion.usdoj.gov/21cfr/21usc/

Deiana, S., & Zamberletti, E. (2018). Cannabidiol as a potential novel therapeutic agent for psychotic disorders. In M. T. Compton & M. W. Manseau (Eds.), *The complex connection between cannabis and schizophrenia* (pp. 309–339). Elsevier/Academic Press.

DeVitt-Lee, A. (2019). *Project CBD releases educational primer on cannabinoid-drug interactions.* Project CBD. https://www.projectcbd.org/how-to/cbd-drug-interactions

Doenni, V. M., Gray, J. M., Song, C. M., Patel, S., Hill, M. N., & Pittman, Q. J. (2016). Deficient adolescent social behavior following early-life inflammation is ameliorated by augmentation of anandamide signaling. *Brain, Behavior, and Immunity, 58,* 237–247. https://doi.org/10.1016/j.bbi.2016.07.152

Drug Enforcement Administration. (2015). *DEA eases requirements for FDA-approved clinical trials on cannabidiol.* https://www.dea.gov/press-releases/2015/12/23/dea-eases-requirements-fda-approved-clinical-trials-cannabidiol

Duprey, R. (2019). *Rite aid: E-Cigs bad, tobacco and CBD rad.* The Motley Fool. https://www.fool.com/investing/2019/04/22/rite-aid-e-cigs-bad-tobacco-and-cbd-rad.aspx

Eichler, M., Spinedi, L., Unfer-Grauwiler, S., Bodmer, M., Surber, C., Luedi, M., & Drewe, J. (2012). Heat exposure of *Cannabis sativa* extracts affects the pharmacokinetic and metabolic profile in healthy male subjects. *Planta Medica, 78*(7), 686–691. https://doi.org/10.1055/s-0031-1298334

ElSohly, M. A., Mehmedic, Z., Foster, S., Gon, C., Chandra, S., & Church, J. C. (2016). Changes in cannabis potency over the last 2 decades (1995–2014): Analysis of current data in the United States. *Biological Psychiatry, 79*(7), 613–619. https://doi.org/10.1016/j.biopsych.2016.01.004

Esposito, G., De Filippis, D., Carnuccio, R., Izzo, A. A., & Iuvone, T. (2006). The marijuana component cannabidiol inhibits β-amyloid-induced tau protein hyperphosphorylation through Wnt/β-catenin pathway rescue in PC12 cells. *Journal of Molecular Medicine, 84*(3), 253–258. https://doi.org/10.1007/s00109-005-0025-1

European Commission. (2019). *Plants: Specific legislation.* https://www.ec.europa.eu/food/plant/plant_propagation_material/legislation/specific_legislation_en.

Fasinu, P. S., Phillips, S., ElSohly, M. A., & Walker, L. A. (2016). Current status and prospects for cannabidiol preparations as new therapeutic agents. *Pharmacotherapy, 36*(7), 781–796. https://doi.org/10.1002/phar.1780

Foldy, C., Malenka, R. C., & Sudhof, T. C. (2013). Autism-associated neuroligin-3 mutations commonly disrupt tonic endocannabinoid signaling. *Neuron, 78*(3), 498–509. https://doi.org/10.1016/j.neuron.2013.02.036

Food and Drug Administration. (2019). *FDA regulation of cannabis and cannabis-derived products: Q&A.* https://www.fda.gov/news-events/public-health-focus/fda-regulation-cannabis-and-cannabis-derived-products-questions-and-answers

Fraguas-Sánchez, A. I., Fernández-Carballido, A., & Torres-Suárez, A. I. (2016). Phyto-, endo-and synthetic cannabinoids: Promising chemotherapeutic agents in the treatment of breast and prostate carcinomas. *Expert Opinion on Investigational Drugs, 25*(11), 1311–1323. https://doi.org/10.1080/13543784.2016.1236913

Garcia, Alise, and Karmen Hanson. (2019). *State medical marijuana laws.* www.ncsl.org/research/health/state-medical-marijuana-laws.aspx

Giacoppo, S., Gugliandolo, A., Trubiani, O., Pollastro, F., Grassi, G., Bramanti, P., & Mazzon, E. (2017). Cannabinoid CB2 receptors are involved in the protection of RAW264. 7 macrophages against the oxidative stress: An in vitro study. *European Journal of Histochemistry, 61*(1), 2749. https://doi.org/10.4081/ejh.2017.2749

Giacoppo, S., & Mazzon, E. (2016). Can cannabinoids be a potential therapeutic tool in amyotrophic lateral sclerosis? *Neural Regeneration Research, 11*(12), 1896. https://doi.org/10.4103/1673-5374.197125

Gottlieb. (2018). *Office of the Commissioner, Statement from FDA Commissioner Scott Gottlieb, M.D., on Signing of the Agriculture Improvement Act and the Agency's Regulation of Products Containing Cannabis and Cannabis-Derived Compounds*. U.S. Food and Drug Administration. www.fda.gov/news-events/press-announcements/statement-fda-commissioner-scott-gottlieb-md-signing-agriculture-improvement-act-and-agencys

Grayson, L., Vines, B., Nichol, K., & Szaflarski, J. P. (2018). An interaction between warfarin and cannabidiol, a case report. *Epilepsy & Behavior Case Reports, 9*, 10. https://doi.org/10.1016/j.ebcr.2017.10.001

GW Pharmaceuticals. (2019). *GW Pharmaceuticals and U.S. Subsidiary Greenwich Biosciences to Present Data on EPIDIOLEX® (Cannabidiol) Oral Solution at the American Epilepsy Society Annual Meeting*. ir.gwpharm.com/news-releases/news-release-details/gw-pharmaceuticals-and-us-subsidiary-greenwich-biosciences-5

Hammell, D. C., Zhang, L. P., Ma, F., Abshire, S. M., McIlwrath, S. L., Stinchcomb, A. L., & Westlund, K. N. (2016). Transdermal cannabidiol reduces inflammation and pain-related behaviours in a rat model of arthritis. *European Journal of Pain, 20*(6), 936–948. https://doi.org/10.1002/ejp.818

Hemp Business Journal. (2017). *The U.S. hemp industry grows to $820mm in sales in 2017*. https://www.hempbizjournal.com/size-of-us-hemp-industry-2017/

Hemponair. (2019). *These New York City coffee shops are serving CBD in their lattes*. https://hemponair.com/2019/01/11/these-new-york-city-coffee-shops-are-serving-cbd-in-their-lattes/

Hill, M. N., Ho, W. S., Sinopoli, K. J., Biau, V., Hillard, C. J., & Gorzalka, B. B. (2006). Involvement of the endocannabinoid system in the ability of long-term tricyclic antidepressant treatment to suppress stress-induced activation of the hypothalamic-pituitary-adrenal axis. *Neuropsychopharmacology, 31*, 2591–2599. https://doi.org/10.1038/sj.npp.1301092

Horth. R. Z., Crouch, B., Horowitz, B. Z., Prebish, A., Slawson, M., McNair, J., Elsholz, C., Gilley, S., Robertson, J., Risk, I., Hill, M., Fletcher, L., Hou, W., Peterson, D., Adams, K., Vitek, D., Nakashima, A., & Dunn, A. (2018). Notes from the field: Acute poisonings from a synthetic cannabinoid sold as cannabidiol—Utah, 2017–2018. *Morbidity and Mortality Weekly Report, 67*(20), 587–588. https://doi.org/10.15585/mmwr.mm6720a5

Hughes, B., & Herron, C. E. (2019). Cannabidiol reverses deficits in hippocampal LTP in a model of Alzheimer's disease. *Neurochemical Research, 44*(3), 703–713. https://doi.org/10.1007/s11064-018-2513-z

Hussain, S. A., Zhou, Z., Jacobsen, C., Weng, J., Cheng, E., Lay, J., Hung, P., Lerner, J. T., & Sankar, R. (2015). Perceived efficacy of cannabidiol-enriched cannabis extracts for treatment of pediatric epilepsy: A potential role for infantile spasms and Lennox-Gastaut syndrome. *Epilepsy & Behavior, 47*, 138–141. https://doi.org/10.1016/j.yebeh.2015.04.009

Indiana University. (2019). *Flockhart Table™—drug interactions*. https://drug-interactions.medicine.iu.edu/Home.aspx

Iseger, T. A., & Bossong, M. G. (2015). A systematic review of the antipsychotic properties of cannabidiol in humans. *Schizophrenia Research, 162*(1–3), 153–161. https://doi.org/10.1016/j.schres.2015.01.033

James, P. (2019). *The top 6 hemp growing countries: USA now ranks number 3*. Ministry of Hemp. https://ministryofhemp.com/?s=top+hemp+countries

Jamontt, J. M., Molleman, A., Pertwee, R. G., & Parsons, M. E. (2010). The effects of Δ9-tetrahydrocannabinol and cannabidiol alone and in combination on damage, inflammation and in vitro motility disturbances in rat colitis. *British Journal of Pharmacology, 160*(3), 712–723. https://doi.org/10.1111/j.1476-5381.2010.00791.x

Katsidoni, V., Anagnostou, I., & Panagis, G. (2013). Cannabidiol inhibits the reward-facilitating effect of morphine: Involvement of 5-HT1A receptors in the dorsal raphe nucleus. *Addiction Biology, 18*(2), 286–296. https://doi.org/10.1111/j.1369-1600.2012.00483.x

Kwiatkoski, M., Guimaraes, F. S., & Del-Bel, E. (2012). Cannabidiol-treated rats exhibited higher motor score after cryogenic spinal cord injury. *Neurotoxicity Research, 21*(3), 271–280. https://doi.org/10.1007/s12640-011-9273-8

La Porta, C., Bura, S. A., Negrete, R., & Maldonado, R. (2014). Involvement of the endocannabinoid system in osteoarthritis pain. *European Journal of Neuroscience, 39*(3), 485–500. https://doi.org/10.1111/ejn.12468

Lande, A. (1962). The single convention on narcotic drugs, 1961. *International Organization, 16*(4), 776–797. https://doi.org/10.1017/S0020818300011620

Linge, R., Jiménez-Sánchez, L., Campa, L., Pilar-Cuéllar, F., Vidal, R., Pazos, A., Adell, A., & Díaz, Á. (2016). Cannabidiol induces rapid-acting antidepressant-like effects and enhances cortical 5-HT/glutamate neurotransmission: Role of 5-HT1A receptors. *Neuropharmacology, 103*, 16–26. https://doi.org/10.1016/j.neuropharm.2015.12.017

Lotan, I., Treves, T., Roditi, Y., & Djaaldetti, R. (2014). Cannabis (medical marijuana) treatment for motor and non-motor symptoms of Parkinson disease: An open label observational study. *Clinical Neuropharmacology, 37*(2), 41–44. https://doi.org/10.1097/WNF.0000000000000016

Maa, E., & Figi, P. (2014). The case for medical marijuana in epilepsy. *Epilepsia, 55*(6), 783–786. https://doi.org/10.1111/epi.12610

Malfait, A. M., Gallily, R., Sumariwalla, P. F., Malik, A. S., Andreakos, E., Mechoulam, R., & Feldmann, M. (2000). The nonpsychoactive cannabis constituent cannabidiol is an oral anti-arthritic therapeutic in murine collagen-induced arthritis. *Proceedings of the National Academy of Sciences, 97*(17), 9561–9566. https://doi.org/10.1073/pnas.160105897

Massi, P., Solinas, M., Cinquina, V., & Parolaro, D. (2013). Cannabidiol as potential anticancer drug. *British Journal of Clinical Pharmacology, 75*(2), 303–312. https://doi.org/10.1111/j.1365-2125.2012.04298.x

McAllister, S. D., Soroceanu, L., & Desprez, P. Y. (2015). The antitumor activity of plant-derived non-psychoactive cannabinoids. *Journal of Neuroimmune Pharmacology, 10*(2), 255–267. https://doi.org/10.1007/s11481-015-9608-y

Mechoulam, R., Peters, M., Murillo-Rodriguez, E., & Hanuš, L. O. (2007). Cannabidiol–recent advances. *Chemistry & Biodiversity, 4*(8), 1678–1692. https://doi.org/10.1002/cbdv.200790147

Mei-Tal, V., Meyerowitz, S., & Engel, G. L. (1970). The role of psychological process in a somatic disorder: Multiple sclerosis 1. The emotional setting of illness onset and exacerbation. *Psychosomatic Medicine, 32*(1), 67–86. https://doi.org/10.1097/00006842-197001000-00006

Millar, S. A., Stone, N. L., Yates, A. S., & O'Sullivan, S. E. (2018). A systematic review on the pharmacokinetics of cannabidiol in humans. *Frontiers in Pharmacology, 9*, 1365. https://doi.org/10.3389/fphar.2018.01365

Morales, P., Hurst, D. P., & Reggio, P. H. (2017). Molecular targets of the phytocannabinoids: A complex picture. *Progress in the Chemistry of Organic Natural Products, 103*, 103–131. https://doi.org/10.1007/978-3-319-45541-9_4

More, S. V., & Choi, D. K. (2015). Promising cannabinoid-based therapies for Parkinson's disease: Motor symptoms to neuroprotection. *Molecular Neurodegeneration, 10*(1), 17. https://doi.org/10.1186/s13024-015-0012-0

Naftali, T., Schleider, L. B. L., Dotan, I., Lansky, E. P., Benjaminov, F. S., & Konikoff, F. M. (2013). Cannabis induces a clinical response in patients with Crohn's disease: A prospective placebo-controlled study. *Clinical Gastroenterology and Hepatology, 11*(10), 1276–1280. https://doi.org/10.1016/j.cgh.2013.04.034

Nagarkatti, P., Pandey, R., Rieder, S. A., Hegde, V. L., & Nagarkatti, M. (2009). Cannabinoids as novel anti-inflammatory drugs. *Future Medicinal Chemistry, 1*(7), 1333–1349. https://doi.org/10.4155/fmc.09.93

Nakano, Y., Tajima, M., Sugiyama, E., Sato, V. H., & Sato, H. (2019). Development of a novel nanoemulsion formulation to improve intestinal absorption of cannabidiol. *Medical Cannabis and Cannabinoids, 2*, 35–42. https://doi.org/10.1159/000497361

National Conference of State Legislators. (2019). *State medical marijuana laws*. http://www.ncsl.org/research/health/state-medical-marijuana-laws.aspxpowers#amdt10_hd4

National Institute of Food and Agriculture. (2019). *Industrial hemp*. https://nifa.usda.gov/industrial-hemp

Neelakantan, H., Tallarida, R. J., Reichenbach, Z. W., Tuma, R. F., Ward, S. J., & Walker, E. A. (2015). Distinct interactions of cannabidiol and morphine in three nociceptive behavioral models in mice. *Behavioural Pharmacology, 26*(3), 304–314. https://doi.org/10.1097/FBP.0000000000000119

Olah, A., Toth, B. L., Borbiro, I., Sugawara, K., Szollosi, A. G., Czifra, G., Pál, B., Ambrus, L., Kloepper, J., Camera, E., Ludovici, M., Picardo, M., Voets, T., Zouboulis, C. C., Paus, R., & Biro, T. (2014). Cannabidiol exerts sebostatic and anti-inflammatory effects on human sebocytes. *Journal of Clinical Investigation, 124*(9), 3713–3724. https://doi.org/10.1172/JCI64628

Pacher, P., Bátkai, S., & Kunos, G. (2006). The endocannabinoid system as an emerging target of pharmacotherapy. *Pharmacological Reviews, 58*(3), 389–462. https://doi.org/10.1124/pr.58.3.2

Parker, L. A., Rock, E. M., & Limebeer, C. L. (2011). Regulation of nausea and vomiting by cannabinoids. *British Journal of Pharmacology, 163*(7), 1411–1422. https://doi.org/10.1111/j.1476-5381.2010.01176.x

Pisanti, S., Malfitano, A. M., Ciaglia, E., Lamberti, A., Ranieri, R., Cuomo, G., Abate, M., Faggiana, G., Proto, M. C., Fiore, D., Laezza, C., & Bifulco, M. (2017). Cannabidiol: State of the art and new challenges for therapeutic applications. *Pharmacology & Therapeutics, 175*, 133–150. https://doi.org/10.1016/j .pharmthera.2017.02.041

Poleg, S., Golubchik, P., Offen, D., & Weizman, A. (2018). Cannabidiol as a suggested candidate for treatment of autism spectrum disorder. *Progress in Neuro-Psychopharmacology and Biological Psychiatry, 8*(89), 90–96. https://doi.org/10.1016/j.pnpbp.2018.08.030

Potter, J. (2009). The propagation, characterization and optimization of Cannabis sativa l as a phytopharmaceutical (Doctoral thesis). https://www.scribd.com/document/214031988/ The-Propagation-Characterisation-and-Optimisation-of-Cannabis-Sativa-l-as-a-Phytopharmaceutical

Reddy, D. S., & Golub, V. M. (2016). The pharmacological basis of cannabis therapy for epilepsy. *Journal of Pharmacology and Experimental Therapeutics, 35*(1), 45–55. https://doi.org/10.1124/jpet.115.230151

Rianprakaisang, T., Gerona, R., & Hendrickson, R. G. (2019). Commercial cannabidiol oil contaminated with the synthetic cannabinoid AB-FUBINACA given to a pediatric patient. *Clinical Toxicology Open Access.* https://www.tandfonline.com/toc/ictx20/current

Rock, E. M., Bolognini, D., Limebeer, C. L., Cascio, M. G., Anavi-Goffer, S., Fletcher, P. J., Fletcher, P. J., Mechoulam, R., & Parker, L. A. (2012). Cannabidiol, a non-psychotropic component of cannabis, attenuates vomiting and nausea-like behaviour via indirect agonism of 5-HT1A somatodendritic auto-receptors in the dorsal raphe nucleus. *British Journal of Pharmacology, 165*(8), 2620–2634. https:// doi.org/10.1111/j.1476-5381.2011.01621.x

Russo, E. B. (2008). Cannabinoids in the management of difficult to treat pain. *Therapeutics and Clinical Risk Management, 4*(1), 245. https://doi.org/10.2147/TCRM.S1928

Russo, E. B. (2017). Cannabidiol claims and misconceptions. *Trends in Pharmacological Sciences, 38*(3), 198–201. https://doi.org/10.1016/j.tips.2016.12.004

Russo, E. B., & Hohmann, A. G. (2013). Role of cannabinoids in pain management. In T. R. Deer, M. S. Leong, A. Buvanendran, V. Gordin, P. S. Kim, S. J. Panchal, & A. L. Ray (Eds.), *Comprehensive treatment of chronic pain by medical, interventional, and integrative approaches* (pp. 181–197). Springer.

Russo, E. B., & Marcu, J. (2017). Cannabis pharmacology: The usual suspects and a few promising leads. In D. Kendall & S. P. H. Alexander (Eds.), *Cannabinoid pharmacology* (Vol. 80). Elsevier.

Schoedel, K. A., Szeto, I., Setnik, B., Sellers, E. M., Levy-Cooperman, N., Mills, C., Etges, T., & Sommerville, K. (2018). Abuse potential assessment of cannabidiol (CBD) in recreational polydrug users: A randomized, double-blind, controlled trial. *Epilepsy & Behavior, 88*, 162–171. https://doi.org/10.1016/j .yebeh.2018.07.027

Sharman, H., Singh, N. P., Zumbrun, E. E., Murphy, A., Taub, D. D., Mishra, M. K., Price, R. L., Chatterjee, S., Nagarkatti, M., Nagarkatti, P. S., & Singh, U. P. (2017). Fatty acid amide hydrolase (FAAH) blockade ameliorates experimental colitis by altering microRNA expression and suppressing inflammation. *Brain, Behavior, and Immunity, 59*, 10–20. https://doi.org/10.1016/j.bbi.2016.06.008

Sharman, M. J., Verdile, G., Kirubakaran, S., Parenti, C., Singh, A., Watt, G., Karl, T., Chang, D., Li, C. G., & Münch, G. (2019). Targeting inflammatory pathways in Alzheimer's disease: A focus on natural products and phytomedicines. *CNS Drugs, 33*(5), 457–480. https://doi.org/10.1007/s40263-019-00619-1

Siniscalco, D., Cirillo, A., Bradstreet, J., & Antonucci, N. (2013). Epigenetic findings in autism: New perspectives for therapy. *International Journal of Environmental Research and Public Health, 10*(9), 4261–4273. https://doi.org/10.3390/ijerph10094261

Solinas, M., Massi, P., Cantelmo, A. R., Cattaneo, M. G., Cammarota, R., Bartolini, D., Cinquina, V., Valenti, M., Vicentini, L. M., Noonan, D. M., Albini, A., & Parolaro, D. (2012). Cannabidiol inhibits angiogenesis by multiple mechanisms. *British Journal of Pharmacology, 167*(6), 1218–1231. https://doi .org/10.1111/j.1476-5381.2012.02050.x

Song, C., Stevenson, C. W., Guimaraes, F. S., & Lee, J. L. (2016). Bidirectional effects of cannabidiol on contextual fear memory extinction. *Frontiers in Pharmacology, 7*, 493. https://doi.org/10.3389/ fphar.2016.00493

Statista. (2016). *U.S. medical marijuana users that would recommend cannabis to friends and family, as of 2016, by gender.* https://www.statista.com/statistics/587034/medical-marijuana-users -recommend-friends-family-cannabis/

Stott, C. G., White, L., Wright, S., Wilbraham, D., & Guy, G. W. (2013). A phase I study to assess the single and multiple dose pharmacokinetics of THC/CBD oromucosal spray. *European Journal of Clinical Pharmacology, 69*(5), 1135–1147. https://doi.org/10.1007/s00228-012-1441-0

The Thistle. (2000). *The people's history*. https://www.mit.edu/~thistle/v13/2/history.html

USDA. (2019). *USDA update on farm bill implementation progress*. www.usda.gov/media/press-releases/2019/04/12/usda-update-farm-bill-implementation-progress

Vogelstein, F. (2017). *One man's desperate quest to cure his son's epilepsy with weed: Boy interrupted*. Wired. https://www.wired.com/2015/07/medical-marijuana-epilepsy/

Vuolo, F., Petronilho, F., Sonai, B., Ritter, C., Hallak, J. E., Zuardi, A. W., Crippa, J. A., & Dal-Pizzol, F. (2015). Evaluation of serum cytokines levels and the role of cannabidiol treatment in animal model of asthma. *Mediators of Inflammation, 2015*, 538670. https://doi.org/10.1155/2015/538670

Wade, D. T., Robson, P., House, H., Makela, P., & Aram, J. (2003). A preliminary controlled study to determine whether whole-plant cannabis extracts can improve intractable neurogenic symptoms. *Clinical Rehabilitation, 17*(1), 21–29. https://doi.org/10.1191/0269215503cr581oa

Ward, S. J., McAllister, S. D., Kawamura, R., Murase, R., Neelakantan, H., & Walker, E. A. (2014). Cannabidiol inhibits paclitaxel-induced neuropathic pain through 5-HT1A receptors without diminishing nervous system function or chemotherapy efficacy. *British Journal of Pharmacology, 171*(3), 636–645. https://doi.org/10.1111/bph.12439

Weiss, L., Zeira, M., Reich, S., Slavin, S., Raz, I., Mechoulam, R., & Gallily, R. (2008). Cannabidiol arrests onset of autoimmune diabetes in NOD mice. *Neuropharmacology, 54*(1), 244–249. https://doi.org/10.1016/j.neuropharm.2007.06.029

Wilkinson, J. D., & Williamson, E. M. (2007). Cannabinoids inhibit human keratinocyte proliferation through a non-CB1/CB2 mechanism and have a potential therapeutic value in the treatment of psoriasis. *Journal of Dermatological Science, 45*(2), 87–92. https://doi.org/10.1016/j.jdermsci.2006.10.009

Williams, S. (2019). *9 major retailers that are selling CBD products*. The Motley Fool. https://www.fool.com/investing/2019/06/03/9-major-retailers-that-are-selling-cbd-products.aspx

World Health Organization. (2017). *Cannabidiol (compound of cannabis): Online Q&A*. https://www.who.int/features/qa/cannabidiol/en/

Yamaori, S., Ebisawa, J., Okushima, Y., Yamamoto, I., & Watanabe, K. (2011). Potent inhibition of human cytochrome P450 3A isoforms by cannabidiol: Role of phenolic hydroxyl groups in the resorcinol moiety. *Life Sciences, 88*(15–16), 730–736. https://doi.org/10.1016/j.lfs.2011.02.017

Yamaori, S., Kushihara, M., Yamamoto, I., & Watanabe, K. (2010). Characterization of major phytocannabinoids, cannabidiol and cannabinol, as isoform-selective and potent inhibitors of human CYP1 enzymes. *Biochemical Pharmacology, 79*(11), 1691–1698. https://doi.org/10.1016/j.bcp.2010.01.028

5

Cannabis Science: Reviewing Trends

Carey S. Clark, PhD, RN, AHN-BC, RYT, FAAN,
Rachel A. Parmelee, MSN, RN, CRRN, and
Barbara J. Ochester, MSN, BSN, RN

CONCEPTS AND CONSIDERATIONS

In this chapter, the reader is invited to learn more about the current state of evidence of cannabinoid medicine and specific illnesses. The National Council of State Boards of Nursing (NCSBN, 2018) stated that nurses must be educated about cannabis pharmacology and the research associated with medical use of cannabis. Therefore, this chapter reviews the current state of evidence focusing on what we have learned about medical use of cannabis since the publication of National Academies of Sciences, Engineering, and Medicine's (NASEM, 2017) landmark report entitled *The Health Effects of Cannabis and Cannabinoids: The Current State of Evidence and Recommendations for Research.* This chapter is included in this textbook as it supports the call by the NCSBN (2018) for nurses to be educated regarding the body of evidence: "The nurse shall have an understanding of cannabis pharmacology and the research associated with the medical use of cannabis."

The NASEM report may be viewed as a go-to source when considering the state of cannabinoid medicine science evidence. The full NASEM (2017) report can be accessed at http://nationalacademies.org/hmd/reports/2017/health-effects-of-cannabis-and-cannabinoids.aspx.

With over 30,000 publications in PubMed related to the medicinal use of cannabis, it becomes important to stay up-to-date in regard to the body of evidence, as cannabis care nurses should be using the latest evidence to support their patients' knowledge acquisition and coaching needs. This chapter explores some of the more recent evidence that has emerged since the 2017 NASEM report, while also providing the reader with examples of how cannabis science evidence can be reviewed.

Learning Outcomes

Upon completion of this chapter, the learners will:

- Become familiar with some of the current state of evidence of cannabinoid therapeutics' effectiveness for specific illness or disease states.
- Engage with the literature review process as a means to launch their knowledge around and experience with analyzing the body of cannabinoid medicine research.
- Consider the future of cannabinoid therapeutic research.

THE NATIONAL ACADEMIES OF SCIENCES, ENGINEERING, AND MEDICINE REPORT: SUMMARY

The NASEM (2017) report was a landmark comprehensive study culling together and reviewing research findings dating back to 1999 related to the health effects of recreational and medical use of cannabis. The review not only summarizes the current state of evidence about what is known about the therapeutic effects of cannabis, it also considers some of the potential health risks of cannabis use related to certain cancers, diseases, mental health issues, and injuries.

The report findings regarding the current levels of evidence of cannabinoid therapeutics effectiveness with specific disease or illness states are summarized in Table 5.1.

Cannabis is one of the most researched plants with over 30,000 published research articles in the PubMed database; however, because of the prohibition effect, most of

TABLE 5.1.	Summary of NASEM report findings		
Conclusive or substantial evidence	Moderate evidence	Limited evidence	Insufficient evidence
• Adult chronic pain • MS/spasticity • Chemotherapy-induced nausea/vomiting • Intractable seizures • Dravet and Lennox-Gastaut syndromes (CBD)	• Sleep disturbances related to pain, MS, fibromyalgia, sleep apnea • Decreasing intraocular pressure in glaucoma	• Dementia • Parkinson's • Schizophrenia symptoms • PTSD symptoms • Appetite/weight issues HIV/AIDS • Traumatic brain injury • Anxiety (CBD) • Tourette's syndrome	• Depression • Addiction abstinence • IBD symptoms • Cancer treatment • Cancer-associated anorexia • ALS symptoms • Dystonia

ALS, amyotrophic lateral sclerosis; CBD, cannabidiol; IBD, inflammatory bowel disease; MS, multiple sclerosis; NASEM, National Academies of Sciences, Engineering, and Medicine; PTSD, posttraumatic stress disorder.

Based on MacCallum, C. A., & Russo, E. B. (2018). Practical considerations in medical cannabis administration and dosing. *European Journal of Internal Medicine, 49,* 12–19. https://doi.org/10.1016/j.ejim.2018.01.004; National Academies of Sciences, Engineering, and Medicine. (2017). *The health effects of cannabis and cannabinoids: The current state of evidence and recommendations for research.* The National Academies Press. https://doi.org/10.17226/24625

the research has been limited to in vivo, in vitro, and animal (mouse or other) studies. There are challenges with standardizing research using whole plant cannabis and controlling for variables. We also know that there is a plethora of cannabis patient "anecdotal" data, or data from patient stories of success with using cannabis in order to palliate or heal themselves. Though one can often see medical cannabis patient stories highlighted via social media platforms, it would be wise for the field to begin to recognize these data as "qualitative" in nature. Perhaps these data are a potential rich source of the patient experience that has yet to be broadly culled and analyzed for themes and patterns that could inform our knowledge base and our care of medicinal cannabis patients; a few studies have been done analyzing the patient experience using sources like social media postings. It is likely that in the near future, efforts can be made to create a nationwide repository of patient's medical cannabis experiences so that we can move toward creating patient-informed practices based in a body of qualitative evidence.

The following sections summarize the NASEM findings and explore some of the newer findings that we found in the current database 2017 to 2019. In Chapter 6, there is an example of how nurses can analyze research articles, and we undertook a similar process here, which aligns with the Johns Hopkins approach to critiquing the evidence:

- The basic process was to use search engine tools to look for recent research articles related to the specific disease processes, using terms like the disease or illness state and cannabis, cannabis research, and so on.
- Articles were reviewed for relevancy, authorship, research methodology, findings, and limitations.
- We not only strived to select high-quality research articles but also included articles that may be of broad interest to cannabis care nurses.
- Owing to limitations in space, we recognized that the articles chosen provide just a small snapshot of the landscape of the body of evidence related to cannabinoid medicine.
- We also recognize that new evidence is continually emerging and that readers should take this evidence as a springboard to supporting their skill development at inquiring about the latest evidence when supporting, educating, and coaching patients and their caregivers. Nurses should become adept at both analyzing research findings and sharing those findings clearly with those they serve.

BODY OF EVIDENCE

The following sections review some of the latest findings related to medicinal cannabis use. A most recent review of cannabis qualifying conditions, via reviewing state medical cannabis registries across the United States, found that chronic pain (67.7%) is the main reason for using medical cannabis, followed by multiple sclerosis (MS) (27.4%), cancer (10%), and irritable bowel syndrome (5.7%) (Boehnke et al., 2019). Interestingly, Boehnke and colleagues found that 85.5% of all medical cannabis patients in the United States are using cannabis for conditions that the NASEM (2017) reported as having substantial or conclusive evidence of effectiveness. This, however, does not mean that the evidence in those areas remains stagnant, as new findings will continue to emerge.

The areas selected to explore in this chapter are adult chronic pain, posttraumatic stress disorder (PTSD), cancer care, addiction/substance abuse, glaucoma, irritable bowel disease, and the neurologic issues of MS/spasticity, intractable seizures, Parkinson's disease (PD), and traumatic brain injury (TBI).

ADULT CHRONIC PAIN

After their review of cannabis use among chronic pain patients, the authors of NASEM (2017) found that there is substantial evidence that cannabis flower is effective for the treatment of pain. The report further stated that more exploration is needed regarding the various routes of cannabis medicine administration and the issues of efficacy, dosing, and potential side effects when using cannabis for relief of pain.

The PubMed database was used to search for recent studies about cannabis use and chronic pain issues. A search was conducted using the words "cannabis" and "pain" for articles published between 2017 and 2019. From the 488 results obtained, three high-quality studies were chosen to be reviewed here, considering their significance to the work of the cannabis care nurse. The sheer amount of results makes it clear that this is a "hot" research topic, and we know that chronic pain is one of the top reasons why people use cannabis medicinally.

Tetrahydrocannabinol: Cannabidiol Oromucosal Spray

Article: Ueberall, M. A., Essner, U., & Mueller-Schwefe, G. H. (2019). Effectiveness and tolerability of THC: CBD oromucosal spray as add-on measure in patients with severe chronic pain: Analysis of 12-week open-label real-world data provided by the German Pain e-Registry. *Journal of Pain Research, 12*, 1577–1604. https://doi.org/10.2147/JPR.S192174

Authors: All of the authors work in Germany for institutions such as the Institute of Neurological Sciences and the Interdisciplinary Center for Pain and Palliative Medicine.

Purpose: To evaluate the safety and effectiveness of a tetrahydrocannabinol-cannabidiol (THC-CBD) oromucosal spray (Sativex) as an adjunctive treatment for patients diagnosed with severe chronic pain.

Methodology: This study was noninterventional, as it reviewed previously collected cohort data. The data were anonymized and collected from a national pain treatment registry German Pain e-Registry (GPR), where doctors electronically enter the self-reported data that they receive from their patients. Of the over 30,000 GPR patient's data, 800 were reviewed to determine whether the use of a one-part THC to one-part CBD oromucosal spray was effective for three different categories of pain: nociceptive, mixed, or neuropathic. Patients could also use any other pain medicines deemed necessary for managing their pain.

A 7-item version of a valid PainDETECT Questionnaire was used with patients self-reporting on their pain intensity, pain-related disabilities/functionality, sleep, overall well-being, quality of life (QoL), and psychological factors (depression, anxiety, and stress). Descriptive and inferential statistics were used to evaluate the various data points. Limitations to the study include lack of a control group, lack of randomization of participants, and the relatively short trial period of 12 weeks. A strength was that no compensations were made to physicians or participants.

Participants: Participants generally followed the recommended dosing for Sativex, starting with an initiation phase of a 2- to 4-week time period and culminating with a recommended dose of 8 to 12 sprays/day (for a generalized total 22 to 32 mg THC:20 to 30 mg CBD). Patients' use was not closely monitored, therefore these totals could vary to some degree. Eight hundred GPR participants were found to meet the criteria of using the spray, though the 12-week attrition rate was 18.1% (n = 145). In all, 57% were female, 43% male. The age range was 19 to 77 years, with a median age of 47 years. The participants were also evaluated for duration of pain issues, with nearly 70% having pain for more than 12 months. Nearly all patients had used non-opioid medications (99.8%), antidepressants (72.5%), mild opioid analgesics (70.9%), and/or antiepileptic medications (65.5%). 87.6% also had used non-medication pain treatments, such as transcutaneous electrical nerve stimulation, acupuncture, physiotherapy, and/or psychological care.

Findings: One of the interesting findings was related to the self-titration process. In addition to the regular medication regime, patients started with an average of 2.6 sprays per day and they continued to titrate up until about week 9, when a plateau was reached of 7.0 sprays/day. By the end of the 12 weeks, patients were averaging 19.2 mg THC and 17.8 mg CBD/day. Furthermore, 67.5% of the patients reported a 50% or more improvement from their baseline day 0 pain scores. The majority of patients also noted a 50% or more improvement for the other areas measured, including stress, pain intensity, depression, overall well-being, anxiety, disabilities in daily life, sleep, and physical and mental disabilities. The researchers found no evidence of abuse or "overdose" among the participants. There were no deaths.

Discussion and implications for cannabis care: According to the NASEM (2017) report, more exploration of the various routes, dosing, and side effects of cannabis are needed; the authors of this study provided supporting evidence in these three areas. The findings show that cannabinoid medicines may offer adequate relief for some patients suffering from chronic pain. The combination of THC-CBD and inclusion of terpenes and flavonoids in the medicine may have also had a significant impact on the effectiveness of the pain treatment when we consider how these components together may impact the endocannabinoid system. In addition, the self-titration dosing process did allow for the patients to, on average, stay within the MacCallum and Russo's (2018) recommended guidelines for dosing and thereby also avoid problematic side effects.

Safety and Efficacy

Article: Sagy, I., Bar-Lev Schleider, L., Abu-Shakra, M., & Novack, V. (2019). Safety and efficacy of medical cannabis in fibromyalgia. *Journal of Clinical Medicine, 8*(6), 807. https://doi.org/10.3390/jcm8060807

Authors: This study was done in Israel. The authors work at various reputable institutions in Israel, including large medical institutions, and the Cannabis Clinical Research Institute. Two of the four authors have affiliations with universities as faculty members.

Purpose: To consider the safety, characteristics, and effectiveness of medical cannabis use with fibromyalgia patients. Chronic pain is an aspect of fibromyalgia that cannabis might help, and these patients also suffer from sleep issues, cognitive impairment, and psychiatric and somatic ailments. Two to 8% of the population suffers from this disorder, and it is the most common cause of generalized pain among women globally. A complex illness, fibromyalgia is often managed with a polypharmacy approach (antidepressants, pain medications/opiates, and anticonvulsants) and lifestyle modifications (exercise, cognitive-behavioral techniques, and dietary changes).

Methodology: In Israel, medical patients go through an approval process where their dose is determined through the Israel Medical Cannabis Agency, which is a division within the Israeli Ministry of Health. Patients then work with a certified nurse in the cannabis field to start the titration process. Retrospectively, data were abstracted from the records of patients with a fibromyalgia diagnosis accessing cannabis through the provider Tikun Olam from 2015 to 2017. Institutional Ethics Committee approval was granted from the Soroka University Medical School. A certified nurse educated patients regarding regulatory issues, routes of administration, chemovar choice (14 chemovars available), delivery methods, dose and titration process, and adverse effects. Patients were given specific guidance about very gradual titration processes starting with one drop of 15.2% THC-rich cannabis three times daily and to gradually, drop-by-drop increase their dosage until symptom relief was attained. Alternately, patients could inhale cannabis from a cannabis cigarette with 0.75 g of cannabis at the rate of 1 puff every 3 to 4 hours. If adverse effects occurred, patients were told to drop back down to the last well-tolerated dose. 20.2% of participants used oil drops only, 67.3% inhaled whole plant cannabis flower, and 12% used both methods of ingestion. Overall, a median of five other medications were used, with a median of just one medication used specifically for fibromyalgia.

Patients had access to 24/7 telephonic support, and they were followed up with at the 1- and 6-month marks, at which time their data were recollected and dosages and cannabis medication regimes were reviewed. Quantitative data analysis approaches included a multivariate analysis using SPSS software.

Questionnaire data included demographics, daily habits, medical history, concurrent medications, history of substance abuse, symptoms checklist, QoL assessment using a Likert scale from very bad to very good, and fibromyalgia symptoms. At the 6-month point, fibromyalgia symptoms were assessed using an 8-point Likert scale (from 1 = severe symptomatic deterioration to 8 = maximal symptom improvement). The study was not randomized (it was observational), there was no control group, and it was difficult to monitor compliance.

Participants: There were 367 potential participants, with a mean age of 52.9 years (the majority of the patients were 40 to 60 years), of whom 82% were female. Twenty-eight patients stopped treatment prior to 6-month follow-up, 28 stopped medical treatment prior to the 6-month follow-up, 4 switched to a different medical cannabis supplier, and 2 died. Of the remaining 298 patients, the 6-month response rate was 70.8% or 211 respondents. The median length of fibromyalgia pain was 7 years, with 87% of patients stating they had daily constant pain, with pain being the main motivator for treatment. 45.2% of participants had experience with using recreational cannabis in the past.

Findings: Pain intensity, measured on a scale of 0 to 10, dropped from a precannabis use median score of a 9 to a 6-month median score of a 5, with 81.1% of the 239 participants experiencing positive treatment response. Initially, patients reporting a pain level of 8 to 10 prior to treatment were 52.5%. At the 6-month checkup, only 7.9% reported a pain level of 8 to 10.

About 92.9% of patients also experienced improvement in sleep (73.4% improved; 13.2% resolved), with 80.8% of patients who suffered from depression also showing improvement in depression-related symptoms. QoL scores went from a pretreatment rate of only 2.7% of participants reporting good or very good up to 61.9% reporting QoL to be good or very good. QoL scores included sleep, appetite, and sexual activity.

Being over age 60 and having concerns about cannabis treatment were associated with treatment failure, whereas previous cannabis use and spasticity were associated with treatment success. Patient median cannabinoid use at the 6-month mark was factored to be 140 mg THC and 39 mg CBD per day. Side effects included dizziness (7.9%), dry mouth (6.7%), nausea and vomiting (5.4%), and hyperactivity (5.5%). Patients also reported stopping or decreasing their other prescribed medications, such as opioids and benzodiazepines.

Discussion and implications for cannabis care: Pain is a complex experience, and the researchers looking beyond simply measuring pain to include issues of sleep and QoL are commendable and point toward a holistic approach. This study demonstrates not only a clear process to support patient's titration of cannabis medicines but also that the medicine is effective at addressing pain and other issues associated with homeostasis related to fibromyalgia. Using nurses to coach and educate the patients supports an emerging role for cannabis nurses and approaches to supporting the cannabis research process. Using standardized cannabinoid medicine helped to make effective dosing and determining therapeutic ranges of THC:CBD, though there is an unknown that if different strains were used, would the same results and dosing emerge? The NASEM (2017) recommended more short-term efficacy studies for populations with conditions that will likely benefit from cannabis should be conducted, and this study meets these recommendations.

Cannabinoids and Pain: A Meta-Analysis

Article: Yanes, J. A., McKinnell, Z. E., Reid, M. A., Busler, J. N., Michel, J. S., Pangelinan, M. M., Sutherland, M. T., Younger, J. W., Gonzalez, R., & Robinson, J. L. (2019). Effects of cannabinoid administration for pain: A meta-analysis and meta-regression. *Experimental and Clinical Psychopharmacology, 27*(4), 370–382. https://doi.org/10.1037/pha0000281

Authors: Most of the authors are all affiliated as researchers at various universities in the Southeastern United States.

Purpose: The authors stated that previous meta-analysis reviews have had competing conclusions, with some stating that cannabis is effective for pain management, and some stating that cannabis has a null effect. Furthermore, "meta-analyses present powerful opportunities to coalesce conventional effect size estimates across published studies, providing clarification regarding results and permitting assessments not possible within the original, single report" (Yanes et al., 2019, p. 373). In other words, when several similar or comparable studies' findings are pooled, we can see a larger pooled-effect size across specific end points or alternatively to make comparisons between two or more drug administration approaches.

Methodology: The authors did a meta-analysis and meta-regression of 25 peer-reviewed studies that looked at pain reduction with the use of cannabinoids versus a placebo control. The meta-analysis was performed to look at drug-induced pain reduction outcomes between cannabinoids versus placebos. The meta-regression allowed the researchers to further examine the relationships between various variables (sample size, age, sex, experimental design, specific pain population), drug administration, and pain reduction. The authors posited that cannabis would be more effective than placebo and that study-level characteristics would be associated with pain reduction standardized effect sizes.

Using a variety of search terms, the researchers looked for literature via the search engines PubMed and Web of Science related to pharmacologic studies that assessed for cannabinoid (whole plant cannabis, whole plant cannabis extracts, and synthetic cannabinoids such as Dronabinol) induced changes in subjective pain ratings compared to placebo approaches. The researchers did not consider non-human research and non–peer-reviewed/nonoriginal research studies were also excluded, with the meta-analysis restricted to randomized controlled trials. The studies had to compare baseline to end point and include a control group that did not include drug-induced pain reduction measures (eg, use of ibuprofen). The articles analyzed were published through the year 2018.

The researchers undertook an in-depth meta-analysis approach to extract data from the 25 studies, including baseline pain severity scores, endpoint pain severity scores, and associated variance estimates to determine the study-level standardized mean-gain effect size. The authors also performed a meta-regression using exploratory fixed-effects multiple linear regression to look at the relationships between continuous categorical outcome variables (sample size, age, sex composition) and continuous outcome variables (study-level standardized effect).

Participants/studies examined: Across the 25 studies analyzed, there were 2,248 participants with a mean age of 52.09 years, and 51.57%, on average, were women. The populations from the studies included neuropathic pain (n = 7), cancer (n = 4), diabetes (n = 3), MS (n = 3), abdominal pain (n = 1), arthritis (n = 1), chronic pain (n = 1), fibromyalgia (n = 1), HIV (n = 1), postoperative pain (n = 1), and "various" types of pain (n = 1).

Five studies used whole plant cannabis, 11 utilized whole plant cannabis extracts, and 9 studies examined synthetic cannabinoids.

Findings: Across the studies, cannabinoids were associated with having a medium to large effect on reducing pain, whereas placebos were found to have a small to medium effect. Overall, cannabinoids were associated with greater pain reduction as compared to placebo administration. The findings held up under meta-regression analysis, with the researchers further determining that the studies with a smaller sample size and those having more female participants were linked with greater pain reduction.

Discussion and implications for cannabis care: The researchers concluded that cannabinoids do lead to changes in self-reported pain and that the placebo effect does have an impact on self-reported pain. The authors called for further research in several areas, including outcomes differences between single-dose use versus longer term use of cannabinoids for pain, the complex interactions between other pain medicines and cannabinoids, and considerations of cannabis substance abuse as access continues to broaden. For cannabis care nurses, these are important points to consider, as many patients will use multiple medications to manage pain, and we do need to consider the well-being of populations as access to cannabis escalates.

The ability to share both the two previous studies and this large-scale meta-analysis demonstrates that there is indeed a good deal of quality research being done around cannabis and cannabinoid therapeutics for chronic pain, as recommended by the NASEM (2017) report.

> **APPLIED LEARNING**

Pain Issues

Do a search for chronic pain and cannabis in an online search engine like PubMed, limiting the search to the past year.
- How many articles were found?
- How could you limit this search further?
- Do the articles seem to be human based or in vivo, in vitro, or animal studies?
- Choose one article to analyze and share within a small group. What was the quality of the article, and what did it add to the knowledge base? Discuss if researchers are making progress in building the body of evidence regarding cannabinoid science and pain.

POSTTRAUMATIC STRESS DISORDER

PTSD diagnostic criteria include exposure to a traumatic event and exhibition of ongoing psychologically distressing symptoms related to the traumatic event exposure. In the NASEM (2017) report, the committee stated that they did not identify any good- or fair-quality systematic reviews of PTSD and cannabis medicine, and they reviewed only one fair-quality randomized crossover trial that showed some evidence of improvement of PTSD symptoms with 10 participants. Clearly, with PTSD being one of the greatest reasons why people seek medical cannabis, more study is needed in this area. Patient experience should be driving our research efforts.

Since the publication of the NASEM (2017) report, more efforts have been made to gather evidence and create systematic reviews focusing on PTSD and cannabis. One thing for cannabis care nurses to consider is the value of the human experience in tandem with the gold standard of randomized controlled clinical trials.

Posttraumatic Stress Disorder: A Systematic Review

Article: Hindocha, C., Cousijn, J., Rall, M., & Bloomfield, M. A. P. (2019). The effectiveness of cannabinoids in the treatment of post-traumatic stress disorder (PTSD): A systematic review. *Journal of Dual Diagnoses, 3,* 1–20. https://doi.org/10.1080/155 04263.2019.1652380

Authors: All authors are from the United Kingdom or the Netherlands. Four of the authors work in university/research settings, and one author works in a clinic that cares for traumatic stress patients.

Purpose: To systematically review the quality of PTSD-cannabis evidence.

Methodology: The authors gathered articles through 2018 where a validated instrument was used to determine reduction in PTSD symptoms, with the population of PTSD patients who were "prescribed" medical cannabis. The authors included randomized controlled trials, observational studies, case studies, and retrospective reports. The authors assessed for bias and quality using validated tools. Ten studies that matched the inclusion criteria were selected.

Findings: The authors stated that every study had a medium to high risk for bias, and all were categorized as "low quality." The authors did conclude that cannabis use may help reduce PTSD sleep disturbance issues and nightmares.

Discussion and implications for cannabis care: The researchers concluded that there is still lack of high-quality trials when it comes to looking at cannabis use and PTSD because most studies are small and of low quality. However, the minimal evidence points toward the need for larger, randomized controlled clinical trials to support the notion that cannabinoids can help manage PTSD symptoms, which is similar to the NASEM (2017) report findings.

Mitigation of Posttraumatic Stress Symptoms

Article: Passie, T., Emrich, H. M., Karst, M., Brandt, S. D., & Halpern, J. (2012). Mitigation of post-traumatic stress symptoms by cannabis resin: A review of the clinical and neurobiological evidence. *Drug Testing and Analysis, 4*, 649–657. http://dx.doi.org/10.1002/dta1377 (Note, older study, not included in NASEM 2017 report).

Authors: No acknowledgments noted, and no funding or conflict of interest indicated. This study's authors were from Hanover Medical School in Hanover, Germany.

Purpose: This article is a review of the evidence that cannabinoids can mitigate some of the symptoms of PTSD. Part of the article is a case study that examined one patient and how he decided to address his PTSD. Some of the potentially beneficial properties of cannabis as related to PTSD include altering fear conditioning and memory systems, with reduction of dream recall, general central nervous system (CNS) arousal, and anxiety mitigating mood and sleep disturbances.

Background: It is known that some PTSD patients turn to recreational drugs to help them cope with their symptoms. There are some effects of cannabis that may be appealing to victims of PTSD, including reduction of anxiety, sleep induction, some sedation, and relaxation. It is known that many PTSD patients are using cannabis to alleviate symptoms. In the adolescent population, with those who have experienced a traumatic event, the number of cannabis users is higher versus those who have not had childhood trauma.

The authors of this article found a strong correlation between the severity of sleep disturbances in PTSD patients and the increased use of cannabis. There is some question as to the actual sleep enhancement properties of cannabis, or if enhanced sleep emerges because there is a reduction of other bothersome symptoms as well. Of interest is the fact that well over one half of patients who start the use of cannabis do so at approximately the same time that the PTSD event occurs.

Clinical case report: This is a case study of a young man who, from the time he was 4 years of age, was sadistically sexually abused by his father and uncle. This abuse continued until this young man was 15 years old, at which point he made two suicide attempts. The patient was not diagnosed with PTSD and did not receive specific services for years: specialized services might have been offered earlier had he been given a correct diagnosis.

The case study begins with the person undergoing an acute hospitalization for stabilization when he began having flashbacks and severe panic attacks and impulses for self-mutilation. This patient was treated with traditional medications (lorazepam). During acute flashback episodes, he would throw himself on the floor, thrash about, and completely lose control. He was stabilized fairly quickly and moved back to his in-patient clinic. After a short time, he experienced marked improvement. His next blood work was negative, except for a positive THC result. He explained that he had learned to smoke cannabis resin from other patients. The patient felt much more in control, had much less anxiety, and less involvement with his flashbacks. Of note is that patient purchased cannabis resin in Turkey. There was no analysis of this product.

Discussion and implications for cannabis care: Although this is an older study, it was not included in the NASEM (2017) report. However, capturing the human experience with cannabis care is an important contribution to the body of evidence, and qualitative research with cannabis patients remains minimal. It is included because of the value of the case report that the authors presented. From more recent studies, it is clear that cannabis is used by many PTSD patients to cope with their symptoms. The case study presented here was a patient with a grave pathology who could handle his symptoms much better and kept his flashbacks at bay with cannabis use. Cannabis has been used as a psychopharmacologic agent for hundreds of years; however, there may be side effects, including mild dependency or worsening of some psychological symptoms. Case studies are often valuable because they point toward the actual human experience of using a medication.

Posttraumatic Stress Disorder and Coping Among Recent Veterans

Article: Elliott, L., Golub, A., Bennett, A., & Guarino, H. (2015). PTSD and cannabis related copping among recent veterans in New York City. *Contemporary Drug Problems, 42,* 60–76. https://doi.org/10.1177/0091450915570309

Authors: This research was supported by grants from the National Institute on Alcohol Abuse and Alcoholism and the Peter F. McManus Charitable Trust. The researchers are from the National Development and Research Institutes in New York City (NYC).

Purpose: To study coping mechanisms of veterans who have returned from Iraq or Afghanistan and to review the coping strategies used to combat PTSD and related side effects.

Methodology: This study looked at veterans who had returned to their New York neighborhood after combat and subsequent separation from the armed services as described earlier. The veterans participating were drawn from two studies. The groups were initially separated into two groups. A focus groups of participants was recruited to look at substance use among returning veterans who lived in NYC. An interview group of participants was recruited from another study, and these veterans were identified as PTSD patients who used cannabis.

Participants: Veterans formerly enlisted, serving after September 11, 2001, and separated from the armed services for at least 24 months before the time of recruitment for the study.

Focus groups: This study was initiated to look at mental health and substance use issues of returning veterans who met the study criteria. There were two groups of 10, with 6 men and 14 women. Racial distribution included African Americans, Hispanics, Caucasians, and Asians. These veterans identified as PTSD patients who either had a formal diagnosis or had self-diagnosed. The 2-hour focus group asked open-ended questions about reintegration, such as finding employment, housing, medical care, and living with mental health issues. The follow-up questions concerned how pharmaceuticals or illicit substances either helped or hindered them in dealing with these reintegration issues. There was much discussion about the advantages of using cannabis for pain, PTSD, and depression.

In-depth interviews: Once the main themes of the focus groups were determined, a smaller subset of the parent study (focus group) were patients suffering from PTSD who were also using cannabis. The field staff that had enrolled patients and conducted the focus groups made recommendations for those who should be included in the interviews. These patients were contacted, the study explained, and contact numbers of the researchers were provided should the veterans want to participate. The participants were screened once again for cannabis use and continued PTSD symptoms. Researchers checked a military PTSD checklist to ensure that each subject has some of the required PTSD symptoms.

Interviews were scheduled, and they averaged about 80 to 120 minutes in length. The interviews focused on three topics: history of PTSD, history of cannabis use, and the subject's experience with cannabis in relationship to PTSD. Thirty-one participants were included in the analysis portion of the study and were compensated $40 for participation in focus groups or interviews. This study was approved by the institutional review board (IRB) of the National Development and Research Institutes.

Findings: A team of three researchers were charged with developing themes using the principles of grounded theory. The predominant research question asked if attempts by veterans with PTSD to medicate with alcohol or other illicit substances are a form of avoidance or escapist behavior versus this behavior being a normal, controlled coping mechanism for PTSD symptoms. There are clearly limitations to the study because of size; however, there was profound feedback from many of the patients. One patient offered the powerful metaphor of "a return to ground zero." The majority of the group agreed that avoiding memories and feelings about one's trauma is dangerous and prolongs resolution. Cannabis speeds along the journey toward resolution by providing a calm and focused mental state. It was concluded that those who use cannabis as part of an ongoing effort to confront their traumatic event and to get support from others may well have better outcomes than those who are using cannabis as an avoidance or escape mechanism, which may in fact delay or block their recovery or resolution.

Discussion and implications for cannabis care: It is important to keep in mind that there are adverse events that can be attributed to cannabis; in a clinical setting, there are likely mechanisms to deal with any severe adverse events. However, the vast majority of veterans who use cannabis do so in an unsupervised environment. With the lack of abundant empirical data regarding who should use cannabis, when to use cannabis, and how to use it, it becomes incumbent on both the veterans and the nongovernmental employees to help answer these types of questions. It is important that sympathetic clinicians and those in the industry that are familiar with appropriate usage develop educational materials and identify support systems for veterans with PTSD.

> ### ▶ APPLIED LEARNING POINTS
>
> **Posttraumatic Stress Disorder**
> This is an opportunity to do some research.
> - How many veterans currently suffer from PTSD?
> - What are some primary goals for treating PTSD symptoms with the veteran population?
> - What are the current common medications and medical treatment regimens for veterans diagnosed with PTSD? How is their effectiveness measured?
> - What challenges do veterans face when trying to access cannabis?

CANCER CARE

Since 2017, one of the authors of this chapter has traveled the country discussing cannabis care with oncology nurses. Over these past several years, what stands out to her is that oncology nurses are educating themselves about patient medicinal cannabis use and helping to end the stigma associated with cannabis use (Clark, 2018).

Along with a cancer diagnosis that requires extensive treatment, cannabis care nurses should always be considering and planning for palliation: cancer patients' outcomes are better when palliation begins upon diagnosis. Cannabis can be a large part of that palliative care plan because it addresses the myriad aspects of oncology patient needs, including nausea, pain, sleep disturbance issues, and spiritual distress. Opioids tend to be a mainstay of treatment for oncology patients, yet they have many side effects and carry risk of addiction, therefore having alternatives and integrative therapies available that can be supportive of palliation and successful completion of treatment is called for. Oncology patients also remain dissatisfied with their emetogenic care, and cannabis offers an alternative for managing nausea and vomiting associated with moderate-to-highly emetogenic chemotherapy treatments. Despite optimal antiemetic prophylaxis, up to 50% of chemotherapy patients experience chemotherapy-induced nausea and vomiting (CINV) (Mersiades et al., 2018). In addition, there is a keen interest in exploring how cannabinoid therapeutics may support healing from cancer, as cannabis supports the body in the apoptosis and autophagy processes of renewing cells and reminding cancer cells to die. One of the greatest issues of studying the effectiveness of cannabis care with cancer/oncology patients is that the prohibition effect has deterred the ability of researchers to perform standardized, randomized controlled clinical trials with substantial numbers of the population in order to generate evidence.

The following sections review some of the latest findings about cancer care and use of cannabinoids for palliation and healing.

Guidelines for Cannabis Use and Chemotherapy

Article: Makary, P., Parmar, J. R., Mims, N., Khanfar, N. M., & Freeman, R. A. (2018). Patient counseling guidelines for the use of cannabis for the treatment of chemotherapy-induced nausea/vomiting and chronic pain. *Journal of Pain & Palliative Care Pharmacotherapy, 32*(4), 216–225. https://doi.org/10.1080/15360288.201 9.1598531

Authors: All of the authors are affiliated with universities/colleges, and they have graduate degrees, including MSc, PhD, and MD.

Purpose: To develop guidelines to help pharmacists educate patients and providers about the use of cannabis in oncologic care.

Methodology: A literature review was performed using Medline, PubMed, and Google Scholar in order to review common practices for cannabinoid treatment for cancer patients with chemotherapy-induced nausea, vomiting, and chronic pain, as well as examining adverse effects of cannabinoid therapeutics. Search terms used included cannabinoid's adverse effects, cannabis, CINV, medical cannabis, natural cannabinoids, and THC. The authors looked at articles from 2015 to 2018 and found four publications in PubMed matching some of the search terms and eight articles in Google Scholar. After reviewing the literature, the authors applied the American Society of Health Systems Pharmacists patient counseling guidelines to develop their guidelines.

Participants: "Participants" in this case would be the total number of all participants culled from the literature analyzed, which consisted mostly of meta-analyses of current studies. In some studies, researchers will cull the total number of participants from all of the studies analyzed, but in this case, the researchers instead summarized the meta-analysis findings of other researchers and did not provide a total number for all studies reviewed.

Findings: The researchers note that smoked and ingested cannabis are not well studied, whereas Cesamet, Sativex, and Marinol have many more randomized controlled clinical studies in place. The authors were able to create a table, showing how each of these medicines works in the following areas: use/expected benefits or actions, expected onset of action, route/dosage form/dosage/administration, precautions, common and severe adverse effects, contraindications/pregnancy, and interactions such as drug to drug, drug to food, and drug to disease. The guidelines are written in such a way as to demonstrate how they can be used to counsel patients.

Discussion and implications for cannabis care: The general problem with this study, and the resultant table for counseling patients, demonstrates that there is still far too little evidence generated for the smoked and orally ingested whole plant cannabis, and there is a potential bias toward synthetic forms of cannabis. This work also becomes less useful in the real life of coaching cannabis patients, as most patients will likely not have access to the synthetic forms of cannabinoid medicines, but they will be able to access the plant forms. The article provides a beginning platform for educating patients about their options while clearly demonstrating the supporting evidence.

Pediatric Oncology Cannabis Care

Article: Skyprek, M. M., Bostrom, B. C., & Bendel, A. E. (2019). Medical cannabis certification in a large pediatric oncology center. *Children, 6*(79), 1–8. https://doi.org/10.3390/children6060079

Authors: All the three authors are physicians who work in the pediatric hematology and oncology department at Children's Hospital of Minnesota (CHM), Minneapolis, Minnesota.

Purpose: To begin to explore the use of medicinal cannabis with pediatric oncology patients. There is a dearth of knowledge and research related to this vulnerable population and their use of cannabis to palliate symptoms, as the majority of the studies of cancer and cannabis use are based on adult populations. The American Academy of Pediatrics current policy opposes cannabis use in pediatric population through young adulthood, unless there is a life-threatening or severely debilitating condition that traditional therapies are failing to address. The authors state that only one other study of pediatric oncology and cannabis use has been performed, and it focused on the pediatric providers' knowledge, attitudes, and barriers related to the use of medical cannabis in the pediatric population. That study found that their providers have an ongoing bias toward pediatric population medical cannabis use, with cannabis used primarily for those pediatric patients with advanced-stage illnesses and/or for palliation (vs as a regular option in routine care or routine palliation for pediatric oncology patients).

Methodology: The study was approved by the IRB of the CHM. The researchers reviewed the records of providers within the pediatric hematology-oncology department at CHM who were certified to write medical cannabis recommendations for pediatric patients. The researchers extracted data from July 2015 through February 2019. Data analyzed included diagnosis/subtype of diagnosis (brain tumors, leukemia, lymphoma, malignant solid tumors mast cell activation), date of diagnosis, indication or reason for medical cannabis certification, date of relapse of tumor(s), and date of death. Statistical analysis was performed using SPSS software.

Participants: Retrospective data were drawn from patient charts. One hundred and one patients were certified over the 3-year time period. The age range was 1.4 to 28.7 years, with the median age 15.3 years, and the makeup was 56% male, 44% female.

Findings: The median time period from diagnosis to medical cannabis certification was 8.9 months; however, 94% of patients received medical cannabis certification as first-line treatment along with diagnosis (to be used in conjunction with allopathic treatments). The primary reason for certification with patients with leukemia, lymphoma, and brain tumors was for chemotherapy-induced nausea; for solid tumor patients, the primary reason was for intractable pain. Seventy-six percent of patients who received a medical cannabis recommendation went on to access medical cannabis. The brain tumor population hoped that cannabis would also have an antitumor effect based on recent studies in this area. The authors stated that compliance with chemotherapy for teenagers and young adults increased with the use of medical cannabis.

Discussion and implications for cannabis care: The authors did not have a clear data as to why about 24% of patients given a medical recommendation for cannabis did not follow through, though they believe cost may be an issue to consider. The authors further hoped that their data would encourage other oncologists to consider supporting pediatric oncology patients to pursue medical cannabis certification at time of diagnosis to begin palliative efforts with diagnosis and chemotherapy treatment, versus waiting until the end-of-life period to recommend cannabis. Although this is a relatively small study, it is very important because it looks at the vulnerable pediatric population and begins to strive to end the stigma around children accessing medicine that can palliate and support compliance with oncologic treatments. If patients have better compliance with oncology treatments via the safe use of cannabis, this treatment should be more widely considered by pediatric oncologists. This article adds to the need for more research in age-related populations for conditions treated with cannabis, as the NASEM (2017) report indicated.

Glioma and Cannabidiol: A Case Study

Article: Dall'Stella, P. B., Docema, M. F. L., Maldaun, M. V. C., Feher, O., & Lancelotti, C. L. P. (2019). Case report: Clinical outcome and image response of two patients with secondary high-grade glioma treated with chemoradiation, PCV, and cannabidiol. *Frontiers in Oncology, 8,* 1–7. https://doi.org/10.3389/fonc.2018.00643

Authors: Four of the authors are affiliated with a department of oncology at a major hospital in Brazil. The other author is associated with a department of pathology in Brazil. This is an open-access article and was reviewed by two leading cannabinoid science researchers. The other authors declared that the research was free from any commercial or financial conflict of interest.

Purpose: To determine whether CBD can potentially enhance the effectiveness of chemoradiation and impact survival length and QoL for glioblastoma patients.

Methodology: Two 38-year-old male patients with grade III/IV glioblastoma underwent subtotal resection of the tumors, approximately 1 year of monthly chemotherapy with temozolomide (TMZ), undertook chemoradiation, and followed this up with a 6-month regime of a chemotherapy cocktail known as PCV (procarbazine + lomustine + vincristine) and use of CBD (one patient used 300 to 450 mg/day, the other used 100 to 200 mg CBD/day; all CBD was given in 50-mg capsules). The study lasted for 2 years with the two participants. The patients were also inhaling THC and, of course, other cannabinoids/terpenes from whole plant cannabis during the first year of treatment in order to alleviate symptoms from chemotherapy.

Participants: The two participants completed a consent form that was submitted to the highest regulatory body in Brazil, called the Anvisa. The authors stated that this precluded them from having to receive approval from the local ethics committee.

Findings: The researchers stated that it is not possible to cure high-grade glioma patients; therefore, the aim of all treatment is to prolong life and prevent deterioration of QoL. The researchers revealed that both cases showed a positive response to the cannabis treatment, with no evidence of disease progression during the 2-year treatment period. One patient did have a recurrence two and half years after diagnosis. Even with large amounts of CBD, neither patient demonstrated impacts on hepatic or cardiac functioning. Neither patient used steroids continually during the study, and neither of them suffered from fatigue, loss of appetite, or nausea. Both participants were able to maintain their routines of work and sports activities. Up to approximately one-third of PCV patients have to stop treatment due to severe medication side effects, including hepatotoxicity, hematologic toxicity, neurotoxicity, nausea, and severe rashes; therefore, CBD may be important in preventing such issues from emerging.

Discussion and implications for cannabis care: The authors state that previous studies have shown that a combination of multiple cannabinoids (THC and CBD) has a greater antitumor effect and impact on survival than CBD or THC alone. Owing to the prohibition effect, the researchers were not able to attain medicine with high percentage of THC. The authors called for large-scale, randomized, placebo-controlled trials to confirm their findings. As this is one of the deadliest forms of cancer, this is the type of research that should be replicated to determine whether cannabinoids could be effective as standardized aspects of treatment for glioblastoma patients. In addition, the idea of greater QoL and adequate palliation for these patients should perhaps even supersede the idea of cannabinoids supporting a cure for this type of cancer.

This concludes the review of just a few recent research articles on cannabis and cancer care. There is much more research that needs to be done to support our understanding of how cannabinoid therapeutics can be used to effectively support the palliation needs of oncologic patients, including enhancing the ability to complete challenging chemotherapeutic regimes.

> **APPLIED LEARNING**

Cancer Care

Consider the patient experience with cannabis use during oncology treatment.

■ Do a web search or comb through social media to review cancer patient reports of using cannabis during oncology treatments.

■ What are patients saying about the use of cannabis to support palliation and healing during oncologic treatments?

■ Look for some common themes across patient experience.

■ How can nurses best use patient experience as a form of evidence to inform cannabis care practice? What are the challenges and/or drawbacks with doing this?

CANNABIS AND OPIOIDS: PAIN AND ADDICTION

As reviewed earlier, cannabis is known to treat pain; however, there is much we need to learn in this area. We must also consider that although cannabis has a low addiction rate of about 10% versus opioids addiction rate of up to 30%, its improper use can be a concern for some people with substance abuse disorders. Meanwhile, though still considered to be controversial, cannabis can also be used as a harm reduction tool, assisting folks to completely taper off, or reduce, the use of opioids. The following section explores some of the latest research findings of cannabis use and opioids.

Opioid Users Cannabis Motivations

Article: Clem, S. N., Bigand, T. L., & Wilson, M. (2019). Cannabis use motivations among adults prescribed opioids for pain. *Pain Management Nursing*, 19, S1524. https://doi.org/10.1016/j.pmn.2019.06.009

Authors: Two of the authors are registered nurses with doctoral degrees who work at Washington State University. One author is a BSN-prepared nurse who presumably was a student at Washington State University during the research process.

Purpose: To examine why those who use prescribed opioids for persistent pain (PP) may also use cannabis and compare it with those who use cannabis and have opioid use disorders (OUDs). Previous studies suggest that this population of opioid users may benefit from cannabis use by using less opioids, suffering less side effects from opioid use, having better pain relief, and decreasing the risks for opioid overdose. By examining this population more closely, clinicians can begin to understand why cannabis use is desirable to this population and begin to better identify their unmet health needs. The concern for risk for addiction and having sound policies in this area is noted. Legal cannabis states have a 25% lower annual opioid-related deaths.

Methodology: The researchers used data collected from a previously published study. The original study sample included 300 cannabis using participants: 150 were from the OUD population, and 150 were prescribed opioids for PP. Participants were issued a survey that asked them to rank their pain, depression, anxiety, self-efficacy, and cannabis use. The Marijuana Motives Measure (MMM) scale was used to ascertain motivations for cannabis use. Answers were analyzed using descriptive statistics.

Participants: The final sample of 243 participants was recruited from two outpatient opioid-treatment centers and three pain clinics in Seattle, Washington. Cannabis was adult-use legal at this time of data collection in 2016 to 2017. Age range was 19 to 77 years (mean 41.1 years old), respondents were 59.7% female and 40.3% male. All participants signed informed consent, and the study was approved by the IRB of the researchers' university.

Findings: Across the study, there was no significant difference across the two populations when it came to using cannabis for pain, as both the OUD and PP ranked pain as a motivator for cannabis use. However, OUD patients were more likely to report opiate-withdrawal symptoms as a reason for using cannabis (OUD = 33% vs. PP = 9%).

All participants further stated that cannabis use was also related to addressing recreational/social needs, sleep issues, and anxiety/stress. This points toward clinicians' need to better address these health-related issues with the PP and OUD populations and the idea that current treatment regimens are not adequately addressing these issues. For the PP group, cannabis was found to improve pain functional outcomes, enhance QoL, and support significant reductions in opioid consumption and related side effects. For the OUD patients, they were more likely to use cannabis for "enhancement" or the euphoria as compared to the PP population, and they were more likely to be motivated to use cannabis to prevent or manage opioid-withdrawal symptoms.

Limitations to the study include self-reporting, cross-sectional nature of the data, the sample being primarily older Caucasian women, and the nature of cannabis use reasons overlapping (making it challenging to differentiate among the reasons).

Discussion and implications for cannabis care: The researchers did conclude that pain patients/opioid users are using cannabis in order to meet their current unmet symptom management needs, and therefore, healthcare professionals need to do a better job of assessing their health needs and how they can best be met. In addition, we need to focus more on how cannabis can best support OUD patients and their symptom management needs. Cannabis may support better adherence to overall treatment, reducing the risk of relapse and fatal overdoses. It is important to once again acknowledge that this research was completed by nurses, and it provides an example of how nurses can become part of the cannabis science evidence-building process.

Cannabis Laws and Opioid Use

Article: Segura, L. E., Mauro, C. M., Levy, N. S., Khauli, N., Philbin, M. M., Mauro, P. M., & Martins, S. S. (2019). Association of US medical marijuana laws with nonmedical prescription opioid use and prescription opioid use disorder. *JAMA Network Open, 2*(7), e197216. https://doi.org/10.1001/jamanetworkopen.2019.7216

Authors: All of the authors are employed by Columbia University's Mailman's School of Public Health sector in various departments, including epidemiology, biostatistics, and sociomedical sciences. Two authors are educationally prepared with master's in public health, one author has an MPH and MD, two authors have PhDs, and one author has an MD and PhD degrees.

Purpose: To determine whether enactment of medical cannabis laws in individual states is associated with changes in nonmedical prescription opioid use disorders (NMPOUDs) and prescription opioid use disorders (POUD). The authors also correlated age and racial/ethnic group.

Methodology: This was a cross-sectional study, examining the data from the 2004 to 2014 National Survey on Drug Use and Health. Interview data were originally collected by trained interviewers. The study was completed in 2018, and data from 627,000 individuals were examined. Data from the time periods before and after medical cannabis laws were compared. The study was granted IRB exemption by Columbia University as data were de-identified.

Participants: Data were obtained from 627,000 participants. Age range was 12 to 50 years, 51.51% were female. Participants self-identified as being 66.97% Caucasian, 11.83% black, 14.47% Hispanic, and 6.73% "Other."

Findings: The findings of the analysis showed only small differences in both populations from enactment of medical cannabis laws: POUD prevalence decreased slightly, though it was not statistically significant. NMPOUD increased slightly. Outcomes were similar when age and race/ethnicity were considered.

Limitations included self-reporting of participant data; lack of data from 2015 to 2017; lack of consideration of populations such as the homeless, incarcerated, and active military personnel; lack of differentiation in medical cannabis programs across states (ie, does the state have medical cannabis dispensaries, allow for growing of cannabis at home, etc.); and no controls for legal recreational cannabis use states.

Discussion and implications for cannabis care: The authors called for more detailed exploration of how medical cannabis laws could potentially reduce the harm from OUDs. The authors state that if their findings are replicated, we need to continue to suggest cannabis-specific approaches and policy interventions (pain clinic laws, prescribing practice laws) to address this issue. What the authors failed to consider was perhaps the lack of education of both providers and those patients diagnosed with substance use disorder around how cannabis may be used to decrease opioid intake. In addition, many statewide cannabis laws fail to include OUD as a state-level cannabis recommendation qualifying medical condition, and many pain and substance use disorder clinics refuse to allow for concurrent use of cannabis, so this patient population may be challenged in accessing medical cannabis and being supported and coached through the process.

Literature Review: Cannabis and the Opioid Crisis

Article: Vyas, M. B., LeBaron, V. T., & Gilson, A. M. (2018). The use of cannabis in response to the opioid crisis: A review of the literature. *Nursing Outlook, 66*, 56–65. https://doi.org/10.1016/j.outlook.2017.08.012

Authors: Two of the authors are nurses with graduate degrees, employed by the University of Virginia. One author is a social worker with a graduate degree and affiliated with the Pain and Policy Studies Group/World Health Organization (WHO) Collaborating Center at University of Wisconsin-Madison.

Purpose: The authors were striving to examine the potential correlation between state-level medical cannabis laws and policies and prescription opioid use and related harms.

Methodology: This was a systematic review of the literature. The researchers used PubMed, Medline, CINAHL, and Cochrane databases to find articles published between 2010 and 2017, completing two searches, one focused on opioids and one on cannabis. The results of the two searches were combined to find articles that included both areas of interest. The terms included opioid, opioid analgesic, opioid-related disorders, prescription drug misuse, OUD, opioid policy, overdose, prescription pain medication, cannabis, medical marijuana, cannabis and pain, cannabis and opioids, alternative therapies, substance use disorder, cannabis use disorder, and cannabis policy. All articles were peer reviewed, based in the United States, and included policy issues including analyses of states after cannabis laws were enacted. Using a process of elimination, the researchers were able to start from a baseline of 11,513 articles and work their way down to just 10 articles to include in the literature review.

Findings: The researchers provided an in-depth analysis of the findings across the studies and provided comparative summaries. Ultimately, all 10 studies showed a correlation between medical cannabis laws and reduced harm from prescribed opiate-based medications. The key outcomes measured included opioid-related overdoses, fatalities, prescribed opioid medication abuse, hospitalizations, use, and cost. States with active legal medical cannabis dispensaries showed lower prescription opiate overdose mortality. The states with medical cannabis legality also showed decreases in prescription opioid use, cost-savings around prescribing drugs for which cannabis could be the alternative choice, decreases in opioid-positivity tests in fatally injured drivers, and reduced prescription opioid hospitalizations. Limitations to the study include study design (with some of the 10 studies relying on self-reporting survey data), all of the studies being strictly descriptive, and the inability to differentiate between medical cannabis and recreational use.

Discussion and implications for cannabis care: The researchers state that one explanation for the findings might be related to the similarities between opioid and cannabinoid receptor systems (both are coupled G-protein receptors expressed through brain reinforcement circuitry). This study makes a strong case for medical cannabis being used as a harm reduction tool. The authors called for more research around opiate harm reduction through the exploration of integrative and alternative therapies. They do caution that the long-term risks of medical cannabis legalization are unclear.

> ## ▶ APPLIED LEARNING
>
> ### Harm Reduction
> Review the following questions and discuss with classmates or colleagues.
> - Define the model of harm reduction in relationship to the current opioid crisis.
> - What are some currently applied holistic strategies for opioid harm reduction beyond use of medications?
> - What makes cannabinoid therapy attractive as a harm reduction tool?
> - What other recent peer-reviewed articles did you find that support use of cannabis as an opioid harm reduction tool?

GLAUCOMA

Immediately apparent when conducting research on cannabis and glaucoma is that there are a good number of articles from the late 1990s and early 2000s, then there is a reasonable gap in research with some becoming available from 2014 and forward. The NASEM (2017) report stated that there is still a lack of high-quality clinical trials related to cannabinoids and glaucoma, with many trials showing only short-term effectiveness of cannabinoids helping to manage this illness. The following section reviews some of the latest research in this area.

Facts Versus Fiction

Article: Katz, J., & Costarides, A. P. (2019). Facts vs fiction: The role of cannabinoids in the treatment of glaucoma. *Current Ophthalmology Reports, 7,* 177–181. http://dx.doi.org/10.1007/s40135-019-00214-z

Authors: The researchers are independent and declare no conflict of interest.

Purpose: To evaluate the latest research related to the role of cannabinoids in the treatment of glaucoma and determine whether the evidence in this area is evolving.

Methodology: A review of a number of studies focused on the benefits of cannabis in the treatment of glaucoma.

Findings: The researchers stated that the mechanism of action of cannabis in relation to glaucoma treatment remains poorly understood. The researchers reviewed a study using rabbits and confirmed that there was a reduction in the production of aqueous humor by affecting sodium transport across cells.

Another study reviewed focused on postmortem human subjects and found that there are CB1 receptors in the human eye, including the ciliary body, corneal epithelium, endothelium trabecular meshwork, and Schlemm's canal. The presence of the CB1 receptors throughout the eye demonstrates that the endocannabinoid system regulates the production and transport of the aqueous humor. There continue to be questions about the mechanism of action of cannabis in relation to glaucoma; however, there are several thoughts regarding possible mechanisms, including a decrease in the production of aqueous humor, an increase in the uveoscleral flow, contraction of ciliary muscles to enhance outflow, and a prostaglandin pathway through the cannabinoid breakdown process.

Discussion and cannabis care implications: It is well known that THC is lipophilic and so any ophthalmologic preparation and/or delivery system must have oil-based solutions or emulsions. Studies are ongoing working with different solutions, each hoping to increase absorption and potentially increase the effects: for instance, some researchers are now working with hydrogels to prolong contact and increase absorption of the cannabinoids.

> ### ▶ SIDE NOTES: HUMAN HISTORY, GLAUCOMA
>
> Robert Randall was diagnosed with advanced open-angle glaucoma. He was 24 years old, and doctors told him he would be blind by the time he turned 30. None of the medications that the doctors prescribed lowered his intraocular pressure (IOP). Smoking marijuana with a friend one evening, Robert noted that his vision improved and the halos that surrounded objects within his vision disappeared. This discovery set Robert on a long path fighting the government to gain the right to use marijuana to treat his glaucoma. Randall successfully used a medical necessity defense when he was charged with illegal possession of cannabis to treat his glaucoma. The case, *United States v. Randall*, is "The first successful articulation of the medical necessity defense in the history of the common law, and indeed, the first case to extend the necessity defense to the crimes of possession or cultivation of marijuana."
>
> Ultimately in 1981, Randall and his long-time partner, Alice O'Leary, founded the Alliance for Cannabis Therapeutics (www.marijuana-as-medicine.org/alliance.htm), the first nonprofit organization focused on changing the federal law prohibiting medical access to marijuana. Robert's widow, Alice O'Leary-Randall, continues to fight for patients' rights to access cannabis and has actively served nurses as a founder of the American Cannabis Nurses Association.

Treating Glaucoma in a Legalized City

Although this study was published prior to the NASEM (2017), it is of interest to our readers because it delves into the actual patient experience of using cannabis to palliate symptoms. Many scientists are not adept at looking at patient experience, and this study made great efforts to consider how patients perceive the effectiveness of the cannabinoid treatments.

Article: Belyea, D. A., Allhabshan, R., del Rio-Gonzalez, A. M., Chadha, N., Lamba, T., Golshani, C., Merchant, K., Passi, N., & Dan, J. A. (2016). Marijuana use among patients with glaucoma in a city with legalized medical marijuana use. *JAMA Ophthalmology, 134*(3), 259–264. https://doi.org/10.1001/jamaophthalmol.2015.5209

Authors: The authors are all associates within a large university school of medicine. The research took place at an academic-based glaucoma clinic. No conflicts of interest were disclosed.

Purpose: The purpose was to determine patients' intentions to use cannabis for glaucoma treatment and, using a linear regression analysis, determine associated factors related to patient's intentions to use cannabis for glaucoma.

Methodology: This was a cross-sectional, survey-based study of 204 patients with glaucoma or suspected glaucoma. The participants were given a survey that gathered demographics and then focused on the individual's perceived severity of glaucoma, prior knowledge about using cannabis for glaucoma, previous cannabis use, perceptions of cannabis use (ie, legal issues, adverse/side effects, safety, effectiveness, false beliefs), satisfaction with current glaucoma management, relevance of treatment costs, and intentions to use cannabis to manage glaucoma.

Participants: Two hundred and four patients completed the survey, about 50% were female, and most were white (40.2%).

Findings: The researchers found that perceptions around legality of cannabis, false beliefs regarding cannabis, satisfaction with current glaucoma care, and glaucoma treatment costs all influenced participants' intentions to use cannabis.

Discussion and implications for cannabis care: Interestingly, the authors called for more ophthalmologists to be educated around cannabis in order to be able to educate their patients. They believed that with increased acceptability, more patients were likely to use cannabis, despite the limited evidence around the effectiveness of cannabis in helping to manage glaucoma. For cannabis care nurses, this points toward the idea that patients need to be educated around the choices that they make, but we may also consider that patients' experiences need to be valued, and that despite greater acceptance of cannabis, there remains a great need for patients to be supported and coached through the process of making informed medical treatment choices.

Tetrahydrocannabinol Versus Cannabidiol: Implications in Glaucoma Care

Article: Miller, S., Daily, L., Leishman, E., Bradshaw, H., & Straiker, A. (2018). Δ-9 Tetrahydrocannabinol and cannabidiol differentially regulate intraocular pressure. *Investigative Ophthalmology and Visual Science, 59*(15), 5904–5911. https://doi.org/10.1167/iovs.18-24838

Authors: All authors are affiliated with a large university research center.

Purpose: To differentiate how both THC and CBD interact with known cannabinoid receptors in lowering IOP.

Methodology: This study was done on mice; however, it is an important work that creates some of the foundational groundwork on how cannabis may impact glaucoma patients in consideration of cannabis and the endocannabinoid system.

Participants: The researchers looked at the effects of topical THC and CBD on live mice.

Findings: The researchers found that THC lowers IOP of mice for at least 8 hours by acting at CB1 and GPR18 sites, though the researchers did note much stronger reactions in male mice. CBD, on the other hand, had very differing effects on the mice: mild mice experienced an increase in IOP, whereas knockout mice experienced a decrease in IOP when CBD was applied. In addition, when CBD and THC were used in a 1:1 ratio, CBD seemed to prevent positive IOP effects of THC, and IOP remained the same. The researchers did not assess the pharmacokinetics. The researchers caution that CBD can potentially elevate IOP, and this needs to be considered as CBD is so widely available.

Discussion and implications for cannabis care: The researchers claim that position statements declaring cannabis as ineffective in treating glaucoma (there are several ophthalmology organizations that declare glaucoma patients should not use cannabis) as being premature and that their study has great implications for how we study cannabinoids and glaucoma in the future. For now, we know that males may experience more benefit from cannabis when managing their glaucoma and that high percentage THC cannabis may be more effective, whereas CBD may have a null effect or even potentially increase IOP. More human studies need to replicate these findings, and more attention should be paid to the physiology of how cannabis interacts with the endocannabinoid system and across genders. This animal study was included as it points toward the future of human studies.

> **▶ APPLIED LEARNING**
>
> **Glaucoma**
> - In how many states is glaucoma listed as a qualifying condition for a medical cannabis recommendation?
> - What kind of research needs to be done to build the body of evidence regarding the effectiveness of cannabis in plaiting glaucoma symptoms?
> - What are the barriers to doing this research?

INFLAMMATORY BOWEL DISEASE (SYNDROME)

The NASEM (2017) reported that approximately 11% of the world's population suffers from inflammatory bowel disease (IBD) symptoms, including abdominal cramping and changes in bowel patterns. IBD can be categorized as IBD with diarrhea, IBD with constipation, IBD mixed, and IBD unclassified. Although the NASEM reported that there are CB1 receptors in the gastrointestinal (GI) tract mucosal cells and there is potential for cannabinoids to help with IBD, there is still insufficient evidence to clearly support or refute any conclusions that cannabinoid medicines are effective in managing IBD symptoms. The following section looks closely at new studies emerging in this area.

NATIONWIDE STUDY

Article: Desai, R., Patel, U., Rimu, A. H., Zalavadia, D., Bansal, P., & Shah, N. (2019). In hospital outcomes of inflammatory bowel disease in cannabis users: A nation-wide propensity matched analysis in the United States. *Annals of Translational Medicine, 7*(12), 1–9. https://doi.org/10.21037/atm.2019.04.63

Authors: The authors are all affiliated with various medical universities in the United States.

Purpose: To determine the impact of recreational cannabis use on Crohn's disease (CD) and ulcerative colitis (UC) patients and to determine whether cannabis use creates distinct outcomes with this population.

Methodology: Undertaking a retrospective propensity-matched analysis, the authors reviewed Nationwide Input Sample data sets from 2010 to 2014, looking specifically for *ICD-9-CM* codes associated with CD and UC to determine whether there were links between recreational cannabis use and in-hospital complications, discharge disposition, mean length of stay, and hospital charges. Using standard statistical approaches, categorical and continuous variables were compared with propensity-matched cohorts.

Participants: The propensity-matched cohorts consisted of 6.022 CD (2,999 cannabis users and 3,003 nonusers) and 1,481 UC (742 cannabis users and 739 nonusers).

Findings: Cannabis using CD patients showed lower prevalence for cancer, parental nutrition, and anemia, whereas fistulizing abscesses/intra-abdominal abscess, lower GI bleed, and hypovolemia were of greater incidence. In addition, the mean hospital stay for CD cannabis users was shorter, with significantly less hospital charges incurred.

UC cannabis users faced a higher incidence of fluid and electrolyte disorders and hypovolemia, but had lower postoperative infections, shorter mean hospital stays, and significantly fewer overall costs.

Discussion and implications for cannabis care: The findings from this study are positive and warrant further investigation. It is noted that the researchers looked only at the patients identified as recreational cannabis users, so there was no data collected regarding the type of cannabis used, dosage, frequency, ingestion route, and so forth. Other medications the patients were on were also not considered. However, this large study does create a call for further research with this population.

Patient Profiles

Article: Kerlin, A. M., Long, M., Kappleman, M., Martin, C., & Sandler, R. S. (2018). Profiles of patients who use marijuana for inflammatory bowel disease. *Digestive Diseases and Sciences, 63*, 1600–1604. https://doi.org/10.1007/s10620-018-5040-5

Authors: All authors are affiliated with college or university medical departments.

Purpose: To determine the benefits IBD patients perceive from using medical or recreational cannabis.

Methodology: The authors accessed participants the IBD Partners (formerly known as the Crohn's and Colitis Foundation of America Partners) online research network of the University of North Carolina School of Medicine. IBD Partners goal is to bring together IBD patients and researchers so that treatments can be optimized. IBD Partners members complete a baseline survey and then provide updates every 6 months. The researchers used several different validated instruments: the Simple Clinical Colitis Activity Index to determine disease activity; the Short Inflammatory Bowel Disease Questionnaire to determine QoL; and the Patient-Reported Outcomes Measurement Information System (PROMIS) to measure anxiety, depression, sleep, pain, and social satisfaction. The authors also hypothesized that the participants would have greater access to recreational cannabis instead of getting medical recommendations in order to access medical cannabis. Analyses were performed using standard statistical approaches for each measurement tool.

Participants: The researchers opened this study to 2,357 potential participants residing in the 25 states where cannabis was medically legal, and 1,666 members took the survey.

Findings: In medical cannabis states, about 12.8% of participants (n = 214) asked their doctor about medical use of cannabis for IBD. Eighty-three participants had been recommended/"prescribed" cannabis and 73 participants (or 4.4% of the study population) were currently using cannabis. Of the 1,666 respondents, 234 reported that they lived in recreational cannabis states, and 20.9% of those patients (n = 40) reported using cannabis legally, but without a medical recommendation. A total of 114 respondents stated they were using cannabis legally (combined recreational and medical users) for the purpose of managing IBD.

The participants noted improvement in pain (68%), appetite (49%), anxiety (48%), fatigue (26%), stool frequency (23%), weight gain (20%), and blood in stool (5%). Nineteen percent of participants note no symptom relief. The cannabis users reported significantly more anxiety, depression, pain, and lower social satisfaction. The medical cannabis users reported having more surgeries and poorer quality of health overall.

Discussion and implications for cannabis care: The researchers noted that those patients who received a recommendation to use cannabis may likely have more issues with poorly controlled symptoms that conventional medicine was not addressing well. The authors did not capture dosing and methods of administration, and active disease was self-reported versus objectively defined. This does bring to mind that cannabis may still be looked as a palliative measure and that its use is often delayed until patients have run out of other allopathic/conventional treatment options.

Inflammatory Bowel Disease: Teens and Young Adults

Article: Hoffenberg, E. J., McWilliams, S. K., Mikulich-Gilbertson, S. K., Murphy, B. V., Langeaux, M., Robbins, K., Hoffenberg, A. S., de Zoeten, E., & Hopfer, C. J. (2018). Marijuana use by adolescents and young adults with inflammatory bowel disease. *The Journal of Pediatrics, 199*, 99–105. https://doi.org/10.1016/j.jpeds.2018.03.041

Authors: Most of the authors are affiliated with the University of Colorado School of Medicine. One author lists the Children's Hospital of Colorado as affiliation. This study was funded by the Colorado Department of Public Health and Environment.

Purpose: To define the value of medical cannabis in pediatric participants and describe their IBD course, their cannabis use patterns, and their perceptions of harm and benefit. There are no previous studies about IBD and cannabis use in the pediatric population.

Methodology: This was a descriptive, cross-sectional study. Cannabis users were compared to noncannabis users. Participants self-reported data on appetite, pain, QoL, depression, anxiety, and cannabis use through various research tools and validated questionnaires. Cannabis use was measured, and perceptions defined through asking various questions adapted from other research tools that investigated non-medical opiate use, cannabis and alcohol consumption motives, as well as unique questions that also had to be validated.

Serum levels of THC/CBD were measured upon enrollment into the study, and participants were asked about their past 6-month history of cannabis use, including route, quantity, dates, and times. Both cannabis and noncannabis users were compared for demographics, IBD disease characteristics, and perceptions of risk related to cannabis smoking.

Participants: Ninety-nine pediatric participants, age 13 to 23, were drawn from those enrolled at Children's Hospital of Colorado. Sixty-three percent had CD, 27% had UC, and 10% indeterminate colitis. Fifty-seven percent of participants were male, and 83% had mild disease. The cannabis users were 32% of the total participants, and the never-use group was 68% of the participants.

Findings: Both the cannabis users and never users were similar for sex, race, disease type, disease activity, pain levels, appetite, QoL, and anxiety. The perception of cannabis being a no to low risk of harm medicine was much higher in the cannabis-use group (80%) versus the never-use group (25%). Of the cannabis users, 31% used daily, 52% used weekly, and only four participants had medical cannabis recommendations cards.

Most of the cannabis users obtained their cannabis through friends and on the black market. Eighty-three percent reported smoking, 50% consuming edibles, 40% dabbing, and 30% vaping. Fifty-three percent of participants used cannabis to relieve physical pain, whereas cannabis consumers also used it to relax (60%), to feel good (50%), and/or to have a good time with friends (47%). Thirty-seven percent reported problems with cannabis use, including cravings or strong desire to use cannabis, needing to use more cannabis to get the same effect, and using larger amounts for longer than intended.

Discussion and implications for cannabis care: This study is quite small and may really be considered to be more of a pilot study with only 32 active cannabis using IBD adolescent teens surveyed among the 99 respondents. Most of the participants had inactive or very mild IBD. The researchers state that they were concerned about the participants' perceptions that cannabis is safe and beneficial, which alludes to the idea that we have not educated our vulnerable youth about the risks of cannabis use, particularly when using THC-based products on a regular, daily basis.

> ### APPLIED LEARNING
>
> **Inflammatory Bowel Disease**
> Journal or discuss with classmates or colleagues about the following questions.
> - What IBD-specific populations might be good candidates for medicinal cannabis use?
> - How can IBD patients be supported to upregulate their endocannabinoid systems through integrative modalities?
> - How can nurses best educate young vulnerable patients who would like to try cannabis for palliation?

MULTIPLE SCLEROSIS

MS is an autoimmune disease that is neuroinflammatory and neurodegenerative in nature. Although the exact etiology is unknown, research efforts have revealed the complexity of the pathophysiologic process, thought to be genetically and environmentally provoked. Categorized into four subgroups, demyelination of neurons along the axon is where the damage occurs. Treatment is often based on symptom presentation. Prominent symptoms (though not all-inclusive) are muscle weakness, spasticity, pain, fatigue, and bladder dysfunction (Gado et al., 2018).

The 2017 NASEM report acknowledged the existence of substantial evidence in patient-reported symptoms supporting nabiximols, oral cannabis extract, and orally administered THC for MS-related spasticity; however, the passive range of motion test for muscle spasticity performed by clinicians (Ashworth Scale [AS]) was inconsistent. Worldwide, 30 countries declared regulatory approval of nabiximols, the drug known as Sativex; the United States is *not* one of them. Nonetheless, many U.S. states recognize MS spasticity as a qualifying condition for medicinal cannabis use. Statistically, Boehnke et al. (2019) declared that MS-related spasms ranked second amid the United States' most reported qualifying condition for state-approved cannabis use. The following articles are a small snapshot of the current research for MS-related spasticity, characteristics of MS patient's cannabis use, and bladder function treated with cannabis-based medicines.

Sativex and Multiple Sclerosis

Article: Markovà, J., Essner, U., Akmaz, B., Marinelli, M., Trompke, C., Lentschat, A., & Vila, C. (2019). Sativex® as add-on therapy vs. further optimized first-line anti-spastics (SAVANT) in resistant multiple sclerosis spasticity: A double-blind, placebo-controlled randomized clinical trial. *International Journal of Neuroscience, 12*(2), 119–128. https://doi.org/10.1080/00207454.2018.1481066

Authors: The investigators for this study were from multiple countries: Praha, Czechia; Hamburg, Germany; Reinbek, Germany; and Barcelona, Spain. They all have either worked full-time, been sponsored by, or served as consultants for Almirall, a pharmaceutical company based out of Barcelona, Spain. GW Pharmaceuticals carry the license for Sativex. Almirall conducted independent research and ultimately offered Sativex to their patient network.

Purpose: To examine if MS patients find relief by adding Sativex (one-part THC:one-part CBD oromucosal spray) to their established antispasmodic medication regimen versus increasing existing medication alone.

Methodology: This was a double-blind, placebo-controlled, randomized clinical trial with two phases. Participant screening occurred at visit 1. Treatment began the following week (visit 2), marking the start of the single-blinded phase A, which lasted 28 days. About one-third of the subjects did not experience more than a 20% improvement on the Numerical Rating Scale (NRS) and were excused as nonresponders. At visit 3, the patients were instructed to discontinue Sativex, but may otherwise continue their normal routine. Lasting for 28 days, the pause in treatment is to limit carry-over effects of Sativex, also known as a washout period. Randomization of treatment occurred at visit 4, marking the beginning of the double-blind phase 2. One group received Sativex, and the other group received a placebo. Patients were instructed to titrate the dose according to their preference, but not to exceed 12 sprays per day. Participants were screened 28 days later at visit 5. The trial continued another 28 days, and participants returned for the visit 6 screening. Final assessments during visit 7 (also 28 days later) concluded the trial. The Sativex group had 50 of 53 participants, and the placebo group had 46 of 53 patients complete the full trial period.

Measures included the Modified Ashworth Scale (MAS) score, Expanded Disability Status Scale (EDSS), the NRS for spasms, and the NRS for pain. The researchers increased the clinically relevant percentage from 20% to 30%. In other words, the results were only considered significant if a patient experienced at least a 30% improvement from baseline numbers.

Participants: Criteria included having an MS diagnosis, moderate-to-severe spasticity experienced longer than a year, being over 18 years old, and lacking adequate relief from at least two antispasmodic medications taken for at least 3 months. Disqualification factors were previous use of Sativex; consumption of cannabis in any form in the past 30 days; psychiatric disorders; cardiac, kidney, or liver impairments; history of dependence disorders; pregnancy or currently breastfeeding; and, finally, botulinum toxin treatment to spastic muscles in the past 6 months.

Findings: Sativex participants (77.4%) demonstrated significant improvements over placebo participants (32.1%). In addition to the overall relief, there were substantial improvements in pain, spasticity, and MAS. More specifically, spasm severity and interrupted sleep improved with Sativex. Each spray contains 2.7 mg THC and 2.5 mg CBD. The average number of sprays for the Sativex group was 7.3 per day (19.71 mg THC and 18.25 mg CBD per day), whereas the placebo group averaged 8.5 sprays per day. Despite 19.4% of the patients in the Sativex group reporting adverse events in phase A, only 9.4% claimed an adverse event in phase B; all of which were mild and not life-threatening.

Discussion and implications for cannabis care: What makes this study interesting is the significance in the objective clinician-measured MAS. The NASEM (2017) study found substantial evidence that the patient-reported (subjective) measures of cannabis for MS spasticity improved; however, the objective measures were not significant. The AS or MAS is a quick test performed without additional equipment. The test is a simple measure using passive motion from a resting position and does not account for spasms specifically prominent in everyday activity with varying degrees of muscle velocity (Balci, 2018). The validity and reliability of this test are questionable and, in many cases, shown to be insufficient (Fleuren et al., 2010; Mutlu et al., 2008). When evaluating research findings, it is wise to understand the strength of the tools or methods used. A combination of patient reports and physical tests, in addition to biomechanical and electrophysiologic evaluations, is ideal for spasticity measures (Balci, 2018).

In addition to significant improvements in the MAS, the results are congruent with NASEM's (2017) patient-reported findings. This study, however, added the additional washout phase to ensure results were not influenced by other factors. This study supported adding on a cannabis-based medicine as it provided superior relief over increasing existing medication dosage alone. As chronic illnesses progress, medicine efficacy may change, ultimately requiring an increase in dosage. Many patients may potentially reach their max dosage, leaving them vulnerable and out of options when using this medicine. In contrast, tolerance to the adverse effects of cannabis-based medicines can also develop (represented in this study), but the benefits remain consistent (MacCallum & Russo, 2018).

Cannabis Use Characteristics: Patients With Multiple Sclerosis

Article: Wienkle, L., Domen, C., Shelton, I., Sillau, S., Nair, K., & Alvarez, E. (2019). Exploring cannabis use by patients with multiple sclerosis in a state where cannabis is legal. *Multiple Sclerosis and Related Disorders, 27*, 383–390. https://doi.org/10.1016/j.msard.2018.11.022

Authors: Five of the authors were from the University of Colorado School of Medicine. The departments listed were cell and developmental biology, neurosurgery, and neurology. One author listed the department of clinical pharmacy from the University of Colorado Skaggs School of Pharmacy and Pharmaceutical Sciences.

Purpose: To examine cannabis use characteristics among patients with MS in a recreational and medical-legal state.

Methodology: The study was performed between October 2017 and April 2018 at the Rocky Mountain Multiple Sclerosis Center. Patients with a previous diagnosis of MS between the ages of 18 and 89 years were approached during visits and asked to fill out an electronic voluntary survey. Provided on a computer tablet, the survey entries were anonymized and formatted in four separate sections:

1. Personal opinions regarding cannabis
2. Characteristics of cannabis use (*omitted if the participant identified as a nonuser*)
3. MS-related history and sociodemographics
4. Patient-reported health outcomes:
   a. Patient Disease Determined Steps (PDDS)
   b. PROMIS-10
   c. Short Form version 1.0 of the Quality of Life in Neurological Disorders Applied Cognition—General Concerns (Neuro-QoL, ACGC).

Chi-square/Fisher's exact association test measured categorical outcomes. t-tests/analysis of variance analyzed scaled results.

Participants: The MS patient population for this study was recruited at the Rocky Mountain Multiple Sclerosis Center in Colorado. Patients were categorized as cannabis users (N = 96; 38%) and nonusers (N = 155; 62%). Cannabis users were those who admittingly used cannabis in the past year and would consider it for MS-related symptom relief. Participants who would never consider cannabis for MS and those who would consider cannabis user, but also denied cannabis use in the past year were categorized as nonusers. All sociodemographic and clinical data between the users and nonusers were equal, except cannabis users had a higher disability score (PDDS = 2) than the nonusers (PDDS = 1).

Findings: Although the following is not a complete capture of measurements from this study, essential highlights between *strictly medicinal* use and *recreational/medicinal* use were recognized. The medicinal-only users preferred the combination (CBD:THC; 52%) followed by CBD only (31%), and ingestion methods of vaporizing (28%) or edibles (25%). Recreational/medicinal users preferred a combination of cannabinoids (CBD:THC; 46%) followed by THC only (20%), and they preferred combustion/smoking (56%) for ingestion. Other measures between the groups were comparable. Both groups chose to purchase cannabis from a dispensary, they typically spent less than $50 per month, and they mostly used cannabis occasionally at one to six times a year or very frequently at one to three times per day. Regardless of category, patients with MS reported using cannabis for pain relief, inadequate sleep, and spasticity. No side effects were claimed by 79% of users; whereas 21% indicated mild side effects. Although tolerable, slowed thinking, weight gain, and decreased attention were mentioned the most.

The authors retrospectively reviewed 4,008 MS patient charts to compare typical medications prescribed for the same reported symptoms for cannabis use. Medications included baclofen (28%), gabapentin (24%), and dalfampridine (13%).

Discussion and implications for cannabis care: These patients with MS used cannabis (38%) more than traditional treatments. Consistent availability of quality cannabis in a legalized adult-use state gives individuals more options and control of their desired treatment. Allowing time to adjust cannabis therapy may relieve multiple symptoms, while simultaneously reducing the need for other pharmaceuticals.

Another consideration is that the greater the disability, the less likely the patient is to smoke cannabis, and this could indicate several things. As the disease progresses, dexterity, sensation, strength, and stability may begin to decline, causing some methods of consumption more difficult to prepare independently. The process of vaporizing, or eating edibles from a dispensary, could be, in some cases, more convenient. Cannabis care nurses should undoubtedly consider the current evidence, but equally as important, attention should be paid to assessing the patient's physical capabilities and how that effects their cannabis use, access, and ease of care.

Cannabinoids and Multiple Sclerosis–Related Overactive Bladder

Article: Maniscalco, G. T., Aponte, R., Bruzzese, D., Guarcello, G., Manzo, V., Napolitano, M., Moreggia, O., Chiariello, F., & Florio, C. (2018). THC/CBD oromucosal spray in patients with multiple sclerosis overactive bladder: A pilot prospective study. *Neurological Sciences, 39*(1), 97–102. https://doi.org/10.1007/s10072-017-3148-6

Authors: Eight authors represented various departments (multiple sclerosis, urology, and neurology) at the "A Cardarelli" Hospital located in Naples, Italy. The ninth author was from the department of public health at the University of Naples, also located in Naples, Italy. Two authors, Maniscalco and Florio, received compensation for public speaking and advisory boards from TEVA and Merk Serono. Maniscalco also received compensation from Novartis, Genzyme, and Biogen.

Purpose: Primarily, the authors wanted to evaluate how THC/CBD oromucosal spray affected MS patients' overactive bladder symptoms of urgency, frequency, nighttime urination, and stress incontinence (bladder contracts forcing urine past the sphincter randomly). Secondary outcomes evaluated postvoid residuals (PVRs; indicates if patient completely empties), bladder volume at first desire (volume triggering the urge), maximum detrusor pressure (measures flow in relation to bladder pressure), cystometric capacity (how much urine causes extreme urge to void), leakage volume, and bladder compliance (ability to fill without excessive detrusor tightening).

Methodology: Before treatment and after 4 weeks of use, participants were assessed using the EDSS, the MAS, the NRS; a 25-ft walking test (T25-WT), and Overactive Bladder Symptom Score (OABSS) Questionnaire. Urodynamic tests completed according to standards, with room temperature 0.9% NaCl saline, rectal tube, and a double-lumen catheter. The treatment began after the first assessment. Participants were asked to slowly self-titrate to their tolerable optimal dose during the first 2 weeks, but not to exceed 12 sprays per day. Improved OABSS of at least 20% indicated significance. The secondary measures were also considered significant if there was a change of 20% or more. Statistics were analyzed according to the type of variable. Numbers reflected as median, and categories displayed as percentage or frequency. The Wilcoxon's test was used to measure overall. Significance was $p \leq 0.05$. This study is considered a prospective observational pilot.

Participants: The study included patients with MS who had moderate-to-severe overactive bladder symptoms and resistance to first-line medications (for at least 3 months of use). Exclusion criteria were urinary tract infection, cannabis use in the past 7 days, use of medicines for urinary symptoms, pregnancy, structural abnormalities (ie, prolapse), stroke, diabetes, kidney or liver impairments, cerebrovascular or neurologic (other than MS) disease, and severe cardiovascular disorder. Ultimately, only 15 patients were analyzed, which makes for a small number in this study.

Findings: Collectively, there were significant improvements in overactive bladder symptoms (OABSS; $p = 0.001$), PVRs ($p = 0.016$), walking-time (T25-WT; $p = 0.027$), and patient-reported spasticity improved by 1.93 points (NRS; $p = 0.001$). Despite an improvement in the other measures, they were not significant. The authors noted that 14 patients' NRS improved by at least 20%, and the average number of sprays was 3.8 per day. The data, however, were not provided for each individual. The authors also reported no significant change in the MAS but failed to reveal actual measurements. Although the number of subjects, length of study, and missing data hinder the quality of this study, the results do indicate improvements in clinician- and patient-measured outcomes.

Discussion and implications for cannabis care: Although this study was limited, the potential of cannabis-based medicine may extend beyond the typical indications.

Often in the rehabilitation setting, the nurse works with physical and occupational therapists to elevate independence. Bowel and bladder programs are introduced to help combat incontinent episodes. Bladder dysfunction may lead to urinary tract infections and renal damage and, ultimately, impact QoL. The goal for any patient is to improve symptoms with the least amount of pharmacologic interventions as possible. For MS patients, cannabis has a high safety profile with the potential to treat pain, spasticity, sleep, and overactive bladder, which are conditions frequently treated with more than one medication at a time.

> ### ▶ APPLIED LEARNING
>
> **Multiple Sclerosis**
>
> Do a Google or social media search and determine what online resources are readily available to MS patients on their journey toward learning about safe and effective cannabis use.
>
> ■ Examine two to three online resources and determine their legitimacy by exploring such things as who the authors are, the accuracy of the content, and the ease of use.
> ■ What sort of information or resources would you add in or delete to enhance the credibility of one of the websites?

SEIZURE DISORDER

Many patients suffering from intractable seizures have turned to medicinal use of cannabis in order to eradicate or decrease their seizure frequency (SF). The NASEM (2017) report acknowledged that both CBD and THC prevent seizures in animal models and that there are millions of people who suffer from epilepsy, with fully one-third of them still experiencing seizures, even when treated. The NASEM report clearly stated that there is a lack of high-quality clinical trials when it comes to epilepsy treatment with cannabinoid therapeutics. The following section reviews some of the more recent studies in this area.

Cannabidiol for Drug-Resistant Seizures With Dravet Syndrome

Article: Devinsky, O., Cross, J. H., Laux, L., Marsh, E., Miller, I., Nabbout, R., Scheffer, I. E., Thiele, E. A., & Wright, S. (2017). Trial of cannabidiol for drug-resistant seizures in the Dravet Syndrome. *The New England Journal of Medicine*, 692–699. https://doi.org/10.1056/NEJMoa1611618
Authors: The investigators for this study were from multiple cities/countries and institutions in London, England, Paris, France, and Melbourne, Australia. This study was funded by GW Pharmaceuticals, Clinical Trials.gov number. NCT02091375.
Purpose: To compare different cannabinoid doses versus placebo to determine SF when added to routine antiepileptic medication(s) versus antiepileptic medication(s) alone. Numbers of seizures were self-reported, and patients were assessed using The Caregiver Global Impression of Change (CGI), which was developed for use in NIMH-sponsored clinical trials to provide a brief, stand-alone assessment of the

clinician's view of the patient's global functioning prior to and after initiating a study medication.

Methodology: In this study, Devinsky et al. (2017) conducted a double-blind, placebo-controlled trial with 120 children and young adults who were randomly assigned to either placebo or an oral CBD solution at a dose of 20 mg/kg of body weight in addition to their standard antiepileptic medications. The primary end point was to determine whether there was a reduction in the frequency of convulsive-seizure activity over a 14-week treatment period when compared to the patients' 4-week baseline period.

Participants: One hundred and seventy-seven patients screened from 23 centers culminating in 120 participants randomized into trial. One hundred and eight patients completed trial. A total of 12 patients withdrew from trial, 9 in the CBD group and 3 from the placebo group. Of 108 who completed trial, 105 went on to the extension study.

Results: The frequency of convulsive seizures per month decreased from 12.4 to 5.9 when subjects used CBD with their standard antiepileptic treatment, compared with a decrease from 14.9 to 14.1 without the addition of CBD to their regimen. There is a 95% confidence interval. The percent of patients who had at least 50% reduction in SF was 43% in patients with CBD and 27% with the placebo. Patient's overall condition improvement was improved by at least one category in 62% of the patients in the CBD group as compared with 34% of the placebo group. The frequency of total seizures of all types was significantly reduced, with no reduction in nonconvulsive seizures. The percent of patients who became seizure free was 5% in the CBD group and 0% for the placebo group. There were more withdrawals from the CBD group of patients than the placebo group. Finally, there were more frequent adverse events from the CBD group than in the placebo, including diarrhea, vomiting, fatigue, pyrexia, somnolence, and abnormal results on liver function tests.

Limitations: Side effects and elevated liver enzyme results when using this medication with Dravet patients warrants more study.

Discussion and implications for cannabis care: There was a clear reduction in the frequency and number of seizures experienced when using this study's standardized CBD medication. However, there were side effects, including somnolence, loss of appetite, and diarrhea, at significantly greater rates versus placebo. Note that GCI is an excellent tool commonly used in evaluating epilepsy patients, but it also is a subjective evaluation tool.

Better Seizure Response With Pharmaceutical Grade Cannabidiol

Article: Skflarsky, J., Hernando, K., Bebin, M., Gaston, T. E., Grayson, L. E., Ampah, S. B., & Moreadith, R. (2019). Higher cannabidiol plasma levels are associated with better seizure response following treatment with pharmaceutical grade cannabidiol. *Epilepsy and Behavior, 95*, 131–136. https://doi.org/10.1016/j.ybeh.2019.03.042

Authors: These researchers from the neurology and pediatric departments worked in collaboration with the University of Alabama Epilepsy Center to identify patients who continued to be treatment resistant to conventional epilepsy treatment.

Purpose: To determine the relationship between CBD dose, CBD plasma levels, and seizure control in a large, open-label, single-center study. University of Alabama's expanded access program works with epilepsy patients.

Methodology: This study was conducted during a weekly research clinic visit. Participant weight was collected at each visit and adjustments made as necessary. Time between study visits was eventually stretched to 12 weeks as long as no adjustment was necessary. An oral formulation of highly purified CBD in sesame oil (Epidiolex) was started at 5 mg/kg/day with adjustments made based on weight and seizure response. At each visit, participants reported any seizure activity: seizure free versus not seizure free since the last visit.

There was also a reporting mechanism for tolerability, indicating adverse events versus no adverse events. There were some participants who reached a daily dosage of 50 mg/kg/day, raising their individual doses to 5,000 mg/day. There were adverse events reported, including diarrhea by up to 30% of the participants and sedation in 14% of participants. Both these adverse events caused dose limiting, but no other dose-limiting events were reported. Other adverse events such as cold, allergies, and dizziness were not thought to be related to CBD dosage but were monitored as part of the study.

Participants continued in the study for approximately 6 months. At each visit, participants provided seizure diaries and had a neurologic and general physical examination. The diaries were reviewed with participant and/or caregiver for accuracy by the study physician. SF was documented and used as a comparator with previously collected baseline activity. SF was collected at each visit. SF was recorded for the previous 12 weeks and averaged over each 14-day period. This was regardless of what type of seizure activity was experienced.

Subjects/Participants: Participants were referred for participation by providers, or self-referred after meeting inclusion criteria. The study was looking for patients who remained treatment refractory. Both children and adults were recruited as subjects and treated with highly purified grade CBD (Epidiolex). The subjects in this study had to also be a part of a parent study looking at seizure activity and CBD; thus, all patients had already been started on CBD. Once patients qualified, agreed to, and entered into the parent study, an additional IRB consent form had to be signed to include the drawing of CBD plasma levels and other routine data collected. CBD dosing was stable for 14 days prior to entry. All other antiepileptic drugs (AEDs) were maintained at a stable dose during study period. Dosages were weight based and could be increased by 5 mg/kg/day up to a maximum dosage of 50 mg/kg/day. Doses were dependent on patient tolerance and seizure control. CBD plasma levels were calculated at each visit, and seizure counts were recorded for each 2-week period. Patients were scheduled consecutively, allowing plasma levels to be drawn from patients at 4 hours postdosing.

Findings: Wilcoxon's rank summary and Pearson's chi-square test were used for categorical variables. The participant group was divided into responders versus nonresponders. Responders were considered those who had a 50% or greater reduction in SF as compared with baseline frequency. When comparing baseline data, there was no substantial difference owing to age or SF at baseline. However, responders did receive higher doses of CBD and had higher CBD plasma levels. There was no difference in the number of AED used by participants. Using statistical software, it was determined that the higher the dosage, the higher the plasma level and the lower the frequency of seizure activity. The authors stated that there is no longer any question as to whether CBD is efficacious when used for reduction of seizures; the question that needs further study is whether it is better for patients when used in combination with other AED or if CBD products can stand alone.

Limitations: As is consistent with all studies that collect participant reported data, there is the need to correct for mistaken or forgetful reporting, but these errors are consistent in all participants and so are deemed nonsignificant. Continued study is suggested to account for the food intake status and individual medication absorption rates, neither of which were monitored in this study. Understanding that CBD is highly lipophilic, monitoring food intake is important, as a diet high in fatty food is likely to increase bioavailability. It is known that oral availability of cannabis is limited in humans to less than 10% with other routes of administration decreasing bioavailability even more.

Discussion and implications for cannabis care: It is clear that adding CBD to other AEDs serves to reduce SF. Questions still remain regarding the use of additional cannabinoids, flavonoids, and/or terpenes. Comparison of whether the efficacy of synthetic versus plant-derived cannabinoids for the treatment of seizures or other neurologic disorders is suggested, and we need to consider then idea of how the cannabis plant's hundreds of chemical components interact with our own endocannabinoid system.

Artisanal Cannabis for the Treatment of Epilepsy

Article: Sulak, D., Saneto, R., & Goldstein, B. (2017). The current status of artisanal cannabis for the treatment of epilepsy in the United States. *Epilepsy & Behavior, 70,* 328–333. http://dx.doi.org/10.1016/j.yebeh.2016.12.032

Authors: Two authors are doctors who run companies where patients can come for medical cannabis recommendations and received expert medical support. One author works for a large university medical center.

Purpose: To report the retrospective data on efficacy and adverse effects of artisanal cannabis in patients with medically refractory epilepsy with mixed etiologies in Washington State, California, and Maine.

Methodology: This was a retrospective study with a chart review of patients from a children's hospital in Washington State and a private cannabinoid medical practice in California. The additional four case studies were from a private cannabinoid medical practice in Maine. Two of these were Dravet patients who were extremely complicated each trying several radical traditional treatments.

Participants: This study had 272 patients from California and Washington. An additional four longer case reports about patients in Maine were included as more in-depth studies, illustrative of clinical responses.

Findings:

- 14% of the patients (n = 37) found cannabinoid medicines to be ineffective at reducing seizures.
- 15% found (n = 29) they experienced a 1% to 25% reduction in seizure activity.
- 18% (n = 60) had a 26% to 50% reduction in seizure activity.
- 17% (n = 45) experienced a 51% to 75% reduction in SF.
- 28% (n = 75) had 76% to 99% reduction in seizures.
- 10% (n = 26) reported that their seizure activity had resolved (a complete clinical response).

Overall, 86% of patients received some clinical benefit from using cannabinoids that were sourced from artisanal sources (meaning that they were not standardized preparations normally considered for research studies, and patients procured the cannabinoid medicines in the community, which is legal in the states where the study took place). Some of the challenges with accessing medicine this way are availability and consistency of supply.

Discussion and implications for cannabis care: Although randomized controlled clinical studies of cannabinoid therapeutics are much needed, this study clearly addresses the issue that medical cannabis patients are accessing "unregulated" or artisanal cannabis medicines in the community in efforts to manage their illnesses. We must consider how they can benefit from having access and also think about safety, availability, and consistency with cannabinoid medicines for patients who need them to best manage their serious health conditions.

▶ APPLIED LEARNING

Seizures

CBD does seem to help with treating seizures.

- What are some challenges patients and families might face when accessing CBD products?
- How might your cannabis care assessment for a pediatric seizure patient differ from that of an adult seizure patient?
- What are the priority educational needs for seizure patients interested in using cannabis?

PARKINSON'S DISEASE

PD is characterized as a chronic neurologic condition affecting movement and usually emerges later in life. In simple terms, neuronal damage (genetic and environmental) causes decreased levels of dopamine in the brain. Although there is no cure once symptoms emerge, slowing progression and symptomatic treatment have become the focus of PD treatment. PD typically presents as rigidity, tremors, slowed movement, and instability. Treatment often begins with the drug levodopa, which can cause dyskinesia or involuntary movements.

The NASEM (2017) report concluded that the evidence was insufficient for the use of cannabinoids as a treatment in PD. The report described several trials using variations of oral preparations, including Cannador, Nabilone, and CBD capsules with poor results. However, in a study conducted in 2014, Lotan and colleagues investigated the effects 30 minutes after 0.5 g smoked cannabis and found significant improvements in pain, sleep, and motor symptoms, including tremor, rigidity, and bradykinesia (as cited in NASEM, 2017). The trials evaluated by NASEM ultimately fell short. Lack of controls, number of subjects, and length of study continued to be a significant concern.

Preclinical studies are connecting links between the endocannabinoid system and neurologic health. In a multimodal manner, the endocannabinoid system plays an integral part in maintaining and protecting portions of our neurologic system; thus, creating more interest in how the system can be manipulated by cannabis medicine to treat incurable neurologic diseases. In 2004 and 2016, Russo demonstrated disturbances or deficiencies of endocannabinoids in those suffering from conditions such as PD (as cited in Russo, 2018), offering a lead in related research. Unfortunately, at the time this publication went to press, very few clinical trials of cannabis, and PD were published since the NASEM's report in 2017. The following section examines some of those limited findings.

Thermal Measures and Parkinson's Disease

Article: Shohet, A., Khlebtovsky, A., Roizen, N., Roditi, Y., & Djaldetti, R. (2017). Effect of medical cannabis on thermal quantitative measurements of pain in patients with Parkinson's disease. *European Journal of Pain, 21*(2017), 486–493. https://doi.org/10.1002/ejp.942

Authors: The authors are faculty of medicine at the Tel Aviv University in Israel. In addition, the Movement Disorder Clinic, Department of Neurology at the Rabin Medical Center—Beilinson Hospital, Petach Tikva, Israel, provided the location for the study. No conflicts of interest were declared.

Purpose: The main objective was to determine whether cannabis (both short and long term) alters movement and pain symptoms in patients with PD.

Methodology: Assessments of the 20 patients occurred before the consumption of cannabis (1 g) and 30 minutes after. Measurements included:

1. Unified Parkinson's Disease Rating Scale (UPDRS) for motor function by two physicians; one blinded for reliability
2. Pain Rating Index (PRI) and Visual Analog Scale (VAS). Both are patient-reported pain scores
3. Thermal Quantitative Sensory Test (QST) measures communication from sensory nerves to the brain using a thermode, beginning at 32 °C. The temperature is adjusted up or down accordingly, by 1 degree/second. Patients are instructed to press a button as soon as they feel a hot or cold sensation (repeated four times). The process for the pain sensation test is identical, except the patient is asked to press the button when they think the temperature change is painful. An average between the two tests is analyzed. For validity, patients without cannabis complete the QST.

Long-term assessments were scheduled at least 10 weeks later. Patients were instructed to use a daily dose of 1 g of cannabis and return for the all but the UPDRS assessments.

Participants: Twenty patients with PD with approval for cannabis use were recruited the Movement Disorders Clinic in Israel. Two of those 20 had diabetes and did not participate in thermal tests due to impaired sensation concerns. The treatment group's medications were levodopa (n = 14), anticholinergics (n = 5), dopamine agonists (n = 6), amantadine (n = 3), and rasagiline (n = 5). Eighteen participants smoked cannabis and two used a vaporizer. The participants brought their cannabis medication from home. The cannabis was not analyzed nor did patients indicate the type and strength of the cannabis products they were ingesting.

Findings: Thirty minutes after cannabis consumption, the UPDRS (38.1 to 30.4), PRI (27 to 9.7), and VAS (6.4 to 3.6) showed significant improvements. The QST cold threshold 30 minutes after smoked cannabis improved significantly (19.5 to 15.6); the QST heat threshold after 10 weeks also improved (43.7 to 40.9). The long-term PRI (15.6) was not substantial; however, the VAS (3.2) was.

Discussion and implications for cannabis care: Without relying on patient-reported measures alone, this study reveals how cannabis impacts pain threshold by using thermal instruments and by blinding one rater for the mobility assessment. The use of a more objective tool was used to validate patients' perception of effect through threshold measures in different pain-signaling pathways. Findings suggested that cannabis may work immediately with sudden pain and cold sensations. Conversely, cannabis use over time may impact delayed pain and heat sensations. Previous studies indicate CB1 receptors are responsible for cold sensation, whereas TRPV1 receptors are accountable for noxious heat sensation (as cited in Shohet et al., 2017). The limitations include the various types of cannabis that patients consumed, small sample size, and the cannabis's effects could have slowed reaction time. Nevertheless, this study is supportive of improved motor and pain symptoms after cannabis administration in patients with PD.

Parkinson's Patients' Cannabis Experiences

Article: Balash, Y., Bar-Lev Schleider, L., Korczyn, A. D., Shabtai, H., Knaani, J., Rosenberg, A., Baruch, Y., Djaldetti, R., Giladi, N., & Gurevich, T. (2017). Medical cannabis in Parkinson's disease: Real-life patients' experience. *Clinical Neuropharmacology, 40*(6), 268–272. https://doi.org/10.1097/WNF.0000000000000246

Authors: The authors have various clinical backgrounds from the Tel Aviv University, Rabin Medical Center, and the Tel Aviv Sourasky Medical Center. Conflicts of interest include one author is an employee of Tikun Olam Co., an international cannabis pharmaceutical company based in Israel. Another author is the head of the Israeli Ministry of Health program for Medical Use of Cannabis in addition to a CSO of a company dedicated to cannabis research for medical purposes.

Purpose: The authors intended to discover the effects of medical cannabis experienced in a population of patients with PD.

Participants: Patients with PD receiving treatment from the Movement Disorders Clinics (two facilities in separate locations) in Israel. Each patient received the approval to use medical marijuana from the Ministry of Health after their neurologist makes a formal recommendation. Participants were deemed nondemented. The age demographics were 39 to 55 (19.1%), 56 to 65 (31.9%), 66 to 75 (34.1%), and 76 to 87 (4.19%). There were more men (40) than women (7), and all participants had the diagnosis of Parkinson's for at least 2 years.

Methodology: This was a retrospective observational study, completely voluntary, and interviews by phone were arranged ahead of time. The calls took about 30 minutes. The survey questions included the effects on activities of daily living, motor, and nonmotor symptoms measured by the Clinical Impressions Scale (similar to a 5-point Likert scale). Moreover, the patients answered questions of disease characteristics, other health concerns, demographics, cannabis use details, and perception of cannabis-associated changes. Results were analyzed as means or median. The data before and after were compared for dependent variables. The significance was rated in three levels: *small* ≤0.5, *moderate* 0.5 to 0.8, and *large* ≥0.8 in terms of effect strength. The higher the number, the stronger the improvement was.

Findings: A total of 47 participants completed the questionnaire. Most participants preferred cannabis cigarettes (91.3%), followed by oil ingestion (8.7%). The average daily dose was between 0.2 and 2.25 g/day (the THC:CBD ratio/dosages were not specified). The only improvement above a moderate effect size was fall occurrence (0.89), recorded as a yes/no if falls occurred before and after cannabis (however, use caution with these findings, as it does not factor in other lifestyle changes, awareness postfall, nor possible rehabilitation sessions). With no reports of worsening, improvements reported by the number of treated include tremors (n = 30), muscle stiffness (n = 32), and dyskinesias (n = 14). Gait disorder improved for 23 patients but worsened in three cases. Nonmotor symptoms improved in pain (n = 35), with no reports of worsening. Depressed mood improved in 35 patients; however, it further exacerbated for one participant. Similarly, insomnia also improved (n = 32), but one participant reported worsening. Provided that smoking was prevalent in this group, it is no surprise that coughing was the main adverse effect (35%), behind any kind of psychotropic effect (38%).

Discussion and implications for cannabis care: Searching for high-quality research related to cannabis effects in PD often leads to reviews, animal trials, and preclinical data. This study adds a refreshingly human element to the existing literature, but a few red flags emerge. For example, were answers collected before cannabis therapy began or were patients forced to recall their symptoms from at least 3 months prior? The authors noted that there was some concern for memory and concentration without a neurocognitive assessment.

The daily doses did not indicate if the calculation was for total weight or dosage strength of THC or CBD. In addition, this research provides no guidance for cannabis types/chemovars that this population preferred. It could indicate that the patients' products were not labeled, or the question about products was not asked. Owing to the many variations, the cannabis chemovar profile may be useful for future research directions with specific populations. The authors suggested that only after other treatments fail, should cannabis be considered for this patient population.

Cannabis Use Patterns: A Survey

Article: Kindred, J. H., Li, K., Ketelhut, N. B., Proessl, F., Fling, B. W., Honce, J. M., Shaffer, W. R., & Rudroff, T. (2017). Cannabis use in people with Parkinson's disease and multiple sclerosis: A web-based investigation. *Complementary Therapies in Medicine, 33,* 99–104. https://doi.org/10.1016/j.ctim.2017.07.002

Authors: The authors list associations with the Colorado State University, University of Colorado Denver, or University of Colorado Health Systems. Kindred has authored several journal articles about cannabis use and neurologic conditions for the past few years. Four of the authors are doctors. Shaffer disclosed working as a consultant/speaker for EMD Serono, Acorda, TEVA, Genzyme, and Mallinckrodt. Otherwise, no other disclosures were reported.

Purpose: The study compared self-reported characteristics in patients with MS or PD that use cannabis versus noncannabis users.

Methodology: An anonymous survey remained open and was displayed on multiple sites in 2016 from February to October. Along with characteristics of use, demographic data and cannabis efficacy were measured. For condition specifics, Guy's Neurological Status Scale (GNDS), Nottingham Health Profile (NHP), Fatigue Severity Scale (FSS), Activities of Balance Confidence (ABC), and the International Physical Activities Questionnaire (IPAQ) were included in the survey.

Participants: The survey was available to anyone with access to the link. After removing those who identified with a condition other than MS and PD, 538 participants completed 100% of the survey. The focus here includes PD measures only, although the study included both MS and PD. Participants with PD averaged at 61 years old, 57.9% were men, 20.3% were classified as obese, and 58.4% had a 4-year degree or higher in education.

Findings: The PD cannabis use details include past use (66.3%), current use (36.6%), medicinal use (72.3%), possess cannabis medical card (38.4%), reduced other medications (47.8%), smoked only (40.9%), edibles only (6.3%), combination of smoking and edibles (19.5%), and have used longer than a year (69.8%). Cannabis use averaged 4.6 days/week, and efficacy on an 8-point Likert scale averaged at 6.2 (0 to 7 scale; 7 = very helpful). Ninety-seven percent of nonusers would consider using cannabis if cannabis was proven to be beneficial. Cannabis users identified as having lower disability ratings and less fatigue, and there was no difference between users and nonusers in physical activity (moderate to vigorous), walking, sitting, or balance confidence.

Discussion and implications for cannabis care: The results of this study revealed contrasting data for what cannabis has previously been believed to affect negatively. For instance, weight gain, decreased physical activity, impaired memory, and depression among cannabis users are often a topic of concern; however, this research suggested otherwise. As the researchers noted, some of the adverse effects are weaker than expected and should warrant further investigation through controlled trials. Moreover, the online nature of the survey may have been representative of those with higher cognitive function. As the authors emphasized, patients are using cannabis regardless of the clinical data; therefore, healthcare professionals should have a working knowledge of the endocannabinoid system's interactions with various diseases.

> ▶ **APPLIED LEARNING**
>
> **Parkinson's Disease**
> Discuss in a small group: What kind of research would be needed to support Parkinson's patients need for more evidence on cannabis efficacy?

TRAUMATIC BRAIN INJURY

Reviews such as *Cannabis Therapeutics and the Future of Neurology* (Russo, 2018); *Endocannabinoids: A Promising Impact for Traumatic Brain Injury* (Schurman & Lichtman, 2017); and the *Review of the Neurological Benefits of Phytocannabinoids*

(Maroon & Bost, 2018) offer a glimpse of the complex neurologic benefits that phytocannabinoids have on the endocannabinoid system. Although we anticipate future studies as the collection of preclinical data, animal studies, a few human observational studies combined with the pathologic processes, molecular characteristics, and chemical properties of the endocannabinoid system have converged, the future of cannabis care in neurology appears promising. The reviews describe many types of neurologic conditions impacted by cannabinoid therapeutics; however, clinical trials examining cannabis medicine for TBIs are nearly nonexistent. In the observational, retrospective chart reviews identified by NASEM (2017), there was limited evidence that cannabis improved TBI and intracranial hemorrhage (ICH) survival outcomes. Nevertheless, the research presented includes a survey and an experimental trial with mice, and efforts in building the body of evidence in this area are ongoing.

Cannabis Use and Traumatic Brain Injury: A Survey

Article: Hawley, L. A., Ketchum, J. M., Morey, C., Collins, K., & Charlifue, S. (2018). Cannabis use in individuals with spinal cord injury or moderate to severe traumatic brain injury in Colorado. *Archives of Physical Medicine and Rehabilitation, 99*(8), 1584–1590. https://doi.org/10.1016/j.apmr.2018.02.003

Authors: The authors are all from the research department at Craig Hospital in Englewood, Colorado. The Traumatic Brain Injury Model Systems National Data and Statistics Center, also in Englewood, Colorado, is also noted by one of the authors. Hawley has a master of science in social work and is a certified brain injury specialist trainer with 30 years of experience in rehabilitation and brain injury.

Purpose: This study examined the cannabis use patterns in those with a spinal cord injury (SCI) or TBI.

Methodology: Approved by the IRB, a mixed-method observational approach was used. For convenience, participants who had follow-up appointments were mailed an information sheet explaining the study. After the patient's appointment, those who agreed answered questions on a written form, which was completed in approximately 5 minutes. Results were presented in frequency, percentages, and means, including standard deviation.

Participants: The initial focus group of 10 participants was recruited, consisting of adults (21 years or older) who received services from Craig Hospital. TBI participants were intentionally left out because physicians asked those patients to refrain from using cannabis. The population surveyed included 51 individuals with an SCI and 65 individuals with a history of TBI. All participants had previously received in-patient care from Craig Hospital. Eighty percent were male and were injured 1 to 5 years before the study.

Findings: The initial focus group indicated reasons for use were pain, spasticity, sleep, relaxation, stress, and to decrease other prescription medications. One explained the side effects of other drugs were "wicked," and another stated, "cannabis is the least scary drug." Other comments included cannabis "saved my life," "takes the edge off," and "allows me to be more present." The adverse effects of cannabis were stigma, cost, no directions for dosing, fatigue, palpitations, fogginess, and lowered muscle control. However, the group acknowledged that they could get quality cannabis and have more control over how much THC versus CBD they desire since legalization.

The survey including both SCI and TBI patients indicated that 70% used cannabis before their injury, and only 48% admitted using after their injury. For TBI, 42% used cannabis before and after; 23% reported no use at all, 32% used before but not after, and only 3% indicated they only began using after their injury. The TBI group reported reasons for use were recreational (72%), stress/anxiety (62%), and sleep (55%). Multiple methods included smoking (90%), edibles (59%), and vaping (45%). Among those with TBI, side effects included lack of motivation (28%), feeling hazy (21%), and fatigue (21%). Of those employed, 38% reported daily use, whereas 25% of the unemployed used daily.

Discussion and implications for cannabis care: Representative of where the research stands and the most recent progress examining TBI and cannabis in the human population, this article indicates patients with TBIs use cannabis. Although it may be appropriate to advise patients to avoid certain activities after discharge, the fact is that patients may not adhere to those recommendations. Cannabis use in patients with a TBI decreased after injury, and recreational use was chosen more than medicinal. The recreational use in this population could have resulted from the SCI-only focus group; failure to include symptoms related to TBI (ie, anger or mood swings) could have limited their responses. The authors also suggested accessibility may impact use because some patients require supervision or support from a caregiver on a more long-term basis. The noted decline in cannabis use post-TBI should be examined further in addition to cognitive effects of cannabis in this population.

Cannabidiol and Allodynia

Article: Belardo, C., Iannotta, M., Boccella, S., Rubino, R. C., Ricciardi, F., Infantino, R., Pieretti, G., Stella, L., Paino, S., Marabese, I., Maisto, R., Luongo, L., Maione, S., & Guida, F. (2019). Oral cannabidiol prevents allodynia and neurological dysfunctions in a mouse model of mild traumatic brain injury. *Frontiers in Pharmacology, 10*(352), 1–11. https://doi.org/10.3389/fphar.2019.00352

Authors: The authors at the University of Campania Luigi Vanvitelli, Naples, Italy, are from the department of experimental medicine (provided funding for publication fees) and the department of plastic surgery. Enecta Group provided CBD, located out of Bologna, Italy. An added contributor from the Drug Addiction Unit (SerT), Naples, Italy, is also noted.

Purpose: Examining behavioral tasks and biochemical evaluations, the researchers aim to analyze CBD effects on TBI-related emotional and cognitive changes in mice.

Methodology: The mice were anesthetized for the precise TBI induction. After the initial healing period, CBD (10%) dissolved in hemp seed oil, and natural fat-soluble alcohols were administered from day 1 to 14 and from day 50 to 60. Blinded observers reported treatment and biochemical characters. Tests included tactile allodynia (measures central pain by withdraw from stimulus), Rotarod test (motor coordination), open-field test (measures general locomotion or willingness to explore), resident-intruder (reaction to other mice in territory), three chambers sociability (socialization), tail suspension test (measures depression through motivation), and microdialysis (measures neurotransmitters after infusion). Finally, their brains were assessed.

Participants: The "participants" were, in fact, mice. Although not ideal, there are many reasons this testing has not been performed in humans. An adequate foundation of preclinical and animal model data must present strong support for the worthiness of expanding related research. It was comforting knowing the author's used techniques to reduce suffering in as few animals as possible. The study followed the Italian and European Commission regulations and was approved by the Animal Ethics Committee of University of Campania in Naples, Italy. Six male mice, weighed 18 to 20 g, were used in this study.

Findings: Tactile allodynia (oversensitive central pain) was reduced in CBD-treated mice at 14 and 21 days. Rearing was reduced in CBD-treated mice with TBI. Fourteen days after sustaining a TBI, mice show increased attacks; however, the CBD-treated mice had a significant reduction versus the control mice. Long-term effects of a TBI in mice (60 days) are depression and reduced sociability, but CBD treatment reduced immobility and withdrawn behaviors compared to the control group. Correspondingly, CBD normalized extracellular glutamate, D-aspartate, and GABA levels.

Discussion and implications for cannabis care: Although this study is based on a mouse model, it reveals biochemical behavioral-associated changes using CBD after a TBI in a controlled environment. There were several benefits of CBD as potential pharmacologic treatment; however, quality of CBD may remain an issue. If there is a possibility of benefit without undue harm, CBD after a TBI may prove worthy for multiple reasons. This study is suggesting that CBD may improve aggression, oversensitivity to pain, anxiety, mobility, and sociability, and normalize various neurotransmitters affected by TBI.

> **▶ APPLIED LEARNING**
>
> **Traumatic Brain Injury and Education**
> TBI sufferers may benefit from CBD use. What are some considerations of CBD access the cannabis care nurse should focus on during educational or coaching sessions?

CONCLUSION

Cannabis is one of the most studied medicinal plants, and the NASEM's (2017) rigorous report provided a foundation for researchers to move forward with future studies as they continue to explore the efficacy of this plant, as there is still a long way to go in building a solid evidence base around cannabis being used for the many disease states discussed here. Chapter 6 delves into the NASEM (2017) report in relation to the nurse's role and explores how researchers need to focus future cannabis science evidence-building efforts. As we move out of the cannabis prohibition era and toward an era of regulation, there may be more opportunities for high-quality research to emerge, with more efforts to capture the patients experience in meaningful ways. Meanwhile, patients who are suffering will continue to access cannabis, whether the evidence is present or not.

It remains important for nurses to stay abreast of the latest findings related to medical cannabis research and the populations they care for. It will likely be years before NASEM issues another report on the status of cannabinoid therapeutic research, so nurses should be using sources like the CannaKeys website (https://cannakeys.com)

to stay abreast of current cannabinoid research. In addition, cannabis care nurses must consider how we can best contribute to the ever-expanding research efforts, and not only support high-quality research projects, but undertake them ourselves. Ethically, the healthcare profession is obligated to continue to generate evidence through randomized controlled trials, but as professionals, we also must not negate the importance of the patient experience and the qualitative data they can provide around their use of cannabinoid medicines for healing and palliation. Using evidence and considering the value of the patient-informed approaches are key aspects of the nurse's work in coaching patients toward wellness with use of cannabinoid therapeutics.

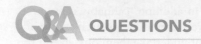 **QUESTIONS**

1. You see an article on social media with a popular magazine reporting about a new cannabis science finding. The news about this finding is going viral, and one of your patients asks if the findings are true. Your best response to the patient is:
   A. It is probably true, otherwise it would not be shared so widely.
   B. A lot of new stuff comes out about cannabis, so I do not really know yet.
   C. Sometimes, the media take just snippets from research journals; I will see if I can find the original research article and let you know.
   D. I would not worry about it until the study has been replicated a few times.

2. In reviewing a recent peer-reviewed research article, you note that the researchers have support from a cannabinoid pharmaceutical company. This means that:
   A. The evidence they generated is likely biased.
   B. As you review the evidence, you should remain alert for any biases.
   C. Since this was disclosed, bias is likely not an issue.
   D. There is no potential for bias, as it is published in a peer-reviewed journal.

3. A patient tells you that they know cannabis will cure them because of all the patient accounts they have read about on the web. What is your *best* response?
   A. "Those accounts may not be true and are likely unreliable."
   B. "Let's take a closer look at research related to cannabis and your illness."
   C. "What else have you heard about cannabis and your illness?"
   D. "I consider so much of patient's sharing about cannabis to be helpful to inform my practice."

4. You are speaking with a colleague about a patient who is using cannabis for pain control. They flippantly state, "Well, it seems like somehow magically cannabis is good for everything nowadays even though we don't have any good research." A good response to this might be:
   A. "I know it can seem that way, but there are over 30,000 studies related to cannabis on PubMed. It's the most studied plant on the planet."
   B. "Let's take a look at the 2017 NASEM report and see what the levels of evidence are around pain control and cannabis."
   C. "I think many patients turn to cannabis regardless of the body of evidence. Let's look for recent evidence around cannabis and pain control that we could share with the patient."
   D. All of the above.

5. Consider qualitative and quantitative approaches to cannabis research. Describe a research study you would like to see done in relation to cannabis and a specific disease or illness process, and how it could best be addressed by researchers: population, research methodology, minimum number needed, and how participants would be recruited.

ANSWERS

1. **Answer: C.** Sometimes, the media take just snippets from research journals; I will see if I can find the original research article and let you know.

2. **Answer: B.** As you review the evidence, you should remain alert for any biases.

3. **Answer: B.** "Let's take a closer look at research related to cannabis and your illness."

4. **Answer: D.** All of the above.

References

Balash, Y., Bar-Lev Schleider, L., Korczyn, A. D., Shabtai, H., Knaani, J., Rosenberg, A., Baruch, Y., Djaldetti, R., Giladi, N., & Gurevich, T. (2017). Medical cannabis in Parkinson's disease: Real-life patients' experience. *Clinical Neuropharmacology, 40*(6), 268–272. https://doi.org/10.1097/WNF.0000000000000246

Balci, P. B. (2018). Spasticity measurement. *Archives of Neuropsychiatry, 55*, S49–S53. https://doi.org/10.29399/npa.23339

Belardo, C., Iannotta, M., Boccella, S., Rubino, R. C., Ricciardi, F., Infantino, R., Pieretti, G., Stella, L., Paino, S., Marabese, I., Maisto, R., Luongo, L., Maione, S., & Guida, F. (2019). Oral cannabidiol prevents allodynia and neurological dysfunctions in a mouse model of mild traumatic brain injury. *Frontiers in Pharmacology, 10*(352), 1–11. https://doi.org/10.3389/fphar.2019.00352

Belyea, D. A., Allhabshan, R., del Rio-Gonzalez, A. M., Chadha, N., Lamba, T., Golshani, C., Merchant, K., Passi, N., & Dan, J. A. (2016). Marijuana use among patients with glaucoma in a city with legalized medical marijuana use. *JAMA Ophthalmology, 134*(3), 259–264. https://doi.org/10.1001/jamaophthalmol.2015.5209

Boehnke, K. F., Gangopadhyay, S., Clauw, D. J., & Haffajee, R. L. (2019). Qualifying conditions of medical cannabis license holders in the United States. *Health Affairs, 38*(2), 295–302. https://doi.org/10.1377/hlthaff.2018.05266

Clark, C. S. (2018). Medical cannabis: The oncology nurse's role in patient education about the effects of marijuana on cancer palliation. *Clinical Journal of Oncology Nursing, 22*(1), E1–E6. https://doi.org/10.1188/18. CJON.E1-E6

Clem, S. N., Bigand, T. L., & Wilson, M. (2019). Cannabis use motivations among adults prescribed opioids for pain. *Pain Management Nursing, 19*, S1524. https://doi.org/10.1016/j.pmn.2019.06.009

Dall'Stella, P. B., Docema, M. F. L., Maldaun, M. V. C, Feher, O., & Lancelotti, C. L. P. (2019) Case report: Clinical outcome and image response of two patients with secondary high-grade glioma treated with chemoradiation, PCV, and cannabidiol. *Frontiers in Oncology, 8*, 1–7. https://doi.org/10.3389/fonc.2018.00643

Desai, R., Patel, U., Rimu, A. H., Zalavadia, D., Bansal, P., & Shah, N. (2019). In hospital outcomes of inflammatory bowel disease in cannabis users: A nation-wide propensity matched analysis in the United States. *Annals of Translational Medicine, 7*(12), 1–9. https://doi.org/10.21037/atm.2019.04.63

Devinsky, O., Cross, J. H., Laux, L., Marsh, E., Miller, I., Nabbout, R., Scheffer, I. E., Thiele, E. A., & Wright, S. (2017). Trial of cannabidiol for drug-resistant seizures in the Dravet syndrome. *The New England Journal of Medicine, 377*, 692–699. https://doi.org/10.1056/NEJMoa1611618

Elliott, L., Golub, A., Bennett, A., & Guarino, H. (2015). PTSD and cannabis related copping among recent veterans in New York City. *Contemporary Drug Problems, 42*, 60–76. https://doi.org/10.1177/0091450915570309

Fleuren, J. F., Voerman, G. E., Erren-Wolters, C. V., Snoek, G. J., Rietman, J. S., Hermens, H. J., & Nene, A. V. (2010). Stop using the Ashworth scale for the assessment of spasticity. *Journal of Neurology, Neurosurgery, and Psychiatry, 81*(1), 46–52. https://doi.org/10.1136/jnnp.2009.177071

Gado, F., Digiacomo, M., Macchia, M., Bertini, S., & Manera, C. (2018). Traditional uses of cannabinoids and new perspectives in the treatment of multiple sclerosis. *Medicines, 5*(3), 91–112. https://doi.org/10.3390/medicines5030091

Hawley, L. A., Ketchum, J. M., Morey, C., Collins, K., & Charlifue, S. (2018). Cannabis use in individuals with spinal cord injury or moderate to severe traumatic brain injury in Colorado. *Archives of Physical Medicine and Rehabilitation, 99*(8), 1584–1590. https://doi.org/10.1016/j.apmr.2018.02.003

Hindocha, C., Cousijn, J., Rall, M., & Bloomfield, M. A. P. (2019). The effectiveness of cannabinoids in the treatment of post-traumatic stress disorder (PTSD): A systematic review. *Journal of Dual Diagnoses, 3*, 1–20. https://doi.org/10.1080/15504263.2019.1652380

Hoffenberg, E. J., McWilliams, S. K., Mikulich-Gilbertson, S. K., Murphy, B. V., Langeaux, M., Robbins, K., Hoffenberg, A. S., de Zoeten, E., & Hopfer, C. J. (2018). Marijuana use by adolescents and young adults with inflammatory bowel disease. *The Journal of Pediatrics, 199*, 99–105. https://doi.org/10.1016/j.jpeds.2018.03.041

Katz, J., & Costarides, A. P. (2019). Facts vs fiction: The role of cannabinoids in the treatment of glaucoma. *Current Ophthalmology Reports, 7*, 177–181. http://dx.doi.org/10.1007/s40135-019-00214-z

Kerlin, A. M., Long, M., Kappleman, M., Martin, C., & Sandler, R. S. (2018). Profiles of patients who use marijuana for inflammatory bowel disease. *Digestive Diseases and Sciences, 63*, 1600–1604. https://doi.org/10.1007/s10620-018-5040-5

Kindred, J. H., Li, K., Ketelhut, N. B., Proessl, F., Fling, B. W., Honce, J. M., Shaffer, W. R., & Rudroff, T. (2017). Cannabis use in people with Parkinson's disease and multiple sclerosis: A web-based investigation. *Complementary Therapies in Medicine, 33*, 99–104. https://doi.org/10.1016/j.ctim.2017.07.002

MacCallum, C. A., & Russo, E. B. (2018). Practical considerations in medical cannabis administration and dosing. *European Journal of Internal Medicine, 49*, 12–19. https://doi.org/10.1016/j.ejim.2018.01.004

Makary, P., Parmar, J. R., Mims, N., Khanfar, N. M., & Freeman, R. A. (2018). Patient counseling guidelines for the use of cannabis for the treatment of chemotherapy-induced nausea/vomiting and chronic pain. *Journal of Pain & Palliative Care Pharmacotherapy, 32*(4), 216–225. https://doi.org/10.1080/15360288.2019.1598531

Maniscalco, G. T., Aponte, R., Bruzzese, D., Guarcello, G., Manzo, V., Napolitano, M., Moreggia, O., Chiariello, F., & Florio, C. (2018). THC/CBD oromucosal spray in patients with multiple sclerosis overactive bladder: A pilot prospective study. *Neurological Sciences, 39*(1), 97–102. https://doi.org/10.1007/s10072-017-3148-6

Markovà, J., Essner, U., Akmaz, B., Marinelli, M., Trompke, C., Lentschat, A., & Vila, C. (2019). Sativex® as add-on therapy vs. further optimized first-line anti-spastics (SAVANT) in resistant multiple sclerosis spasticity: A double-blind, placebo-controlled randomized clinical trial. *International Journal of Neuroscience, 12*(2), 119–128. https://doi.org/10.1080/00207454.2018.1481066

Maroon, J., & Bost, J. (2018). Review of the neurological benefits of phytocannabinoids. *Surgical Neurology International, 26*(9), 91–136. https://doi.org/10.4103/sni.sni_45_18

Mersiades, A., Tognela, A., Haber, P., Stockler, M. R., Lintzeris, N., McGregor, I., Olver, I., Allsop, D. J., Gedye, C., Kirby, A., Morton, R. L., Tran, A. T., Briscoe, K. P., Fox, P., Clarke, S. J., Aghmesheh, M., Wong, N., Walsh, A., Hahn, C., & Grimison, P. S. (2018). Pilot and definitive randomised double-blind placebo-controlled trials evaluating cannabinoid-rich THC/CBD cannabis extract for secondary prevention of chemotherapy-induced nausea and vomiting. *Journal of Clinical Oncology, 36*(15). https://doi.org/10.1200/JCO.2018.36.15_suppl.TPS10128

Miller, S., Daily, L., Leishman, E., Bradshaw, H., & Straiker, A. (2018). Δ-9 Tetrahydrocannabinol and cannabidiol differentially regulate intraocular pressure. *Investigative Ophthalmology and Visual Science, 59*(15), 5904–5911. https://doi.org/10.1167/iovs.18-24838

Mutlu, A., Livanelioglu, A., & Gunel, M. K. (2008). Reliability of Ashworth and modified Ashworth scales in children with spastic cerebral palsy. *BMC Musculoskeletal Disorders, 9*(44), 1–8. https://doi.org/10.1186/1471-2474-9-44

National Academies of Sciences, Engineering, and Medicine. (2017). *The health effects of cannabis and cannabinoids: The current state of evidence and recommendations for research.* The National Academies Press. https://doi.org/10.17226/24625

National Council of State Boards of Nursing. (2018). The NCSBN national nursing guidelines for medical marijuana. *Journal of Nursing Regulation, 9*(2), S1–S60.

Passie, T., Emrich, H. M., Karst, M., Brandt, S. D., & Halpern, J. (2012). Mitigation of post-traumatic stress symptoms by cannabis resin: A review of the clinical and neurobiological evidence. *Drug Testing and Analysis, 4*, 649–657. http://dx.doi.org/10.1002/dta1377

Russo, E. B. (2018). Cannabis therapeutics and the future of neurology. *Frontiers in Integrative Neuroscience, 12*(51), 1–11. https://doi.org/10.3389/fnint.2018.00051

Sagy, I., Bar-Lev Schleider, L., Abu-Shakra, M., & Novack, V. (2019). Safety and efficacy of medical cannabis in fibromyalgia. *Journal of Clinical Medicine, 8*(6), 807. https://doi.org/10.3390/jcm8060807

Schurman, L. D., & Lichtman, A. H. (2017). Endocannabinoids: A promising impact for traumatic brain injury. *Frontiers in Pharmacology, 8*(69), 1–17. https://doi.org/10.3389/fphar.2017.00069

Segura, L. E., Mauro, C. M., Levy, N. S., Khauli, N., Philbin, M. M., Mauro, P. M., & Martins, S. S. (2019). Association of US medical marijuana laws with nonmedical prescription opioid use and prescription opioid use disorder. *JAMA Network Open, 2*(7), e197216. https://doi.org/10.1001/jamanetworkopen.2019.7216

Shohet, A., Khlebtovsky, A., Roizen, N., Roditi, Y., & Djaldetti, R. (2017). Effect of medical cannabis on thermal quantitative measurements of pain in patients with Parkinson's disease. *European Journal of Pain, 21*(2017), 486–493. https://doi.org/10.1002/ejp.942

Skflarsky, J., Hernando, K., Bebin, M., Gaston, T. E., Grayson, L. E., Ampah, S. B., & Moreadith, R. (2019). Higher cannabidiol plasma levels are associated with better seizure response following treatment with pharmaceutical grade cannabidiol. *Epilepsy and Behavior, 95*, 131–136. https://doi.org/10.1016/j.ybeh.2019.03.042

Sulak, D., Saneto, R., & Goldstein, B. (2017). The current status of artisanal cannabis for the treatment of epilepsy in the United States. *Epilepsy & Behavior, 70*, 328–333. http://dx.doi.org/10.1016/j.yebeh.2016.12.032

Ueberall, M. A., Essner, U., & Mueller-Schwefe, G. H. (2019). Effectiveness and tolerability of THC:CBD oromucosal spray as add-on measure in patients with severe chronic pain: Analysis of 12-week open-label real-world data provided by the German Pain e-Registry. *Journal of Pain Research, 12*, 1577–1604. https://doi.org/10.2147/JPR.S192174

Vyas, M. B., LeBaron, V. T., & Gilson, A. M. (2018). The use of cannabis in response to the opioid crisis: A review of the literature. *Nursing Outlook, 66*, 56–65. https://doi.org/10.1016/j.outlook.2017.08.012

Wienkle, L., Domen, C., Shelton, I., Sillau, S., Nair, K., & Alvarez, E. (2019). Exploring cannabis use by patients with multiple sclerosis in a state where cannabis is legal. *Multiple Sclerosis and Related Disorders, 27*, 383–390. https://doi.org/10.1016/j.msard.2018.11.022

Yanes, J. A., McKinnell, Z. E., Reid, M. A., Busler, J. N., Michel, J. S., Pangelinan, M. M., Sutherland, M. T., Younger, J. W., Gonzalez, R., & Robinson, J. L. (2019). Effects of cannabinoid administration for pain: A meta-analysis and meta-regression. *Experimental and Clinical Psychopharmacology, 27*(4), 370–382. https://doi.org/10.1037/pha0000281

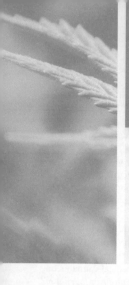

6

The Nurse's Role: Providing Cannabis Care

Carey S. Clark, PhD, RN, AHN-BC, RYT, FAAN

CONCEPTS AND CONSIDERATIONS

This chapter is written as an exploration of the role of the registered nurse in providing cannabis care. The chapter addresses several of the six essential National Council of State Boards of Nursing (NCSBN, 2018) nurse recommendations for working with patients using cannabis for palliation and healing; notably, the nurse will identify safety considerations for patients' use of cannabis and approach the patient without judgment regarding the patient's choice of treatment.

This chapter reviews how nursing theory, specific holistic tools, and the nursing process can support a truly holistic approach to working with medicinal cannabis patients. In addition, an approach to how nurses can evaluate cannabis science evidence is provided. The chapter intends to support the learner in gaining confidence when providing cannabis care and ensuring patients' safe and effective use of cannabinoid therapeutics. The chapter will also bolster the nurse's ability to act as an advocate for medicinal cannabis patients effectively.

Learning Outcomes

Upon completion of this chapter, the learners will:

- Have a baseline knowledge of how to effectively work with medicinal cannabis patients.

Specifically, from the NCSBN essential areas of knowledge, the learners will:

- Identify the safety considerations for patient use of cannabis.
- Be able to approach the patient without judgment regarding the patient's choice of treatment or preferences in managing pain and other distressing symptoms.

In addition, the learners will:

- Consider the holistic role of the nurse when providing cannabis care.
- Gain confidence in their ability to support patients' use of medicinal cannabis therapeutics with vulnerable populations in need of healing by applying the nursing process.
- Focus on the ability to evaluate the body of evidence related to cannabinoid therapeutics.

CANNABIS NURSING: WHAT IS IT?

A cannabis care nurse may work in diverse settings with a variety of patients and their support systems to help facilitate the patient's health and well-being through the safe and effective use of cannabinoid medicines and supporting the upregulation of the endocannabinoid system (ECS). According to the *Scope and Standards of Practice for Cannabis Nurses* (American Cannabis Nurses Association [ACNA], 2019), an evolving document that strives to define cannabis care nursing, the cannabis care nurse has extensive knowledge about:

- The human ECS
- Cannabis and cannabinoid medicine pharmacokinetics and pharmacodynamics
- The cannabis plant and cannabinoid therapeutics
- The current body of cannabis and cannabinoid science evidence
- The history of cannabis as a sacred plant
- Holistic modalities as self-care techniques that upregulate the ECS
- The lived experience of enacting self-care on a regular basis to best role model self-care for patients, caregivers, and colleagues
- The ability to create caring-healing spaces with patients through the application of Human Caring Theory
- The skills of educating and coaching cannabis patients through the medicinal cannabis use process, including the specific state-based recommendation procedures, medical cannabis self-titration techniques, and therapeutic maintenance routines
- Cannabis advocacy skills that can be applied to support cannabis care professionals and patients
- Federal, state, and local laws and legislative processes related to the role of cannabis advocacy work
- How to address the stigma associated with cannabis prohibition through education and advocacy
- Applied ethics related to supporting the patient's right to autonomy and freedom of choice regarding what they ingest for healing (ACNA, 2019)

CANNABIS CARE NURSING: WHAT IS IT?

Who: Cannabis care nurses may be professional licensed vocational nurses, registered nurses, or advanced practice nurses.

What: Cannabis care nurses have knowledge and formal training regarding the physiology of the human ECS, cannabinoid pharmacodynamics/pharmacokinetics, the body of scientific evidence related to cannabinoid effectiveness, and advocacy approaches. They educate and support patients to use cannabis safely and effectively, and they also provide coaching around the upregulation of the ECS. They act as advocates for patients to have access to safe, tested cannabinoid medicines. Cannabis care nurses focus on educating and coaching patients toward maximizing the health potential of the ECS and obtaining homeostasis.

Where: Cannabis care nurses work in a variety of settings where cannabis may be part of the patient's plan for healing and palliation of symptoms. This may involve many specialty nursing areas with patients across the life span. As new evidence emerges regarding cannabinoid therapeutics effectiveness for various illnesses, the "where" of cannabis nursing expands. Cannabis care nursing happens where the patient is at, when there is recognition that the human ECS needs to be upregulated in order to support homeostasis. This recognition comes from the patient who is interested in accessing cannabis for healing and/or from the nurse who recognizes people and populations who could benefit from cannabinoid therapeutics and lifestyle changes that upregulate the ECS.

When: Cannabis care nursing happens when the patient is ready to access healing and palliation and has a desire to maximize their health potential, and when the nurse is prepared to support, educate, and coach the patient through the process. It happens when the nurse is able to create a caring-healing environment with patients so that education and coaching are best received.

Why: The nursing profession is ethically obligated to care for those in need. The NCSBN (2018) also issued a call that all nursing students must be educated around six essential areas of knowledge and skill development to best care for medical cannabis patients. As the cannabis prohibition era ends, and more patients are accessing cannabis for healing and palliation, we become ethically obligated to support their autonomy in choice of treatment and ensure that they can access cannabis and use it safely and effectively.

How: The nurse advances their education in the areas of the science of ECS therapeutics, cannabis pharmacology, ethics, caring-healing theory, coaching, and advocacy in order to provide the best care for the populations who are using medicinal cannabis.

Every cannabis care nurse wants to see the cannabis prohibition-era stigma end so that patients may feel free to discuss their cannabis use, be coached toward safe and effective use of this herbal plant medicine, and access medicines that are safe and tested.

Until the publication of this book, cannabis care nurses have generally had to find their way through a slew of information. They had to make choices from many commercial, educational products to do basic self-education to be prepared to work with vulnerable populations who were looking to use healing cannabinoid medicines. Pioneering cannabis care nurses have had to learn to analyze the body of cannabis scientific evidence and educate themselves about everything from the human ECS to how to be politically active to advocate for patients. Cannabis care nurses have stood up, despite the prohibition-era stigma, to become spokespersons for those who cannot speak for themselves, and they have learned how to best share this wealth of information with others. Cannabis care nurses are leaders in creating change: they will continue to advocate for positive change that supports patients' rights to autonomy in healing, even as we enter this cannabis post-prohibition era and move into an era of cannabis regulation. Cannabis care nurses are called to be caring, compassionate, social justice warriors to ensure that all patients in need have the opportunity to access cannabis therapeutics along their palliative and healing journeys.

Almost every cannabis care nurse that I have met brings with them a beloved "ghost" or two (a dead loved one or patient who could have benefited from the use of cannabis, but could not or would not access it out of fear or ignorance) who provides the cannabis care nurse with the motivation to keep moving forward, despite the ongoing stigma and discrimination. Some of us have lost loved ones who could have greatly benefited from cannabis use to palliate symptoms while going through intensive medical treatments; others have seen patients suffering, unnecessarily, when they could have had relief using cannabis, but they were too afraid to try the herb. Some of us have had loved ones imprisoned for cannabis possession or use, and some nurses may have even spent time in jail or prison themselves for merely possessing a plant that they chose to help them heal themselves or their loved ones.

From a personal perspective, I have worked with many oncology nurses, traveling the country to provide brief overviews of the ECS, information on how cannabis works in the body, and approaches to how they can support patients' safe and effective use of cannabis. It is sad to say that oncology patients suffer when undergoing oncologic treatments, with 80% experiencing chemotherapy-induced nausea and vomiting, not to mention pain, fatigue, depression, and spiritual distress. Yet, we have an amazing herbal plant that could potentially help support oncology patients' exact palliative care needs while undergoing treatment for a life-threatening illness (Aggarwal, 2016). At a certain point as cannabis care nurses, we have come to realize that the ethical issues related to supporting patients' access to safe tested cannabinoid medicines extend beyond patient autonomy to make decisions about their treatment and encompasses all of the ethical concepts we as nurses are charged with enacting: nonmaleficence, beneficence, justice, fidelity, and principles of totality and integrity. Ethics will be discussed in greater detail in Chapter 8.

Other nurses have needed cannabis to support their healing, and they may have lost a job or been forced to quit because of their choice to ingest cannabis for healing.

Nurses have lost jobs or had their licenses threatened because of their cannabis advocacy. Nurses are people too, and if we consider the wounded healer theory of nurses in need of healing for themselves (Clark, 2014), we can begin to assume that nurses are interested in supporting other's healing, even as they should also be on a healing journey themselves. Part of the nurse's healing journey might include the use of cannabinoid medicines. Still the prohibition effect has dramatically impacted many nurses' ability to access the medicine and keep the nursing job they may love.

Cannabis care nurses primarily work with patients by providing education and coaching. Current laws in the American states prohibit nurses from directly handling cannabinoid medicines when working with patients, and the NCSBN (2018) has clearly stated that nurses may not handle cannabinoid medicines unless their state laws allow them to do so. These laws create some space between patient and nurse at the time of the herbal ingestion. Yet, the nurse's coaching and education interventions are paramount to ensure that patients have access to safe medicines and use them without encountering adverse effects. In Israel, the nurse may assist the patient with cannabis ingestion, and indeed, they can handle the plant directly.

Patients should feel supported in a world where accessing cannabis medicines can feel strange or foreign. Use of cannabinoid medicines generally breaks from the usual routine of the doctor or APRN calling in a prescription to the pharmacy, then the patient picking it up at their leisure, with a feeling of certainty or expectation that they will be provided the right dosage and the proper instructions for how to take the medicine. With the herb cannabis, patients are often left on their own to self-titrate the medicine. Cannabis care nurses help fill this void by sharing knowledge, guiding the patient while using evidence, and coaching the patient. The cannabis care nurse may work with the patient from the exploration phase, to receiving a recommendation, through the self-titration process, and on to more of a regular medicinal cannabis use maintenance phase.

The beauty and the challenge of cannabis plant medicine lurk in this magical area where patients are primarily in charge of discovering the right medicine, the right dose, and the right ingestion methods to support their healing. The nurse also further supports the patient by educating and coaching them on how best to upregulate their ECS so that their personal minimal effective amount of cannabis used can support maximal ECS potentiation. Lifestyle choices can also influence the tone of the ECS, and the cannabis care nurse must be knowledgeable in coaching patients in how to potentiate the ECS. This holistic approach reduces the risk of cannabis side or adverse effects. It lessens the financial burdens that patients may face, as currently, most insurance will not cover the cost of cannabis medicines.

The following sections help prepare you to enact the nursing process with cannabis care patients. The nursing theoretical background provides the platform from which all cannabis care is provided.

NURSING THEORETICAL BACKGROUND

In the development of the *Scope and Standards of Practice for Cannabis Nurses* (ACNA, 2019), Watson's Theory of Human Caring was used to support the role of the cannabis care nurse. While many nursing theories can guide the work of the cannabis care nurse, the reason why Watson's theory was chosen to help guide cannabis care nurses is its fit with the evolving role of the cannabis care nurse as well as the need for cannabis care nurses to create a caring-healing presence with those they serve. In addition, Human Caring Theory (Watson, 2012) is particularly helpful in supporting our caring-healing practices in ways that honor the sacredness of the feminine cannabis plant (it is generally the female cannabis plant that is used for healing). This section briefly reviews how Watson's theory can support nurses' work with cannabis patients.

Watson's Theory

Watson's Theory of Human Caring is complex and abstract for many nurses: it is deeply rooted in the humanities, Eastern philosophy, and transpersonal psychology. Meanwhile, contemporary nursing education is generally still deeply rooted in the sciences. When Watson talks about a caring-healing moment where the nurse meets the patient, what she is referring to:

> is a sort of deep, intentional, consciousness-based caring that the nurse calls forth in conjunction with the patient's willingness to move into this healing space that is created during the transpersonal experience and it provides us with a way of considering how we can learn to care deeply, creating nursing interactions that are meaningful for both the patient and the nurse. This deep caring that emerges in a transpersonal human caring moment aligns with the call to be a nurse and to support others on their healing journey (Clark, 2016, p. 3–4).

When we enter into a transpersonal caring moment, moving beyond the ego-self, we are then able to "read the field," moving beyond the patient's outer appearance and behaviors, and connecting with the patient on a spiritual level (Watson, 2012). Human caring is the guiding moral idea and ideal of nursing. As humans, we attempt to connect deeply with others to enhance their well-being, protect them, and preserve their dignity and humanity, as they strive to find meaning in illness, pain, suffering, and the process of being a human (American Nurses Association, 2015; Watson, 2012). The connections that we create can be described as spiritual in nature, as we move out of our ordinary states of being and create new states of being where our spirits meet the spirits of those we care for. This is important because truly effective caring promotes healing, health, individual/family growth, a sense of wholeness, forgiveness, evolved, consciousness, and an inner peace that transcends or goes beyond, our fears/anxieties related to disease, illness, trauma, and crises (Watson, 2012). Caring promotes health and well-being, and it aligns so well with being called to provide cannabis care for patients, since these patients are often vulnerable as they undertake on their healing journeys.

Watson's theory has Ten Caritas Processes that are listed here (Watson Caring Science Institute [WCSI], 2019) and further aligned with the art and skills of cannabis care nursing.

1. "Sustaining humanistic-altruistic values by practice of loving-kindness, compassion, and equanimity with self/others" (WCSI, 2019). In this process, we are called to provide cannabis care from a place of love and compassion, and loving-kindness (which is a Buddhist meditative and applied practice that begins with first loving and caring for oneself and then extending that love and care to the other).

2. "Being authentically present, enabling faith/hope/belief system; honoring subjective inner, life-world of self/others" (WCSI, 2019). The nurse providing cannabis care views each individual as unique: the nurse is present to the others' needs, even as they are aware of their experience. This requires that the nurse is also self-aware and on their own healing journey to best support others.

3. "Being sensitive to self and others by cultivating own spiritual practices; beyond ego-self to transpersonal presence" (WCSI, 2019). By cultivating our spiritual practice, we can better meet patients in the place of transpersonal space where deep caring takes place. Spiritual practices can be very different from religious practices, and they may include things like yoga, chanting, walking in nature, reading spiritual texts, and so on. We also know that many spiritual practices may help reduce stress and upregulate the ECS.

4. "Developing and sustaining loving, trusting-caring relationships" (WCSI, 2019). This means we approach patients with love, trust, and care. It may help to think of the one we are caring for as the beloved of another human being (somebody's mother, father, child, etc.), or as an element of our connections within the grand universe. Cannabis care nurses may also develop a personal relationship with the cannabis plant that assists them as they care for those using the same healing plant.

5. "Allowing for expression of positive and negative feelings—authentically listening to another person's story" (WCSI, 2019). Many spiritual practices also prepare us to listen to others. This can take time to learn: the art of being with the other and investing time just listening to a patient. We can eventually reap the time back as our care for patients become authentic, and we move in synchronicity. We must know the patient's story to support them with the safe and effective use of cannabis.

6. "Creatively problem-solving-'solution-seeking' through caring process; full use of self and artistry of caring-healing practices via the use of all ways of knowing/being/doing/becoming" (WCSI, 2019). Our previous experiences inform our current care approaches. What often starts as a set of technical skills we learn in nursing school morphs into an applied art as we learn from our patients, reflect, and grow into our practice expertise. Given the complexity of cannabis care nursing, problem-solving is a regularly applied skill.

7. "Engaging in transpersonal teaching and learning within context of caring relationship; staying within other's frame of reference-shift toward coaching model for expanded health/wellness" (WCSI, 2019). We need to learn about creating transpersonal states (going beyond the ego-self and meeting the patient where they are) as we coach our patients toward wellness. The coach model goes beyond "educating" and moves toward applying tools like motivational interviewing (MI) and problem-solving to support patients' healing journeys. Cannabis patients benefit greatly from experiencing transpersonal caring with their cannabis care nurse.

8. "Creating a healing environment at all levels; subtle environment for energetic authentic caring presence" (WCSI, 2019). This is about nurses creating environments where patients can truly heal. In other words, you the nurse become the place of healing; to do this, you must be on your own healing journey. Patients know when we geniunely care and this space of caring comes from the heart center.

9. "Reverentially assisting with basic needs as sacred acts, touching mindbodyspirit of spirit of other; sustaining human dignity" (WCSI, 2019). This means that even the most boring or mundane tasks, like bathing and changing linens, become an opportunity to honor the true spiritual nature of those we care for. With cannabis care, we honor the mindbodyspirit by assisting patients in using tools to upregulate the ECS and enter into a state of wellness known as homeostasis.

10. "Opening to spiritual, mystery, unknowns-allowing for miracles" (WCSI, 2019). Believe in miracles. In providing cannabis care, you will see them every day. (Used with permission from Watson, Jean, Watson Caring Science Institute [2019]. Link to WCSI: www.watsoncaringscience.org).

Although we can recognize that there is likely much more to be said about applying nursing theory, keep in mind that patients in need of cannabis care are often vulnerable patients: elderly, children with cancer or seizures, and patients who have become so frustrated with their health, that they have given up on allopathic medicine or they recognize that allopathic approaches do not have all of the answers for them. We have a duty to care for these populations deeply.

When nurses provide cannabis care, they must also be caring for themselves, for how can we ask patients to focus on enhancing their ECS when we may be suffering from poor ECS tone? The art and practice of self-care, therefore, becomes a means to both providing the best care for patients and providing the best care for self; the science of psychoneuroimmunology supports this idea (Clark, 2014). Self-care and caring for others are connected and united, as self-care allows us to provide the best possible cannabis care, where our own ECS is upregulated, and we can role model for patients what a healthy ECS looks like. "The cannabis nurse is a leader in supporting patients toward wellness and health as they support patients toward a maximal state of homeostasis. The cannabis nurse practices self-care to maintain a professional and caring presence with patients" (ACNA, 2019, p. 6).

We must also consider the role mirror neurons play in working with cannabis care patients (Clark, 2014). Communication is key to successful nurse–patient interactions, and much of our communication is nonverbal. The research on mirror neurons helps us to comprehend how patterns arise from the communicating dyad (nurse–patient): the speaker (nurse) may impact the listener's (the patient) neuronal pathways (Silbert et al., 2010). The neuronal pathways of the listener (the patient) are directly impacted by the neuronal state of the speaker (the nurse), with the dyad members both evoking the same brain state (Silbert et al., 2010).

> Mirror neurons help us to understand not only another's physical actions or speech but also another's mind and their intentions. In other words, on an unconscious neurologic level, patients are able to gage the nurse's mindset and their intentions; if the nurse is there to get their paycheck and make it through the shift, the patient knows this via neurologic wisdom; conversely, if the nurse is there with the intention of being a source of caring, compassion, love, and healing for the patient, this is also conveyed. In addition, the nurse's stress state is easily communicated via mirror neurons to the patient, potentially causing harm as the stress-related neural pathways to be physiologically mirrored and replicated in the patient. (Clark, 2014, p. 149)

This has been a brief overview of the importance of using caring theory with vulnerable cannabis care populations. It can be challenging to learn to apply complex nursing theories, but it is essential that the cannabis care nurse recognizes the primacy of care when working with patients. In the future, there will likely be more research on how the caring environment and transpersonal connections with others impact the tone of the ECS and, therefore, potentiates homeostasis. If we think back to Florence Nightingale, she suggested that it was the environment that supported the patient to heal themselves, and we still have much to explore in this area.

> ### ▶ APPLIED LEARNING
>
> **Human Caring Theory**
> 1. What is your comfort level with applying Watson's Human Caring Theory? What resources are available to help you learn more about this theory?
> 2. Discuss with classmates or colleagues the challenges with creating caring-healing spaces in your current workplace or clinical setting. How does your self-care relate to these challenges?
> 3. Are there other nursing theories that could be used to provide the framework for supporting cannabis care?

THE CANNABIS CARE NURSE'S TOOLS

The next sections focus on the specific knowledge and skills cannabis care nurses should have in place before enacting the nursing process with medicinal cannabis patients. These proceed the section on using the nursing process with cannabis care patients because they are foundational to the cannabis care nurses' work and are embedded within the skills that the cannabis care nurse must possess. An understanding of how the ECS can be upregulated through holistic modalities is essential for nurses to share with patients because cannabis care includes coaching patients toward caring for their own ECS. Coaching and MI are some of the vital tools employed while enacting the nursing process in order to best support the patient in setting and meeting their healing goals.

HOLISTIC MODALITIES: THE CARE AND FEEDING OF THE ENDOCANNABINOID SYSTEM

One grand aspect of the cannabis care nurse's approach is summarized in the following statement: "The cannabis nurse considers patients' holistic needs (body, mind, spirit) when designing plans of care. The nurse is cognizant that in addition to supporting patient's use of cannabis for health and healing, the nurse is also obligated to promote the patient's knowledge of endocannabinoid system function and the ability to create homeostasis; therefore, evidence-based use of holistic-integrative modalities should be utilized as needed" (ACNA, 2019, p. 7).

The following section looks at how holistic or integrative modalities may help to upregulate or potentiate the ECS by assisting people in producing more endocannabinoids. Furthermore, these modalities may help people reduce stress levels, making it easier for the ECS to maintain homeostasis. For purposes of this chapter, holistic modalities fall into the categories of mind–body medicine, body-manipulation practices, biologic–physiologic practices, and energy medicine. Holistic modalities may also be known as nonconventional or complementary (used together with conventional/allopathic modalities), alternative (used in place of conventional/allopathic medical modalities), or integrative (brings together the conventional and complementary treatments) approaches that are employed by holistic nurses to support the whole person. The American Holistic Nurses Association (AHNA, 2019) further clarified that it is the use of the modality with the *intention* to support the person's holistic health and well-being that makes a modality holistic, versus simply using a modality to address only the physiologic needs of the patient. This is a key concept for nurses to consider as they support the patient; this herb has the potential to be used holistically and the work goes beyond the supporting of physiologic health and moves toward the fullest potentiation of the patient's holistic mindbodyspirit.

Dietary: The Feeding of the Endocannabinoid System

It may seem odd at first to consider diet to be a holistic modality. Still, when one moves beyond the allopathic world and enters the world of lifestyle medicine, diet becomes one of the primary focuses. It is a modality that can be manipulated or intended for the healing of the patient, and therefore, it can be viewed through the lens of holism. The salient homeostatic roles of ECS are to help us to relax, sleep, eat, forget, and protect (McPartland et al., 2014). What we eat also has an impact on the ECS.

Endocannabinoid system and food control

The endocannabinoids anandamide and 2-arachidonoylglycerol (2-AG) are produced on demand by the ECS. They are derivatives of arachidonic acid formed from dietary linoleic acid, which belongs to the n-6 family of fatty acids. It is clear that dietary intake and certain approaches to food consumption (such as short-term fasting) can help increase anandamide and 2-AG production (Maccarronne et al., 2010). Many factors can impact dietary intake, and metabolism is influenced by the ECS, with CB1 receptors colocalizing with many receptors in the hypothalamus (which synthesizes both catabolic and anabolic proteins to control energy stores). This further suggests that the endocannabinoids are part of our nutritional regulation system, and they function to influence both our homeostatic and hedonic food intake, hunger levels, appetite regulation, satiety, and even dietary preferences (Maccarronne et al., 2010). It is also of interest to note that if we can inhibit fatty acid amide hydrolase (FAAH), which breaks down endocannabinoids we make, we can help sustain endocannabinoid levels in our systems, and potentially further support homeostasis.

Dietary intake to support the endocannabinoid system

The ECS is complex and so is our need for specific nutritional components to best support the ECS. Our Western diets tend to be high in omega-6 fatty acids and lower in omega-3 fatty acids. For optimal functioning, the ECS requires a balance between the two, and for some people, supplementation with omega-3 fatty acids (found in flax, hemp, and chia seeds as well as in cold-water fish) may be beneficial to the ECS (Lafourcade et al., 2011; McPartland et al., 2005).

Flavonoids are the colorful polyphenolic components found in plants (such as berries, citrus fruits, apples, grapes, chocolate, legumes, onions, broccoli, peppers, and tea). They are also crucial for the health of the ECS as they upregulate CB2 receptors and inhibit FAAH breakdown of anandamide (Gertsch et al., 2010).

Furthermore, eating an anti-inflammatory diet helps to support the health of the ECS; therefore, avoiding processed foods, trans-fats, sugar, and environmental toxins becomes essential. Pesticides such as chlorpyrifos and diazinon are known to alter ECS function, so eating organic foods whenever possible is postulated to promote the health of the ECS and help maintain homeostasis (McPartland et al., 2014). Probiotics and prebiotics may help upregulate CB1 receptors (Gioacchini et al., 2017). Acute alcohol in very small amounts may upregulate the ECS, but chronic use or binge drinking may lead to decreased CB1 density (McPartland et al., 2014). In a small clinical trial, large amounts of caffeine (4 to 8 cups/day) were shown to downregulate the ECS. The researchers postulated that the caffeine's propensity to increase stress in the body leads to the lowered production of endocannabinoids (Cornelis et al., 2018). Although there is still much to be studied about caffeine and the ECS, moderation of caffeine is suggested. Stress and the ECS are discussed with more detail in the next section.

The overall takeaway when it comes to dietary lifestyle habits and the ECS is that: a diet balanced in omega-3 and omega-6 fatty acids, rich in flavonoids from whole fruits and vegetables, and low in pesticides, processed foods, sugar, caffeine, and alcohol supports the upregulation and homeostatic capacity of the ECS.

Lifestyle: Holistic Stress Management

The stress response is activated by both the autonomic nervous system (ANS) and the neuroendocrine system. Threats are perceived by the thalamus and primary sensory cortical centers, which then transmit the information to the amygdala, which further detects preconscious threat through cross-talk with the medial prefrontal cortex and the hippocampus (Morena et al., 2015). The ANS response includes stimulation of the sympathetic nervous system and hormonal outputs through descending neural circuits from preautonomic control centers, resulting in catecholamines being released in the brain and the circulatory system (Morena et al., 2015).

Managing our stress is crucial, and the ECS is an integral regulator of our stress responses: we know that stress exposure reduces anandamide, increases 2-AG, and downregulates CB1 receptors (Morena et al., 2015). The decline in anandamide leads to a further manifestation of stress response and increased activation of the hypothalamic–pituitary–adrenal (HPA) axis, leading to the release of corticosteroids, while an increase in 2-AG leads to changes in pain perception, memory, and synaptic plasticity (Morena et al., 2015). The functioning of the ECS related to stress has implications for psychiatric conditions, such as anxiety, depression, and post-traumatic stress disorder (PTSD). Chronic exposure to the same stressors may lead to overall lower levels of anandamide (which support the initiation and manifestation of the stress response and increased anxiety, activation of the HPA axis, decreased neurogenesis, decreased fear extinction, anhedonia, and increased memory consolidation), higher levels of 2-AG (which may buffer against increased anxiety and facilitate termination of the stress response, HPA response termination, HPA axis habituation, modulation of synaptic plasticity, decreased memory retrieval, and decreased pain), downregulation of the CB1 receptor, and increased levels of FAAH (Morena et al., 2015).

It stands to reason that if we can better manage our stress, we can support the health and functioning of the ECS, as it is sensitive to stress exposure. The following sections look specifically at holistic modalities that support the health of the ECS and decrease the stress response.

Exercise

Exercise may be considered to be a holistic modality because it generally remains outside the prescribed allopathic world, while also being a way to care for the mind-bodyspirit. Our bodies were made to move and be active, and when we fail to do so, we may be impacting the health of the ECS.

Research on sustained voluntary medium- to high-intensity aerobic activity has demonstrated that this type of exercise increases CB1 density and the release of anandamide (Brellenthin et al., 2017; McPartland et al., 2014). The "runner's high" that we used to link to endorphins seems now to be more closely related to the ECS and release of anandamide. In addition, when stressed experimental mice are given access to a running mill, ECS deficits seem to be repaired through exercise (Rossi et al., 2008).

Yoga may be viewed as both an exercise and a mind–body practice, as one focuses on the breath and being in the poses while taking an asana. We know that deep breathing helps to elicit the relaxation response, and yoga also increases GABA and dopamine while flooding the body with anandamide (Telles et al., 2017). Regular yoga practice may increase pain tolerance and help make the parasympathetic nervous system the driver of our responses to stress. Although yoga and the ECS need much more study, there is good evidence to show that yoga reduces stress and helps to manage depression and symptoms of PTSD. The connection with the ECS seems evident, even though we lack specific evidence-based data and clinical trials related to ECS health and yoga participation. There are some small studies underway looking at the levels of anandamide and 2-AG with yoga practice.

Acupuncture

Acupuncture is a treatment derived from ancient Chinese medicine where the body is influenced by the insertion of needles into the specific points on the human body known as "acupoints." The Chinese word for acupuncture is *Zhenjiu*, and the two Chinese characters 针灸 represent "metal needle" and "heating," which indicate that acupuncture includes techniques beyond the insertion of metal needles, such as heat, pressure/massage, electroacupuncture, and even coherent laser light treatments (Evidence Based Acupuncture, 2019).

Over the past two decades, the body of evidence related to the effectiveness of acupuncture has emerged with over 13,000 studies conducted in countries from around the globe, focusing on acupuncture's effectiveness with issues such as pain, cancer, pregnancy, stroke, mood disorders, and sleep disorders (Evidence Based Acupuncture, 2019). The Acupuncture Evidence Project (McDoanld & Janz, 2017) examined the literature, specifically meta-analyses and systematic reviews of acupuncture's effectiveness. They determined that acupuncture has a positive effect with eight conditions, including "migraine prophylaxis, headache, chronic low back pain, allergic rhinitis, knee osteoarthritis, chemotherapy-induced nausea and vomiting, postoperative nausea and vomiting, and post-operative pain" (McDoanld & Janz, 2017, p. 2). Moderate evidence was found for acupuncture's effectiveness with 38 conditions, and there was weak/positive proof of effectiveness for 71 other conditions (McDoanld & Janz, 2017).

There is emerging evidence that acupuncture also helps to upregulate the ECS, which begins to make sense as we consider the many illnesses that acupuncture can help address and how the ECS is involved with homeostasis and overall health:

- A study by Su et al. (2012) found that electroacupuncture activates peripheral CB2 receptors and reduces both inflammation and proinflammatory cytokines. The researchers further noted that this technique might enhance nociception of pain, which aligns with increased anandamide levels in the skin (McPartland et al., 2014; Su et al., 2012).
- Chen et al. (2009) found that electroacupuncture increased anandamide in inflamed skin tissues and also activated CB2 receptors.
- Wang et al. (2009) determined that electroacupuncture could protect the brain from ischemia via activation of CB1 receptors and the release of endocannabinoids.
- The activation of the ECS via acupuncture helps with analgesia and supports neuroprotection through stimulation of endocannabinoids and activation of CB1 receptors (Hu et al., 2017).

Hu et al. (2017), in their meta-analysis, summarized that ECS activation and acupuncture treatments have similar effects around creating homeostasis. Acupuncture and the ECS produce many of the same biologic effects, including maintenance of energy balance and regulation of immune, respiratory, and gastrointestinal (GI) system effects. The authors concluded that a better understanding of the links and correlations between acupuncture and the ECS could help increase the clinical efficacy of acupuncture while also enabling patients to lower their doses of cannabinoid therapeutics, enhance the effectiveness of cannabinoid medicines, and lower the risk of side or adverse effects from cannabinoids.

Osteopathy

Osteopathy is performed by Doctors of Osteopathic Medicine (DO) who are physicians practicing in all areas of medicine, emphasizing a whole-person approach to treatment and care. DOs strive to support patients holistically, and they have specialized training in the interconnection between the musculoskeletal system and the nervous system (American Osteopathic Association, 2019).

McPartland et al. (2005) found that after osteopathic treatment, serum anandamide increased 168% from pretreatment levels, whereas 2-AG did not change. Patients receiving the sham treatment demonstrated no changes in endocannabinoid levels. Patients may want to consider osteopathy as a way to help realign the body, reduce pain, and support homeostasis.

Singing

In a small study (n = 9 females, postmenopausal, age 57 to 61) seeking to find ways beyond exercise to enhance circulating endocannabinoid levels, Stone et al. (2018) determined that participants who had prior experience singing in a group/chorus setting had an increase of blood plasma anandamide by 42% after 30 minutes of group singing. Although this study was small, it is important to note that the singers enjoyed singing and had experience singing in groups, so the effect of ECS enhancement and anandamide increases may relate to a subset of people. Patients who have experience with chorus or group singing may benefit by being supported to continue or return to enjoying this type of experience.

Essential Oils/β-Caryophyllene

As noted in Chapters 2 and 3, the essential oils in the cannabis plant, or terpenes, interact to help support the health of the ECS. Indeed, the terpenes in many essential oils may help support the health of the ECS, but the cannabis plant alone has over 200 aromatic terpenes, which may serve the purpose of helping to protect the plant from bacteria and fungi. In addition, terpenes work with the limbic system and impact receptors and neurotransmitters. They may also serve to decrease the intoxicating effects of tetrahydrocannabinol (THC). Terpenes found in the plant may play a role in the differentiating therapeutic values of various cannabis chemovars.

Beta-caryophyllene (BCP) is an essential oil/terpenoid found not only in the cannabis plant but also in various essential oils and many spices and food plants. BCP is found in basil, black pepper, black caraway, hops, oregano, lavender, lemon, rosemary, cinnamon, clove, thyme, tamarind, wild parsnip, sage, parsley, cilantro, coriander, mugwort, celery, ylang-ylang, copaiba, frankincense, and myrrh (Natural Medicine Plants, 2015).

BCP has been found to selectively bind at the CB2 receptor and act as a CB2-receptor agonist (Gertsch et al., 2008); therefore, it is both a cannabinoid and terpenoid. A study by Jung et al. (2015) found that BCP helped suppress melanoma tumor growth and lymph node metastasis in mice. It is also known to act as an anxiolytic (lowers anxiety), antidepressant, anti-inflammatory, neuroprotective agent, and antinociception (decreases pain perception) agent.

In addition, several essential oils or terpenes found in nature may also help support the health of the ECS. Table 6.1 is an example of some common terpenes that may also support how the ECS functions.

TABLE 6.1.	Benefits of terpenes			
α-Pinene	Linalool	β-Caryophyllene	Myrcene	Limonene
Anti-inflammatory Bronchodilator Memory Antibacterial	Anesthetic Anticon-vulsant Analgesic Antianxiety Calming Sedation	Anti-inflammatory Analgesic GI cell protectant Antifungal	Sedative effects Sleep aid Muscle relaxant Calming Antispasm	Treats acid reflux Antianxiety Antifungal Antibacterial Anticarcino-genic
Also found in pine needles	Also found in lavender	Also found in black pepper; other herbs and spices, cloves	Also found in hops Smells like cloves	Also found in citrus Smells like citrus
Counteracts effects of THC; helps with memory		Activates CB2 receptors	Most common one found in cannabis; increases THC psychoactivity	Usually second to fourth most present

GI, gastrointestinal; THC, tetrahydrocannabinol.
Adapted from Boyar, K. (2016). Beyond aroma: Terpenes in Cannabis. 2016. https://www.sclabs.com/beyond-aroma-terpenes-in-cannabis/

Sleep

Patients need to be supported toward creating healthy sleep regimes, with the average adult needing between 7 and 9 hours of sleep per night. When people do not get enough sleep, they go into stress response, which stresses the ECS as it strives to maintain homeostasis. There is some emerging data around how the ECS is involved with the sleep cycle: "Among the modulatory properties of the endocannabinoid system, current data indicate that the sleep-wake cycle is under the influence of endocannabinoids since the blocking of the CB1 cannabinoid receptor or the pharmacological inhibition of FAAH activity promotes wakefulness, whereas the obstruction of anandamide membrane transporter function enhances sleep" (Murillo-Rodriguez et al., 2017, p. 370).

Sleep is one of the areas that need to be more fully studied when it comes to cannabis use as many of the studies related to cannabis and sleep were performed in the 1970s, with most results finding that cannabis helps people to fall asleep more easily, though it may impact the quality of rapid eye movement (REM) sleep and create a sense of grogginess the next day. From a holistic perspective, we can say that nurses should continue to support healthy sleeping habits and proper sleep hygiene when caring for medicinal cannabis patients. If cannabis seems to be disrupting sleep, changes in how the medicine is used may be called for.

Patient and Nurse Considerations

The nurse providing cannabis care is obligated to support patients to maximize the health of their ECS. It is also helpful if the nurse has experience in these areas so that they can also roll out the yoga mat and lace-up the jogging shoes. As you gain experience in upregulating your ECS, you can best coach patients on how to implement these modalities.

> **APPLIED LEARNING**

Upregulate Your Endocannabinoid System
1. What is your knowledge about, and experience with, holistic modalities?
2. What is your plan for learning more about holistic modalities?
3. What steps are you willing to take to create a plan to upregulate your ECS using holistic modalities?

CANNABIS AS SPIRITUAL CARE AND HEALING: THE NURSE'S ROLE

"Entheogen" is a word used to describe substances that "generate the divine within" and create mind-manifesting experiences. They help us to remember and connect with our divine nature. Cannabis is an entheogen (Gray, 2016).

Cannabis had a historical role in many well-known religious traditions, including Hinduism, Taoism, Sikhism, Buddhism, Zoroastrianism, and Judaism. When cannabis is used with the "proper intention and practices, it can help us dissolve our head-sourced beliefs and drop down into direct and intuitive heart perception and wisdom of the body ... it can help us enter deeply into the present ... and awaken to the illusion of separateness that has permeated the lives of the vast majority of people" (Gray, 2016, p. 3–4). One core aspect of using cannabis on the spiritual path is the ability of the plant to help us relax and let go into a sense of inner stillness, awareness, and peace where we can awaken to the nature of love (Gray, 2016).

From a holistic perspective, physical and spiritual healing are interwoven. Cannabis care nurses need to coach cannabis care patients around addressing their spiritual needs for healing. Though nursing has a long history of providing spiritual care, this can be a new skill-set for many nurses: our nursing curricula tend to focus on evidence-based practice techniques and critical-thinking skills, often toward the exclusion of learning about the process of supporting patients' spiritual healing. Patients may need support if they experience discomfort or confusion when entering an altered state of consciousness while using cannabis. Nurses must be skilled at helping patients learn how to be in the sense of inner stillness that cannabis brings forth. As cannabis changes perceptions around time and space, it can take some getting accustomed to altered states of consciousness to fully embrace the plant's holistic healing powers. This is just another reason for patients to start low with THC-based dosing of cannabis and gradually increase doses as they become accustomed to the plant's power.

Cannabis can be seen as a flexible plant ally. Despite its power, it can also be gentle in its ability to open one to a sense of awakening on the path toward healing and enlightenment. Entheogens such as cannabis have a long history of supporting and producing genuine spiritual and mystical experiences. Cannabis used for spiritual growth and healing may require the proper set, setting, and context to summon an appreciation for life, stimulate the imaginative centers, and enter into the spiritual state of inner stillness. Gray (2016) provided some steps that create context around the use of cannabis for spiritual healing:

- Set: This refers to what the individual brings to the cannabis healing experience, including history, personality, psychospiritual foundation, intention, and preparation for using the medicine via a spiritual approach (ie, having a spiritual practice or practices in place). The person's set that they bring with them prior to ingestion has an impact on how they will respond to the spiritual awakening that the plant can bring forth.
- Setting: This is the actual environment and conditions in which one partakes of the plant's gifts. Is the environment peaceful, comfortable, and uplifting? The setting for cannabis care patients using the plant with a spiritual intention can, for many people, become a key aspect of the healing process.
- Creating ritual: How are intentions, set, and ritual created and used? A brief "thank you" or expression of gratitude toward the medicine, a prayer, taking a few deep breaths, or lighting a candle can all be ways to create a meaningful ritual before ingestion of the plant medicine. The ritual helps to make the mind more present, and sets the tone for the creation of the nonordinary spiritual space.

Undertaking spiritual practice with the use of the cannabis plant may include the following activities:

- Focus on the breath: This is a simple way to practice meditation and focus the mind after ingesting cannabis. As the mind wanders away from the breath focus, it can then be brought gently back again.
- Other breath practices such as square breathing or yogic-based pranayama techniques may be used.
- Guided imagery or visualization practices
- Yoga
- Sacred chant or prayer
- Dance
- Tai chi
- Listening to or making music
- Reading spiritual texts
- Walking in nature
- Receiving healing touch via massage or other techniques

Assessing the patient's need for spiritual healing can be as simple as asking them about their religion and spiritual practices and how they relate to their spiritual care needs and physical healing. If the cannabis care patient has spiritual needs, coaching them about ways to use the medicine in peaceful ways can be helpful. Though many would say this area of the spiritual nature of ingesting cannabis lacks scientific evidence, the thousands of years of cannabis use in spiritual and religious gatherings informs us of its potential to support spiritual healing.

> **APPLIED LEARNING**

Spirituality
1. What is your comfort level with supporting and coaching patients regarding the use of cannabis to enhance spiritual healing?
2. What are some approaches you can use as part of your assessment of cannabis patients' spiritual needs? Role-play a cannabis care spiritual assessment with a colleague or classmate and discuss what worked well and what you might do differently.

Spiritual Healing: Feminine Energy of Cannabis

Generally, the female species of the cannabis plant is what is ingested by humans. Patients interested in using cannabis for spiritual healing may take the time to get to know the plant, her history, and relate to her from a spirit-based perspective. Cannabis allows us to change perspective and see things differently for a while, creating a liminal time or space (limen being the place between known places). This liminal space that cannabis creates can offer the patient some time to contemplate, understand, or appreciate the mysteries of life and their place in it, as the observer or inner eye is awakened (Harrison, 2016).

Some cultures may also believe that plants can help us to learn and that plants as allies in healing can take on a persona of their own: in some historical cultures, cannabis was seen or felt like a deity or being, and the ancient Chinese referred to her as "Ma," with a connotation of the plant being the one who nurtures, clothes, and binds communities together (Harrison, 2016).

It has been suggested that creating a ritual around the use of cannabis can also support the ability to access the entheogens healing powers, as the plant can facilitate understanding and help us first to observe, and then release, patterns that bind us up too tightly (Harrison, 2016). Cannabis can help us to create a worldview that is softer, one where the interconnection of species becomes clear.

As nurses, if the cannabis care patient expresses the need for spiritual healing, we can help coach them to gain a deeper understanding of the cannabis plant. We can begin by exploring if patients have a personal ritual around the cannabis plant's use (it can be as simple as expressing gratitude for the plant's healing powers), how or if they set the intention for healing to emerge, and how they allow for time and space to get to know the plant ally. As cannabis care nurses, we can respect the power of this plant species and ensure that new cannabinoid therapeutics are developed. I believe that it is imperative in this era of regulation that we never lose sight of the spiritual nature of the plant and that we support the patients' ability to create a conscious connection with the plant.

This idea of cannabis as an entheogen is not new, and yet many nurses may question this concept of using a herbal medicine to support spiritual healing: after all, there are no randomized clinical controlled trials addressing cannabis as a tool for spiritual health. However, thousands of years of cannabis being used as a cultural and spiritual tool that can also inform our practice. Spiritual distress is also not a qualifying condition for the recommendation of medicinal cannabis, yet many physical or chronic conditions may have spiritual components. Cannabis is proving to be very beneficial for end-of-life care, which is often mired in spiritual concerns. Nurses are often under-educated regarding providing spiritual care, and cannabis care provides us with the keen opportunity to grow our spiritual care skills.

MOTIVATIONAL INTERVIEWING: A SKILL FOR GOAL SETTING

MI allows for the cannabis care nurse to become a coach and assistant to the patient as they undertake the change process. MI was originally designed to help people with addiction change unhealthy behaviors (Droppa, 2014). One key aspect of MI is that it calls for the nurse to accept where the patient is in the present moment. MI has the goal of helping patients resolve their ambivalence that can deter acquisition of goal attainment (Miller & Rollnick, 1991). MI has its foundations in Carl Rogers' Humanistic Theory of Personality, with an emphasis on optimism and self-actualization. By moving beyond the concept of nurse-driven information sessions, MI helps nurses to be patient-centered as they engage patients in conversations that highlight where the patient is at now and where they would like to be in the future (Droppa, 2014). What are the patient's current concerns, how can we help them manage their ambivalence and motivate them to make changes in behavior (Droppa, 2014)? Motivation to change should not be imposed upon people, rather elicited from them (Substance Abuse and Mental Health Services Administration [SAMHSA], 2018).

MI strategies tend to be persuasive and supportive. Some general strategies of MI include:

1. Express empathy through reflective listening.
2. Develop or highlight discrepancies between clients' goals or values and their current behavior.
3. Avoid argument and direct confrontation.
4. Roll with the resistance. Adjust to client resistance rather than opposing it directly.
5. Support self-efficacy and optimism (Droppa, 2014; Miller & Rollnick, 1991).

Empathy

Empathy allows us to demonstrate respect for and acceptance of patients and their feelings, while also encouraging a nonjudgmental, collaborative relationship as we strive to support the patient. Empathy helps us to listen, rather than telling, and it helps us to persuade and support patients in both setting and meeting their goals (Miller & Rollnick, 1991). By using reflective listening as we practice nonjudgmental acceptance, we can rephrase the patient's comments in a way that conveys a sense of understanding and determination to understand the patient's point of view. Showing the patient warmth, respect, and understanding will help them on the path toward change (SAMHSA, 2018).

Develop and Highlight Discrepancy

We can help patients understand the gap or distance between where they are now and where they would like to be. Patients can gain a sense of motivation by understanding the gap between where they are at now and where they would like to be (Droppa, 2014).

Resistance

Instead of arguing directly with the patient about the need for change or the change process, when using MI techniques, it is better to accept the resistance. Know that part of the process of change is moving through ambivalence (Droppa, 2014).

Self-Efficacy

Support the patient's optimism so that they can undertake the change process (Droppa, 2014). Patients need to know that they can commit to positive behavioral changes, and that things can get better for them. Highlighting the patient's past small or large successes with creating change can help raise their self-confidence and support self-efficacy (Droppa, 2014).

OARS TECHNIQUE FOR MOTIVATIONAL INTERVIEWING

MI can be implemented using the OARS technique. The OARS technique is:

- **O**pen-ended questions are used to garner depth of explanation and create a deeper sense of contemplation.
- **A**ffirmations are used to create positive experiences and feelings throughout the process.
- **R**eflections back to the patient demonstrate that the cannabis care nurse truly has heard and now understands the patient.
- **S**ummaries can be generated from simple reflections to foster the patient's momentum and generate even greater interest in the change process (Droppa, 2014).

As the nurse works with applying the MI process with the cannabis care patient, they should resist the righting reflex (offering a solution to every problem and avoiding imposing a personal perspective) (Droppa, 2014). This can be difficult for nurses, who often know what the "right thing to do" is; however, telling a patient what to do versus supporting them to problem solve and reach their personal solution allows us to empower the patient and partner with them versus being more paternalistic in our efforts. As they listen intently, the cannabis care nurse should strive to truly understand and reflect the patient's reasons for making behavioral changes. The cannabis care nurse can still share knowledge and experiences that might help guide the patient, but this is different from the righting reflex.

Ultimately, the goal of using MI is to empower the cannabis care patient in the change process (Droppa, 2014). Why is it so crucial that cannabis care nurses use empowering techniques when working with cannabis care patients? Unfortunately, both cannabis care patients and nurses must overcome the stigma that generations of Reefer Madness have created. If we use a truly holistic approach to providing cannabis care, we will be supporting patients to do more than use cannabis to create homeostasis; we will also be coaching them to engage in behavioral changes that upregulate the ECS, and this can be part of the hard work of healing. As cannabis care nurses, we have a vested interest in patients using cannabinoid medicines in ways that side effects are minimized, finances are managed, and the health of the ECS is potentiated. Arguably, the only way to help patients upregulate the ECS consistently is to use MI and coaching techniques to support patients making meaningful and sustainable lifestyle changes.

> **▶ APPLIED LEARNING**
>
> **Motivational Interviewing**
>
> Partner with a classmate, colleague, or friend who is willing to discuss a lifestyle change they would like to make. Apply MI techniques, such as the OARS approach. Reflect on what was challenging, and how this was different from the way you normally would approach this situation. What do you need to do to grow your MI skills?

THE NURSES ROLE: APPLYING THE NURSING PROCESS

We have reviewed some of the key components foundational to enacting the nursing process with cannabis care patients, including nursing theory, holistic approaches to upregulating the ECS, spiritual approaches to the use of cannabis, and MI. The nursing process can be applied by nurses providing consultation, education, and coaching for cannabis patients and nurses working in more allopathic settings. The nursing process helps us to use a systematic approach so that we can identify specific patient problems, pertinent nursing diagnoses, and how to evaluate patient outcomes. The five steps in the process are assessment, diagnosis, planning, interventions, and outcomes. A note to APRN's: your process is a bit different related to your expanded role, so please refer to that process in the APRN role in Chapter 7.

Assessment

The nurse performs the initial assessment of the patient using a holistic approach, with both objective and subjective data gathered. Objective data may include full medical history, labs, vital signs, pertinent diagnostic test findings, intake/output if applicable, and a complete head-to-toe holistic assessment. Medical diagnoses are considered, body systems are reviewed, and subjective data are also gathered. Gathering subjective data is an essential aspect of the nurse's work, and this can be further enhanced by practicing techniques like MI and creating an intentional caring-healing space with the patient while applying Watson's Caritas Processes.

In addition to the usual standards of nursing practice applied with all patients, the nurse becomes more curious about the patient's cannabis knowledge and assesses for:

- Patient's current knowledge base around the use of cannabis as a palliative/ healing tool. This assessment of patient's knowledge may include their understanding of how cannabis works in the body and their familiarity with the body of evidence related to the effectiveness of cannabis for their specific qualifying conditions and health concerns. This will help direct the nurse in planning educational support.

- Where the patient gets their information about cannabis from. Are they relying on the experience of other cannabis patients, knowledge gleaned from friends or relatives, social media?
- Current and previous/historical patterns of cannabis use. Has the patient had any previous substance use disorders or concerns?
- Patient's baseline knowledge of cannabis ingestion methods and dosing approaches
- Current medical recommendation to use cannabis. Do they know how to obtain a medical recommendation? Do they have a qualifying medical condition? (Consider the legal status of cannabis in the state). This may not be needed to legally access cannabis in some states where adult-recreational use is allowed; however, there may still be distinct benefits to having a medical recommendation (ie, being able to access medical cannabis in other states that offer a reciprocal medical cannabis program or lower tax rates when purchasing from a dispensary).
- Patient's baseline knowledge of cannabis laws in the state and how cannabis can be procured and used. In some states, patients are not allowed to smoke cannabis, some states allow for cannabidiol (CBD) use only, and so on.
- Patient's beginning ideas around their healing and palliative goals with the use of medicinal cannabis: physical, psychological, mental, and spiritual needs considered
- Patient's support system around the use of cannabis. Are the patient's family members or caregivers supportive and knowledgeable?
- Patient's financial ability to pay for cannabis and available financial resources
- Knowledge about safety, side effects, adverse effects, and medication or drug–drug interactions
- Knowledge about and current use of modalities that support ECS health (see holistic modalities). This may include assessment of dietary, exercise, sleep habits, and so on.

The nurse approaches the patient by forming a caring-healing environment as they enact Watson's Caritas Processes. The nurse uses a nonjudgmental attitude as they build rapport and trust during the assessment process.

Diagnoses

Any number of nursing diagnoses may apply, and it is important that the nurse knows the patient's initial goals and how cannabis might help the patient achieve these goals. Any number of the over 240 NANDA-approved nursing diagnoses may apply, with this list culling together many likely to apply to patients who are looking to use cannabis for palliation and healing:

- Activity intolerance
- Anxiety
- Comfort, impaired
- Coping, ineffective
- Deficient knowledge
- Disturbed energy field
- Dry mouth, risk for

- Falls, risk for
- Fatigue/activity intolerance
- Fear
- Health literacy, readiness for enhanced
- Imbalanced nutrition: more than body requirements
- Imbalanced nutrition: less than body requirements
- Impaired resilience
- Ineffective coping/readiness for enhanced coping
- Ineffective role performance
- Insomnia/sleep deprivation/readiness for enhanced sleep
- Moral distress
- Pain, acute
- Pain, chronic
- Nausea
- Nutrition, readiness for enhanced
- Powerlessness
- Readiness for enhanced health management
- Readiness for enhanced self-concept
- Risk for injury
- Role anxiety
- Self-care, readiness for enhanced
- Sleep deprivation
- Sleep pattern disturbed
- Spiritual distress
- Spiritual well-being, readiness for enhanced
- Stress overload (Herdman & Kamitsuru, 2014).

The nurse can also share the nursing diagnoses with the patient, and together, they can further refine their goals.

Planning

During the planning phase, the nurse works closely with the patient and any involved caregivers/significant others to plan for the resources the patient will need to use medicinal cannabis effectively and safely.

The nurse considers what the patient has in place and what they need in place for the patient to access cannabis and meet their goals. The nurse may act as educator and coach to support the patient's ability to safely and effectively access cannabinoid therapeutics.

The nurse uses evidence as they coach the patient through:

- The medical recommendation process as applicable to the patient's state of residence
- Use of holistic modalities (see previous section) to upregulate ECS
- How cannabis works in the body
- The body of evidence related to the patient's specific health concerns

- Inpatient restraints on the use of cannabis (know your state law and your facility's policies; for more information, see Special Considerations)
- Ingestion methods: What products are available that will work with patient's needs? What has the patient tried in the past, and was it effective? Consider inhalation (smoking, vaping, aerosolized), topical, transdermal, oromucosal, edibles, tinctures, oral, and rectal.
- Cannabis chemovars: How will the patient determine the best chemovar for them? Consider how they will interact with dispensary/caregiver to select cannabis products that will be of most benefit.
- Dosing and titration strategies
- Side effects, adverse effects, and how they can be managed
- Reviewing the process of keeping a cannabis diary should include the date, time, route, strain, dose, effects, and side effects.
- Consider how to use cannabis as a spiritual tool for healing, if this aligns with patient goals.

Interventions/Implementation

Based on the findings from the assessment and goal-setting stage, the nurse may need to provide ongoing education, coaching, and support. Patients need assistance with using cannabis safely and effectively and upregulating their ECS.

Cannabis coaching

Coaching is a bit different from educating regarding the nurse's role in working with patients. If we think of a coach, we might think of someone who walks hand in hand with us as we strive toward our goals: they empower and motivate us toward success. Nurse coaching starts with a partnership with the patient, where they are viewed as their own expert, and the nurse works creatively to generate a skilled, purposeful, and results-oriented client/patient interaction, having the ultimate purpose of patients achieving their goals (Dossey & Hess, 2013). Nurse coaches have the knowledge and skills to support behavioral and lifestyle changes that enhance overall health, well-being, and personal growth (Dossey & Hess, 2013). Nurse coaches recognize that they are addressing the biopsychosocial–cultural–environmental dimensions of health:

> Effective nurse coaching interactions involve the ability to develop a coaching partnership, to create a safe space, and to be sensitive to client issues of trust and vulnerability, as a basis for further exploration, self-discovery, and action planning related to desired outcomes. It builds on the client's strengths rather than attempting to "fix" weaknesses. Nurse coaching interactions are based on research findings related to positive psychology and flow theory, and learned optimism as it relates to transformational change (Dossey & Hess, 2013, p. 12).

Coaching begins with the assessment process, establishing goals, and providing coaching interactions; it continues through evaluation of goal attainment. Patients should have a clear plan and established goals before beginning the cannabis ingestion and titration process. By keeping a cannabis diary, the patient is then able to follow up with the nurse about what is working and what might need to be modified, what side effects may be experienced, and the effectiveness of the strain.

General self-titration education and coaching

MacCallum and Russo (2018) recommended the following information for patients learning to titrate their medicinal use of cannabis. Having access to safe medicine that is clearly labeled with THC mg content makes this process possible, and this is likely only available to patients in legalized states with access to dispensaries or providers/caregivers who have their medicine tested. As nurses, we can educate and coach patients through the process, using established guidelines that we can share with them so they can self-titrate the medicine safely and effectively. Keep in mind that nurses are not prescribing or telling patients what their dosing should be, rather giving them evidence-based information and offering support around the process.

MacCallum and Russo (2018) stated that if medicinal cannabis is legal where the patient resides, a trial with whole-plant medicine is the best approach over using synthesized cannabinoids. Dosing should "start low, go slow, stay low" when it comes to THC content of the plant used, keeping in mind that THC causes both the euphoria or "high" and the side or adverse effects. In addition, in most states at the time of this publication, nurses may not administer or handle cannabis products when interacting with patients (know your state laws, regulations, and nurse practice acts). As described earlier, patients should keep a cannabis diary (may include the date, time, symptom, cannabis strain, route, dose, onset, effectiveness, duration, side effects).

Inhalation

- One inhalation, wait 15 minutes. Proceed with one inhalation every 15 to 30 minutes until symptoms are relieved. Slowly titrate to avoid side effects. Duration 2 to 4 hours.
- Use CBD dominant to avoid side effects of THC.
- Euphoria state is not needed for relief of symptoms (MacCallum & Russo, 2018).

Oral Preparations

- Start with oral preparations at bedtime. Consider the patient may experience drowsiness, hence the bedtime approach.
  - Days 1 to 2: 1.25 to 2.5 mg THC
  - Days 3 to 4: increase by 1.25 to 2.5 mg THC
  - Days 5 to 6: increase again by 1.25 to 2.5 mg THC every 2 days until symptom relief
  - Side effects experienced: reduce back to best-tolerated dose
  - Proceed to daytime strategy, dose two to three times/day (BID/TID):
  - Days 1 to 2: 2.5 mg THC/once/day
  - Days 3 to 4: 2.5 mg THC/BID
  - Increase as tolerated up to a maximum of 15 mg THC, divided BID or TID
  - THC doses greater than 20 to 30 mg/day may increase adverse effects or cause tolerance with no increase in efficacy.
  - Include CBD: 5 to 20 mg, divided BID or TID (MacCallum & Russo, 2018).

Example of a cannabis diary

Date	Time	Symptom	Strain	Route	Dose	Onset	Effect	Duration	Side effects
January 15, 2020	12:12 pm	Pain, "8"/10	Jack Frost	Inhala-tion	2 puffs	5 min	Pain down to a "4"/10	3 h 3:30 need more med?	Dry mouth
January 15, 2020	4:00 pm	Pain "6"/10	Jack Frost	Inhala-tion	3 puffs	6 min	Pain "2"/10	4 h	Dry mouth, Sleepy

> ### APPLIED LEARNING
>
> **Nurse's Role with Titration**
> The cannabis care nurse works closely with patients and coaches them toward success with titration processes.
> - What is the best way for you to grow your coaching skills and gain confidence in supporting patients' self-titration process? Consider role-playing the process with a classmate or colleague.

Special considerations for cannabis administration: policy development

Because of cannabis federal Drug Enforcement Administration (DEA) level I scheduling, many hospitals and facilities, even in legal states, do not allow for cannabis to be consumed in their settings; however, some states do allow for medicinal cannabis patients to use cannabis in their settings, and hospitals and facilities may then develop their policies around patient use of medicinal cannabis.

This was the case in Minnesota: when medicinal cannabis became legal, the Minnesota Hospital Association (MHA) came up with three sample policies that align with three different stances that hospitals can take (American College of Physicians [ACP], 2019). The MHA created a medical cannabis committee made up of physicians, nurses, pharmacists, and representatives from state-based organizations and medical cannabis manufacturers.

The three Minnesota statewide policy options and templates that hospitals can choose from are summarized as follows:

- Cannabis not be allowed at all in the hospital.
- Registered cannabis patients may self-administer cannabis in the hospital with their personal supply, which should be securely stored.
- Medical cannabis can be administered by a nurse upon clinician approval, and the cannabis must be stored securely in the facility (ACP, 2019).

For registered nurses, when it comes to facilities and policy development, we should be concerned about the ethical implications of patient autonomy and the patient's ability to access medicines that will best support their healing, as recommended by a physician or APRN. Nurses should have the knowledge, skills, and attitudes to properly assist medicinal cannabis patients' use of cannabinoid therapeutics in the inpatient setting if both their state laws and hospital policies state as such. Although this may be a strange-new land for most nurses, we are obligated to educate ourselves on how we can end the stigma and support patient access to safe cannabinoid therapeutics.

> **APPLIED LEARNING**

Your Facility and Cannabis

Know your facility's or setting's cannabis care policies. If there is not one in place, consider how you can advocate for the development of patient-centered cannabis care policies? Are other facilities or organizations in your area also needing to address this issue?

Evaluation

The final step in the nursing process is the evaluation step. The nurse as coach would help the client review the goals they set during the planning phase, determine what is working well, and decide together what might need to change in the plan of care.

- Is the patient experiencing any side effects or drug–drug interactions?
- Which goals were attained? Which might need to be modified or reconsidered?
- Are nursing diagnoses resolved?
- Is the patient able to use the medicine safely and effectively?
- Is the patient able to adhere to the statewide cannabis policy constraints around the medicinal use of cannabis?
- Is the patient getting the most benefit from the plant?
- Is the patient able to undertake steps to upregulate the ECS?
- Is the patient able to afford the current and projected medicinal cannabis costs?
- Is the patient able to keep THC doses low?

Evaluation also provides us a way to return to the care plan, revisit our assessment findings, and support the patient's striving for their goals.

> **APPLIED LEARNING**

Growing Your Skills

Cannabis care is holistic care that occurs in the space of caring-healing atmosphere created by the nurse. Consider patients' needs for cannabis to support healing and changes in lifestyle to upregulate the ECS. Set some goals for your knowledge and skill acquisition in this area.

Evaluating the Evidence: The Nurse's Role

The NCSBN (2018) issued a recommendation that *The nurse shall have an understanding of cannabis pharmacology and the research associated with the medical use of cannabis.* As nurses start considering this, it is quite a tall order, with over 30,000 cannabis-based published studies on the PubMed website, how is the nurse to gain an understanding of the research associated with cannabis and, more specifically, with cannabis care? One approach is to familiarize yourself with the cannabis science body of evidence related to the patients you work with. There are also some useful articles that do meta-analyses of cannabis science findings. Those articles and ones like them can help the nurse get a grasp of the evolving body of knowledge related to cannabis science and the implications for specific disease states.

A good place to start evaluating the body of cannabis science evidence is with The National Academies of Sciences, Engineering, and Medicine (NASEM) published consensus report from 2017 titled The *Health Effects of Cannabis and Cannabinoids: The Current State of Evidence and Recommendations for Research.* The goal of this work was to update the original review of the evidence that was completed in 1999, as the field of cannabis has dramatically expanded despite the prohibition effect. "This report summarizes the current state of evidence regarding what is known about the health impacts of cannabis and cannabis-derived products, including effects related to therapeutic uses of cannabis and potential health risks related to certain cancers, diseases, mental health disorders, and injuries. Areas in need of additional research and current barriers to conducting cannabis research are also covered in this comprehensive report" (NASEM, 2017).

The report has a lot of depth. The short version of the findings and levels of evidence available for specific disease/illness categories can be found at https://www.nap.edu/resource/24625/Cannabis-conclusions.pdf, and the full content of the report can be accessed for free at https://www.ncbi.nlm.nih.gov/books/NBK423845/.

The levels of evidence for specific illness/disease issues are summarized in the following table.

Levels of evidence of efficacy	Conclusive or substantial evidence	Moderate evidence	Limited evidence	Insufficient evidence
Benefits	• Adult chronic pain • Multiple sclerosis (MS)/spasticity • Chemotherapy-induced nausea/vomiting • Intractable seizures • Dravet and Lennox-Gastaut syndromes (CBD)	• Sleep disturbances related to pain, MS, fibromyalgia, sleep apnea • Decreasing intraocular pressure in glaucoma	• Dementia • Parkinson's • Schizophrenia symptoms • PTSD symptoms • Appetite/weight issues with HIV/AIDS • Traumatic brain injury • Anxiety (CBD) • Tourette's syndrome	• Depression • Addiction abstinence • IBS symptoms • Cancer treatment • Cancer-associated anorexia • ALS symptoms • Dystonia

This report provides cannabis care nurses with knowledge of what needs to be studied and a baseline of what is known about the evidence-based effectiveness of cannabis. This report defined the current state of barriers to performing cannabis research including:

- Regulatory issues related to DEA/Food and Drug Administration (FDA) and the current federal cannabis prohibition issues
- Access to cannabis plant medicine issues, with access to cannabis only being available in the United States from the National Institutes of Drug Abuse (NIDA), whose mission on studying drug use/addiction is contradictory to examining the therapeutic benefits of cannabis
- All varieties of cannabis plant medicine provided for research in the United States come from the University of Mississippi, and they are known to be of poor quality and low potency in comparison to strains of cannabis available in medicinal dispensaries in medicinal/legalized states in the United States. There are issues regarding quality, type, and quantity of cannabis plant materials available.
- Funding for cannabis research is so limited that the amount of research done now cannot adequately inform healthcare or public practice. Only about 10% of NIDA's budget is allocated to supporting research regarding the therapeutic properties of cannabis. The NASEM has called for consideration that funding strategies may need to move to being more squarely National Institutes of Health (NIH) and disease-specific focused. Diversity around funding is necessary.
- Drug delivery issues, with issues related to how to best deliver whole-plant medicine to be studied. Although smoking or vaporizing may be a preferred route for many cannabis users, funding for this type of research may be limited because of safety and replicability issues. Currently, much of the cannabinoid therapeutics research is done around oral doses of single-isolated synthetic cannabinoids, such as dronabinol or CBD, and not the whole-plant medicine that contains over 400 components that may interact with our ECS.
- Lack of good placebo or control medication for randomized clinical controlled studies to compare the effects of cannabinoid medicines to placebo or control
- Participants have issues with accurately reporting prior substance use and exposure to cannabinoids. This is a complex issue, but basically, it is difficult to rely on people accurately recalling their previous cannabis use and experiences. Yet, we need to strive to obtain useful baseline data of participants' historical cannabis use.
- There is a need for improvements with standardization and research methodologies (NASEM, 2017).

The NASEM (2017) went on to call for recommendations that support and improve research around cannabis. In a few nutshells, they recommended:

- The development of a national cannabis research agenda, including basic research studies aimed at minimizing the harm and maximizing the benefits of cannabis, with a goal of maximizing population health impact of cannabis-related research
- Health policy and public health research related to the effects of broader social use and associated behavioral and health status changes

- Translational research techniques should be used to ensure that findings are practical and can be used to inform healthcare practice, the creation of public health priorities, national and state policies, and public safety standards.
- Clinical and observational research should the health effects of cannabis on vulnerable populations, investigating the pharmacokinetic and pharmacodynamic effects of cannabis, determining the health benefits/harms related to the various ways cannabis can be ingested, and the unstudied and understudied benefits/risks of high-priority health issues (namely, PTSD, pediatric epilepsy, pediatric and adult cancers, and cannabis adverse reactions).
- Investigate the national and state economic impacts of medicinal and recreational cannabis use, including the impact on healthcare systems, insurance providers, and patients.
- Identify gaps and deficiencies in cannabis-related knowledge and healthcare providers' skills among public health professionals (NASEM, 2017).

Ultimately, the NASEM (2017) report calls for developing a conclusive body of evidence related to both the harms and benefits regarding the short- and long-term health effects of cannabis use. The report calls for the U.S. Department of Health and Human Services, NIH, and Centers for Disease Control and Prevention to jointly fund a workshop that would "develop a set of research standards and benchmarks to guide and ensure the production of high-quality cannabis research" (NASEM, 2017, p. 388). Lastly, "The Centers for Disease Control and Prevention, National Institutes of Health, U.S. Food and Drug Administration, industry groups, and nongovernmental organizations should fund the convening of a committee of experts tasked to produce an objective and evidence-based report that fully characterizes the impacts of regulatory barriers to cannabis research and that proposes strategies for supporting development of the resources and infrastructure necessary to conduct a comprehensive cannabis research agenda" (NASEM, 2017, p. 389).

Although cannabis science is still emerging, nurses need to look at this research process from a nonreductionistic perspective. The NASEM report calls for more in-depth approaches to looking at both positive and negative implications of the broader use of cannabis. Chapter 5 explores specifics about the current body of evidence and cannabis effectiveness, expanding on the NASEM (2017) report, and reviewing the current state of the evidence.

EXAMPLE OF HOW TO REVIEW THE SCIENTIFIC EVIDENCE

I have heard from many nurses who do not feel comfortable examining the research, though there are many approaches and tools available to nurses to support this process. The journal *American Nurse Today* (Kaplan, 2012) recommended using a basic systematic approach as follows:

- Does the title describe the article accurately?
- Is the abstract representative of the article?
- Does the opening clearly define the purpose of the article?
- Is there a theoretical framework?
- Is the literature review relevant and comprehensive?

- Does the methods section relate to answering the research question?
- Is the analytical approach aligned with the study and research design?
- Are the results presented clearly? Do the tables and figures make sense?
- What is the level and quality of the evidence?

Although this is one basic approach to determining whether the article is sound, the lived experience of diving into an analysis of a cannabis science article can be very daunting and time-consuming. It can also be enlightening and rewarding when one takes the time to take a more in-depth look at that evidence. If you are passionate about cannabis science, I suggest taking that deeper dive into some of the body of evidence related to your interests.

LIVED EXPERIENCE: REVIEWING THE EVIDENCE

In the spring of 2019, as is known to happen, a near viral posting about some cannabis-related research findings was making it away across social media platforms. The concern? That use of high-potency cannabis was leading to first-time psychosis diagnoses. There has been a long history related to the evocation of fear based in the findings from cannabis studies, dating back to at least the Reefer Madness era of the late 1930s, when it was anecdotally propagated that the use of the devil's weed would lead one to go insane.

The following section provides the learner with an exemplar of a critical appraisal process to comprehensively analyze the aforementioned viral article about first-time psychosis and high-potency cannabis. This section looks closely at the paper, provides insights to both understand the scientific findings and analyze their value. This analysis was originally shared on the Nurse Manifest website. This process is appropriate to share in this chapter, as it aligns with the NCSBN (2018) call that nurses must know the body of evidence. To truly know the evidence, we also need to be clear on how to evaluate the evidence. This section is geared more to the learner who is new to evaluating the evidence, though more experienced learners may also find it interesting. As this is about the lived experience of evaluating research, I have included some of my reflective and critical-thinking processes.

The article evaluated is listed as follows, and it may be accessed for free online: https://www.thelancet.com/journals/lanpsy/article/PIIS2215-0366(19)30048-3/fulltext
(Be sure to download the appendix as well, for following along!).
Full APA citation of the article being reviewed:

> DiForti, M., Quattrone, D., Freeman, T. P., Tripoli, G., Gayer-Anderson, C., Quigley, H., Rodriguez, V., Jongsma, H. E., Ferraro, L., Cascia, C. L., Barbera, D. L., Tarricone, I., Beradi, D., Szöke, A., Arango, C., Tortelli, A., Velthorst, E., Bernardo, M., Del-Ben, C. M., … Murray, R. M. (2019). The contribution of cannabis use to variation in the incidence of psychotic disorder across Europe (EU-GEI): a multicenter case-control study. Lancet Psychiatry, 6(5): 427–436. https://doi.org/10.1016/S2215-0366(19)30048-3

Although I was concerned about the viral nature of this article in the spring of 2019, and social media postings about the dangers of psychosis and cannabis use proliferated, I am pro-patient and pro-safe use of cannabis, so I strived to undertake an honest analysis. The applied critical appraisal method is the same that I would use in my work with my RN-BSN students; going through each area of the research and using an approach to express my concerns that all healthcare professionals can understand.

All levels of nursing education should have some foundational experiences with analyzing evidence; for some readers, this process will be a review, and for others, it might be a more foundational experience. In general, one wants to review each aspect of the research presented, including authors (affiliations and funding), the journal (reputation: scholarly vs. predatory), problem statement/research question/ or hypothesis (well-written, logical), literature review (depth and quality along with relevancy and being current), research methodology (appropriate choice; will it help answer the research question; the "n" aligning with the method), findings (sound, proper statistical or qualitative analyses used), limitations, and conclusions/ discussions.

Title: The contribution of cannabis use to variation in the incidence of psychotic disorder across Europe (EU-GEI): A multi-center case-control study. This was a long title, but fairly clearly depicts what the study is about. The article is open access, which makes it accessible to many.

Journal: *Lancet Psychiatry*. This is a reputable journal. *The Lancet* is a peer-reviewed medical journal and is among the oldest (began publishing in 1823), most prestigious, and best-known general medical journals. The journal is owned by Elsevier. It has the second-highest impact score after *The New England Journal of Medicine*. The *Lancet Psychiatry* is a specialty journal published by *The Lancet*.

Authors: The authors/researchers have lots of credentials here, with a mix of MDs and PhDs. There are over 30 authors, which I found interesting. Sometimes, this is a good thing; sometimes, it does not mean much.In the field of nursing, 30 authors would be quite extensive; in the world of physics, hundreds to even thousands of authors can get credit; one might wonder, are they all truly authors? Occasionally, if somebody reviews a draft, edits, and/or makes suggestions, they may be listed as an author. With a multisite study like this, having over 30 authors/researchers is reasonable. The link that discusses this issue of having many listed authors is https:// physicstoday.scitation.org/doi/10.1063/PT.3.1499.

Funding: This was funded by a number of different groups, including the Medical Research Council, the European Community's Seventh Framework Grant, Sao Paulo Research Foundation, the National Institute for Health Research Biomedical Research Center, Maudsley NHS Foundation Trust (South London and University College London), Kings College London, and Wellcome Trust. At least five of the authors report funding from pharmaceutical companies, though stating that they were funded for other studies, not this study. You may review the full list at the end of the article.

Getting funded is part of the researchers' job. It is just one of those little tidbits to keep in mind that certain loyalties and biases may be playing a part in the research. "Big pharma" can be viewed as having vested interests in people using cannabinoids (which they may eventually produce cannabinoid medicines on a mass market level), or people sticking with their traditional allopathic medicines, or creating pharmaceuticals that treat psychosis. It is possible that the researcher's funding sources from other projects may have influenced their work here.

Problem: At the beginning of the article, the authors state that with legalization movements, we may have "an increase in cannabis use and associated harm, even if the later only affects a minority of patients" (p. 1) and they go on to state that several studies "support a causal link between cannabis use and psychotic disorder" (p. 1).

Ideally, I would have time to thoroughly analyze each of the five cited studies in the first paragraph. As this is time-intensive, I went to the fifth article cited because the researchers' claim that the research may "support a causal link."

And it turns out that "support" is very important. When I reviewed the aforementioned fifth article cited (Gage et al., 2016), I found that it was entitled "Association Between Cannabis and Psychosis: Epidemiological Evidence." The researcher's conclusions lead me to believe that they did *not* determine causation. Gage et al. looked at the evidence from several longitudinal studies. In their findings, they distinctly refrained from making a "causal" statement: "Overall, evidence from epidemiological studies provides strong enough evidence to warrant a public health message that cannabis use can increase the risk of psychotic disorders. However, further studies are required to determine the magnitude of this effect, to determine the effect of different strains of cannabis on risk, and to identify high-risk groups particularly susceptible to the effects of cannabis on psychosis."

DiForti et al. (2019) in the introduction go on to state that there is a rising incidence of schizophrenia in the world: "Differences in the distribution of risk factors for psychosis, such as cannabis use, among the populations studied might contribute to these variations" (p. 1).

This rise in schizophrenia may or may not be related to cannabis use. I reviewed the articles DiForti et al. cited to support this idea, and the rise in incidence appears to have more to do with income, urbanicity, migrant status, age, race/ethnicity, and whether or not the person owned their home versus cannabis use. We should be careful as readers and consumers of evidence to pay very close attention to the subtle ways that data can be cited and perhaps even manipulated to support ideas. I determined that what DiForti et al. stated is that they think cannabis should be examined in light of rising schizophrenia diagnoses, not that the studies they cited indicated that cannabis was a cause for this. In addition, some of the literature I read as part of this process (of going down the rabbit hole of evidence) stated that schizophrenia is not rising, rather it is *falling* as we do a better job of differentiating and diagnosing schizophrenia. This is one dilemma nurses face in reviewing and analyzing cannabis-related and other research articles; people can pick and choose from a variety of available evidence that best suits their needs, and they may end up with a bias. Evidence can also be misconstrued.

In a box on page 2 of DiForti et al.'s article, the authors summarized some of the previous work done in this area. I found their review of the literature a bit compelling; they only found three articles that matched their criteria for psychotic disorders in combination with specific terms such as "high-potency cannabis," "skunk-super skunk," or "high THC cannabis." Two of the articles were from the researchers' work. The third article was much older, going back to 1965 to 1999 London, where increasing rates of schizophrenia "might be related" to cannabis use in the previous year.

I think the literature review reads thin, but that could be related to the lack of research in this area, which may be the case with many cannabis science articles.

Doing some more exploration on the issue of rising schizophrenia rates, I stumbled upon several significant issues with the diagnostic criteria for schizophrenia, how it was historically diagnosed, and the argument that there may be some issues around valid *Diagnostic and Statistical Manual of Mental Disorders* (*DSM*) criteria for the various types of schizophrenia (https://www.ncbi.nlm.nih.gov/pmc/articles/PMC5103459/). The *DSM* has a history of sparking controversies.

"Psychotic disorders" are pretty much undifferentiated in the *DSM*, and this is why the researchers used this term versus choosing a more definitive diagnosis such as perhaps bipolar or schizophrenia, which may be a more difficult diagnosis to make and may take time to differentiate. According to the NIH/National Institutes of Mental Health (NIMH), "psychosis" describes conditions where the person has a "mind" condition. They have lost contact with reality. Psychosis can be a sign of a mental illness or physical illness, it can be caused by medications/alcohol/drug abuse, 3% of the population experiences it, and symptoms include hallucinations, delusions, paranoia, and disordered thoughts/speech. One can review the link at https://www.nimh.nih.gov/health/publications/raise-fact-sheet-first-episode-psychosis/index.shtml

One fact stood out for me from the NIMH publication: studies show that it is common for people to have psychosis symptoms for more than a year prior to diagnosis. This is extremely important to note because DiForti et al. (2019) looked at cases of first-time psychosis. Still there appears to be no follow-up regarding if these were "temporary" diagnoses or if the persons were eventually diagnosed with schizophrenia or bipolar diseases. They did use *International Classification of Diseases*, 10th revision (*ICD-10*) criteria to define the psychosis population eligible for the study: https://www.icd10data.com/ICD10CM/Codes/F01-F99/F20-F29/F20

One might wonder if ongoing use of cannabis for a (potential) year after symptoms emerged helped or worsened the condition.

It is known that the adverse effects of cannabis can be hallucinations and paranoia: I clarified that in this study if the patient's symptoms were from acute cannabis intoxication, the person was not included in the study.

Participants: Participants were those aged 18 to 64 years and were diagnosed using the *ICD-10* criteria for psychosis (which envelops a lot, see previous link). Control groups were randomly selected from the same geographical area using postal address, age, race, gender, ethnicity, and lack of psychotic symptoms as the control criteria. The researchers had participants in the 17 areas of England, France, the Netherlands, Italy, Spain, and Brazil. The researchers were striving to assess 1,000 first-time psychosis and 1,000 controls. The "n" for each group was good: control = 1,237, first-time psychosis cases = 901.

Cannabis use was not confirmed by a urinalysis or blood test; therefore, the study relied on self-reported use of cannabis. This concerns me, as we do not know if the cannabis was contaminated with other substances, including other illicit drugs, pesticides, mold, fungus, or heavy metals, all of which could also play a part in first-time psychosis diagnosis.

Methods: DiForti et al. (2019) asked the participants about six measures of cannabis use: lifetime use (whether or not they ever used cannabis), current use, age at first use, lifetime frequency (pattern or most consistent use), and money spent weekly (or during most consistent use period). The researchers then used data from the European Monitoring Centre for Drugs and Drug Addiction (EMCDDA) 2016 report to determine cannabis potency by THC (http://www.emcdda.europa.eu/publications/edr/trends-developments/2016_en). The data available at the time were from 2018. I am assuming the researchers likely used 2016 data, as their article was published in the first few months of 2018 (http://www.emcdda.europa.eu/data/stats2018/ppp_en).

DiForti et al. did not ask the patients what specific cannabis cultivars/chemovars they were using, nor did they test the cannabis the patients used; instead, they conjectured from the data. Data from patients beyond frequency of use that demonstrated that they were actually, truly consuming high-potency cannabis would have been helpful or testing the most recently consumed cannabis might have yielded some interesting data.

Another discovery in the EMCDDA report demonstrated a downtrend in cannabis use in Europe, particularly in the three countries that previously were high prevalence cannabis use countries such as Germany, Spain, and the United Kingdom. Although cannabis may be getting stronger in THC content, its use has dropped off significantly since the year 2000 in these three countries (which perhaps goes against the researchers' thoughts that cannabis use is on the rise and poses a higher risk for psychosis) (EMCDDA, 2016).

Refocusing on the method for this research, I was directed to the appendix to investigate further how the researchers determined "high potency," which can be downloaded from *The Lancet* site. The appendix has a lot of great details and crucial data.

The researchers defined low-potency cannabis as less than 10% THC and high-potency cannabis as more than 10% THC. Participants were asked to report the type of cannabis used in their own language, and potency was estimated based on the data from EMCDDA. The participants seemed to give what I can only categorize as broad terms for the cannabis they were using, including U.K. home-grown skunk/sensimilla; U.K. super-skunk; Italian home-grown skunk/sensimilla; Italian super-skunk; the Dutch Nederwiet, Nederhasj, and geïmporteerde hasj; the Spanish and French Hashish (from Morocco); Spanish home-grown sensimilla; French home-grown skunk/sensimilla/super-skunk; and Brazilian skunk. *Sensimilla* refers to a high-potency cannabis plant that does not produce seeds and it does not refer to a particular cultivar/chemovar.

To clarify, in the United Kingdom, "skunk" is a term used for all high THC% cannabis plants; however, I could not find a clear definition for "skunk" in terms of chemovars or precisely what the cutoff is for a plant to be called skunk.

This process of asking data-based questions of patients experiencing first-time psychosis brought up red flags for me: first, asking patients who are in first-time psychosis what "type" of cannabis the participants' were using seems potentially unreliable. The problem with patients and participants self-reporting data is well known. The researchers had questions about the use of other intoxicants (this will be revisited in the Results section).

Second, the actual cannabis consumed was never tested for accurate potency (back to the idea of the researchers claiming these patients used high-potency cannabis, but the only evidence of them doing so was that they might have consumed cannabis in a geographical area where high-potency cannabis is available), nor was there any indication that the patients were tested for THC (granted they could have tested negative and last use could have been some months before the episode).

It is my opinion that until researchers start testing the cannabis that patients in these types of studies are using, they will not be doing good science. Granted, we know that THC is responsible for many of the side and adverse effects of cannabis, but to state that the issue with cannabis is that it has become high in THC% is far too reductionistic. There is no specific proof that this one cannabinoid alone is the issue regarding the relationship between cannabis and new the onset of psychosis. The researchers stated that they opted not to test patients' cannabis because it provides only a snapshot of a moment of cannabis use in the person's history. However, relying on reports of what cannabis is available in the area also leaves too much of a gap in determining what patients are consuming. Cannabis is a complex plant with over 500 chemicals. Still a few simple tests could provide a wealth of information for determining whether high-potency THC cannabis truly does play a role in the onset of psychosis, or if something else is going on here.

If the researchers were to test the cannabis consumer, the tests could minimally include the cannabinoid and terpene profiles, in addition to testing for heavy metals, molds, fungus, and pesticides. Although this would have some associated costs, it could have let the researchers know if the chemovar profile of the previous cannabis used could be very enlightening.

Another consideration with testing cannabis is that there is a long history of concern when it comes to the role of heavy metal ingestion and the onset of psychiatric symptoms (Attademo et al., 2017; Orisakwe, 2014). Cannabis plants can easily become contaminated with heavy metals when grown in soils containing heavy metals. Pesticides can also contaminate cannabis, and the consideration of pesticides as both endocrine disruptors and possible contributing factors to schizophrenia/psychosis has also been researched over the years (Maqbool et al., 2016).

As a side note: What if what we need to regulate or worry about is not the cannabis plant and THC potency, so much as contaminants that are in the plant? In my thought process, this becomes an ethical question of what we are researching and what might bring harm to patients and vulnerable populations. One of the issues related to the end of cannabis prohibition and the beginning of the regulation era of cannabis should be that people have access to herbal medicine that is tested and safe, so people know what they are consuming. Beneficence and autonomy come to mind as ethical concerns related to this issue. Testing would encourage safe products to be produced, help people with their healing quests, and help them to be a more informed consumer.

Participants: There was a good split between male/female participants, with the median age of 36 years for control and 31 years for case. The median age coupled with the wide range of ages (18 to 64) included in the study was just a bit concerning, because we know that first-time psychosis tends to happen in the early to mid-20s. The vast majority of all participants were white, with at least some college or vocational training and full-time employment. It was also clear between case and control participants that there was much more use of cigarettes, cannabis, and other "drugs" (stimulants, hallucinogens, ketamine, etc.) by the case group. Alcohol was not included in the summary data table, but in the body of text, the researchers stated there was no difference in alcohol consumption among the case versus control groups.

And this points to another issue: that it is really hard to control these types of studies because most people who are using "drugs" tend to use many different types of substances. It is hard to determine which drug or drug contaminant is having the impact, particularly as there can be short- and long-term implications. Could the issue of poly-substance abuse perhaps be the larger issue to study versus just looking at the THC% in cannabis?

The International Early Psychosis Association published research by Nielsen et al. (2016) that found that alcohol, cannabis, and other drugs increase the risk of developing schizophrenia later in life. This was a large retrospective study with the Danish population. The full paper can be accessed at https://pdfs.semanticscholar.org/1d58/2eaad2f2f9b61f5952f2ecf696bb81a55c7e.pdf

It has the diagnosis of substance abuse that correlates with the risk of being diagnosed with schizophrenia sixfold. Indeed, both cannabis and alcohol greatly increase the risk for an eventual schizophrenia diagnosis. Still Nielsen et al. are careful to state that they cannot say alcohol and substance abuse caused the schizophrenia in this large-scale retrospective study.

DiForti et al. (2019) also found in their population that most people who have a substance abuse disorder do not use one substance alone. The case participants in most of the drug-use categories rated themselves as using nearly twice as many substances as the control group. This is concerning because it could be that poly-substance use is the contributing factor with this issue versus high-potency cannabis-use alone. DiForti et al. did not address this possibility.

Self-medicating is also not addressed in this article, but were the participants asked about why they used cannabis? Since most people with psychosis have at least one year of symptoms before being diagnosed with the new-onset psychosis, they may be self-medicating with many different substances during that year of onset of symptomology.

Areseneault et al. (2004) in their meta-analysis of five other research articles found that while youthful cannabis use may create a twofold increased risk factor for psychosis and may be responsible for up to 8% of the world's schizophrenia diagnoses, it also is just one part of the contributing "complex constellation of factors." Vulnerable youth should avoid the use of cannabis.

Overall Findings: The statistical analysis seems logical and well run.

Simply stated, the findings relate the concepts of starting use of cannabis before age 15, using high-potency cannabis (>10% THC), and the daily use of cannabis as having the greatest relationship to psychosis. One should keep in mind that causation is not proven here: almost all of the case participants had also indulged in other substance use at much higher rates than the control group, the issue of possible contamination of ingested cannabis, and the lack of knowledge about the full cannabinoid and terpene profile of the cannabis used.

Conclusions: This study did little to change my mind about cannabis and its safety profile, nor change my overall thoughts on the safe use of cannabis, including the idea that cannabis should likely not be used recreationally by young people in their teens and early 20s: people need education about the safe and effective use of cannabis, the risks involved, and they should have access to safe, tested cannabis plant medicines.

For most people using cannabis medicinally, a high-potency THC cannabis is likely not needed; however, having safe tested cannabis helps people make informed decisions about the quality of cannabis they are ingesting and the amount of THC they are consuming. High-potency THC cannabis, or escalating doses of THC, may indeed be risky for some people, including young people, those with a predisposition to addiction or history of familial psychotic episodes or diagnosis of mental health issues, those with childhood trauma, people with familial history of substance abuse, and people who currently are poly-substance users.

The following are my final thoughts and recommendations upon reviewing this article:

- Avoid using cannabis (and all "drugs" and alcohol) until one is in the mid-20s and the brain is well developed. This does not account for the idea that teens will use substances, but they should still avoid poly-substance use, and cannabis is generally safer than alcohol. Alcohol is far more readily available for teens to access, and it too is a significant risk factor for psychosis (and immediate death if one becomes too intoxicated, whereas one cannot die from cannabis ingestion).
- Use tested cannabis that is free from heavy metals, pesticides, fungus, and mold.
- Know the potency of the cannabis medicine. Avoid long-term use of "high-potency THC cannabis," or better yet know your THC consumption in mg and limit it to 15 mg max/day (divided into TID doses), balanced with CBD (up to 20 mg/day) and terpenes from whole-plant medicine (MacCallum & Russo, 2018).
- Take regular cannabis breaks. For the recreational consumer, avoid daily use and avoid regular use of high-potency THC strains. For the medicinal consumer, consider working with your healthcare provider to determine what a break schedule might look for you, and use lower THC strains if they are still effective at managing symptoms.
- For young people who may benefit from the use of medicinal cannabis, support the use of lower THC strains if effective.
- Medicinal users of cannabis: start low, go slow with the THC dosing. One does not need to be "high" to feel relief of symptoms, and with cannabis being a biphasic medication, sometimes less is more. For specific dosing guidance, see MacCallum and Russo (2018).
- For nurse researchers: as cannabis prohibition ends and we move toward an era of cannabis regulation, let us find ways to create the best body of evidence available when it comes to the benefits and risks associated with this herbal medication. Let us base our public policy and educational efforts on sound science. Let us not jump from correlation to causation, which means we will have to approach the study of this plant through a lens of complexity.

> ### ▶ APPLIED LEARNING
>
> ■ Evaluating the evidence can be time-consuming and is not always a linear process. Although it takes time to do a thorough evaluation, the efforts are often enlightening.
> ■ Our research evaluation processes help us advocate for better research processes that look at the complexity of cannabis use and health outcomes.
> ■ In a group, choose a recent medical cannabis article to evaluate, perhaps dividing the sections up. Do you agree that the researchers' conclusions were generated from a sound scientific process?

NOW WHAT? SHARING THE EVALUATION

It took me several hours over several days to fully evaluate this research article. My nursing colleagues encouraged me to reach out to *The Lancet Psychiatry* to share my rebuttal of the findings. Unfortunately, this journal only allows for 400-word rebuttals, so I took on the challenge of trying to find the most influential points I made here and whittling my response down to the word limit.

The following rebuttal was published in *The Lancet Psychiatry* in June 2019:

Clark, C. S. (2019). High-potency cannabis and incident psychosis: correcting the causal assumption. Lancet Psychiatry. 6(6), e14. doi: 10.1016/S2215-0366(19)30178-6

Carey S. Clark

Psychosis has many different causes, and I have concerns with the methods used in the article by Marta DiForti and colleagues, which aimed to correlate the use of cannabis of high THC percentage with the onset of psychotic disorders.

The researchers did not test the cannabis plants used by the case group for actual cannabinoids and for dangerous contaminants. What if the plants consumed were contaminated with heavy metals, or pesticides, which have also been related to the onset of psychosis?

Furthermore, most people with a substance use disorder use more than one substance. In their research, the first-time psychosis case group had significantly more lifetime users of other drugs, such as ketamine ($p = 0.0002$), hallucinogens ($p < 0.0001$), and stimulants ($p < 0.0001$), than the control group. Nielsen and colleagues found in their large population-based retrospective study that it was the diagnosis itself of having substance use disorder that increased the likelihood of a schizophrenia diagnosis later in life, with both alcohol consumption and cannabis use linked to the diagnosis. Focusing on just cannabis use is very reductionist and adds little to the body of evidence in determining the complex underlying mechanisms of psychosis causation.

Assuming that a complex constellation of factors relates to a diagnosis of psychosis is far more responsible. Researchers should remain diligent to not be reductionist in defining the manifold causations of psychosis.

(https://www.thelancet.com/journals/lanpsy/article/PIIS2215-0366(19)30178-6/fulltext)

CONCLUSION

The role of the cannabis care nurse is a challenging one. It requires the nurse to be committed to gaining knowledge, expertise, and skills in a variety of areas, including cannabinoid science, research, and therapeutics; the ability to create caring-healing spaces with patients, using MI; becoming adept at coaching; and supporting the use of holistic modalities and advocacy skills. The cannabis care nurse remains committed to supporting patients' healing processes and potentiating their ECS, all while considering the latest evidence-based findings. The cannabis care nurse is adept at communicating, educating, coaching, and advocating for positive cannabis regulation that supports patients' capacity to use the cannabis plant.

Most importantly, the cannabis care nurse is passionate about supporting healing and palliation through the upregulation of the ECS. Cannabis care nursing includes support for the patient with coaching and education about the safe and effective use of cannabis; it revolves around guiding the patient to make lifestyle changes that support the health of the ECS, coaching them to embrace holistic modalities that upregulate the ECS, and providing navigation as they achieve homeostasis to live their best life possible.

The nurse providing cannabis care becomes aware that supporting the patient through the creation of caring-healing spaces and walking with them on their spiritual-healing journey are the very rewarding aspects of cannabis care nursing. Cannabis patients are often discouraged by the failure of allopathic medicines to address all of their complex healing needs, they are looking for ways to heal, and they should be able to rely on nurses' caring skills and compassion. Cannabis care nursing is truly a holistic approach to supporting patients toward their full health potential.

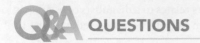 **QUESTIONS**

1. The cannabis care nurse is working with a patient who is interested in using cannabis for sleep. The patient lives in a medical cannabis use state and is 40 years old. The nurse's first step is to:
   A. Discuss the state's laws regarding the use of cannabis by pulling up the program online and reviewing with the patient.
   B. Consider all of the medications the patient currently takes and how they may impact sleep.
   C. Assess the patient's current sleep patterns and sleep hygiene patterns by gathering subjective and objective data.
   D. Encourage the patient to try allopathic medications first.

2. The cannabis care nurse gets a call from a patient who states that they may be took too much cannabis the other day because they felt "so much anxiety" and "too high." The cannabis care nurse's first step would be to:
   A. Encourage the patient to have some CBD on hand in case this happens again.
   B. Review the cannabis diary with the patient, to see consumption patterns and what took place on the day they had this experience.
   C. Tell the patient to call the cannabis care nurse if it happens again, and the cannabis care nurse will coach them through the experience.
   D. Coach the patient to go back to the best-tolerated dose experienced during the titration process.

3. In working with a patient who wants to access medical cannabis, the nurse determines that they have an ailment that may qualify them for medical cannabis recommendation in their state. The nurse tells the patient:
   A. "You are in luck, you will qualify for a medical cannabis recommendation based on your diagnosis."
   B. "I think medical cannabis would be a good option for you, as your diagnosis is listed as a qualifying condition in the state."
   C. "Let's see if we can find you somebody to write your medical recommendation for cannabis use."
   D. "It looks like you do have a condition that might qualify you for a medical cannabis recommendation in this state. We will need to explore this further."

4. The patient brings their medical cannabis candy to the floor with them when they check in prior to surgery. The patient states, "I wanted you to know that I brought these. We are in a state where cannabis is legal for adults, and I need them to manage my pain. I'll just keep them in my bedside table." The nurse should:
   A. Review the hospital's policy and procedure on cannabis use in the hospital and follow related protocols with the patient.
   B. Tell the patient that it is fine for her to possess them because this is a legal state for adult-use cannabis.

C. Tell the patient to send the candies back home with a relative, because it is not safe to keep them in the hospital and she does not have a medical recommendation.

D. Tell the patient that the nurse must call the patient's doctor and discuss with them the patient's use of cannabis.

5. The cannabis patient has been experiencing a lot of nausea and vomiting, and it actually seems to get worse after ingestion of cannabis. Warm showers help to relieve the symptoms. They symptoms have been present for several days. The cannabis care nurse takes the following steps to provide best care for the patient:

A. Cannabis generally helps with this issue, so encourage the patient to use as needed and get checked for a stomach virus.

B. Tell the patient to stop using cannabis for a few days and, when they start again, see if symptoms return.

C. Provide active listening and compassionate presence. Refer the patient to the emergency department or primary provider, and encourage them to be honest about their symptoms and cannabis use.

D. Assess the patient's food intake and possible exposure to food poisoning.

ANSWERS

1. **Answer: C.** Assess the patient's current sleep patterns and sleep hygiene patterns by gathering subjective and objective data.

   Rationale: The nurse should first gather subjective and objective data from the patient to further define the patient's concern with sleep.

2. **Answer: B.** Review the cannabis diary with the patient, to see consumption patterns and what took place on the day they had this experience.

   Rationale: The cannabis care nurse needs to have a better understanding of the patient's consumption patterns and titration process, as well as symptoms and dosing patterns, before taking the next steps.

3. **Answer: D.** "It looks like you do have a condition that might qualify you for a medical cannabis recommendation in this state. We will need to explore this further."

   Rationale: This is the best answer, as we must consider that having a qualifying condition alone is not enough to determine whether the particular individual patient will benefit from medicinal use of cannabis.

4. **Answer: A.** Review the hospital's policy and procedure on cannabis use in the hospital and follow related protocols with the patient.

   Rationale: The nurse needs to implement the hospital policy and procedure when it comes to inpatient use of cannabis.

5. **Answer: C.** Provide active listening and compassionate presence. Refer the patient to the emergency department or primary provider, and encourage them to be honest about their symptoms and cannabis use.

   Rationale: The patient may have cannabis hyperemesis syndrome, and they should be supported to receive proper medical care.

References

Aggarwal, S. K. (2016). Use of cannabinoids in cancer care: Palliative care. *Current Oncology, 23*(2), S33–S36. https://doi.org/10.3747/co.23.2962

American Cannabis Nurses Association. (2019). Scope and standards of practice for cannabis nurses, 2019 version. https://cannabisnurses.org/Scope-of-Practice-for-Cannabis-Nurses

American College of Physicians. (2019, January). Medical marijuana … in the hospital? https://acphospitalist.org/archives/2017/01/marijuana-policies-hospital.htm

American Holistic Nurses Association. (2019). Nurses and complementary healing modalities. https://www.ahna.org/Home/Resources/Healing-Modalities

American Nurses Association. (2015). *Scope and standards of practice* (3rd ed.). Author.

American Osteopathic Association. (2019). What is a DO? https://osteopathic.org/what-is-osteopathic-medicine/what-is-a-do/

Arseneault, L., Cannon, M., Witton, J., & Murray, R. M. (2004). Causal association between cannabis and psychosis: Examination of the evidence. *The British Journal of Psychiatry, 184*(2), 110–117. https://doi.org/10.1192/bjp.184.2.110

Attademo, L., Bernardini, F., Garinella, R., & Compton, M. T. (2017). Environmental pollution and risk of psychotic disorders. *Schizophrenia Research, 18*, 55–59. https://doi.org/10.1016/j.schres.2016.10.003

Brellenthin, A. G., Crombie, K. M., Hillard, C. J., & Koltyn, K. F. (2017). Endocannabinoid and mood responses to exercise in adults with varying activity levels. *Medicine & Science in Sports & Exercise, 49*(8), 1688–1696. https://doi.org/10.1249/MSS.0000000000001276

Chen, L., Zhang, J. M., Li, F., Qiu, Y., Wang, L., Li, Y. H., Shi, J. M., Pan, H. L., & Li, M. (2009). Endogenous anandamide and cannabinoid receptor-2 contribute to electroacupuncture analgesia in rats. *Journal of Pain, 10*, 732–739. https://doi.org/10.1016/j.jpain.2008.12.012

Clark, C. S. (2014). Stress, psychoneuroimmunology, and self-care: What every nurse needs to know. *Journal of Nursing and Care, 3*, 146. https://doi.org/10.4172/2167-1168.1000146

Clark, C. S. (2016). Watson's human caring theory: Pertinent transpersonal and humanities concepts for educators. *Humanities in Health Professions Education and Practice, 5*(21), 1–12. https://doi.org/10.3390/h5020021

Cornelis, M. C., Erlund, I., Michelotti, G. A., Herder, C., Westerhuis, J. A., & Tuomilehto, J. (2018). Metabolomic response to coffee consumption: Application to a three-stage clinical trial. *Journal of Internal Medicine, 283*(6), 544–557. https://doi.org/10.1111/joim.12737

Dirfotri, M., Quatronne, D., Freeman, T. P., Tripoli, G., Gayer-Anderson, C., Quigley, H., Rodriguez, V., Jongsma, H. E., Ferraro, L., Cascia, C. L., Barbera, D. L., Tarricone, I., Beradi, D., Szoke, A., Arango, C., Tortelli, A., Velthorst, E., Bernardo, M., Del-Ben, C. M., … Murray, R. M. (2019). The contribution of cannabis use to variation in the incidence of psychotic disorder across Europe (EU-GEI): A multicenter case-control study. *The Lancet Psychiatry, 6*(5), P427–P436. https://doi.org/10.1016/S2215-0366(19)30048-3

Dossey, B. M., & Hess, D. (2013). Professional nurse coaching: Advances in national and global healthcare transformation. *Global Advances in Health and Medicine, 2*(4), 10–16. https://doi.org/10.7453/gahmj.2013.044

Droppa, M. (2014). Motivational interviewing: A journey to improve health. *Nursing2014, 44*(3), 40–45. https://doi.org/10.1097/01.NURSE.0000443312.58360.82

European Monitoring Centre for Drugs and Drug Addiction. (2016). European drug report 2016: Trends and development. http://www.emcdda.europa.eu/publications/edr/trends-developments/2016_en

Evidence Based Acupuncture. (2019). Acupuncture overview. https://www.evidencebasedacupuncture.org/present-research/acupuncture-scientific-evidence/

DiForti, M., Quattrone, D., Freeman, T. P., Tripoli, G., Gayer-Anderson, C., Quigley, H., Rodriguez, V., Jongsma, H. E., Ferraro, L., Cascia, C. L., Barbera, D. L., Tarricone, I., Berardi, D., Szoke, A., Arango, C., Trotelli, A., Velthorst, E., Bernardo, M., Del-Ben, C. M., … Murray, R. M. (2019). The contribution of cannabis use to variation in the incidence of psychotic disorder across Europe (EU-GEI): A multicentre case-control study. *The Lancet Psychiatry*. Open Access. https://doi.org/10.1016/S2215-0366(19)30048-3

Gage, S. H., Hickman, M., & Zammit, S. (2016). Association between cannabis and psychosis: Epidemiologic evidence. *Biological Psychiatry, 79*(7), 549–556. https://doi.org/10.1016/j.biopsych.2015.08.001

Gertsch, J., Leonti, M., Raduner, S., Racz, I., Chen, J. Z., Xie, X. Q., Altmann, K. H., Karsak, M., & Zimmer, A. (2008). Beta-caryophyllene is a dietary cannabinoid. *Proceedings of the National Academy of Sciences of the United States of America, 105*(26), 9099–9104. https://doi.org/10.1073/pnas.0803601105

Gertsch, J., Pertwee, R. G., & DiMarzo, V. (2010). Phytocannabinoids beyond the cannabis plant: Do they exist? *British Journal of Pharmacology, 160*(3), 523–529. https://doi.org/10.1111/j.1476-5381.2010.00745.x

Gioacchini, G., Rossi, G., & Carnevali, O. (2017). Host—probiotic interaction: New insight into the role of the endocannabinoid system by in vivo and ex vivo approaches. *Scientific Reports, 7*(1261), 1–12. https://doi.org/10.1038/s41598-017-01322-1

Gray, S. (2016). *Cannabis and spirituality: An explorer's guide to an ancient plant spirit.* Park Street Press.

Harrison, K. (2016). Who is she? The personification of cannabis in cultural and individual experience. In S. Gray (Ed.), *Cannabis and spirituality: An explorer's guide to an ancient plant spirit.* Park Street Press.

Herdman, T. H., & Kamitsuru, S. (Eds.) (2014). *NANDA International, INC. Nursing diagnoses: Definitions and classification 2015-2017* (10th ed.). Wiley Blackwell.

Hu, B., Bai, F., Xiong, L., & Wang, Q. (2017). The endocannabinoid system, a novel and key participant in acupuncture's multiple, beneficial effects. *Neuroscience and Biobehavior Reviews, 77,* 340–357. https://doi.org/10.1016/j.neubiorev.2017.04.006

Jung, J., Kim, E. J., Kwon, G. T., Jung, Y. J., Park, T., Kim, Y., Yu, R., Choi, M. S., Chun, H. S., Kwon, S. H., Her, S., Lee, K. W., Han, J., & Park, J. H. (2015). β-Caryophyllene potently inhibits solid tumor growth and lymph node metastasis of B16F10 melanoma cells in high-fat diet–induced obese C57BL/6N mice. *Carcinogenesis, 36*(9), 1028–1039. https://doi.org/10.1093/carcin/bgv076

Kaplan, L. (2012). Reading and critiquing a research article. https://www.americannursetoday.com/reading-and-critiquing-a-research-article/

Lafourcade, M., Larrieu, T., Mato, S., Duffaud, A., Sepers, M., Matias, I., De Smedt-Peyrusse, V., Labrousse, V. F., Bretillon, L., Matute, C., Rodríguez-Puertas, R., Layé, S., & Manzoni, O. J. (2011). Nutritional omega-3 deficiency abolishes endocannabinoid-mediated neuronal functions. *Nature Neuroscience, 14*(3), 345–350. https://doi.org/10.1038/nn.2736

MacCallum, C. A., & Russo, E. B. (2018). Practical considerations in medical cannabis administration and dosing. *European Journal of Internal Medicine, 49,* 12–19. https://doi.org/10.1016/j.ejim.2018.01.004

Maccarronne, M., Gapseri, V., Catani, M. V., Diep, T. A., Dianese, E., Hansen, H. S., & Avigliano, L. (2010). The endocannabinoid system and its relevance for nutrition. *Annual Review of Nutrition, 30,* 423–440. https://doi.org/10.1146/annurev.nutr.012809.104701

Maqbool, F., Mostafalou, S., Bahadar, H., & Abdollahi, M. (2016). Review of endocrine disorders associated with environmental toxicants and possible involved mechanisms. *Life Sciences, 145,* 265–273. https://doi.org/10.1016/j.lfs.2015.10.022

McDoanld, J., & Janz, S. (2017). *The acupuncture evidence project: A comparative literature review.* Australian Acupuncture and Chinese Medicine Association, LTD. http://www.asacu.org/wp-content/uploads/2017/09/Acupuncture-Evidence-Project-The.pdf

McPartland, J. M., Giuffrida, A., King, J., Skinner, E., Scotter, A., & Musty, R. E. (2005). Cannabimimetic effects of osteopathic manipulative treatment. *Journal of the American Osteopathic Association, 105,* 283–291. https://jaoa.org/article.aspx?articleid=2093088

McPartland, J. M., Guy, G. W., & Di Marzo, V. (2014). Care and feeding of the endocannabinoid system: A systematic review of potential clinical interventions that upregulate the endocannabinoid system. *PloS One, 9*(3), e89566. https://doi.org/10.1371/journal.pone.0089566

Miller, W. R., & Rollnick, S. (1991). *Motivational interviewing: Preparing people to change addictive behavior.* Guilford Press.

Morena, M., Patel, S., Bains, J. S., & Hill, M. N. (2015). Neurobiological interactions between stress and the endocannabinoid system. *Neuropsychopharmacology, 41*(1), 80–102. https://doi.org/10.1038/npp.2015.166

Murillo-Rodriguez, E., Pastrana-Trejo, J. C., Salas-Crisostomo, M., & de la Cruz, M. (2017). The endocannabinoid system modulating levels of consciousness, emotions, and likely dream contents. *CNS and Neurological Disorders, Drug Targets, 16*(4), 370–379. https://doi.org/10.2174/1871527316666170223161908

National Academies of Science, Engineering, and Medicine. (2017). *The health effects of cannabis and cannabinoids: The current state of evidence and recommendations for research.* National Academies Press.

National Council of States Boards of Nursing. (2018). THE NCSBN national nursing guidelines for medical marijuana. *Journal of Nursing Regulation, 9*(2), S5–S46. https://doi.org/10.1016/S2155-8256(18)30098-X

Natural Medicine Plants. (2015). Top plants containing beta-caryophyllene. https://www.naturalmedicinefacts.info/chemical/7164.html

Nielsen, S. M., Toftdahl, N. G., Nordentoft, M., & Hjorthoj, C. (2016). Association between alcohol, cannabis, and other illicit substance abuse and the risk of developing schizophrenia: A nationwide population-based register study. https://pdfs.semanticscholar.org/1d58/2eaad2f2f9b61f5952f2ecf696b-b81a55c7e.pdf

Orisakwe, O. E. (2014). The role of lead and cadmium in psychiatry. *North American Journal of Medical Sciences, 6*(8), 370. https://doi.org/10.4103/1947-2714.139283

Rossi, S., DeChiara, V., Musella, A., Kusayanagi, H., Mataluni, G., Bernardi, G., Usiello, A., & Centonze, D. (2008). Chronic psychoemotional stress impairs cannabinoid-receptor-mediated control of GABA transmission in striatum. *Journal of Neuroscience, 28*, 7284–7292. https://doi.org/10.1523/JNEUROSCI.5346-07.2008

Silbert, L., Stephens, G., & Hasson, U. (2010). Do we click? Speaker-listener neural coupling underlies successful communication. H+ Summit at Harvard. http://www.slideshare.net/humanityplus/silbert

Stone, N. L., Millar, S. A., Herrod, P. J. J., Barret, D. A., Ortori, C. A., Mellon, V. A., & Sullivan, S. E. (2018). An analysis of endocannabinoid concentrations and mood following singing and exercise in healthy volunteers. *Frontiers in Behavioral Neuroscience, 12*. https://doi.org/10.3389/fnbeh.2018.00269

Su, T. F., Zhao, Y. Q., Zhang, L. H., Peng, M., Wu, C. H., Pei, L., Tian, B., Zhang, J., Shi, J., Pan, H. L., & Li, M. (2012). Electroacupuncture reduces the expression of cytokines in inflamed skin tissues through activation of cannabinoid CB2 receptors. *European Journal of Pain, 16*(5), 624–635. https://doi.org/10.1002/j.1532-2149.2011.00055.x

Substance Abuse and Mental Health Services Administration. (2018). Empowering change: Motivational interviewing. https://www.samhsa.gov/homelessness-programs-resources/hpr-resources/empowering-change

Telles, S., Sayal, N., Nacht, C., Chopra, A., Patel, K., Dalvi, P., Bhatia, K., Miranpuri, G., & Anand, A. (2017). Yoga: Can it be integrated with treatment of neuropathic pain. *Integrative Medicine, 4*, 1–2, 69–84. https://doi.org/10.1159/000463385

Wang, Q., Peng, Y., Chen, S., Gou, X., Hu, B., Du, J., Lu, Y., & Xiong, L. (2009). Pretreatment with electroacupuncture induces rapid tolerance to focal cerebral ischemia through regulation of endocannabinoid system. *Stroke, 40*, 2157–2164. https://doi.org/10.1161/STROKEAHA.108.541490

Watson, M. J. (2012). *Human caring science: A theory of nursing* (2nd ed.). Jones & Bartlett.

Watson Caring Science Institute. (2019). Ten Caritas processes®. https://www.watsoncaringscience.org/jean-bio/caring-science-theory/10-caritas-processes/

Advanced Practice Nursing Considerations

Eloise Theisen, MSN, RN, AGPCNP-BC

CONCEPTS AND CONSIDERATIONS

The role of the advanced practice registered nurse (APRN) is evolving. In some states, nurse practitioners (NPs) have gained full practice authority (FPA), allowing them to work independently of physicians. FPA enables NPs to evaluate, diagnose, order, and interpret diagnostic tests; and initiate and manage treatment such as prescribing medications and controlled substances as defined by the state board of nursing (American Association of Nurse Practitioners [AANP], 2018). As more states are adopting FPA for APRNs, APRNs are serving the needs of patients in areas where there are physician shortages. Although there are, as of this writing, 33 states plus the District of Columbia and Guam that allow for FPA, the remaining states allow for reduced or restricted practice. Both reduced and restricted practice limit NPs' scope while requiring career-long regulated collaborative or supervision agreements (AANP, 2018). There is one exception. On December 14, 2016, the Veterans Affairs (VA) ruled in favor of allowing NPs FPA within the VA system regardless of the state's scope of practice (AANP, n.d.).

Legislation in many states continues to push for FPA so that NPs can practice to the full scope of their training and education. Even with the 33 states and the District of Columbia allowing for FPA, APRNs are even more limited when it comes to working with medical cannabis. Currently, only eight states—Hawaii, Maine, Massachusetts, Minnesota, New Hampshire, New York, Vermont, and Washington—allow APRNs to certify patients with a qualifying condition for medical cannabis (NCSBN, 2018). Despite multiple systematic reviews of the research demonstrating that APRNs can provide care comparable to that of physicians without the physicians' oversight, they continue to be held back from practicing to the full extent of their education (Spetz, 2019). APRNs are more likely to spend quality time with patients at much lower costs and often in specialty areas where physicians are not interested in practicing. It comes as no surprise that APRNs would be a natural fit in helping patients who are interested in using medical cannabis as a treatment modality.

Learning Outcomes

Upon completion of this chapter, the learners will:

* Have an understanding of the role of the APRN concerning caring for patients using medical cannabis.
* Demonstrate knowledge of the National Council of State Boards of Nursing (NCSBN) six essential areas of medical cannabis knowledge as applied to the role of the APRN.

THE ROLE OF THE ADVANCED PRACTICE REGISTERED NURSE WITH MEDICAL CANNABIS

As the need to respond to patients' use of cannabis grows, the American Cannabis Nurses Association developed the scope and standards of practice for cannabis nurses and the National Council of State Boards of Nursing issued medical cannabis guidelines for nurses and APRNs. Both organizations recognized that patients are using cannabis and that nurses will need to be educated to care for them. Although the American Nurses Association (ANA) and the individual state boards of nursing have not officially recognized the ACNA and NCSBN guidelines, they provide nurses with a practice framework.

In 2018, the NCSBN released guidelines for prelicensure nurses, registered nurses, and APRNs on caring for patients using cannabis (NCSBN, 2018). The guidelines have created a baseline for competency when providing cannabis care, via defining the essential areas of knowledge. The NCSBN (2018) recommended that all prelicensure, registered nurses, and APRNs gain essential knowledge in six principle areas:

1. The nurse shall have a working knowledge of the current state of legalization of medical and adult-use cannabis.
2. The nurse shall have a working knowledge of the jurisdiction's medical cannabis program.
3. The nurse shall have an understanding of the endocannabinoid system (ECS), the receptors, ligands, enzymes, and the interactions among them.
4. The nurse shall have an understanding of cannabis pharmacology and the research associated with the medical use of cannabis.
5. The nurse shall be able to identify the safety considerations for patient use of cannabis.
6. The nurse shall approach the patient without judgment regarding the patient's choice of treatment or preferences in managing pain and other distressing symptoms.

The role of the APRN with these essential principles will be further defined later in this chapter.

Another challenge for nurses and APRNs is the federal scheduling status of cannabis as Schedule I and the resultant lack of federal oversight and regulation regarding cannabis products. At the time of this writing in late 2019, there are 33 states, plus the District of Columbia, that allow medical cannabis, 11 states that allow adult-use cannabis, and 16 states that allow for cannabidiol (CBD) and low tetrahydrocannabinol (THC) only. Only three states (Idaho, South Dakota, and Nebraska) remain complete prohibition states (National Organization for the Reform of Marijuana Laws [NORML], n.d.). Each state is allowed to develop and implement its cannabis regulation. States can determine whether cannabis is fully legal, for medical use only, decriminalized, or fully illegal. Also, within the states that allow medical cannabis, each state can determine which conditions qualify for use, and whether or not there is moderate- to high-quality evidence to support those conditions. This process, leads to inconsistencies across the nation, and the lack of uniformity may mean that a patient could qualify for medical cannabis use in one state, but not in another.

Minnesota, for example, initially had a very restrictive medical cannabis program. When medical cannabis was approved in Minnesota back in 2014, it was highly criticized for the restrictions on qualifying conditions and patient access to various cannabis products. Minnesota only approved three ratios of THC and CBD, leaving patients with very limited choices. Within the first few years, 86% of registered Minnesota patients using cannabis reported that the cost of medical cannabis was somewhat unaffordable, and 29% stated that using medical cannabis was cost prohibitive (Marijuana Policy Project, 2019). Over the past 5 years, intractable pain, post-traumatic stress disorder (PTSD), obstructive sleep apnea, autism, and Alzheimer's disease have been added to the qualifying conditions list (Minnesota Department of Health, n.d.).

In contrast to Minnesota's medical cannabis program, California voters approved the Compassionate Use Act in 1996. This included a list of 11 qualifying conditions plus text that stated "or any other illness for which marijuana provides relief" (Compassionate Use Act, 1996). That last sentence was deliberately added to allow physicians to qualify patients who may not fit into the 11 qualifying conditions. Over the course of many years, physicians began to create cannabis clinics to certify patients within a matter of minutes. The medical community viewed this approach as problematic, and California's medical program was highly criticized as recreational. Almost anyone could qualify under the Compassionate Use Act, and medical cannabis was not taken seriously.

The stark contrast of medical cannabis programs in Minnesota and California is the result of states having the authority to create and implement their medical cannabis and adult-use programs. Unfortunately, patients are stuck in the middle. Someone living in Kansas with severe PTSD may not be able to use cannabis as a treatment modality, whereas someone in Colorado with PTSD can use cannabis freely, but they may lack clinician oversight. The lack of national standards has led to confusion and poor access for many who would benefit from cannabinoid therapy.

With cannabis remaining a Drug Enforcement Agency (DEA) Schedule I drug, states that have developed medical and adult-use programs have come to find many clinicians are not truly engaging with cannabis as a medication. Years of prohibition and limited ability to study the benefits of cannabis have left clinicians to disregard it as a medicine. However, patients have continued to explore and use the plant, whether their clinician approves of the use or not. As a result, many patients have turned to the internet or friends for advice. Unfortunately, a recent study demonstrated that only 1 out of every 30 cannabis articles published on the internet was written by a medical professional (Boatwright & Sperry, 2018). Without proper medical guidance, using cannabis can pose a risk for harm. Medical professionals must become educated about the benefits and risks of cannabis use. Recognizing that most people look to those they trust for advice and that nurses are the most trusted professionals 17 years in a row, it is no surprise that nurses started a platform to educate and advocate others on cannabis.

THE AMERICAN CANNABIS NURSES ASSOCIATION'S ADVANCED PRACTICE REGISTERED NURSE ROLE COMPETENCIES FOR CANNABIS NURSING RECOMMENDATIONS

The ACNA is a national nursing organization founded in 2012. Its mission is to advance excellence in cannabis nursing practice through advocacy, collaboration, education, research, and policy development. In 2017, ACNA released its first version of the scope and standards of practice for cannabis nurses. The scope and standards of practice document was updated in March 2019 to reflect the NCSBN guidelines and clearly define the APRN's role in cannabis nursing. In line with ACNA's mission to advance excellence in cannabis nursing practice through education, the scope and standards are the first steps toward obtaining certification for cannabis nursing through the ANA. Following the ANA Scope and Standards of Practice Third Edition, the ACNA developed its scope and standards to address the who, what, where, when, how, and why of cannabis nursing practice (ANA, 2015). The scope and standards are a work in process and will continue to evolve as the role of the cannabis nurse/APRN evolves. See Table 7.1 for ACNA's (2019) APRN scope and standard.

THE NATIONAL COUNCIL OF STATE BOARDS OF NURSING'S ADVANCED PRACTICE REGISTERED NURSE ROLE COMPETENCIES FOR CANNABIS NURSING RECOMMENDATIONS

The NCSBN (2018) recognized that patients are using cannabis and that nurses will need to be equipped with practical information to better care for these patients, whether they are consuming medical or adult-use cannabis. Most importantly, the NCSBN made sure to include statements regarding the patient's autonomy to use cannabis and that nurses must put aside any bias and judgment, to provide quality care.

NCSBN (2018) further defined the role of APRNs under the six principles of essential knowledge. The principles are intended to provide the APRN with guidelines that promote patient safety. Whether the APRN is working directly with medical cannabis patients or they simply have patients enquiring about it, the guidelines provide a working framework to help APRNs further define their role.

TABLE 7.1.	ACNA's (2019) APRN scope and standard

Standard 1: Assessment

1. Uses advanced assessment skills during a review of systems to best potentiate the patient's journey toward endocannabinoid system health and wellness. Performs a complete clinical assessment to identify whether a patient has a qualifying condition based on the state MMP guidelines. Considers current and previous mental health and substance use history

2. Initiates appropriate tests and diagnostics related to the endocannabinoid system health status and patient-specific health concerns

3. Reviews current treatment of qualifying conditions and responses to treatment. Reconciles medications

4. Applies current requirements and principles of state MMP and considers the current NCSBN recommendations. Considers if cannabis will be effective for the qualifying condition while considering the current state of evidence related to cannabis and the qualifying condition(s)

Standard 2: Diagnosis

1. Formulates a differential diagnosis or diagnoses based on the assessment, history, physical examination, and diagnostic test findings and results

2. Considers risks to specific vulnerable populations and the current body of scientific evidence related to qualifying cannabis recommendation considerations and effectiveness of cannabinoid medicines

Standard 3: Outcomes identification

1. Ensures that expected outcomes and the patient-centered cannabinoid therapy plan are in alignment

2. Supports the patient titration process plan as per the NCSBN

3. Anticipates results from the implementation of the personalized patient-centered plan, considering current evidence-based science, projected costs to patient and family, clinical effectiveness, and individual patient response

Standard 4: Planning

1. Creates an evidence-based plan in partnership with the patient and interdisciplinary team members

2. Incorporates coaching techniques such as motivational interviewing, appreciative inquiry, and active listening with the patient in efforts to develop a patient-centered holistic plan

3. Develops innovative strategies and utilizes patient-centered tools as part of the planning process to meet the needs of the cannabis patient

4. Demonstrates leadership in the design and implementation of therapeutic interventions, considering all modalities that may support endocannabinoid system health

5. While developing the plan of care, the APRN integrates assessment strategies, diagnostic strategies, and therapeutic interventions that reflect current cannabis evidence-based knowledge and practice

(continued)

TABLE 7.1.	ACNA's (2019) APRN scope and standard (*continued*)

Standard 5: Implementation

1. Supports patient implementation of evidence-based interventions stated in the personalized treatment plan

2. Uses prescriptive authority with pharmaceuticals and recommendation privileges with cannabis and cannabinoid medicines in accordance with state laws and with an awareness of federal laws. Follows state-based MMP guidelines for the cannabis recommendation process. Uses prescriptive authority for procedures, referrals, and treatments and therapies following state and federal law. Educates the patient about evidence-based cannabinoid agents and therapies in accordance with clinical indicators after reviewing the results of diagnostic and laboratory tests

3. Utilizes an integrative approach where cannabis medicine can be incorporated with lifestyle management, holistic modalities, traditional pharmaceutical medications, and herbal therapies or supplements in an appropriate and safe manner to support endocannabinoid system tone. Side effects, adverse effects, variable effects, and safety considerations are explored with the patient/family/caregiver as decisions about cannabis recommendations are made

4. Provides ongoing clinical consultation regarding cannabis medicine, the titration process, and the endocannabinoid system

5. Provides patient/family members/caregivers with relevant and accurate information and guidance on appropriate cannabis dosing, routes of administration, cannabinoid ratios, and terpenes/terpenoids as allowed by practice standards, state MMP mandates, and federal laws

6. Monitors the patient for side effects, adverse effects, and cannabis use disorder

7. Avoids conflicts of interest with the cannabis industry

8. Provides clinical cannabis consultation for healthcare consumers and other professionals related to complex clinical cannabis cases to improve patient care and outcomes

Standard 6: Evaluation

1. Enacts a systematic evaluation process with the goal of enhancing a patient-centered cannabis plan of care effectiveness

2. Considers results of evaluation when making recommended revisions to plan

3. Remains patient-centered and utilizes interdisciplinary team members' insight as the plan is revised

4. Supports patients with recommendations for cannabinoid/terpenoid administration routes, doses, and ratios based on evaluation findings

5. Follows up with patients regarding any changes in the body of scientific evidence related to cannabis and current qualifying condition(s)

6. Makes recommendations for policy, procedure, or protocol revisions based on the evaluation results and patient outcomes

Standard 7: Ethics

1. Acts as a leader in developing cannabis nursing–related policies, procedures, and practices that are evidence based and ethically sound

2. Practices cannabis nursing from a framework of caring ethics and social justice with a nondiscriminatory, caring, and compassionate approach

TABLE 7.1.	ACNA's (2019) APRN scope and standard (*continued*)

3. Participates with interprofessional teams as they address ethical risks, benefits, and outcomes related to cannabis healthcare industry practices

4. Acts as an advocate to end the social stigma related to cannabis use

Standard 8: Culturally congruent practice

1. Acts as a leader within interdisciplinary teams to identify and respond to the cultural needs of patients and communities

2. Works with patients, communities, medical organizations, and lawmakers to create and maintain a focus on cross-cultural partnerships, both within the holistic cannabis medical practice and the population at large

3. Researches holistic and cannabis medicine interventions to improve the quality of life and healthcare outcomes for culturally diverse cannabis patients

4. Develops nondiscriminatory recruitment and retention strategies to achieve a diverse and inclusive workforce in cannabis clinics and dispensaries

5. Works closely with the patient to resolve discrepancies that may exist between cultural preferences and/or patient experiences versus evidence-based cannabis practice; includes the patient in the process of planning, recommending/certifying patients for medicinal cannabis use, and assessing outcomes

Standard 9: Communication

1. Utilizes NVC, focusing on needs and expectations when working with cannabis clients, discussing new legislation with lawmakers, and interfacing with colleagues

2. Leads the charge for patient advocacy and communicates the need for change so that patients have adequate access to cannabis

3. Guides conversations in a forward direction with a positive attitude to facilitate productive discussions and creative solutions in the evolving cannabis healthcare industry

4. Acts as a leader by shaping cannabis environments and conversations that encourage healthy communication

Standard 10: Collaboration

1. Guides interprofessional activities, including endocannabinoid education, consultation, management, technologic development, and research, to enhance positive outcomes

2. Establishes and maintains collaborative relationships among cannabis peers and those seeking cannabis knowledge in efforts to improve patient care

3. Develops protocols and tools to assist cannabis interdisciplinary professionals as they create plans of care for the patient. Provides an open forum with other interdisciplinary cannabis professionals to collaborate in customizing these protocols to meet specific needs

Standard 11: Leadership

1. Participates in, and aligns with, decision-making bodies to increase the effectiveness of patient outcomes and advance professional cannabis nursing practice

(*continued*)

TABLE 7.1.	ACNA's (2019) APRN scope and standard (*continued*)

2. Is an active member of interprofessional healthcare teams

3. Educates policymakers, colleagues, and patients about advanced practice cannabis nursing and role development

4. Provides guidance and counseling to colleagues regarding the acquisition of clinical knowledge, skills, ways of knowing, and judgment about the safe and effective use of cannabis medicine

5. Promotes advanced cannabis nursing practice and supports APRNs in being able to practice within the full scope of, or at the top of, their license. Serves as a role model for other APRNs entering the cannabis nursing specialty

6. Models expert cannabis nursing practice to colleagues, consumers, and interdisciplinary team members

7. Advocates for the continuous improvement of systems that support the advancement and implementation of cannabis medicine

Standard 12: Education

1. Uses current cannabis healthcare research findings and other evidence to expand knowledge, skills, abilities, and judgment to enhance role performance

2. Presents and disseminates cannabis science evidence to professional interprofessional colleagues, communities, and policymakers

3. Educational endeavors incorporate the role of the endocannabinoid system in homeostasis and are inclusive of the integrative modalities that support endocannabinoid system health and self-regulation

Standard 13: Evidence-based practice and research

1. Integrates current cannabis science evidence in all practice settings to enhance the quality of services provided

2. Utilizes current cannabis science evidence to continuously develop knowledge, skills, abilities, role performance, and clinical judgment

3. Uses critical thinking skills to integrate cannabis science evidence and holistic nursing theory to enhance patient-centered practices

4. Contributes to the cannabis nursing knowledge base by conducting cannabinoid science research or synthesizing current cannabinoid science evidence to enhance patient outcomes

5. Encourages other nurses to enhance and grow their research skills

6. Performs rigorous critiques of cannabinoid science to create progressive, evidence-based cannabis nursing practices and protocols

7. Advocates for ethical cannabis science research and translational scholarship with consideration of research participants as protected healthcare consumers

8. Supports a climate of collaborative interprofessional research and clinical inquiry

9. Disseminates research findings through peer-reviewed journal publications, presentations, and consultations

TABLE 7.1.	ACNA's (2019) APRN scope and standard (*continued*)

Standard 14: Quality of practice

1. Examines trends in nursing quality data, especially as it relates to the delivery of cannabis medicine. Explores cultural, ethnic, and population-based considerations when examining the data

2. Designs innovative plans of care with cannabis medicine in accordance with state MMP requirements and consideration of federal laws

3. Provides leadership in the design and implementation of the protocols and processes that support the safe delivery of cannabis medicine

4. Contributes to cannabis nursing knowledge through the pursuit of scientific inquiry

5. Utilizes scientific and qualitative data in system-level decision-making

6. Influences organizational systems that incorporate endocannabinoid medicine because they strive to improve outcomes

7. Obtains and maintains professional or specialty certifications

Standard 15: Professional practice evaluation

No differentiation in APRN role

Standard 16: Resource utilization

1. Considers holistic needs and conditions of the patient using cannabis, the potential for adverse effects, stability of the patient's condition, complexity of the treatment protocol, differences in personal preferences, and responses to initiation of cannabis treatment when creating holistic treatment plans

2. Creates innovative strategies and solutions to effectively manage the use of cannabis medicine resources, while continuously improving quality of care

3. Explores and promotes cost-effectiveness, cost benefits, and strategies for increasing efficiency associated with cannabis nursing practice

4. Connects the patient using cannabis with local cannabis resources, including supportive programs, cannabis educational opportunities, and informational materials

5. Initiates and leads change in cannabis nursing theory, research, education, and practice by assuming advanced leadership roles

6. Utilizes organizational and community cannabis resources when creating holistic interdisciplinary treatment plans

Standard 17: Environmental health

1. Analyzes the impact of social, political, environmental, and economic influences on cannabis plant–based medicine and pharmaceutical production of cannabinoid medicines

2. Creates partnerships that promote environmentally sound and sustainable cannabis plant production

ACNA, American Cannabis Nurses Association; APRN, advanced practice registered nurse; MMP, Medical Marijuana Program; NCSBN, National Council of State Boards of Nursing; NVC, nonviolent communication skills.

Six Principles of Essential Knowledge for Advanced Practice Registered Nurses

1. The APRN shall have a working knowledge of the current state of legalization of medical and recreational cannabis use (NCSBN, 2018).
   a. Practitioners are not allowed to prescribe cannabis while it remains as a Schedule I controlled substance (Drug Enforcement Agency [DEA], n.d.).
   b. Federally funded research for cannabis must come from the University of Mississippi, and applications must go through the U.S. Food and Drug Administration (FDA), the DEA, and the National Institute on Drug Abuse.
   c. Cannabis is legal for medical purposes in over 33 states plus the District of Columbia even though it conflicts with federal law, and Congress has no current intentions of preempting state laws (NORML, n.d.).
   d. Cannabis has been decriminalized in many states and legalized for adult use (NORML, n.d.).
   e. The U.S. Attorney General in 2009 took a position that discourages prosecutors from going after people who distribute or use cannabis for medical purposes as long as they comply with state laws (U.S. Department of Justice, Office of Public Affairs [DOJ], 2009).
2. The APRN shall have knowledge of the jurisdiction's MMP (Medical Marijuana Program) (NCSBN, 2018).
   a. The APRN can find the state's rules and regulations through their Department of Health. It is important for APRNs to be sure that they are reviewing the most up-to-date statute or rules. Cannabis laws and regulations can change rapidly, and there may be different statutes within the state's various counties and cities.
   b. Cannabis cannot be prescribed by *any* healthcare provider. As long as it remains a Schedule I in the Controlled Substances Act (CSA), clinicians can only recommend cannabis.
   c. Qualifying conditions, the certification process, and the type of healthcare provider will be specified in the states' MMP. Not all states will have the same qualifying conditions. Some states will allow for qualifying conditions even if there is not enough moderate- to high-quality evidence to support the use of cannabinoids for that condition.
   d. Some states have different rules for the provider-patient relationship. The APRN must verify whether a preexisting and ongoing relationship is necessary to certify patients.
   e. APRNs who can certify qualifying patients will be listed explicitly in the MMP. Currently, only eight states—Hawaii, Maine, Massachusetts, Minnesota, New Hampshire, New York, Vermont, and Washington—allow APRNs to certify patients with a qualifying condition for medical cannabis (NCBSN, 2018).
   f. Cannabis medicine can be obtained through a licensed dispensary once the patient has been certified and registers with the MMP. As some states transition to adult use from medical use, there is potential for unlicensed dispensaries to operate. This could mean that the products sold in the unlicensed dispensaries are untested and unregulated. A list of state-licensed dispensaries is available on the Department of Health or MMP website for each state.
   g. Patients or their registered caregivers can obtain and administer medical cannabis. Each MMP will specify whether a caregiver is allowed and how to

register as a designated caregiver. Designating and registering a caregiver can be valuable for patients who are homebound or have difficulty traveling outside of the home.

h. Employees of hospice, nursing, or medical facilities, visiting nurses, home health aides, or personal care attendants may qualify as caregivers in some MMPs. In some states, cannabis can be dispensed to patients in assisted living facilities as long as the cannabis is controlled and properly stored.

3. The APRN shall have an understanding of the ECS, cannabinoid receptors, cannabinoids, and the interactions between them (NCSBN, 2018).

a. The ECS is a group of receptors, ligands, and enzymes responsible for the degradation and synthesis of endocannabinoids (Bhattacharyya & Sendt, 2012).

b. The main receptors in the ECS were discovered in 1988 by Dr. Howlett and her team of researchers. The ECS is a regulatory system designed to promote homeostasis and balances our mood, appetite, sleep, pain perception, and memory (Bhattacharyya & Sendt, 2012).

c. The two most studied cannabinoids are THC and CBD. There are over 100 cannabinoids in the cannabis plant. Lesser known cannabinoids such as THCA, CBDA, and cannabigerol (CBG) are showing potential therapeutic effects.

d. There are three types of cannabinoids: endocannabinoids produced within the body, phytocannabinoids found in the plant, and synthetic cannabinoids such as dronabinol.

4. The APRN shall have an understanding of cannabis pharmacology and the research associated with the medical use of cannabis (NCSBN, 2018). The NCSBN guidelines clarify that there is a need for more research and that the use of cannabis as a medicine has outpaced the research. For now, the guidelines focus on the moderate- to high-quality research from randomized placebo-controlled studies to help guide the APRN in making the right decision for certifying qualifying conditions. In addition, the NCSBN guidelines note the lack of clinical studies for using cannabis as an anti-inflammatory, antitumoral, and antibacterial agent.

a. Many patients report using cannabis for symptom relief. Most are using cannabis for insomnia, chronic pain, and anxiety. Although some states allow other qualifying conditions such as Alzheimer's and Parkinson's disease, the NCSBN (2018) listed the following conditions on the basis of the current studies of moderate- to high-quality evidence:

i. Cachexia
ii. Chemotherapy-induced nausea and vomiting
iii. Cancer and/or rheumatoid arthritic pain
iv. Chronic pain
v. Multiple sclerosis and/or peripheral neuropathy
vi. Spasticity

b. Side effects from cannabinoids are influenced by the cannabinoid dose, other medications, metabolism, and comorbidities. Many patients report dizziness, tachycardia, hyperphagia, short-term memory loss, sedation, anxiety, and anticholinergic effects such as constipation, dry mouth, and dry eyes. Most of the side effects are dose dependent, and starting low and slow may help the patient to avoid adverse effects. The APRN needs to be aware of patients with preexisting balance issues, cognitive impairment, or psychosis because cannabinoids, particularly THC, can exacerbate those issues in some patients.

Although a fatal overdose of cannabis is not possible because of the minimal amounts of cannabinoid receptors in the brainstem, patients can overconsume cannabis and experience adverse effects or prolonged impairment (Herkenham et al., 1990).

c. The effects of cannabis will vary depending on the route of administration. Current research related to methods of administration in humans predominantly focuses on inhaled cannabis. Other routes, such as sublingual, oral, topical, transdermal, and vaporized cannabis, have less evidence for onset, duration, and absorption in humans. Inhaled cannabinoids, whether vaped or smoked, can reach peak concentrations in the bloodstream within minutes lasting upto 2 hours (Newmeyer et al., 2016). Oral onset and duration can vary, with onset taking up to 2 hours and duration lasting 5 or more hours (Grotenhermen, 2003). Understanding how the different routes of administration work can help the APRN educate patients on the most appropriate route depending on their condition. For more information on routes of administration and drug-drug interactions, see the various sections on Clinical Implications.

5. The APRN shall be able to recognize the signs and symptoms of cannabis use disorder and cannabis withdrawal syndrome (NCSBN, 2018).

a. According to the *Diagnostic and Statistical Manual of Mental Disorders, Fifth Edition (DSM-5)*, cannabis use disorder is defined as use that is significant enough to cause impairment or distress (American Psychiatric Association [APA], 2013). The APRN needs to recognize when a patient's use is interfering with activities of daily living and/or causing issues in relationships. If the patient's use outweighs any benefit, the APRN must help the patient reduce or eliminate the cannabis use. Patients who have been consuming cannabis daily for long periods may experience withdrawals with abrupt cessation of cannabis. Withdrawals may include irritability, insomnia, headaches, diarrhea, and appetite loss (APA, 2013). It is important to point out that most studies that look at cannabis use disorder have been with THC. Studies evaluating CBD usage are lacking. In general, dosages of 750 mg to 4,500 mg of CBD have been well tolerated in humans (Schoedel et al., 2018). When reducing the cannabis dosages, it is best practice to wean the patient down slowly when appropriate. In a daily user, the cannabinoid half-life can be between 5 and 13 days (Owens et al., 1981). Weaning over 4+ weeks will help reduce or avoid potential cannabis withdrawals.

6. The APRN shall have an understanding of the safety considerations for patients' use of cannabis (NCSBN, 2018).

a. Potential drug-drug interactions with cannabis must be reviewed before, and throughout, the course of cannabis therapy. For more information on how cannabinoids are metabolized with other medications, see the section Identify Drug-Drug Interactions later in this chapter.

b. APRNs need to consider other safety issues such as proper storage and disposal of cannabis products. It is essential to educate the patient to keep cannabis away from children, pets, and nonmedical users. Cannabinoids are sensitive to heat and light and are best stored in a cool, dark place. Most states require child-resistant packaging. The packaging can be difficult to open for older patients or those with disabilities. Some of these patients may need special assistance to open their packages.

c. Educating patients on how to read a label is also vital to the patient's safety. Without proper standardization of medical cannabis products, potency can vary; and patients may not be aware that the dosage of one product is different from that of another product. Many tinctures are expressed in milligrams/milliliter, and edibles may be expressed in milligrams per package. Patients should be able to correctly identify a serving size and the expiration date on any given product.

d. Proper disposal of cannabis products can be handled through the DEA's Disposal Act. Check with your state's MMP to best identify the appropriate way to dispose of cannabis.

Outside of the six essential principles, the NCSBN (2018) guidelines also make further recommendations regarding clinical encounters, informed and shared decision-making, documentation and communication, ethical considerations, and some special considerations when assessing a patient for a qualifying condition. For more information on assessment, see the section Assessment later in the chapter.

Clinical Encounter and Identification of a Qualifying Condition

1. The APRN shall perform a clinical assessment in person and review the diagnostic information necessary to certify a patient under a qualifying condition (NCSBN, 2018).

   a. Assessing a patient in person allows the APRN to conduct a thorough and comprehensive assessment of the patient. The APRN can better identify and qualify a patient for medical cannabis when the assessment is performed in person.

2. The APRN shall review the patient's current treatment plan and how well that patient is responding to the current treatment (NCSBN, 2018).

   a. As with any other treatment modality, qualifying a patient for medical cannabis should not be a different approach. There may be opportunities to identify treatments in addition to or beyond use of medical cannabis. Patients who are noncompliant with their current regimen may not be compliant with a medical cannabis regimen. Addressing the upregulation of the ECS through the use of holistic modalities falls within the APRN's role.

3. The APRN shall reconcile all medications and monitor their state's prescriptive drug program (NCSBN, 2018).

   a. Because there is potential for cannabinoids to inhibit or induce other medications, a thorough review of medications both prescribed and over the counter must be conducted before beginning any medical cannabis program. Patients should also be advised to consult with their APRN any time there is a change in medications. For more information on potential medications interactions, see the section Identify Drug-Drug Interactions later in the chapter.

4. The APRN shall review the patient's health history and identify any history of mental illness, substance abuse, and alcohol intake (NCSBN, 2018).

a. Many clinicians may associate cannabis use with an increased risk of developing a psychiatric condition. Although the National Academy of Sciences, Engineering, and Medicine (NASEM, 2017) committee found substantial evidence of a statistical *correlation* between frequent cannabis use and developing schizophrenia and/or other psychoses, it did not find evidence that cannabis use *causes* schizophrenia and/or psychoses. It is important to remember that correlation does not equal causation.

The question remains whether frequent, heavy cannabis use affects the incidence of psychosis. Most recently, the *Lancet Psychiatry* published a study in May 2019 that found high THC use was associated with an increased risk of developing a psychotic disorder (Di Forti et al., 2019). The study reported that they found daily use of high-potency cannabis increased the odds of developing psychosis fivefold. High-potency THC cannabis was defined as 10% or more, and those values were not measured directly, but rather determined through self-reports from study participants and THC levels in cannabis that had been previously seized. Other components of the cannabis plant or possible contaminants that might contribute to this issue were not considered.

A patient with a history of cannabis abuse and/or other substance use disorders should be closely monitored and may not be a candidate for cannabis use.

5. The APRN shall obtain information on the patient's previous and current cannabis use and education (NCSBN, 2018).

a. Understanding the patient's previous cannabis use can help illuminate challenges and successes with cannabis, and help identify any myths or misconceptions the patient may have about cannabis. For example, if a patient has never consumed cannabis before and they spent their whole life telling their children to stay away from "drugs," that patient may be more reluctant to explore all that cannabis has to offer. Conversely, those who have been using cannabis for decades may not see cannabis as harmful.

Understanding what a patient knows about cannabis and where they are getting that information is also essential. The patient may have inaccurate information, or they may be relying on friends and family to guide their cannabis use. Cannabis is a personalized and individualized medicine, and what works for one person may not be appropriate for another.

6. The APRN shall consider other factors when certifying patients, such as scientific evidence related to the qualifying condition:

a. Potential side effects that may impact the current condition or other comorbidities

b. The unpredictability of cannabis effects

c. Ability to titrate dosages

d. Identifying high-risk/vulnerable patient groups (NCSBN, 2018)

7. The APRN shall continue to monitor and evaluate the patient after certification (NCSBN, 2018).

This is an incredibly vital point. Many patients currently do not receive ongoing support from clinicians once they start cannabis therapy.

INFORMED AND SHARED DECISION-MAKING

Informed and shared decision-making is important for the patient, family members, and the APRN to all be on the same page. It helps avoid confusion and identifies the goals of care.

1. The APRN shall provide information to the patient and family members/caregivers regarding the following:
   a. Cannabis-based scientific evidence regarding the qualifying condition
   b. Potential side effects of cannabis and interactions with other medications
   c. The unpredictability of cannabis, effects especially ingested cannabis products and artisanal products. Even batches from the same producer can vary by as much as 20%.
   d. How to self-titrate cannabinoid dosages
   e. Safety factors
   f. Identifying and clarifying the goals of care. Cannabis is a personalized medicine, and individual responses will vary. Without more double-blind, placebo-controlled clinical studies on dosages, most information provided will be based on empirical data. It is also important that the patient understands that cannabis products are not covered by insurance.
   g. Establishing expectations for ongoing monitoring and evaluation. Be sure to let the patients know when you will follow up with them and how to contact you if they are having an adverse effect. In the event that a patient experiences side effects such as anxiety, paranoia, hallucinations, or tachycardia, it is imperative that they know what to do (NCSBN, 2018).
2. Together, the APRN and the patient shall decide whether to proceed with certifying the qualifying condition (NCSBN, 2018).
   a. Once the patient understands the risks and benefits of cannabis, it is up to them whether theywant to proceed with cannabis as a treatment.

DOCUMENTATION AND COMMUNICATION

1. The APRN shall document the patient assessment, reasoning underlying the therapeutic use of cannabis for the qualifying condition, goals of therapy, means to monitor and evaluate response, and the education provided to the patient (NCSBN, 2018).
   a. Documenting the clinical interaction with cannabis should follow the same expectations as with all other clinical interactions. Cannabis-specific electronic health records (EHRs) are under development. For now, APRNs can document the specifics in their current EHR.
2. The APRN shall communicate the patient's plan of care for the use of medical cannabis to other healthcare team members (NCSBN, 2018).
   a. As more and more patients add cannabis to their regimen, it is crucial that the APRN communicates with other clinicians about the patient's cannabis use, including dosages, cannabinoids, routes of administration, and outcomes when applicable.

ETHICAL CONSIDERATIONS

1. In addition to the ethical responsibilities under the jurisdictional law, the APRN shall approach the patient without judgment regarding the patient's choice of treatment or preferences managing pain and other distressing symptoms (NCSBN, 2018).

   a. For over eight decades, cannabis has been prohibited, and research has been stymied. Many clinicians have been led to believe that as cannabis is a Schedule I drug, it does not have any benefits, and it is dangerous and highly addictive. As patients begin to explore cannabis as a treatment option, APRNs must put aside their biases and help patients navigate the complexity of cannabis. Without proper guidance, patients may experience more harm than benefits.

2. The APRN shall take all appropriate steps to ensure that the APRN is not in a position where there is or may be an actual conflict, or potential conflict of interest between the APRN and a cannabis dispensary or cultivation center (NCSBN, 2018).

   a. APRNs who have a vested financial interest in a cannabis manufacturing company may not be acting in the best interest of the patient. As more cannabis companies come online, it will be essential for the APRN to understand the safety and quality of the products before recommending them to patients. APRNs who are well educated in cannabinoid sciences may be able to serve as a consult to cannabis companies and provide valuable input on product development.

3. The APRN shall not certify an MMP qualifying condition for oneself or a family member (NCSBN, 2018).

   a. To avoid a potential conflict of interest, APRNs should have themselves or a family member certified by another qualified clinician.

SPECIAL CONSIDERATIONS

1. Follow specific employer policies and procedures, terms of the collaborative agreement, standard care arrangement, and facility policy and procedures regarding certifying a qualifying condition (NCSBN, 2018).

   a. Many facilities and institutions are in the process of developing policies and procedures for cannabis care. APRNs should enquire about them and become familiar with them before they begin certifying patients.

ESTABLISHING ROLE COMPETENCY

Establishing role competency for cannabis nurses and APRNs is still under construction. ACNA's (2019) efforts in establishing the scope and standards of practice and the NCSBN (2018) guidelines are the first steps in developing core role competencies for nurses and APRNs working in the field of medical cannabis. It will also be important to gather and maintain support from larger nursing organizations.

In 2016, the ANA issued a position statement on cannabis that supports the review and reclassification of cannabis from Schedule I status to support research that informs patients and providers of the efficacy of cannabinoids. The ANA (2016) statement also supports the following changes in cannabis medicine:

1. Prescribing standards for dosages, routes of administration, indications of use, potential side effects, and guidelines on when to stop other medications
2. Determining evidence-based standards for the use of cannabinoids
3. Decriminalization of cannabis for patients using cannabis appropriately under their state law
4. Healthcare practitioners who use cannabis, dispense, recommend, or administer cannabis in accordance with state and professional standards should be exempt from criminal prosecution, civil liability, or professional sanctioning (ANA, 2016).

The need to define and establish role competency has become necessary because more and more patients are exploring cannabis as a treatment option. Patients are facing many barriers to accessing cannabis as medicine. As patients' use of cannabis continues to grow, nurses need to understand the barriers to cannabis care and address them accordingly. Beyond identifying risks and benefits, potential drug interactions, and appropriate routes of administration, APRNs will need to have an understanding of their states' medical and adult-use programs. The complexity of cannabis as a medicine is vast, and coupled with the intricacies of local and state legislation, it can quickly become overwhelming.

The lack of standardization of roles and education is not unique to cannabis care nursing. Oncology nurses faced similar issues and are still challenged with getting the role of the oncology nurse navigator (ONN) recognized as a nursing specialty by the American Nurses Credentialing Center (ANCC). Many oncology nurses found that their primary role was helping cancer patients navigate the complexity of cancer care. In 2011, the Oncology Nurse Society (ONS) recognized that even though the role had not been clearly defined or recognized, many oncology nurses reported functioning as nurse navigators (Bailey et al., 2018). The ONN core competencies were developed in 2013, which helped define, support, and standardize the role. In 2017, the core competencies were updated to reflect more evidence-based practice. The core competencies will continue to support ONNs as the role evolves.

The undefined role of a cannabis APRN makes it challenging to provide standardized care. Because there is no standard training process for APRNs who want to work with cannabis and cannabis has not been recognized as a specialty practice, it may be several years before nurses and APRNs can be certified in cannabis care as a nursing specialty. Until then, nurses and APRNs who want to learn about cannabis and work in the field must self-educate to provide high-quality cannabis care.

Because there are not enough gold-standard randomized, double-blind placebo-controlled studies, evidence-based research on cannabis as a medicine is lacking. The NASEM (2017) report on the health effects of cannabis does provide an overview of the current levels of evidence and the steps we need to take to grow this evidence. As the legal landscape changes and more research takes place, some of the necessary evidence base will emerge to support ACNA's efforts in gaining ANCC recognition of cannabis care as a nursing specialty. Similar to the ONN, cannabis care nursing will continue to evolve as the barriers to cannabis medicine shift.

THE EDUCATION AND TRAINING PROCESS FOR ADVANCED PRACTICE REGISTERED NURSES

With the wide range of variations in state medical and adult-use cannabis programs, the majority of state boards of registered nursing have not begun to address formal cannabis education or training for nurses and APRNs. Without direction from the various state boards of nursing, nurses are left with no clear official standards, which exposes them to potential legal risks. Some nurses and APRNs are concerned about whether they can even discuss cannabis with their patients, although the NCSBN (2018) clearly states that the nurse's role is to educate patients around the medicinal use of cannabis. Despite the lack of standards, nurses are entering the cannabis industry and creating unique roles that allow them to incorporate their nursing skills.

Currently, nurses working within the cannabis industry are, to a degree, unregulated. To date, there are no recognized board certifications available; however, many educational opportunities are being developed by nurses, doctors, and academicians. As the industry grows, educational programs will pop up. Soon the market will be flooded with cannabis education, making it difficult to discern quality programs, especially if there is no accreditation available for such programs. The ACNA has a core curriculum for nurses developed in 2015; however, that curriculum rapidly became outdated. Recognizing that nurses need accurate, up-to-date information, the ACNA has started to partner with other educational organizations to meet the demands for nursing education even as they develop webinar series addressing the NCSBN's (2018) six essential areas of knowledge.

Cannabis education is not yet required in most schools; it is only recommended. Until the National Council Licensure Examination (NCLEX) and AANP/ANCC include questions regarding the ECS cannabinoid therapeutics, the body of cannabis science, and the nurse's role, academia may be reluctant to develop curricula in this area. In addition, as long as cannabis remains in the DEA Schedule I, there will be many barriers to APRN cannabis care practice, and clinicians will be less likely to recommend cannabis as a treatment option. Currently, patients who want to use cannabis as a treatment modality must rely on clinicians who specialize in cannabinoid therapeutics, and they are not likely to receive any information from their primary care or specialty clinicians.

Even with the ANA statement and the NCSBN (2018) guidelines, most of the state boards of nursing have not taken an official position or defined a scope of practice inclusive of cannabis and cannabinoid therapeutics. At the time of the writing of this chapter, only three states, Oregon, New Hampshire, and Missouri, have issued statements about cannabis, but none have issued practice guidelines. The lack of national official practice standards regarding nurses working with cannabis makes it difficult for nurses and APRNs to clearly understand their role with regard to patients who would like to or need to use cannabis.

The NCSBN (2018) guidelines provided recommendations for cannabis education in APRN programs. Similar to the recommended practice guidelines, medical cannabis education is intended to arm students with information that will provide them with the knowledge to practice safe patient care and reduce patient harm. One difference in the NCSBN student APRN recommendations is that the student shall be mindful of medical cannabis administration considerations. The student APRN needs to understand if, and what types of, cannabis can be administered according to the state's MMP. Even with these guidelines, the majority of APRN programs have not adopted medical cannabis education into their curricula. Some colleges offer cannabis education as a certification separate from the standard nursing curriculum, but there is not yet curricula developed specifically focused on the APRN's role regarding cannabis care.

In addition, there may be few opportunities to train in cannabis care medicine. Some leading clinicians in the field have started to offer preceptorships and/or training programs for healthcare professionals interested in cannabinoid medicine. Until the ANA and the ANCC recognize cannabis as a nursing specialty, education and training will not be uninformed, or standardized, and it may be difficult to discern who is qualified to provide cannabis care.

Assessment

Approaching patients regarding cannabis as a treatment modality should not be treated any differently from other allopathic treatments. APRNs can leverage other evaluation techniques when assessing patients. Before meeting with a patient, it is recommended that the APRN collect, at a minimum, the following information. The collection of the suggested information helps the APRN prepare for the consultation and identify potential concerns before meeting with the patient.

- Medical records related to the illness or condition
- Results of related tests or examinations
- A list of medications and supplements, including indications, dates, type, dosage, and quantity prescribed
- A list of all allergies to medications and foods, and the reaction to the allergen
- Health history, including current and past treatments, comorbidities, family history of mental health issues, history of cannabis use, and potential substance abuse

Once the APRN is ready to meet with the patient, it is important to outline the goals of care and to perform a thorough assessment. Additional considerations listed here can add value to the consultation and help obtain success more quickly. Motivational interviewing techniques can be used to partner with the patient.

- The patient's primary health concerns
- The patient's goal of cannabis therapy
- The number of hours of sleep the patient has each night
- The amount of water, caffeine, and alcohol the patient consumes
- The amount of exercise the patient gets daily
- What stress management techniques the patient uses daily
- Any possible life changes/events within the past year
- The patient's previous and current cannabis experience and use
- The patient's employment status and education level

Identifying Potential Risks and Benefits Through a Thorough Health History

In addition to the abovementioned intake information, the APRN should complete a review of systems. See Table 7.2 taken, with permission, from *Using Cannabis to Treat Cancer-related Pain* (Byars et al., 2019) for cannabis-specific considerations when reviewing systems.

TABLE 7.2.	Cannabis assessment	
System	Assessment parameters	Considerations for cannabis
General	• Presence of allergies • Weight changes • Fatigue level • History of fever or chills • Pain, including rectal, abdominal, gallbladder, head and neck, breast, chest, prostate, vaginal, and oral • Length, quality, and consistency of sleep, and history of sleep apnea • Implanted devices, such as central lines, pacemakers, implanted pain pumps, shunts and drains • Fall risk	• Terpene reactions are usually related to an allergy and can manifest as a rash or as nausea.
HEENT	• Xerostomia and dry eyes • Hearing loss and visual changes, such as blurred vision, double vision, and the need for assistive devices • Vocal changes • Sore throat and mucositis • Taste changes	• Dry eyes can be a side effect produced by high-potency cannabis products. • Inhalation can aggravate the pain and dry mouth associated with mucositis. • Alcohol-based cannabis extracts can aggravate mucositis.
Cardiovascular	• Chest pain, edema, heart palpitations, or arrhythmias • Hypotension and orthostatic hypotension	• Cannabinoid-naive patients have reported tachycardia. Tachycardia is a potential side effect that can resolve after repeated use. • Prolonged cannabis use can lead to decreased blood pressure. • For geriatric patients using an antihypertensive medication, orthostatic BP should be obtained, and safety education should be included in the treatment plan.

TABLE 7.2.	Cannabis assessment (continued)	
System	Assessment parameters	Considerations for cannabis
Respiratory	• Shortness of breath, cough • History of bronchitis and pleural effusions	• Inhaled cannabis can cause bronchial irritation and can aggravate chronic bronchitis or other inflammatory respiratory conditions. In these cases, HCPs should consider a different route of administration. Patients with decreased lung capacity may not be able to properly inhale cannabis.
Musculoskeletal	• Muscle or joint pain • Muscle spasms and stiffness • Numbness, tingling, and the loss of sensation • History of gout, scoliosis, fractures, joint replacements, and arthritis	• CBD can cause dizziness and lightheadedness. • THC can cause decreased BP. • CBD and CBDA do not cause impairment. • THC can cause impairment with high doses. • Consider multiple routes of administration when addressing pain. Pain relief can often take longer to achieve. Plans should include a systematic titration schedule that enables the patient to start at a low dose and slowly titrate up.
Mental health	• Anxiety • Panic attacks • Nervousness • Anger problems • Depression • Suicidal ideation • Substance abuse	• Adults with any diagnosis can be at risk for aggravation of psychiatric disorders.
Renal	• Frequency of urination, h/o UTIs, kidney stones, incontinence, stents and/or kidney disease • Urostomies or stomas or pouches	• The metabolism of oral routes of administration may be affected by kidney disease. If applicable, other routes of administration would be considered.

(continued)

TABLE 7.2.	Cannabis assessment (continued)	
System	**Assessment parameters**	**Considerations for cannabis**
Neurologic	• Cognition and ability to self-administer and self-titrate cannabis • Seizures, blackouts, tremors, or involuntary movements • Numbness, tingling, and loss of sensation • Gait changes • Difficulty walking	• CBD and CBDA do not cause impairment. • THC can cause impairment with high doses. • THCA typically does not cause impairment. • The HCP's baseline assessment will assist in the identification of which routes of administration can be safely self-administered (or which routes the family can safely administer). Assess for other CNS depressants that might contribute to balance issues.
Endocrine	• Diabetes, thyroid disease, and adrenal fatigue • Temperature intolerances to hot and cold	• HCPs should assess for potential drug interactions. THC can affect temperature regulation. Assess for heat and cold intolerances.
Gastrointestinal	• Dysphagia and esophageal strictures • Swallowing dysfunction • Enteral feeding tubes • Stomas • Nausea and vomiting • Dehydration • Constipation • Appetite loss	• The small intestine is the primary area of cannabinoid absorption. Radiation to this field can impact absorption, onset, and duration. • Patients with a h/o gastric bypass for malignant and nonmalignant reasons can have decreased absorption. In these cases, HCPs should consider a different route of administration. • Oil-based products can damage enteral feeding tubes, which are made of rubber. Also, oils can stick to the inside of the tube and the full dose might not reach the stomach. • Ensure that the stoma is patent and well healed, and that there is no diarrhea or constipation. • Ingestion of cannabinoids might not be effective if a patient cannot hold down food or liquids.

TABLE 7.2.	Cannabis assessment (continued)	
System	**Assessment parameters**	**Considerations for cannabis**
Hepatic	• Liver disease • Polypharmacy and potential drug-drug interactions	• Cannabinoids can be an astringent and can contribute to dehydration. • Constipation and dehydration can impact cannabinoid excretion, prolong cannabinoid half-life, and might increase side effects. • THC can stimulate appetite and CBD can decrease appetite. • Liver disease can affect the metabolism of cannabinoids. • Consider routes of administration other than oral in the highly diseased liver. • Cannabinoids can affect drug levels in the plasma (eg, cannabinoids might potentiate the effects of warfarin).
Dermatologic	• Conditions that can alter skin integrity and absorption, such as scarred skin surfaces, keloid areas, acne, and skin excoriation related to radiation, chemotherapy, and targeted therapies • Open wounds, abnormal lumps, new rashes, and itching	• Cannabinoids applied topically might improve skin alteration and promote healing by binding to CB2 receptors in the skin. • Terpene allergies can manifest as a rash. CBD anti-inflammatory effects might improve itchiness and rashes and reduce abnormal lump sizes.

BP, blood pressure; CB2, cannabinoid receptor 2; CBD, cannabidiol; CBDA, cannabidiolic acid; CNS, central nervous system; HEENT, head, eyes, ears, nose, and throat; HCP, healthcare provider; h/o, history of; THC, tetrahydrocannabinol; THCA, tetrahydrocannabinol acid; UTI, urinary tract infection.
Used with permission from Byars, T., Theisen, E., & Bolton, D. (2019). Using cannabis to treat cancer-related pain. *Seminars in Oncology Nursing, 35*(3), 300–309. https://doi.org/10.1016/j.soncn.2019.04.012

A thorough health history and intake will help the APRN identify other co-morbidities where cannabis may help or exacerbate other conditions. It is best if the APRN and patient determine priorities together as part of the shared decision-making process, as defined in the NCSBN (2018) guidelines. Cannabis must be individualized to the patient. There is no one-size-fits-all protocol for cannabis, and patients need to be supported with the self-titration process. Although it may be difficult to establish standardized protocols for different conditions, we can establish best practices on the basis of the collection of observational reports. Starting low and going slow with dosing is the consensus to the best approach with titrating cannabis. Although there are plenty of preclinical studies demonstrating the potential curative effects of cannabis, there is a lack of clinical trials to demonstrate the curative effects of cannabinoids for health conditions. The next section focuses on cannabis for symptom management with pain, anxiety, depression, and sleep.

CLINICAL IMPLICATIONS: PAIN AND CANNABIS APPROACHES

Up until recently, opioids have been well excepted as a treatment for managing chronic pain. Using opioids can pose serious risks for patients. Approximately 130 people die every day from opioid overdose, and the rise in opioid overdose deaths has led to a national epidemic. In response to the epidemic, the Centers for Disease Control and Prevention (CDC) published guidelines in 2016 for prescribing opioids for chronic pain. In the guidelines, the CDC addressed best practices for clinical treatment, which included information about thorough assessment, monitoring risks, how to safely discontinue opioids, and alternative treatment options. In addition, the guidelines address further potential harms associated with chronic opioid use by suggesting an opioid dosing strategy. Opioid dosages for chronic pain should be equal to or less than 50 MME (morphine milligram equivalents)/day and not exceed 90 MME/day unless documentation supports a higher need.

After the guidelines were published, some clinicians felt compelled to reduce the dosages of their opioid-dependent patients to comply with the new recommendations. Although the CDC guidelines have improved clinician prescribing practices, they did not properly address the millions of patients who continue to suffer from chronic pain. Those who relied on opioids to control their pain were forced to lower dosages even if they had no evidence of misuse or abuse. Unfortunately, these patients were offered few alternatives.

With around one-third of Americans suffering from chronic, debilitating pain and the rise in opioid deaths, it is no surprise that patients are exploring cannabis as a treatment option (Johannes et al., 2010). Many clinicians are reluctant to recommend cannabis as an alternative to opioids because of the Schedule I status. Clinicians have commented about the lack of studies regarding cannabis for pain. Contrary to federal government scheduling, research supports that cannabis can be beneficial in conjunction with or in place of opioids for chronic pain.

Studies have demonstrated that cannabis can be efficacious for several types of pain, especially neuropathic pain. In a randomized placebo study of 42 patients with neuoropathic pain, participants were given 2.9% THC, 6.7% THC, or placebo (Wilsey et al., 2016). Researchers found that the lower and higher levels of THC were more effective in alleviating pain than was placebo. In addition, the NASEM (2017) report on the health effects of cannabis concluded that there is substantial evidence that cannabis is effective for chronic pain.

In some cases, opioids may not be enough to manage pain. Cannabis has been shown to work synergistically with opioids. A study with 244 patients found that having access to legal cannabis allowed patients to decrease opioid use by 64% while improving quality of life (Byars et al., 2019). In another randomized, place-bo-controlled, double-blind study, when THC was administered with morphine, patients decreased their morphine dose to a quarter of their typical dose (Russo & Marcu, 2017). Cannabis can produce analgesic effects independent of opioid use (Byars et al., 2019).

Determining the type of pain first guides the APRN on the appropriate canna-binoid regimen. Once the APRN has a better understanding of the pain, cannabis treatment options can be offered.

When assessing for pain, the following should be addressed with patients:

- Location
- Intensity (determining the most intense, least intense, and acceptable pain levels)
- Quality (eg, whether the pain is aching or throbbing or a numbness, whether the pain is sharp or dull, whether the pain is localized or radiates, and so forth)
- Onset, duration, variation, and rhythm
- The manner in which the patient expresses the pain
- Factors that alleviate pain and factors that aggravate pain
- The impact that pain has on the quality of life, especially as related to:
  - Sleep
  - Appetite
  - Physical activity
  - Relationships
  - Emotions

There may be an opportunity for the APRN to address multiple quality-of-life factors after the pain assessment is complete. It is not unusual for pain to affect sleep and mood. In reviewing the patient's health history, the APRN may recom-mend a cannabis treatment plan for pain that starts by focusing on sleep rather than on the pain. For example, if patients report that their pain only allows them to get 2 to 3 hours of sleep at night, they may not be able to participate in other activities of daily living, such as exercise, that would help improve their overall condition.

Determining which cannabinoid is best for pain depends on the type of pain. THC is an effective analgesic at low dosages. The analgesic effects of THC occur through the activation of multiple different receptors—cannabinoid 1 (CB1), CB2, G protein–coupled receptor (GPR) 18, GPR55, and 5-hydroxytryptamine (5-HT) (Brusberg et al., 2009; Jhaveri et al., 2007; Pertwee, 2001). CBD is effective in reducing inflammation, modulating pain, boosting opioid analgesic effects, and shifting the dysphoria associated with pain (Iuvone et al., 2009; Kathmann et al., 2006; Resstel et al., 2009).

Routes of cannabis administration are also important when it comes to addressing pain. Patients with chronic pain will benefit from multiple different routes of administration to manage their pain. Quick-acting methods are best for immediate pain relief. If a patient has varying levels of pain, then a topical preparation or inhalation may provide relief the quickest. A tincture, edible, or transdermal patch can provide between 5 and 12 hours of longer lasting relief.

A topical preparation will work quickly, generally within 15 minutes and last several hours. It is unlikely that the topical will reach the bloodstream, and it may not be effective enough for pain deep in the joints such as the hips, back, or knees. Because the topical does not reach the bloodstream, it does not produce systemic effects, and may be the best option for those who need to avoid any impairment (Byars et al., 2019).

Inhalation is generally the least desired method of administration by patients. Most patients associate inhaling, whether smoking or vaping cannabis, with negative health consequences. In the NASEM (2017) report, the reviewers concluded that there was limited evidence to support an association between smoking cannabis and lung damage. The report also found that there was substantial evidence that smoking cannabis improved airway capacity with acute use. Inhaled cannabis reaches the bloodstream within minutes and can provide immediate relief. Patients can find relief quicker with inhalation, allowing them to find their dose faster and feel more in control of their pain (Byars et al., 2019).

Ingesting cannabis can provide longer lasting relief for those who need consistent relief from pain. Edibles are not advised in a new, inexperienced user because the dosages are difficult to titrate. Overconsumption of THC can lead to unpleasant side effects such as anxiety, paranoia, hallucinations, vomiting, and dysphoria (Byars et al., 2019). The best way to control the cannabis dose, and start low and go slow, is with a tincture.

Transdermal patches provide longest lasting relief. On average, they last for 8 to 12 hours and bypass the liver, thereby avoiding potential drug-drug interactions. The longer lasting effects are ideal for those who struggle with ingesting multiple dosages throughout the day (Byars et al., 2019). Unfortunately, transdermal patches are expensive and may be cost prohibitive for most patients.

Determining the dosages and frequency of various cannabinoids is best when individualized. Depending on the type and severity of pain, the number of medications, and the patient's metabolism, some patients may need once-a-day dosing, and others may benefit from every 4 hours. Keeping a cannabis diary or journal will help inform the patient and clinician how well the current regimen is working and where adjustments need to be made.

Table 7.3 is an equianalgesic chart based on Byars et al. (2019) that can be used to determine target dosages of THC to common opioids. The dosages listed are target dosages and not starting dosages. APRNs can use the chart to help replace or reduce opioids with THC and/or CBD. The chart presumes that 10 mg of THC is similar to 60 mg of codeine (Campbell et al., 2001).

TABLE 7.3.	Equianalgesic chart: THC to common opioids		
Morphine/mg	Codeine/mg	THC/mg	mg of THC per 1/mg morphine
60	200	33.33	0.5555
Hydromorphone	Codeine/mg	THC/mg	mg of THC per 1/mg hydromorphone
7.5	200	33.33	4.444
Meperidine	Codeine/mg	THC/mg	mg of THC per 1/mg meperidine
300	200	33.33	0.1111
Methadone	Codeine/mg	THC/mg	mg of THC per 1/mg methadone
20	200	33.33	1.6665
Oxycodone	Codeine/mg	THC/mg	mg of THC per 1/mg oxycodone
30	200	33.33	1.111
Oxymorphone	Codeine/mg	THC/mg	mg of THC per 1/mg oxymorphone
10	200	33.33	3.333

THC, tetrahydrocannabinol.

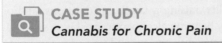

CASE STUDY
Cannabis for Chronic Pain

An 81-year-old retired male, cannabis naive: Reported ongoing pain for 65 years and had 26 orthopedic surgeries starting at the age of 16. The pain was getting progressively worse in the past 6 months. The patient reported an achy, constant pain in the right hip and lower back that varied in intensity depending on activity level. The pain was worse with standing for an extended time or walking long distances—on average, pain level was 8 with activity. Sitting or lying down did not exacerbate the pain. Without activity, pain level was a 3. Current diagnosis of spinal stenosis L4-L5 area. The patient had been receiving steroid injections every 12 weeks, which were becoming less effective over time. Recently, the patient was diagnosed with atrial fibrillation (a-fib) and was started on apixaban and metoprolol. The patient reported using acetaminophen 500 to 2,000 mg daily for pain with little relief. No additional medications.

Owing to the recent a-fib diagnosis, the patient was started on a topical cannabinoid while awaiting approval from the cardiologist. Cannabis can cause tachycardia and a confirmation that the patient's a-fib was stable was essential before proceeding with any oral cannabinoids. The topical did not provide any relief, and after the cardiologist signed off on the a-fib, 5 mg of a THCA tincture three times per day was added. After a week, the patient reported that the THCA tincture was only minimally effective for pain. At that time, the patient was switched to tincture that contained 3 mg CBD, 3 mg CBDA, 3 mg THCA, and 1 mg THC/mL. The tincture was administered three times per day. After a week, the patient reported marked improvement in back pain, down from 8 with activity to 2, and was able to stop acetaminophen use. Pain at rest was negligible. No reported incidences of tachycardia.

CLINICAL IMPLICATIONS: DEPRESSION AND CANNABIS APPROACHES

According to the National Alliance on Mental Illness (NAMI, 2017b), around 16 million American adults suffered from one major depressive event in the past year. When assessing for depression, the Patient Health Questionnaire (PHQ-9) is a tool that the NPs can use to determine whether the patient is suffering from depression. Depression is considered if the patient is experiencing problems in four different areas, more than half the days to nearly every day (Spitzer, 1999). The severity of the depression is determined by the total score, with higher scores correlating with moderate to severe depression. Symptoms such as difficulty with sleep, changes in appetite, lack of energy/motivation, difficulty concentrating, feeling hopeless or guilty, physical pain, or suicidal thoughts have all been associated with depression. The symptoms will vary from person to person, day to day, and if they persist beyond 2 weeks, a diagnosis of depression can be made.

Determining the cause of depression is essential as well. In some cases, there may be multiple contributing factors, and in others, there may be no precipitating factors. The more common causes include traumatic events, genetics, and stressful life events such as marriage, divorce, financial instability, raising a family, medications, and/or substance abuse. In some cases, patients may be using alcohol or cannabis to self-treat their depression. It is important to assess the patient's current and past cannabis use to determine whether cannabis, particularly THC, is contributing to or causing the depression. The NASEM (2017) report concluded that there is moderate evidence that heavy THC users have a small, increased risk of developing depression. If the clinician suspects that THC may be a factor in the patient's depression, it is best to encourage the patient to stop all cannabis use for at least 2 weeks. If the depressive symptoms resolve after 2 weeks, the clinician will need to decide whether cannabis can be resumed. In some cases, changing the cannabinoid profile, dosage, and/or route of administration may be enough to prevent the recurrence of depressive symptoms.

Treatment of depression depends on the severity. In some cases, using multiple methods of treatment may produce the best results. Most patients will benefit from psychotherapy, particularly cognitive-behavioral therapy (CBT), which provides patients with skills to cope with depression. In addition, medications such as antidepressants can be used to help with symptoms of depression. Antidepressants may take between 2 and 4 weeks to take effect and upward of 12 weeks to reach their full potential (NAMI, 2017b).

When it comes to using cannabis for depression, a combination of THC and CBD may produce the best results. Many patients have been self-medicating with high-THC cannabis for depression for decades. A 2016 survey found that 50% of cannabis users sought relief from depressive symptoms (Sexton et al., 2016). THC has been known to produce euphoric effects. Many patients report feelings of well-being, improved mood, and blissfulness when consuming THC. The psychoactive effects of THC occur because it partially binds with the CB1 and CB2 receptors. CB1 receptors can also interact with the 5-HT receptors, thereby increasing the release of serotonin. A 2018 study demonstrated that the ECS plays a large role in regulating mood, and a dysfunctional ECS may contribute to depression (Ibarra-Lecue et al., 2018). We currently have very little data on cannabinoids for the treatment of depression. As research opens up, we may determine which cannabinoids and dosages are most effective for treating depression.

> ### CASE STUDY
> #### Cannabis and Depression
>
> A 72-year-old female with a history of scoliosis and osteoporosis for 14 years. No history of depression or anxiety. Presented with pain in the lower lumbar area and bilateral hips. Pain management started in 2016. Duloxetine was prescribed for pain; patient-reported side effects outweighed benefits and discontinued use after 6 days. The patient received two steroid epidurals to L2-L3 and L5-S1, three lumbar steroid facet injections, six medical branch block/steroid injections, radiofrequency ablation of the lumbar facet medial branch, and an interlaminar steroid injection over a year with relief of the left hip pain only. Surgery was recommended after a year of trying to manage the pain and the patient declined. After two more additional lumbar interlaminar steroid injections that did not address the pain, the patient was prescribed tramadol, acetaminophen, and codeine to help manage the pain. Instead of using the prescribed pain pills, the patient wanted to explore cannabis first to see whether it could address the pain. For the first 6 months, the patient found relief of her right groin pain from a THC-dominant topical. She could apply it one to two times a day and achieve symptom relief without any side effects. As the pain progressed over the next 6 months, her acetaminophen use increased to 3,000 mg/day divided into three doses throughout the day. In an attempt to decrease her acetaminophen use and better address her pain, an oral CBD tincture was recommended. At 10 mg CBD twice a day, the patient reported better pain control, but was not able to decrease her acetaminophen dose. After 4 weeks, THCA was added and the CBD dosage was increased. Total daily cannabinoid intake was 30 mg CBD and 30 mg THCA orally. After 4 weeks, the patient was able to stop acetaminophen intake altogether. Two months into the THCA and CBD regimen, the patient reported feelings of sadness and lack of motivation. She acknowledged that the constant pain, although it was better, may be contributing to her depressed feelings. With no previous history of depression, the THCA was discontinued and the CBD dosages were increased to 100 mg/day. After 2 weeks, the depressive symptoms were resolved. The patient continued to use 100 mg of CBD daily with little relief, and the acetaminophen was increased to 3,000 mg/day. Eventually, the patient decided to stop cannabis use altogether.

CLINICAL IMPLICATIONS: ANXIETY AND CANNABIS APPROACHES

Anxiety disorders represent the most common type of mental health concern in the United States, with around 40 million adults suffering from anxiety (NAMI, 2017a). Although there are several different types of anxiety disorders, including generalized anxiety disorder, social anxiety disorder, panic disorder, and phobias, most people will experience similar emotional and physical symptoms.

The hallmark symptom of anxiety is constant and excessive worry and/or fear. The anxiety and worry are bad enough to affect social, occupational, and physical functioning.

In addition, people can suffer from feelings of dread, irritability, restlessness, tension, tachycardia, sweating, headaches, fatigue, shortness of breath, chest pain, nausea, diarrhea, and urinary frequency. The physical symptoms of anxiety can often lead people to think they may be having a serious health condition, such as a heart attack. Panic attacks can cause someone to visit the emergency room because the physical symptoms are troublesome.

An anxiety diagnosis is generally made 2 to 4 weeks after a patient has experienced excessive worry and fear that was difficult to control and not caused by a medical condition or another substance (Kavan et al., 2009).

Key recommendations for APRN practice in treating general anxiety disorder include assessing for depression in patients experiencing anxiety and recommending CBT, serotonin-norepinephrine reuptake inhibitors (SNRIs), selective serotonin reuptake inhibitors (SSRIs), and/or benzodiazepines (Kavan et al., 2009). Many patients have come to explore more natural or alternative treatments for anxiety. Side effects reported from benzodiazepines, SNRIs, and SSRIs can often lead to noncompliance with some patients, and research has shown a link to benzodiazepine use and an increased risk of dementia (Billioti de Gage, 2012).

Cannabis, particularly CBD, has gained popularity as a potential treatment for anxiety. According to Google's 2018 year-end trend report, "CBD gummies" was the third most popular food-related Google search of the year. CBD has been shown to interact with many of our receptors, particularly the 5-HT_{1A} and transient receptor potential vanilloid 1 ($TRPV_1$), that help regulate fear and anxiety-related behaviors (Blessing et al., 2015). The ECS also plays an important role in mood regulation. A dysfunctional ECS is associated with impaired fear regulation (Blessing et al., 2015).

Cannabinoids show promise as an effective anxiolytic. THC, in low doses, may help reduce anxiety, but in large dosages, it may increase anxiety. In contrast, low doses of CBD can cause anxiety, and larger dosages may reduce anxiety. The bidirectional effects of cannabinoids may cause the patient to experience the opposite intended effect. Specific dosages of CBD and THC in the treatment of anxiety have not yet been established.

Blessing et al. (2015) reviewed clinical CBD studies for anxiety, and oral dosages ranging from 15 to 600 mg. The various studies showed that CBD effectively reduced generalized anxiety, social anxiety, panic disorder, obsessive-compulsive disorder, and PTSD, and that CBD may potentially protect from THC-induced anxiety (Blessing et al., 2015). A study on CBD for anxiety was published by Shannon et al. (2019). It was a retrospective series study that looked at CBD for the treatment of anxiety and sleep. Dosages of CBD ranged from 25 to 175 mg/day. Anxiety responded better to the lower dosages, and sleep responded better to the higher dosages.

Determining cannabinoid dosages and routes of administration must be individualized. If the anxiety is constant, an oral regimen may provide more benefits than a quick-acting method. With panic attacks, inhalation can help the patient achieve relief within minutes and prevent further anxiety. As with any regimen, multiple routes of administration may allow for greater symptom management.

CLINICAL IMPLICATIONS: INSOMNIA AND CANNABIS APPROACHES

According to the American Academy of Sleep Medicine (AASM, n.d.), 33% to 50% of adults experience insomnia at least occasionally. Those with a history of other medical or psychiatric disorders will have higher rates of insomnia ranging from 50% to 75%.

Insomnia is defined by the AASM as difficulty falling or staying asleep that is frequent or persistent. Difficulty sleeping can be a symptom of another condition such as anxiety, chronic pain, depression, or substance abuse. Additional factors such as female sex, age, shift work, unemployment, or lower socioeconomic status can also increase the probability of insomnia. Risks associated with insomnia are increased risk of cardiovascular events, decreased immunity, diabetes, obesity, asthma, and seizures. It is estimated that the cost of insomnia in the U.S. economy is upward of $90 billion a year (AASM, n.d.).

When assessing for insomnia, it is essential to discuss the patient's sleep hygiene. In a position statement released by AASM, they recommend covering specifics such as the patient's presleep habits, sleep-wake cycle, other sleep-related complaints, and how their sleep conditions affect them during the day (Schutte-Rodin et al., 2008). A diagnosis of insomnia can be made if the patient meets specific criteria. AASM diagnostic criteria for insomnia include the following:

1. Complaining of difficulty falling asleep, staying asleep, poor-quality sleep, or early morning wakening
2. Difficulty with sleep occurs even when there are ample opportunities and appropriate circumstances for sleep
3. One or more of the following symptoms occur during the day as a result of difficulty sleeping or poor-quality sleep:
   a. Fatigue
   b. Difficulty with concentration, memory, or attention
   c. Poor performance at school or work
   d. Irritability or mood swings
   e. Daytime sleepiness
   f. Lack of motivation or energy
   g. Susceptible to errors or accidents at work or while driving
   h. Complaints of headaches, gastrointestinal issues with lack of sleep
   i. Worry or anxiety about sleep

Establishing a patient's sleep hygiene is also important. Many patients may be unaware that bad habits such as watching television before bed, drinking excessive alcohol or caffeine, smoking, napping, or drinking fluids before bed may contribute to poor sleep quality.

Some older adults admit to consuming between 14 and 21 alcoholic beverages a day. Often after retirement, alcohol becomes a recreational habit that can greatly contribute to frequent early waking. Older adults who continue to use caffeine late into the day may find it difficult to fall asleep. Although they report that caffeine does not seem to be as stimulating, they may not recognize that their decreased metabolism leads to decreased clearance of caffeine. Identifying some of these risk factors during an assessment can be all that the patient needs to improve their sleep quality. In the incidences where patients are practicing proper sleep hygiene and sleep is still an issue, pharmacologic intervention may be necessary.

Using pharmaceuticals to treat insomnia requires a risk versus benefit analysis. In some instances, the medication side effects may outweigh the therapeutic effects, and choosing the appropriate medication comes after a thorough health history and intake.

Determining the cause of sleep disruption and whether the patient is having a hard time falling and/or staying asleep can help the APRN choose the appropriate cannabinoid regimen. If a patient is having a hard time falling asleep, choosing a method of administration that is quick acting, such as inhalation or sublingual administration, may be most effective in improving sleep latency. In instances where the patient has a hard time staying asleep, a longer lasting route of administration such as an edible or a transdermal patch may provide longer lasting effects. If the patient is having a hard time falling asleep and staying asleep, multiple routes and/or dosages may be required to achieve success.

Currently, most patients will respond to low doses of THC for sleep. THC has known sedative side effects. It can be an effective sleep agent for most patients. On average, a dose of 2.5 to 5 mg of THC will provide patients with the necessary amount of sedation to improve sleep quality with minimal side effects.

CBD has been gaining popularity as a potential sleep agent. Contrary to popular belief, CBD can be stimulating at small dosages and can even counteract the sedating effects of THC. CBD may be sedating if it has high levels of myrcene or if it is taken with other sedation medications such as benzodiazepines (Russo, 2017). Although CBD is well tolerated in higher dosages, most CBD products are more expensive than THC is, and it may become cost prohibitive for patients to find the most effective CBD dosage for sleep.

Cannabinol (CBN) is another cannabinoid that is promoted as an effective sleep agent. Many cannabis companies have promoted CBN as the "sleepy cannabinoid," and they make products that are CBN dominant. Most patients reported that CBN was ineffective or produced intense side effects that forced them to discontinue the regimen. Dr. Tagen, also known as Professor of Pot, wrote a blog in 2018 that delved into the research around CBN. In his blog post, *Cannabinol (CBN)—The Sedative That Isn't?*, Tagen reported that the research does not support CBN as a sedative, and there is little research to support that CBN is effective for sleep (Tagen, 2018a). More studies are needed to support CBN as an effective sedative.

Educating patients on the different cannabinoids and possible side effects will allow them to make more informed decisions about which product to start with for sleep. Have patients start with the lowest dose possible, and titrate the dose gradually until the intended outcome has been reached.

CANNABIS DOSING

Dosing continues to remain a challenge for practitioners and patients. It is one of the biggest questions patients ask clinicians—How much cannabis do I need to take for___? Lack of double-blinded placebo studies makes it difficult to establish dosing in humans, and clinicians do not have standardized protocols to refer to when recommending cannabis. The complexity of the cannabis plant and the makeup of various plant chemovars may also come into play with dosing considerations. Although many observational and retrospective case studies have provided ranges of different cannabinoid dosages for different medical conditions, cannabis is still a personalized experience. Patients are encouraged to start with low doses, go slow with titrating doses up, and record the effects ("start low, go slow"). Keeping a cannabis diary or journal will allow the patient to document the medicine used, route, dosage, how long it took to take effect, how long the effects lasted, side effects, and benefits. Sharing those details with the APRN will allow them to make adjustments accordingly and achieve positive outcomes sooner.

Side effects of cannabinoids are often dose dependent. The biphasic properties of cannabis can produce the opposite effects of the intended outcome. In small doses, cannabis may help with nausea, and a large dose may cause one to vomit. Different cannabinoids, for example, CBD, may be stimulating at low dosages and sedating at higher dosages. An average starting dose can be between 2.5 and 10 mg or 1 and 5 mg for geriatric patients (Byars et al., 2019).

Identify Drug-Drug Interactions

Assessing for drug interactions is within nurses' and APRNs' scope of practice. The more medications a person takes, the higher the risk of a drug-drug interaction. With one medication, there is a 10% chance of an adverse drug event (ADE). Each additional medication increases the chances of ADE by an additional 10%, and if someone is taking 10 medications, there is a 100% chance of an ADE. The use of multiple medications is known as polypharmacy.

Polypharmacy has been defined as five or more medications (Maher et al., 2014). In a study looking at different settings, polypharmacy occurred in the ambulatory setting at a rate of 37.1% with men, and 36% of women, aged 75 to 85 years. In the hospital setting, the number of medications rose significantly, with 41.4% taking between five and eight medications, and 37.2% taking more than nine medications a day. As suspected, a survey of nursing home patients found 39.7% had nine or more daily medications (Maher et al., 2014).

The consequences of polypharmacy can be quite significant and include increased healthcare costs, increased risk of adverse drug effects, possible drug-drug interactions, medication noncompliance, decreased functional status, increased risk of cognitive impairment, increased risk of falls, decreased nutritional intake, and increased urinary incontinence (Maher et al., 2014).

Before adding cannabis to a patient's treatment plan, all medications should be reviewed to determine whether there is a potential drug-drug interaction. All cannabinoids, whether from plant or synthetic sources, can have side effects and interactions with other medications. The most information we have on cannabinoid drug interactions and side effects comes from FDA-approved synthetic THC (dronabinol and nabilone) and plant-based CBD (Epidiolex). GW Pharmaceuticals produces a CBD and THC plant-based tincture approved in over 30 countries, but not in the United States.

Dronabinol (Marinol) is a synthetic cannabinoid Δ-9-THC in sesame oil indicated for the treatment of anorexia in AIDS patients, and nausea and vomiting associated with cancer chemotherapy in those who have failed conventional treatment. Approved in 1985, it is a Schedule III drug. Dosages range from 2.5 to 10 mg three to four times daily. Syndros is a dronabinol oral solution with the same clinical indications as Marinol. It is a Schedule II drug. Dosages range from 2.1 to 4.2 mg four to six times a day. Side effects from dronabinol may include hypotension, tachycardia, central nervous system (CNS) depression, euphoria, dizziness, drowsiness, somnolence, confusion, new or worsening nausea and vomiting, seizures and seizure-like activity, and potential substance abuse (Wolters Kluwer Clinical Drug Information, 2019).

Nabilone (Cesamet) is a synthetic cannabinoid similar in structure to Δ-9-TCH found in *Cannabis sativa* L. It is approved for nausea and vomiting in patients on chemotherapy who have not responded to the standard of care for antiemetics. Dosages range from 1 to 2 mg two to three times a day for a maximum of 6 mg/day. Nabilone is a Schedule II drug. Side effects from nabilone may include tachycardia, orthostatic hypotension, dizziness, drowsiness, hallucinations, ataxia, and potential substance abuse (Wolters Kluwer Clinical Drug Information, 2019).

CBD (Epidiolex) is an FDA-approved liquid derivative from the cannabis plant. It was approved for the treatment of seizures in Lennox-Gastaut syndrome (LGS) and Dravet syndrome in patients aged 2 and older. Dosages start at 2.5 mg/kg twice a day and can be titrated up to 20 mg/kg/day. Epidiolex is a Schedule V drug with low abuse potential. Side effects may include hepatocellular injury, somnolence, sedation, and suicidal ideation (Wolters Kluwer Clinical Drug Information, 2019).

Nabiximols (Sativex) is a Δ-9-THC and CBN, 1:1 (2.7 mg THC and 2.5 mg CBD/ spray) prepared oral mucosal spray derived from the *C. sativa* plant. It has been approved in 25 countries for multiple sclerosis spasticity. It is currently not approved in the United States. Dosages range from 2 sprays up to 12 sprays a day. Side effects may include tachycardia and transient alterations in blood pressure, dizziness, changes in mood, memory, and coordination, and potential substance abuse (GW Pharmaceuticals, n.d.).

According to Russo-Marcu's (2017) *Cannabis Pharmacology: The Usual Suspects and a Few Promising Leads*, synthetic cannabinoid preparations have not led to any black market or addiction treatment issues, despite being available by prescription for decades.

Dronabinol and CBD have limited FDA-approved therapeutic uses, and large studies to assess drug interactions with other medications have not occurred. Without formal studies, most clinicians will need to make an educated guess as to whether cannabinoids will impact other medications. It will also be a while before we see any off-label use of dronabinol or CBD.

Both ingested and inhaled cannabinoids can be metabolized through the cytochrome P450 enzymes. Studies have demonstrated that THC is mostly metabolized by CYP2C9, CYP2C19, and CYP3A4 and is converted into 11-hydroxy-THC (11-OH-THC), and then into 11-carboxy-THC (11-COOH-THC) (Schwope et al., 2011). CBD is metabolized in the liver by the CYP enzymes, mostly by CYP2C19 and CYP3A4, and is converted to 7-hydroxy-cannabidiol (7-OH-CBD) (Zendulka et al., 2016).

There are also genetic variations that can influence how cannabinoids are metabolized. Known as genetic polymorphisms, these variations can provide the clinician with additional information as to how well cannabinoids will be metabolized and whether the patient is at risk for increased or decreased effects related to the cannabinoids. The most common polymorphism for the CYP2C9 enzyme, where THC is primarily metabolized, is CYP2C9*1 (Tagen, 2016). In patients with this polymorphism, the effects of THC may be more pronounced, and even low dosages may produce a strong effect. CYP3A4 metabolizes most medications and is also involved in metabolizing THC and CBD. Patients with the *22 polymorphism may experience stronger and more prolonged effects from the cannabinoids (Tagen, 2018b). Most patients have not had genetic testing done to establish how they will metabolize medications. If the APRN has access to that information, it can be used to determine whether the patients are fast, slow, or regular metabolizers of cannabinoids and whether they are at higher risk for experiencing increased side effects.

Table 7.4 is a guide as to whether there is a potential interaction with other medications when ingesting and/or inhaling cannabis. It is best to look for medications that are metabolized through CYP3A4, CYP2C9, and CYP2C19 because THC and CBD are most likely to be metabolized through those CYP enzymes. Interactions are unlikely with a topical, rectal, or transdermal route, although the literature does not

TABLE 7.4.	Possible cannabis drug-drug interactions			
Drug	Brand name	Metabolism pathway via the liver	Interaction with CBD	Notes
Abacavir/dolutegravir/lamivudine	Triumeq	MRP2/CYP3A4	None known	Monitor
Acamprosate	Campral	Unknown	None known	Monitor
Adalimumab	Humira	Unknown	None known	Monitor
Alemtuzumab	Campath/Lemtrada	Unknown	None known	Monitor
Alosetron	Lotronex	CYP1A2, CYP2C9, CYP3A4	None known	Monitor
Alprazolam	Xanax	CYP3A4	CBD may ↑ effects	Monitor for ↑ side effects of the drug. Use extreme caution with CBD.
Amantadine	Gocovri	OCT2	None known	Monitor
Amitriptyline	Elavil	CYP1A2, CYP2C19, CYP2C9, CYP3A4	None known	Potential for CBD to ↑ effects of amitriptyline
Amoxicillin	Moxatag	Unknown	None known	Monitor
Apixaban	Eliquis	CYP1A2, CYP2C19, CYP2C9, CYP3A4, P-gyp	None known	Monitor for increased bleeding.
Aprepitant	Emend	CYP1A2, CYP2C19, CYP2C9, CYP3A4	Aprepitant has the potential to ↑ the effects of CBD.	Monitor for ↑ the effects of CBD.
Aspirin	Multiple brands	CYP2C9	None known	Monitor
Atorvastatin	Lipitor	CYP3A4, P-gyp	None known	Monitor
Azathioprine	Azasan	Unknown	None known	Monitor
Baclofen	Lioresal, Gablofen	Unknown	May ↑ drug effect	Monitor for ↑ side effects of the drug. Use extreme caution with CBD.

(continued)

TABLE 7.4. Possible cannabis drug-drug interactions (continued)

Drug	Brand name	Metabolism pathway via the liver	Interaction with CBD	Notes
Benztropine mesylate	Cogentin	CYP2D6	None known	Monitor
Bictegravir/emtricitabine/tenofovir alafenamide	Biktarvy	P-gyp	None known	Monitor
Buprenorphine	Belbuca, Probuphine, Buprenex, and Butran	CYP3A4, CYP2A6	May ↑ drug effect	Monitor and consider dosage adjustments with concurrent use.
Buspirone HCl (Buspar)	Anxiolytic	CYP3A4, CYP2A6	May ↑ effect of buspirone	Monitor and consider dosage adjustments with concurrent use.
Carbamazepine	Tegretol, Equetro, and others	CYP3A4, CYP1A2	May ↑ drug effect	Monitor and consider dosage adjustments with concurrent use.
Carbidopa/levodopa	Duopa, Sinemet, Rytary	Unknown	None known	Monitor
Cefuroxime	Zinacef, Ceftin	Unknown	None known	Monitor
Celecoxib	Celebrex	CYP2C9, CYP3A4	None known	Monitor
Citalopram	Celexa	CYP2C19, CYP3A4	None known	Monitor for potential ↑ drug effect with CBD use.
Clonazepam	Klonopin	CYP3A4	CBD may ↑ effects.	Monitor for ↑ side effects of the drug. Use extreme caution with CBD.
Clopidogrel	Plavix	CYP2C19, CYP3A4	None known	Monitor for increased bleeding.
Cyclobenzaprine	Amrix, Fexmid	CYP1A2, CYP3A4	Potential for CBD to ↑ effects of cyclobenzaprine	Monitor and consider dosage adjustments with concurrent use.

TABLE 7.4. Possible cannabis drug-drug interactions *(continued)*

Drug	Brand name	Metabolism pathway via the liver	Interaction with CBD	Notes
Cyclophosphamide	Cytoxan	CYP2C19, CYP2C9, CYP3A4	None known	Available in tablets and IV Monitor
Cyclosporine	Restasis, Sandimmune	CYP3A4, P-gyp	Potential for CBD to ↑ cyclosporine	Monitor
Dabigatran etexilate	Pradaxa	P-Gyp	None known	Monitor for increased bleeding.
Dexamethasone	Ozurdex, Dex-Pak 6	CYP3A4, P-gyp	CBD has potential to ↑ effects of dexamethasone.	Monitor
Dextromethorphan	Multiple, including Tussin Cough (DM only), Scot-Tussin Diabetes CF, Robitussin ER, Tussin Maximum Strength	CYP2C19, CYP2C9, CYP3A4	Unknown	Monitor for potential ↑ drug effect with CBD use.
Diazepam	Valium	CYP1A2, CYP2C19, CYP3A4, CYP2C9	CBD may ↑ effects.	Monitor for ↑ side effects of the drug. Use extreme caution with CBD.
Dimethyl fumarate	Tecfidera	Unknown	None known	Monitor
Diphenoxylate and atropine	Lomotil	CYP1A2, CYP3A	None known	Potential for CBD to ↑ diphenoxylate and atropine. Monitor for increased drug effect.
Disulfiram	Antabuse	CYP1A2, CYP3A	None known	Interaction is clinically insignificant.
Dolutegravir/rilpivirine	Juluca	CYP3A4	None known	Monitor

(continued)

TABLE 7.4. Possible cannabis drug-drug interactions (*continued*)

Drug	Brand name	Metabolism pathway via the liver	Interaction with CBD	Notes
Donepezil	Aricept	CYP3A4	None known	
Doxycycline	Doxy-100, Oracea, Targadox	Unknown	None known	Monitor
Dronabinol	Marinol	CYP3A4 CYP2C9	CBD has the potential to ↓ the side effects from dronabinol but not the effectiveness.	Monitor
Duloxetine	Cymbalta	CYP1A2 CYP2D6	CBD may ↓ drug effect.	Monitor effect.
Edaravone	Radicava	Unknown	None known	Monitor for potential ↑ drug effect.
Efavirenz/emtricitabine/ tenofovir disoproxil fumarate	Atripla	CYP3A4 CYP2C19	CBD may ↑ effects.	Monitor for ↑ side effects of the drug. Use caution with CBD.
Eluxadoline	Viberzi, Truberzi	MULTIPLEMRP2, OAT3	None known	Monitor
Elvitegravir/cobicistat/ emtricitabine/tenofovir alafenamide	Genvoya	CYP3A4	Potential to ↑ the effects of CBD	Monitor for ↑ the effects of CBD. Consider dose reduction of CBD.
Elvitegravir/cobicistat/ emtricitabine/tenofovir disoproxil fumarate	Stribild	CYP3A4 CYP2D6	Potential to ↑ the effects of CBD	Monitor for ↑ the effects of CBD. Consider dose reduction of CBD.
Emtricitabine/rilpivirine/ tenofovir alafenamide	Odefsey	CYP3A4	None known	Monitor

TABLE 7.4. Possible cannabis drug-drug interactions (continued)

Drug	Brand name	Metabolism pathway via the liver	Interaction with CBD	Notes
Emtricitabine/rilpivirine/tenofovir disoproxil fumarate	Complera	CYP3A4	None known	Monitor
Entacapone	Comtan	CYP2A6	CBD may ↑ effects.	Monitor for potential ↑ drug effect with CBD use.
Escitalopram	Lexapro	CYP2C19 CYP3A4	None known	Monitor for potential ↑ drug effect with CBD use.
Eszopiclone	Lunesta	CYP3A4	None known	CBD has the potential to ↑ effects of eszopiclone. Monitor
Etanercept	Enbrel	Unknown	None known	Monitor
Fentanyl	Duragesic	CYP3A4	CBD may ↑ effects.	Monitor for ↑ side effects of the drug. Use caution with CBD.
Fingolimod	Gilenya	CYP3A4	None known	Monitor
Fluoxetine	Prozac	CYP1A2 CYP2C19 CYP2C9 CYP3A4	None known	Monitor for potential ↑ drug effect with CBD use.
Gabapentin	Neurontin	Unknown	Levels of gabapentin may ↑ with CBD.	Monitor
Galantamine	Razadyne	CYP3A4	None known	Monitor
Glatiramer acetate	Copaxone	Unknown	None known	Monitor
Granisetron	Sustol	CYP3A4	CBD has the potential to ↑ the effects of granisetron.	Monitor and use caution.
Haloperidol	Haldol	CYP1A2 CYP3A4	Potential for CBD to ↑ haloperidol.	Monitor

(continued)

TABLE 7.4. Possible cannabis drug-drug interactions (continued)

Drug	Brand name	Metabolism pathway via the liver	Interaction with CBD	Notes
Hydrocodone	Vicodin	CYP3A4	CBD has the potential to ↑ the effects of hydrocodone.	Monitor and use caution. The patient may be able to ↓ hydrocodone with CBD use.
Hydroxychloroquine	Plaquenil	Unknown	None known	Monitor
Hydroxyzine HCl (Vistaril)	Histamine	Unknown	May ↑ effect of hydroxyzine	Monitor
Ibuprofen	Advil, Motrin, many others	CYP2C19 CYP2C9	None known	
Infliximab	Remicade	Unknown	None known	Monitor
Isocarboxazid	Marplan	Monoamine Oxidase	Isocarboxazid may ↑ effects of CBD.	Monitor and consider CBD dose adjustments.
Levetiracetam	Roweepra, Keppra	Unknown	Potential for CBD to ↑ levetiracetam.	Potential for CBD to ↑ levetiracetam. Monitor for increased drug effect.
Linaclotide	Linzess	Unknown	None known	Monitor
Lorazepam	Ativan	Unknown	CBD may ↑ effects of lorazepam.	Use extreme caution with CBD.
Losartan	Cozaar	CYP2C9 CYP3A4	None known	Monitor
Lubiprostone	Amitiza	Unknown	None known	Monitor
Meloxicam	Mobic, Vivlodex	CYP2C9 CYP3A4	None known	Monitor
Mercaptopurine	Purixan	Unknown	None known	Monitor
Methadone	Diskets, Methadone Intensol, Methadone, and Dolophine	CYP2C19 CYP2C9 CYP3A4	CBD may ↑ drug effect of methadone.	Monitor and consider dosage adjustments with concurrent use.

TABLE 7.4. Possible cannabis drug-drug interactions (*continued*)

Drug	Brand name	Metabolism pathway via the liver	Interaction with CBD	Notes
Methotrexate	Otrexup, Xatmep, Trexall	P-GYP	None known	Monitor
Milnacipran (Novantrone)	Savella	Unknown	None known	Monitor
Mitoxantrone	Mitoxantrone	BCRP/ABCG2	None known	Monitor
Mycophenolate	CellCept, Myfortic	Multiple different pathways	None known	Monitor
Nabilone	Cesamet	Unknown	CBD has the potential to ↓ the side effects from nabilone but not the effectiveness.	Monitor
Naltrexone	Vivitrol, ReVia	Unknown	None known	Monitor
Naproxen	Aleve, Naprosyn, many others	CYP1A2 CYP2C9	None known	Monitor
Natalizumab	Tysabri	Unknown	None known	Monitor
Nortriptyline	Pamelor	CYP1A2 CYP2C19 CYP3A4	None known	Potential for CBD to ↑ effects of nortriptyline.
Ocrelizumab	Ocrevus	Unknown	None known	Monitor
Olanzapine	Zyprexa	CYP1A2	Potential for CBD to ↑ olanzapine	Monitor and consider dosage adjustments with concurrent use. Use with caution.
Ondansetron	Zofran	CYP1A2 CYP2C9 CYP3A4	CBD has the potential to ↑ the effects of ondansetron.	Monitor and use caution.

(continued)

TABLE 7.4. Possible cannabis drug-drug interactions (continued)

Drug	Brand name	Metabolism pathway via the liver	Interaction with CBD	Notes
Oxcarbazepine	Oxtellar XR, Trileptal	CYP3A4	None known	Monitor
Oxycodone	Roxicodone, Xtampza, Oxaydo	CYP3A4	CBD has the potential to ↑ the effects of oxycodone.	Monitor and use caution. The patient may be able to ↓ oxy-codone with CBD use.
Palonosetron	Aloxi	CYP1A2 CYP3A4	CBD has the potential to ↑ the effects of palonosetron.	Monitor and use caution.
Paroxetine	Paxil	CYP2D6	None known	Monitor for potential ↑ drug effects with CBD use.
Phenelzine	Nardil	Monoamine oxidase	Phenelzine may ↑ effects of CBD.	Monitor and consider CBD dose adjustments.
Pramipexole	Mirapex	Unknown	None known	Monitor
Prednisone	Deltasone, Rayos	CYP3A4	None known	Monitor
Pregabalin	Lyrica	Unknown	None known	Monitor for potential ↑ drug effects with CBD use.
Propranolol	Inderal LA or XL, Hemangeol	CYP1A2 CYP2C19 CYP3A4	None known	Monitor for ↓ od drug effect
Quetiapine	Seroquel XR and Seroquel	CYP3A4	May ↑ effect of quetiapine.	Monitor for ↑ drug effect. Use with caution.
Quinidine	Nuedexta	CYP2C9 CYP3A4 P-GYP	Unknown	Monitor for potential ↑ drug effects with CBD use.
Rifaximin	Xifaxan	S CYP3A4 P-GYP	None known	Monitor

TABLE 7.4. Possible cannabis drug-drug interactions *(continued)*

Drug	Brand name	Metabolism pathway via the liver	Interaction with CBD	Notes
Riluzole	Rilutek	CYP1A2	None known	Monitor for potential ↓ drug effects with CBD use.
Risperidone	Risperdal	CYP3A4 P-GYP	Potential for CBD to ↑ risperidone	Monitor and consider dose adjustments. Use with caution.
Rivastigmine	Exelon	Unknown	None known	Monitor
Rizatriptan	Maxalt	Unknown	None known	Monitor. May be combined with naproxen in Treximet
Ropinirole	Requip	CYP1A2 CYP3A4	CBD may ↓ drug effect.	Monitor for decreased drug effect.
Rosuvastatin	Crestor	CYP2C9 CYP3A4	None known	Monitor
Selegiline	Eldepryl, Zelapar	CYP1A2 CYP3A4	None known	Monitor
Sertraline	Zoloft	CYP2C19 CYP2C9 CYP3A4	None known	Monitor for potential ↑ drug effect with CBD use.
Siponimod	Mayzent	CYP3A4	None known	Monitor
Sumatriptan	Imitrex and several other brands	Unknown	None known	Monitor
Temazepam	Restoril	CYP2C19 CYP2C9 CYP3A4	None known	CBD has the potential to ↑ effects of temazepam. Monitor
Teriflunomide	Aubagio	CYP1A2	None known	Monitor
Tetrabenazine	Xenazine	CYP2D6	CBD may ↑ increase tetrabenazine.	Monitor

(continued)

TABLE 7.4. Possible cannabis drug-drug interactions (continued)

Drug	Brand name	Metabolism pathway via the liver	Interaction with CBD	Notes
Tolcapone	Tasmar	COMT	Levels of tolcapone may ↑ with CBD.	Monitor for ↑ side effects.
Topiramate	Trokendi XR, Qudexy XR, Topamax	Unknown	Levels of topiramate may ↑ with CBD.	Monitor for ↑ side effects.
Tramadol	Ultram	CYP3A4	None known	CBD may ↑ effects of tramadol. Monitor
Tranylcypromine	Parnate	CYP2A6	Tranylcypromine may ↑ effects of CBD.	Monitor and consider CBD dose adjustments.
Trazodone	Desyrel	CYP3A4 CYP2D6	Unknown	CBD has the potential to ↑ the effects of trazadone.
Trihexyphenidyl	Artane	Unknown	None known	Monitor
Venlafaxine	Effexor	CYP2C19 CYP2C9 CYP3A4 CYP2D6n	None known	Potential for CBD to ↑ venlafaxine.
Warfarin	Coumadin	CYP1A2 CYP2C19 CYP2C9 CYP3A4	CBD may ↑ effects.	Monitor for ↑ side effects of the drug. Use extreme caution with CBD. Potential increased risk for bleeding
Zolpidem	Ambien	CYP1A2 CYP2C19 CYP2C9 CYP3A4	None known	CBD has the potential to ↑ effects of zolpidem. Monitor

CBD, cannabidiol.
↑, increase; ↓, decrease.

establish those routes well. This is not an exhaustive list. Consult a clinical drug information resource or a knowledgeable cannabis healthcare provider who can review medications before starting cannabis therapy, and continue to monitor the patient for the duration of treatment (Wolters Kluwer Clinical Drug Information, 2019).

Important Safety Considerations

According to Byars et al. (2019), certain testing elements should be performed before purchasing any cannabis products. In California-licensed state dispensaries, all products sold must go through testing for potency, pesticides, bacteria, residual solvents, heavy metals, and mycotoxins, as well as for moisture and water activity. The testing parameters for cannabis are determined by each state, and the testing standards information is available through the state's cannabis regulatory board. Third-party testing provides the consumers with the verification they need to be assured that they are consuming a quality product.

CBD that is sold on the internet is not subject to regulatory oversight at this time and may not be tested. In 2017, the *Journal of American Medical Association* (JAMA) released a study that demonstrated 70% of CBD products were mislabeled (Bonn-Miller et al., 2017). The study analyzed various CBD products, such as vaporizer cartridges and tinctures. Of the 70% of mislabeled CBD concentrations in these products, 42% contained more CBD than advertised, and 26% contained less CBD than advertised. It is best to purchase CBD products from a state-licensed dispensary, where they are likely tested and regulated. Check your state, county, and city medical cannabis regulatory boards to locate a licensed dispensary and/or delivery service. Nonlicensed dispensary and/or delivery services should be avoided. If the patient lives in a state or an area where they cannot access CBD or cannabis from a licensed state dispensary, be sure that if they purchase CBD online it has been third-party tested for potency, pesticides, bacteria, residual solvents, heavy metals, mycotoxins, and moisture and water content.

CONCLUSION

Despite the cannabis plant being used for thousands of years by humans, it is relatively new as a medicine. Over the past eight decades, cannabis has been prohibited in the United States, which has stifled our ability to study the medicinal effects of cannabinoids in humans. The discovery of the ECS has led to the science of cannabis medicine. The body of evidence will only continue to grow, and if cannabis is rescheduled or descheduled in the United States, it will open up the flood gates. APRNs are not yet required to learn about cannabinoid sciences. However, as the demand for patient education increases, APRNs who do not know about the ECS, cannabinoids, potential drug-drug interactions, routes of administration, and clinical implications will find themselves unable to answer their patients' questions and provide them with the kind of supportive care they need through coaching and education. As APRNs, we must be ready to address patients' concerns and provide them with the education that helps reduce risks and improves outcomes. If nurses are not educated on cannabis, patients will receive misinformation from the public. Supporting the patients' choice to incorporate cannabis into their regimen will not only help reduce harm, but it also has the potential to improve quality of life with minimal side effects.

Q&A QUESTIONS

1. When assessing a patient with chronic pain who is interested in adding cannabis into the regimen, the clinician knows it is important to include additional quality-of-life factors such as:
   A. Diet, exercise regimen, alcohol intake.
   B. Sleep duration and quality, anxiety, depression, and cannabis experience.
   C. Marital status, recent life changes, and diet.
   D. Mood, sleep, tobacco use.

2. In looking at different routes of administration for chronic pain, the clinician knows if the patient is noncompliant with taking multiple doses, the most effective route may be:
   A. Inhalation.
   B. Suppository.
   C. Edibles.
   D. Transdermal patches.

3. When monitoring a patient with depression who has been consuming Δ-9-THC for symptom relief, which of the following indicates a need to stop the cannabis:
   A. Worsening depression
   B. Decreased alcohol intake
   C. Improved mood
   D. Exercise intolerance

4. Regulating our ECS through CB1 and CB2 activation with cannabinoids has shown to play a role in the management of anxiety- and fear-related behaviors. Which other receptors can cannabinoids activate to help regulate anxiety and fear?
   A. CB3 and GPR55
   B. CB2 and dopamine
   C. 5-HT1A and TRPV1
   D. TRPV8 and GABA

5. When determining an appropriate cannabinoid profile for a patient with insomnia, the clinician knows the following cannabinoid is the least likely to assist with sleep:
   A. Δ-9-THC
   B. CBD
   C. Dronabinol
   D. CBN

6. When assessing for potential drug-drug interactions, the clinician knows the following route is the most likely to cause an interaction:
   A. Inhalation
   B. Ingesting
   C. Transdermal
   D. Rectal

7. When looking for a cannabis product, the clinician knows to educate the patient on which of the following safety considerations of third-party testing that includes:
   A. Residual solvent, heavy metals, mycotoxins, potency, and pesticides.
   B. Alcohol content, heavy metals, molds, and fungus.
   C. Potency, serving size, and mycotoxins.
   D. Cannabinoid content, glycophosphate levels, and mineral content.

ANSWERS

1. **Answer: B.** Sleep duration and quality, anxiety, depression, and cannabis experience
2. **Answer: D.** Transdermal patches
3. **Answer: A.** Worsening depression
4. **Answer: C.** 5-HT1A and TRPV1
5. **Answer: D.** CBN
6. **Answer: B.** Ingesting
7. **Answer: A.** Residual solvent, heavy metals, mycotoxins, potency, and pesticides

References

American Academy of Sleep Medicine. (n.d.) *Insomnia provider fact sheet*. https://j2vjt3dnbra3ps7ll1cl-b4q2-wpengine.netdna-ssl.com/wp-content/uploads/2019/03/ProviderFS_Insomnia_18.pdf

American Association of Nurse Practitioners. (2018). *State practice environment*. https://www.aanp.org/practice/practice-information-by-state

American Association of Nurse Practitioners. (n.d.). *U.S. Department of veterans affairs final rule*. https://www.aanp.org/advocacy/recent-legislative-changes/u-s-department-of-veterans-affairs-final-rule

American Cannabis Nurses Association. (2019). *Scope and standards of practice*. www.cannabisnurses.org

American Nurses Association. (2015). *Scope and standards of practice* (3rd ed.). Author.

American Nurses Association. (2016). *Position statement: Therapeutic use of marijuana and related cannabinoids*. https://www.nursingworld.org/~49a8c8/globalassets/practiceandpolicy/ethics/therapeutic-use-of-marijuana-and-related-cannabinoids-position-statement.pdf

American Psychiatric Association. (2013). *Diagnostic and statistical manual of mental disorders* (5th ed.). Author.

Bailey, K., McMullen, L., Lubejko, B., Christensen, D., Haylock, P. J., Rose, T., Sellers, J., & Srdanovic, D. (2018). Nurse navigator core competencies. *Clinical Journal of Oncology Nurses, 22*(3), 272–281. https://doi.org/10.1188/18.CJON.272-281

Bhattacharyya, S., & Sendt, K. V. (2012). Neuroimaging evidence for cannabinoid modulation of cognition and affect in man. *Frontiers in Behavioral Neuroscience, 6*(22), 272. https://doi.org/10.3389/fnbeh.2012.00022

Billioti de Gage, S. (2012). Benzodiazepine use and risk of dementia: Prospective population based study. *British Medical Journal, 345*, e6231. https://doi.org/10.1136/bmj.e6231

Blessing, E. M., Steenkamp, M. M., Manzanares, J., & Marmar, C. R. (2015). Cannabidiol as a potential treatment for anxiety disorders. *Neurotherapeutics, 12*(4), 825–836. https://doi.org/10.1007/s13311-015-0387-1

Boatwright, K. D., & Sperry, M. L. (2018). Accuracy of medical marijuana claims made by popular websites. *Journal of Pharmacy Practice, 12*, 825. https://doi.org/10.1177/0897190018818907

Bonn-Miller, M. O., Loflin, M. J. E., Thomas, B. F., Marcu, J. P., Hyke, T., & Vandrey, R. (2017). Labeling accuracy of cannabidiol extracts sold online. *Journal of the American Medical Association, 318*(17), 1708–1709. https://doi.org/10.1001/jama.2017.11909

Brusberg, M., Arvidsson, S., Kang, D., Larsson, H., Lindström, E., & Martinez, V. (2009). PPAR and pain and cb1 receptors mediate the analgesic effects of cannabinoids on colorectal distension-induced visceral pain in rodents. *Journal of Neurosciences, 29*(5), 1554–1564. https://doi.org/10.1523/JNEUROSCI.5166-08.2009

Byars, T., Theisen, E., & Bolton, D. (2019). Using cannabis to treat cancer-related pain. *Seminars in Oncology Nursing, 35*(3), 300–309. https://doi.org/10.1016/j.soncn.2019.04.012

Campbell, F. A., Tramer, M. R., Carroll, D., Reynolds, D. J., Moore, R. A., & McQuay, H. J. (2001). Are cannabinoids an effective and safe treatment option in the management of pain. *British Medical Journal, 323*(7303), 13–16. https://doi.org/10.1136/bmj.323.7303.13

Center for Disease Control and Prevention. (2016). *CDC guidelines for prescribing opioids for chronic pain.* https://www.cdc.gov/drugoverdose/prescribing/guideline.html

Compassionate Use Act. (1996). *Prop 215.* https://leginfo.legislature.ca.gov/faces/codes_displaySection.xhtml?sectionNum=11362.5.&lawCode=HSC

Di Forti, M., Quattrone, D., Freeman, T. P., Tripoli, G., Gayer-Anderson, C., & Quigley, H. (2019). The contribution of cannabis use to variation in the incidence of psychotic disorder across Europe (EU-GEI): A multicenter case-control study. *The Lancet Psychiatry, 6*(5), 427–436. https://doi.org/10.1016/S2215-0366(19)30048-3

Drug Enforcement Agency. (n.d.). *Drug scheduling.* https://www.dea.gov/drug-scheduling

Grotenhermen, F. (2003). Pharmacokinetics and pharmacodynamics of cannabinoids. *Clinical Pharmacokinetics, 42*(4), 327–360. https://doi.org/10.2165/00003088-200342040-00003

GW Pharmaceuticals. (n.d.). *Healthcare professionals: Sativex.* https://www.gwpharm.com/healthcare-professionals/sativex

Herkenham, M., Lynn, A. B., Little, M. D., Johnson, M. R., Melvin, L. S., de Costa, B. R., & Rice, K. C. (1990). Cannabinoid receptor localization in brain. *Proceedings of the National Academy of Sciences of the United States of America, 87*(5), 1932–1936. https://doi.org/10.1073/pnas.87.5.1932

Ibarra-Lecue, I., Pilar-Cuellar, F., Muguruza, C., Florensa-Zanuy, E., Diaz, A., & Callado, A. F. (2018). The endocannabinoid system in mental disorders: Evidence from human brain studies. *Biochemical Pharmacology, 157*, 97–107. https://doi.org/10.1016/j.bcp.2018.07.009

Iuvone, T., Esposito, G., De Filippis, D., Scuderi, C., & Steardo, L. (2009). Cannabidiol: A promising drug for neurodegenerative disorders. *CNS Neuroscience Therapeutics, 15*(1), 65–75. https://doi.org/10.1111/j.1755-5949.2008.00065

Jhaveri, M. D., Sagar, D. R., Elmes, S. J., Kendall, D. A., & Chapman, V. (2007). Cannabinoid CB2 receptor-mediated anti-nociception in models of acute and chronic pain. *Molecular Neurobiology, 36*(1), 26–35. https://doi.org/10.1007/s12035-007-8007-7

Johannes, C. B., Le, T. K., Zhou, X., Johnston, J. A., & Dworkin, R. H. (2010). The prevalence of chronic pain in the united states adults: results of an internet-based survey. *Journal of Pain, 11*(11), 1230–1239. https://doi.org/10.1016/j.jpain.2010.07.002

Kathmann, M., Flau, K., Redmer, A., Tränkle, C., & Schlicker, E. (2006). Cannabidiol is an allosteric modulator at mu-and delta-opioid receptors. *Pharmacology, 372*(5), 354–361. https://doi.org/10.1007/s00210-006-0033-x

Kavan, M. G., Elsasser, G. N., & Eugene, J. B. (2009). Generalized anxiety disorder: Practical assessment and management. *American Family Physician, 79*(9), 785–791. https://www.aafp.org/afp/2009/0501/p785.html

Maher, R. L., Hanlon, J., & Hajjar, E. R. (2014). Clinical consequences of polypharmacy in elderly. *Expert Opinion on Drug Safety, 13*(1), 57–65. https://doi.org/0.1517/14740338.2013.827660.

Marijuana Policy Project. (2019). *Minnesota: Legislature fails to act on bills to legalize and regulate cannabis.* https://www.mpp.org/states/minnesota/

Minnesota Department of Health. (n.d.). *Medical cannabis qualifying conditions.* https://www.health.state .mn.us/people/cannabis/patients/conditions.html

National Academy of Sciences, Engineering, and Medicine. (2017). *The health effects of cannabis and cannabinoids: The current state of evidence and recommendations for research.* The National Academies Press.

National Alliance on Mental Illness. (2017a). *Anxiety.* https://www.nami.org/Learn-More/Mental-Health-Conditions/Anxiety-Disorders

National Alliance on Mental Illness. (2017b). *Depression.* https://www.nami.org/Learn-More/Mental-Health-Conditions/Depression/Treatment

National Council of State Boards of Nursing. (2018). Part I: current legislation, scientific literature review, and nursing implications. *Journal of Nursing Regulation, 9*(2), S6–S21. https://doi.org/10.1016/s2155-8256(18)30083-8

National Organization for the Reform of Marijuana Laws. (n.d.). *State laws.* https://norml.org/laws

Newmeyer, M. N., Swortwood, M. J., Barnes, A. J., Abulseoud, O. A., Scheidweiler, K. B., & Huestis, M. A. (2016). Free and glucuronide whole blood cannabinoids' pharmacokinetics after controlled smoked, vaporized, and oral cannabis administration in frequent and occasional cannabis users: Identification of recent cannabis intake. *Clinical Chemistry, 62*(12), 1579–1592. https://doi.org/10.1373/clinchem.2016.263475

Owens, S. M., McBay, A. J., Reisner, H. M., & Perez-Reyes, M. (1981). 125I radioimmunoassay of delta-9-tetrahydrocannabinol in blood and plasma with a solid-phase second-antibody separation method. *Clinical Chemistry, 27*(4), 619–624. https://doi.org/10.1093/clinchem/27.4.619

Pertwee, R. G. (2001). Cannabinoid receptors and pain. *Programmed Neurobiology, 63*(5), 569–611. https://doi.org/10.1016/s0301-0082(00)00031-9

Resstel, L. B. M., Tavares, R. F., Lisboa, S. F. S., Smia, R., Correa, F. M. A., & Guimaraes, F. S. (2009). 5-HT 1A receptors are involved in the cannabidiol-induced attenuation of behavioural and cardiovascular responses to acute restraint stress in rats. *British Journal of Pharmacology, 156*(1), 181–188. https://doi.org/10.1111/j.1476-5381.2008.00046.x

Russo, E. B. (2017). Cannabidiol claims and misconceptions. *Trends in Pharmacological Sciences, 38*(3), 198–201. https://doi.org/10.1016/j.tips.2016.12.004

Russo, E. B., & Marcu, J. (2017). Cannabis pharmacology: The usual suspects and a few promising leads. *Advanced Pharmacology, 80*, 67–134. https://doi.org/10.1016/bs.apha.2017.03.004

Schoedel, K. A., Szeto, I., Setnik, B., Sellers, E. M., Levy-Cooperman, N., Mills, C., Etges, T., & Sommerville, K. (2018). Abuse potential assessment of cannabidiol (CBD) in recreational polydrug users: A randomized, double-blind, controlled trial. *Epilepsy & Behavior, 88*, 162–171. https://doi.org/10.1016/j .yebeh.2018.07.027

Schutte-Rodin, S., Broch, L., Buysse, D., Dorsey, C., & Sateia, M. (2008). Clinical guidelines for the evaluation and management of chronic insomnia in adults. *Journal of Clinical Sleep Medicine, 4*(5), 487–504. https://doi.org/10.5664/jcsm.27286

Schwope, D. M., Karschner, E. L., Gorelick, D. A., & Huestis, M. A. (2011). Identification of recent cannabis use: Whole-blood and plasma free and glucuronidated cannabinoid pharmacokinetics following controlled smoked cannabis administration. *Clinical Chemistry, 57*(10), 1406–1414. https://doi.org/10.1373/clinchem.2011.171777

Sexton, M. L., Cuttler, C., Finnell, J. S., & Mischley, L. K. (2016). A cross sectional survey of medical cannabis users: Patterns of use and perceived efficacy. *Cannabis and Cannabinoid Research, 1*(1), 131–138. https://doi.org/10.1089/can.2016.0007

Shannon, S., Lewis, N., Lee, H., & Hughes, S. (2019). Cannabidiol in anxiety and sleep: A large case series. *The Permanente Journal, 23*, 18–41. https://doi.org/10.7812/TPP/18-041

Spetz, J. (2019). *California's nurse practitioners: How scope of practice laws impact care. California Health Care Foundation Publication.* https://www.chcf.org/publication/californias-nurse-practitioners/

Spitzer, R. L. (1999). *Patient health questionnaire: PHQ.* New York State Psychiatric Institute.

Tagen, M. (2016). *How your genes affect your cannabis high-the case of the CYP2C9 [Blog post]*. http://profofpot.com/genetic-polymorphism-cyp2c9/

Tagen, M. (2018a). *Cannabinol (CBN)-the sedative that isn't? [Blog post]*. https://profofpot.com/cannabinol-cbn-sedative/

Tagen, M. (2018b). *Psychosis risk of THC is determined by your genetics [Blog post]*. http://profofpot.com/genetics-thc-psychosis/

U.S. Department of Justice, Office of Public Affairs. (2009). *Attorney general announces formal medical marijuana guidelines*. https://www.justice.gov/opa/pr/attorney-general-announces-formal-medical-marijuana-guidelines

Wilsey, B., Marcotte, T. D., Deutsch, R., Zhao, H., Prasad, H., & Phan, A. (2016). An exploratory human laboratory experiment evaluating vaporized cannabis in the treatment of neuropathic pain from spinal cord injury and disease. *Journal of Pain, 17*(9), 982–1000. https://doi.org/10.1016/j.jpain.2016.05.010

Wolters Kluwer. (2019). *Wolters Kluwer clinical drug information*. Author.

Zendulka, O., Dovrtelova, G., Noskova, K., Turjap, M., Sulcova, A., Hanus, L., & Jurica, J. (2016). Cannabinoids and cytochrome P450 interactions. *Current Drug Metabolism, 17*(3), 206–226. https://doi.org/10.2174/1389200217666151210142051

8

Legal, Ethical, and Advocacy Concerns: Cannabis From the Federal to State Level

Carey S. Clark, PhD, RN, AHN-BC, RYT, FAAN

CONCEPTS AND CONSIDERATIONS

This chapter on cannabis care ethics, legal issues, and advocacy concerns is essential to building your general cannabis care knowledge. Nursing is consistently noted to be the most ethical of all professions, and there is, of course, a need for applying ethical concepts when working with cannabis patients, particularly given the federal status of cannabis and the issues many advocates and patients face as the nation emerges from the cannabis prohibition era and progresses toward the cannabis regulation era. The National Council of States Boards of Nursing (NCSBN, 2018), as part of its six essential areas of knowledge, called upon nurses to:

- Have a working knowledge of the current state of legalization of medical and recreational cannabis use.
- Have a working knowledge of their jurisdiction's medical marijuana program (MMP).

Many nurses may not have considered what they need to know in order to best support patients' access to safe, tested medical-grade cannabis, and how the legal status of the plant impacts this process. In states where cannabis is not legal, patients have been known to risk their freedom in order to have access to the healing cannabis plant: Historically, many people have been prosecuted for possessing or growing cannabis for healing. Meanwhile, because cannabis is legal in some states and not others, patients have been known to cross state lines to access cannabis and illegally transport the cannabinoid plant products across state lines (which is technically a federal drug trafficking crime). Many people remain imprisoned for the crime of possessing cannabis, although cannabis is now legal (on some level) in the states where they were prosecuted. In both prohibition and legal-regulation states, people are still being prosecuted for possessing cannabis, with their sentencing often being based on the zip code of where they stood when they were apprehended. We need to answer the looming question of how we can, as nurses, help to address some of these social justice issues.

It is imperative that the nurse's work with cannabis care patients be grounded in an ethical base. It is not enough to know that nurses are ethical and to acknowledge when we are faced with ethical dilemmas: We have to be able to link these issues to ethical concepts and use a standardized process to support our ethical decision-making processes.

Learning Outcomes

Upon completion of this chapter, the learners will:

- Be able to explore their state-level medical cannabis laws.
- Apply ethics to guide cannabis care practice.
- Reflect on social justice issues related to the end of cannabis prohibition and the beginning of the cannabis regulation era.
- Understand the legal implications for nurses providing cannabis care.
- Review the nurse's cannabis care advocacy process.

FROM GLOBAL TO STATE LEVEL: CANNABIS LEGAL ISSUES

The NCSBN (2018) report called for nurses to know their state "MMP." This can be challenging, because each state's rules, regulations, and processes all differ to a great degree. Additionally, these laws change frequently. To understand the state-level concerns, a brief overview of the current global and federal-level legal statuses of cannabis should first be considered.

Global Legal Issues

The United Nations Single Convention on Narcotic Drugs (ratified in 1961), the Convention on Psychotropic Substances (1971), and the Convention Against Illicit Traffic in Narcotic Drugs and Psychotropic Substances (1988) all served to keep cannabis manufacturing and distribution on the black market, unregulated, and illicit for many years. Adult use or recreational use of cannabis in most countries remains illegal, with penalties ranging from minor violations for possession (similar to a traffic ticket) in countries that have decriminalized cannabis to years of imprisonment in countries that strictly enforce prohibition.

After many decades of global prohibition of cannabis, many countries are coming onboard with the movement toward ending prohibition and regulating cannabis, thereby making it available for medical and/or adult use and, in some cases, available for exportation to other countries. Canada and Uruguay have fully "legalized" (or perhaps legally regulated is a better term) cannabis, and other countries like the Netherlands and Spain tolerate cannabis sales at certain licensed businesses ("cafes"). At the time of publication of this text, medical cannabis is currently legal in Argentina, Australia, Canada, Chile, Colombia, Croatia, Cyprus, Germany, Greece, Israel, Italy, Jamaica, Lithuania, Luxembourg, North Macedonia, Norway, The Netherlands, New Zealand, Peru, Poland, Switzerland, Thailand, and the United Kingdom. Note that this list will change rapidly because many countries are paving the way toward legalization/regulation. Other countries like Paraguay, Portugal, and Slovenia have decriminalized cannabis. The United States has legal cannabis in various states, although it remains federally illegal.

The implications for legalizing cannabis on a larger scale are enormous. In addition to helping to ensure people have access to safe, tested, and labeled medicines, legalization or regulation could allow for better research processes, development of new cannabinoid therapeutics, and evolution of new global business, trade, and revenue streams. According to Forbes (Kovacevich, 2018), the legalized cannabis industry is set to reach a global economy of approximately 146 billion dollars by the year 2025.

For nurses, as the global landscape shifts, it's important to consider the implications of this movement for patients, particularly around cost, quality, and access. Although there are sure to be many benefits for patients as we move into the regulation era, there may be some drawbacks as well, mainly related to affordable access to quality medicines and the ability to grow one's own medicine. There is a small danger that as cannabis becomes part of the legitimate global economy, the plant gets treated more like tobacco or alcohol, and this could have grave implications for ensuring that its medical potency and natural herbal remedy status is preserved, even if it becomes mass produced or otherwise manipulated for majority population consumption.

FEDERAL LEGAL ISSUES

The NCSBN (2018) report stated that all nursing students should be educated around the "MMP" in their states and be aware of the related federal-level issues. NCSBN stated that the surge in cannabis legalization has outpaced the research related to direct cannabis patient care because of the federal schedule I issues and the restrictions this has created. This can be concerning because public health and evidence-based research inform much needed related policy development.

Additionally, cannabis as a therapeutic agent has not been reviewed or approved by the Federal Drug Administration (FDA), and it is not subject to quality control and safety measures on a federal level. (Some states such as California may require mandatory lab testing of products to be sold to consumers, but this does not address issues with potential black-market products.) Schedule I medications are categorized as such because they have "no accepted medical value" and present at high rates of potential for abuse. Although many cannabis advocates believe that there is enough generation of evidence related to the medical value of cannabis (see Chapter 5 around the current levels of evidence), at the time of publication, cannabis remains a Schedule I drug and is still very hard to study in America, particularly with the "gold-standard" approach of using randomized controlled clinical trials. The process of trying to obtain cannabis for use in controlled studies or federally funded research studies is very challenging. In the year 2020, only one source of cannabis, known for its poor quality and low tetrahydrocannabinol (THC) percentage, can be used for such studies (NCSBN, 2018). At the time of this publication, there is a Drug Enforcement Agency (DEA) pending process regarding how federally funded researchers may grow or source their cannabis supply. Historically, the federal government has been in no measurable way supportive of the United States developing a robust research program around medicinal cannabis benefits, impacts, adverse effects, and policy development. This puts us behind other countries, such as Israel, that are leading the way in developing cannabis/cannabinoid therapeutics.

Although cannabis remains federally illegal at the time of this publication, during 2009–2014 the US Attorney General on multiple occasions via department of justice position papers took a stance that discouraged the federal government from prosecuting people who are using or distributing medical cannabis in alignment with their state laws. However, this stance was changed in 2018, when the US Attorney General took a bit broader stance: Instead of clearly supporting state's rights, federal prosecutors are to focus on weighing relevant considerations, the seriousness of the crime, the potential deterrent effects of prosecuting, and the community impact of the crimes (NCSBN, 2018).

Even as more states come on board with legalization efforts, as of 2020, there were several efforts to move cannabis out of schedule I status at the federal level as well as some to help support cannabis science research, including:

- The 2019 Marijuana Opportunity Reinvestment and Expungement (MORE) Act, HR 3384: removes cannabis from the controlled substances act, provides funding through social equity programs for people and communities impacted by prohibition and the war on drugs, repeals immigration-related penalties for cannabis offenses, and provides for resentencing and expunging of federal records for those with cannabis convictions. This act is unique in that it includes aspects of social and racial justice.
- Ending Federal Marijuana Prohibition Act, HR 2012: amend the controlled substances act to provide that federal law shall not preempt state law.
- Regulate Marijuana Like Alcohol Act, HR 420: regulate cannabis products like alcohol.
- Marijuana Justice Act of 2017, S507 and HR 1456: amend the controlled substances act by removing all marijuana and cannabinoid language.
- VA Medical Cannabis Research Act of 2019, S179 and HR 712: To direct the Secretary of Veterans Affairs to carry out clinical trials regarding the effects of cannabis on chronic pain and posttraumatic stress disorder (PTSD).
- Medical Cannabis Research Act of 2019, HR 601: (as mentioned previously) to increase the number of manufacturers registered in the controlled substances act, so that medical-grade cannabis can be manufactured for research purposes and allow for providers at the Department of Veterans Affairs to provide recommendations to veterans to participate in federally approved cannabis clinical trials and for other medical purposes.

While there is a lot going on at the federal level, movement forward seems to be potentially restrained by lingering stigma, lack of research, poor involvement with policy development, and likely competing political lobbying groups who may lose some financial standing if cannabis is removed from the controlled substances act or de-scheduled.

STATE-LEVEL REGULATION

In some states, the people have voted in medical cannabis access for their qualifying populations, and in other states, the legislature has decided to create laws around medicinal cannabis use. Before I speak about cannabis care to nurses in various states,

I usually look up the specific state laws and strive to share the pertinent information with the audience: where nurses and patients can access the laws and regulations, what conditions qualify for medical cannabis in that state, what the basic process for getting a recommendation looks like, and how patients who have medical cannabis recommendations can access their medicine (grow their own, buy from a dispensary, have a third party "caregiver" grow for them, etc.).

States can change the status of cannabis legality "on a dime," so efforts to list here specific state regulations may prove futile, as surely laws will change before the text even becomes available. At the time of this writing, in 2020, 33 states and Washington, DC have some form of law related to the cannabis legalization process. Eleven states and DC, Guam, Puerto Rico, and the Virgin Islands have adopted laws related to adult legal use. When looking to get a briefing on the status of cannabis across various states, some useful websites are available that support a broad overview. Still, to really get to know your state's medical cannabis laws, you must do a search for the laws in your state by typing in the state name, "marijuana," law. Your state legislative websites should also have information about the cannabis laws in your state.

National Conference of State Legislators

The National Council of State Legislators (NCSL) maintains a website that is up-dated with the most recent state medical cannabis laws. It provides an overview of which states have a full medical cannabis program and which ones have partial or low tetrahydrocannabinol/cannabidiol (THC/CBD) programs. It is updated fre-quently. This website includes links to the actual laws that will help the nurse in their quest to understand the parameters around which their patients can use med-ical cannabis in their states (http://www.ncsl.org/research/health/state-medical-marijuana-laws.aspx).

National Organization for the Reform of Marijuana Laws

National Organization for the Reform of Marijuana Laws (NORML) was founded in 1970 as a nonprofit public policy advocacy group striving to provide a voice in the public policy debate regarding the ongoing prohibition of cannabis. NORML lobbies state and federal legislators to create change in policy and also acts as a clear-inghouse of information and publisher of newsletters, while it creates a platform for activists to interact and engage. "NORML's mission is to move public opinion sufficiently to legalize the responsible use of marijuana by adults, and to serve as an advocate for consumers to assure they have access to high-quality marijuana that is safe, convenient and affordable" (National Organization for the Reform of Marijuana Laws [NORML], 2019). The NORML Foundation is its secondary orga-nization that focuses on educating the public on cannabis policy, providing legal as-sistance to victims of cannabis prohibition and focusing on relevant cannabis policy research (NORML, 2019).

On the NORML webpage, one can click on a link labeled as state info (https://norml.org/states), where a broad overview of state issues may be found. After you have chosen your state of interest, you are then linked to a variety of information. The state laws tab focuses on legal issues and penalties. Additionally, there is information about the congressional representatives for the state and their stance on cannabis reform. This information can be important if you are preparing to support the medical cannabis movement in your state.

Marijuana Policy Project

The Marijuana Policy Project (MPP) is an organization that is committed to creating change in cannabis policy; their main mission is to support state-level policy change while also calling for shifts in federal policy that allow for medical cannabis use to be legal in all states and for cannabis to be regulated for adult use in the same ways that alcohol is. MPP claims responsibility for changing most of the state-level cannabis laws since the year 2000. Although the idea of regulating cannabis like alcohol is unappealing for many reasons (namely, the potential impact related to medicinal cannabis use), MPP does offer some excellent resources around learning about the policy change process and the current laws and regulations within any given state. They are also committed to supporting efforts to enact medical cannabis laws in states where access for patients is still illegal.

By visiting the following link, one can see an overview of the current legal status of cannabis in any given state: https://www.mpp.org/states/. By clicking on any given state, one can be linked to the most recent legislative efforts within that state, and on the far right side of the page, there is a summary of some of the current cannabis laws for that state. For example, even though Colorado is known to be the first adult-use state, it continues to have changes in legislation. In the spring of 2019, the state enacted some new cannabis regulations, allowing for the following:

- Home delivery of cannabis, if it aligns with city/county ordinances (HB 1234).
- Hotels or restaurants to be able to set aside cannabis consumption zones and sell small amounts of cannabis for personal consumption as city/county ordinances allow (HB 1230).
- Capital investment in cannabis companies or business from publicly traded companies (HB 1090).
- Patients may register to use medical cannabis for any condition for which they would be prescribed opiates (SB 13).
- Pediatric patients can be certified for medical cannabis use by any physician (before this law, pediatric patients could be certified for medical cannabis use only by certain specialty physicians) (SB 13).

The webpage also provides links to the actual language included in the bills or laws and this is helpful for any person exploring the current situation of the medical and adult-use cannabis laws in their state.

Getting to know your state medical cannabis laws and regulations is an important and complex step in supporting patients with safely and legally gaining access to medicinal cannabis. The NCSBN (2018) calling for all nursing students to have this knowledge serves to underscore the importance.

As we approach the end of the prohibition era and move into the era of regulation of cannabis, in addition to legal concerns, the nurse should also be aware of the many ethical concerns that may arise.

> ### APPLIED LEARNING
>
> **Medical Marijuana Programs**
>
> Cannabis care nurses must have knowledge of their state "MMP" and both state- and federal-level legislation. Cannabis care nurses must have ways to have input on how these programs impact patients' abilities to access safe, affordable, and high-quality cannabinoid medicine. How does your state MMP impact patient access? Explore social media and other online sources for stories about patients' medical cannabis access in your state or a legal state near you if you live in a cannabis prohibition state.

ETHICAL CONCERNS

This section will help you understand how ethical concepts can guide a nurse's medicinal cannabis care practices. Nursing is consistently viewed as the most ethical of all professions. When it comes to working with cannabis care patients, and/or within the medicinal cannabis industry, nurses must remain guided and supported by ethical concepts. Nurses are expected to recognize ethical dilemmas, take appropriate action when warranted, inform client/staff members of ethical concerns that may impact the care given, follow the code of ethics for registered nurses, and evaluate outcomes of interventions intended to promote an ethical nursing practice. Cannabis care nurses hold the same ethical obligations when caring for medicinal cannabis patients, and they must apply a process to ensure that ethical concerns and challenges are well managed.

Ethical Problem-Solving Process

When faced with an ethical dilemma regarding a cannabis care patient, a clear and well-defined approach should be used to best address the issue.

- The problem must be defined in consideration of the specific circumstances.
- Data should be collected and analyzed regarding the ethical issue and in consideration of the *Code of ethics for nurses with interpretive statements* (American Nurses Association [ANA], 2015), evidence-based approaches, the published literature, and standards of practice. Nurses should consider which specific ethical principles are being violated, and they should be able to clearly articulate these principles.
- Generation of all possible solutions to the ethical concerns. This should include the probability of specific outcomes and implications of each possible solution.
- The best possible solution should be selected and implemented.
- Evaluate results.

This approach seems to align with the nursing process, and it can be used to both help the nurse make the best ethically sound decisions for those they serve and to protect their license. Nurses should become familiar with their hospital policies and procedures around approaching ethics committees when ethical issues seem to be complicated, ethical decision-making is at a standstill, and/or perhaps the delay in making a decision is creating harm to the patient or his or her family/significant others/caregivers. This remains true when caring for medical cannabis patients, who should not be shunned or stigmatized for their desire to be in homeostasis via medical cannabis use.

The Guiding Ethical Principles for Nurses

Nurses should be familiar with the guiding concepts of autonomy (respecting patient wishes even if they differ from one's values or beliefs), beneficence (compassion and doing good for the patient), nonmaleficence (competency in practice and reporting suspected abuse), justice (treating all patients equally and fairly), fidelity (using the virtue of caring to keep commitments to patients), and totality/integrity (considering the entire person) (Butts & Rich, 2015).

ANA's (2015) *Code of ethics* emphasizes nurse's advocacy, collaboration with nurse colleagues and other health care professionals, honoring of patient's dignity, autonomy, right to privacy, avoidance of discriminatory practices, and remaining accountable for safe, competent, high-quality nursing care. The ethical provisions are a set of nonnegotiable ethical standards, and they express nursing's clear commitment to society (ANA, 2015).

Table 8.1 aligns the nine ethical provisions (ANA, 2015, p. 8) with cannabis care concerns and the emerging standards and scope of cannabis nursing practice (American Cannabis Nurses Association [ACNA], 2019).

End the Stigma: A Call Toward Autonomy of Patient Choice

With cannabis care nursing, ethics become even more important because of the lingering "refer madness" propaganda. The NCSBN (2018) clearly stated that nurses must support and not stigmatize the patient's autonomous right to use medicinal cannabis for healing. With cannabis, just as with many other medicines and interventions, the nurse may not agree with the patient's choice but is still obligated to support, educate, and coach the patient regarding the safe and effective use of the plant.

Autonomy can be defined as respect for the right of patients to make their own health care decisions (Butts & Rich, 2015). This includes the right to make decisions without health care providers trying to sway or influence the patient's decision. Nurses can, of course, still educate and support the patient through their decision-making process but should remain neutral regarding the patient's choices.

While supporting patient autonomy sounds easy enough, many nurses, other health care professionals, administrators, and patients have lingering misunderstandings and knowledge deficits regarding the medicinal benefits of cannabis. Even use of slang or unscientific terms for cannabis (marijuana, weed, pot, chronic, dope, tea, bud, etc.) can serve to further stigmatize patients and their choices. As nurses who have garnered knowledge through this textbook, we become additionally obligated to share our knowledge to ensure that the people we care for are well educated in their autonomous choice to use medicinal cannabis for healing. Additionally, nurses need to ensure that undereducated health care professionals and colleagues, particularly those suffering from the ongoing propagandization of the cannabis herb, no longer stigmatize cannabis patients regarding their choices to utilize a medicine that has a high level of safety and supports homeostasis.

TABLE 8.1.	American Nurses Association ethical provisions and cannabis care nursing ethical concerns	
	American Nurses Association provision	**Cannabis care nursing ethical concerns**
Provision 1	The nurse practices with compassion and respect for the inherent dignity, worth, and unique attributes of every person.	• This is expressed clearly in the cannabis care nurse's application of human caring theory. • Creating caring-healing spaces for patients. • Focus on holistic health needs to potentiate the endocannabinoid system.
Provision 2	The nurse's primary commitment is to the patient, whether an individual, family, group, community, or population.	• Cannabis care nurses must be patient focused. • This may become a concern if a nurse becomes financially involved with the cannabis industry.
Provision 3	The nurse promotes; advocates for; and protects the rights, health, and safety of the patient.	• Cannabis care nurses are obligated to help patients maximize their healing potential through upregulation of the endocannabinoid system. • Acts as an advocate for patients' rights to access safe, effective, and texted quality cannabinoid medicines. • Patients should be educated by nurses about cannabis safety concerns.
Provision 4	The nurse has authority, accountability, and responsibility for nursing practice; makes decisions; and takes action consistent with the obligation to promote health and to provide optimal care.	• Cannabis care nurses are accountable for education and coaching provided to maximize patient health. • There is an understanding that medicinal use of cannabis and coaching patients to take steps toward upregulating the endocannabinoid system are indicative of the health promotion efforts of the cannabis care nurse.
Provision 5	The nurse owes the same duties to self as to others, including the responsibility to promote health and safety, persevere wholeness of character and integrity, maintain competence, and continue personal and professional growth.	• Cannabis care nurses practice self-care and make efforts toward potentiating their own endocannabinoid system in order to best role model holistic health for patients and communities. • Patients are supported by cannabis care nurses to use medicinal cannabis in a safe and effective manner. • Cannabis care nurses maintain competence by staying up to date on relevant cannabis science evidence, as well as continuing their education as lifelong learners. • Personal and professional growth may be linked as cannabis care nurses learn to act as advocates and agents of change, while creating healthy and constructive personal-professional patterns.

(continued)

TABLE 8.1.	American Nurses Association ethical provisions and cannabis care nursing ethical concerns (*continued*)	
	American Nurses Association provision	**Cannabis care nursing ethical concerns**
Provision 6	The nurse, through individual and collective effort, establishes, maintains, and improves the ethical environment of the work setting and conditions of employment that are conducive to safe quality health care.	• The cannabis care nurse is called upon to ensure ethical concepts are considered when addressing patient (and/or workplace) safety and health issues.
Provision 7	The nurse, in all roles and settings, advances the profession through research and scholarly inquiry, professional standards development, and the generation of both nursing and health policy.	• Creation of evidence-based projects, particularly focusing on data around patient outcomes, is an aspect of the work of the cannabis care nurse. • Cannabis care nurses develop and offer expertise around supporting and advocating for sound federal, state, local, and facility policies related to cannabinoid medicines and cannabis care. • The cannabis care nurse as the generator of evidence is an emerging role.
Provision 8	The nurse collaborates with other health professionals and the public to protect human rights, promote health diplomacy, and reduce health disparities.	• The cannabis care nurse works to educate other health care professionals, by sharing their expertise and knowledge to create positive medicinal cannabis experiences for patients. • Global health policy advocacy around the future of cannabinoid medicines and patient-population access to whole plant medicines is a focus of the cannabis care nurse.
Provision 9	The profession of nursing, collectively through its professional organizations, must articulate nursing values, maintain the integrity of the profession, and integrate principles of social justice into nursing and health policy.	• American Cannabis Nurses Association is the 501c3 nonprofit professional nursing organization focused on developing and evolving the role of the nurse around cannabinoid medicine therapeutics and potentiation of the endocannabinoid system through lifestyle changes and holistic approaches/integrative modalities. American Cannabis Nurses Association strives to support cannabis care nursing as an emerging specialty within the field. • As the world transitions out of the cannabis prohibition era and toward an era of cannabis regulation, cannabis care nurses remain concerned with ensuring that social justice and human rights issues are addressed via the creation of new guiding policies and laws, as well as with addressing historical human rights–based concerns.

Adapted from American Nurses Association. (2015). *Code of ethics for nurses with interpretive statements.* Author. https://www.nursingworld.org/coe-view-only and American Cannabis Nurses Association. (2019). *Scope and standards of practice for cannabis nurses.* https://cannabisnurses.org/Scope-of-Practice-for-Cannabis-Nurses

Additionally, nurses and other health care providers who provide cannabis care or use cannabis for their own healing have been historically penalized for their stances and/or their efforts to upregulate their endocannabinoid system (ECS). There are multitudes of stories of nurses losing jobs related to either their cannabis advocacy efforts or their use of cannabinoid medicines for healing. Nurses have lost their jobs simply because they were present at a medical cannabis conference and their pictures showed up on social media or because they tested positive for THC on a random drug test when they were using products that they mistakenly thought were CBD isolate only, but that actually had trace amounts of THC in them.

When it comes to nurses' medical or adult-use cannabis, as with any other medicine that can alter perception and coordination (such as alcohol, opiates, benzodiazepines, and even some over-the-counter drugs like Benadryl or cold medications), one should not be in the workplace if one feels impaired or unable to meet the job requirements around ensuring safe nursing practice, appropriate clinical decision-making, creating patient caring-healing spaces, collaborating, and meeting of standards of care. The nurse should not be impaired at work, whether from substances, lack of sleep, or emotional distress. That being said, the nurse should also have the ability to use a supplemental herb that supports their homeostasis if they are deficient in endocannabinoids. The idea that one needs to be "high" or impaired to be healed with cannabis is also a false assumption, yet as THC is stored in adipose tissue in the body, people can test positive for THC for weeks or sometimes months after using it. THC positive tests do not indicate intoxication or impairment on their own. All nurses should be educated around knowing if they are fit for work or not, whether the issues are related to health or use of impairing substances.

The following case study will support your learning around applying the concept of autonomy with cannabis care situations.

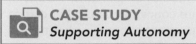

CASE STUDY
Supporting Autonomy

Kiki is a 62-year-old female oncology patient who is being treated for stage 3A lung cancer. Kiki completed her surgical and chemotherapy regimens, and now, a few months later, she is getting brachytherapy radiation treatment for a recurring cancerous lesion. She tells the oncology nurse navigator that she would like to use medicinal cannabis to help her "cope better" with the treatments.

- What should the nurse navigator explore with the patient during the assessment phase?
- What questions will help the nurse to best support Kiki through this process?

During the assessment phase, the nurse navigator finds that Kiki is well informed about how cannabis might palliate her symptoms, but she needs education around the ECS, current state laws, the MMP in the state where she lives (which is a medical cannabis state), side effects, potential medication interactions, financial considerations, and proper dosing and titration strategies.

As Kiki's oncology nurse navigator, you want to encourage, educate, coach, and support her process of exploring the use of medicinal cannabis for cancer palliation.

- During a team meeting, when you bring up the patient's desire to use medical cannabis for palliation, the oncologist states that she knows nothing about that, she cannot recommend it to the patients, and she thinks the patient should try other medications for pain, nausea, and sleep before exploring cannabis use. What is your best response to the oncologist in light of the ethical principle of autonomy and current body of evidence related to effectiveness of cannabis for palliation? How could you support your response with evidence?
- A fellow nurse navigator colleague, Karen, also hears that Kiki wants to try medical cannabis for palliation. Karen rolls her eyes and says, "Nowadays, all of the patients just want to get high and forget about what they need to do to get better." She adds with a laugh, "all of the patients have gone to pot since this state made it legal to use weed." What is your best, most caring-compassionate reply to your colleague Karen, inclusive of a focus on patient autonomy and justice?

Kiki decides to seek her medical cannabis recommendation from a cannabis nurse practitioner who is able to write cannabis recommendations in their state. The nurse practitioner, on completion of a thorough intake including Kiki's health history and a focused physical exam and assessment, determines that Kiki could benefit from medicinal cannabis. However, Kiki's daughters, who help with her care, are concerned about her choice and that the oncologist still wants Kiki to use more allopathic pharmaceutic drugs for palliation.

- In consideration of the principle of autonomy, how can you best support Kiki's daughters in understanding their mother's right to choose this medicine?
- How could you apply the ethical problem-solving process to this scenario, focusing on autonomy? Are there other ethical concepts you might consider?

Hopefully, this case study sparked some good insight into the complexity of supporting patients' autonomy. When it comes down to it, the nurse must be able to confidently and fully support patients' rights to use cannabis medicinally when deemed appropriate by a health care provider if cannabis is legal in the state where you are providing care. The nurse must also support the patient through education and coaching.

Beneficence: The Art of Doing Good

Beneficence is the ethical concept of doing the good and right thing and also connotes a sense of caring, kindness, and compassion on the part of the nurse. The nurse is always obligated to support the well-being of the patient. Kinsinger (2009, p. 46) stated that

> *Health care professionals have a duty of care that extends to the patient, professional colleagues, and to society as a whole. Any individual professional who neither understands nor accepts this duty is at risk for acting malevolently and violating the fiduciary principle of honoring and protecting the patient.*

As we care for our patients, nurses are ethically bound to favor the client's well-being and to do nothing that promotes harm; we must weigh the risks and benefits of interventions to ensure that the patient is well informed during their decision-making processes. When nurses apply and understand the concept of beneficence, we have the power to address the greater good for the patient and society.

Practicing Beneficence: End of Life Example

The nurse may know that hospice patients can benefit from the use of cannabis at end of life by potentially decreasing the reliance on pharmaceuticals (note that cannabis can be safely used with opioids) that have a number of side effects that can impact quality of life. A hospice patient living in an adult/recreational legal state like Colorado or California may be able to access cannabis without a medical recommendation to support management of their pain, anxiety, sleep, fatigue, appetite, and/or spiritual needs at end of life. Hospice patients can benefit from use of cannabis at the end of life, potentially avoiding some pharmaceutical side effects, as it can impact quality of life and provide symptom control (Cyr et al., 2018).

There are many challenges to patients using cannabis at the end of life, even in legalized states, particularly related to access and cost. Additionally, clinicians are poorly trained around initiating use and evaluating the effectiveness of cannabinoid medicines, with few clinical frameworks available to guide the practice, and stigma and public/political opinions creating ongoing obstacles (Cyr et al., 2018). We know that with cancer care in legal states, patients are fairly likely to use cannabis (24% used cannabis within the last year as cited in Cyr et al., 2018). Cannabis care has yet to enter the hospice setting in meaningful ways on a broad scale, despite the fact that it could reduce harm and enhance the well-being of end of life care patients, thereby doing good for the patient.

> ### ▶ APPLIED LEARNING
>
> #### Exploring Beneficence, Cannabis, and End of Life. A Learning Opportunity
> When we consider the principle of beneficence, it becomes clear that we want patients to experience "more good than harm" when it comes to their end of life care. If cannabis can help support quality of life at end of life, despite the lack of phase II/III clinical trials, shouldn't the

hospice team or physician be ethically obligated to suggest the use of cannabis for palliation at end of life?

Reflect on the following questions in a small group setting or via a reflective journal:

- If you were working in a legal cannabis state, where hospice patients can access medicinal cannabis at end of life, how might you use the ethical principle of beneficence, in combination with your knowledge of cannabinoid therapeutics, to guide your conversations with health care providers, the hospice team, patients, and caregivers?

- What sort of frameworks, education, and policies need to be in place in order for beneficence related to the use of cannabis to be enacted at end of life within specific facilities or hospice settings? (Hint, see Cyr et al., 2018).

- If you live in a legal state, it may be of interest to professionally explore whether cannabis is allowed or supported by the local hospices or other settings where end of life care is common. Do these organizations have written policies or accepted practices when it comes to patients' use of cannabis? Do your findings suggest that cannabis use at end of life is generally supported, tolerated, or ignored? How does this relate to the principle of beneficence?

Nonmaleficence: Avoiding Harm

When it comes to nonmaleficence, avoiding harm is a key aspect of this ethical concept; whether it is about doing the least amount of harm or avoiding harm altogether, the cannabis care nurse is obligated to make ethical decisions that have beneficial outcomes for the patient.

I have done a lot of educating with oncology nurses interested in learning about cannabinoid therapeutics and supporting oncology patients' safe and effective use of medical cannabis. A frequent concern that I hear from oncology nurses is that patients who are distrustful of allopathic medicine, fearful of chemotherapy, and/or experiencing severe adverse effects or complications from oncologic treatments may want to turn to cannabis for a cure (and not as a palliative medicine). However, despite the widely available patient-reported (unanalyzed qualitative data) body of evidence that cannabinoid medicines can support healing from cancer or being cancer free, there are no strong studies that provide evidence for this being the case.

Justice: Social Justice

When we consider the idea of treating all patients and populations equally and fairly, cannabis care nurses have a lot to consider.

Many people who used cannabis medicinally during the "war on drugs" and prohibition era were imprisoned for lengthy mandatory sentences. Some may be still serving sentences in states where cannabis has been made legal for adult use. Nurses should be active in supporting the call for release of these people who may remain

---

CASE STUDY
For Group Discussion: Nonmaleficence

In small groups, in online discussions, or a debate setting, discuss the following case study:

The 72-year-old patient Kaitlyn has stage II uterine cancer that is currently being treated with chemotherapy. Kaitlyn lost all of her hair after the first chemotherapy infusion. She has abdominal pain that radiates to the back, and it is managed with a combination of opioids and low doses of cannabis at around 5 mg THC TID via whole plant medicine (ie, it includes terpenes and other cannabinoids). Kaitlyn is frequently nauseated and fatigued and complained that she has ongoing anxiety and depression. She says that the chemotherapy is ruining her life, and she heard that cannabis care using full extract cannabis oil (FECO) could cure her so she could enjoy being with her grandchildren again. She wants to quit chemotherapy and comes to you as the nurse to help her have the conversation with her oncologist to terminate chemotherapeutic treatment.

- How would you apply the ethical decision-making process in light of nonmaleficence? What further information might you need to gather from the patient and other sources? How would you best use motivational interviewing techniques here?
- Does the decision-making process change if the person is a minor or otherwise deemed to be a vulnerable person?
- Do the ethical issues change if the diagnosis, staging of the cancer, and/or long-term prognosis change?
- Do the ethical issues change if the patient's symptoms are different?
- What is your group's decision about how to best support Kaitlyn from the standpoint of nonmaleficence?

---

suffering in prison for cannabis possession charges related to crimes that posed no harm to others.

When we consider patients being treated fairly and equally, we must recognize that as of the writing of this text, access to medicinal cannabis in the United States is based largely on one's zip code. This precludes patients and whole populations from having equal and fair access to safe, tested cannabinoid medicines that may support their healing by upregulating the ECS.

Social justice issues related to cannabis include racial, economic, and access issues. Historically, people of color, and those living in lower-income neighborhoods, have been targeted for drug law enforcement actions at considerably higher rates and with greater legal consequences than have wealthier Caucasians. Women are the fastest-growing segment of the prison population (Drug Policy Alliance [DPA], 2018), and 25% of all incarcerated women within state prisons have been convicted of drug-related offenses (vs. 15% of incarcerated males), whereas 61% of all female federal prisoners are incarcerated for drug offenses (vs. 50% of men) (DPA, 2018). All drug use occurs at equal rates across the racial spectrum, yet black women are twice as likely to be incarcerated for drugs as white women; Latina women are 20% more likely to be imprisoned for drugs versus white women (DPA, 2018). In recent history, over half of all of the drug arrests in the United States were related to cannabis, with 88% of these arrests being for simple possession of cannabis (American Civil Liberties Union [ACLU], 2013). As far as we know, the "war on drugs" has not changed the rate of drug use, although it has served to increase the prison population in the United States.

There are many economic and social justice issues related to the medicinal use of cannabis, including the fact that most people need to pay for medical cannabis out of pocket because insurance does not cover the costs of herbal medicines. This precludes fairness when it comes to accessing cannabis for healing, because people without the finances to pay for the medicine may not be able to afford access to safe, tested cannabis. Lastly, there are disparities within the cannabis industry, with women and people of color being vastly underrepresented. However, there is some hope that we are seeing a shift in fairness and disparities related to cannabis. For example, the Massachusetts Cannabis Control Commission, in preparation for legalizing adult-use cannabis, developed a Social Equity Program to address such disparities (Cannabis Control Commission, Commonwealth of Massachusetts, 2019), and this is an excellent example of steps that can be taken to enhance fairness.

Social justice: criminal status

In 2017, even as cannabis legality grew on the state level, there was an increase in cannabis arrests, with one arrest happening every 48 seconds (Federal Bureau of Investigation [FBI], 2018). Arrests for cannabis possession were much greater than for heroin, cocaine, synthetic drugs, and other nonnarcotic dangerous drugs. Total drug-related arrests in the United States equaled about 15% of all arrests in the country, with cannabis making up 40% of those total drug possession arrests (FBI, 2018). Despite growing legalization/regulation, there was a small but meaningful upward shift in cannabis-related arrests in the United States; 659,700 in 2017, compared with 653,249 in 2016 (FBI, 2018).

At any given time in the United States, there are 4.5 million people either on parole or probation, which is about twice the number of people who are incarcerated, and equals one in every 55 adults or 2% of the population (The Pew Charitable Trusts [PEW], 2018). Of those on parole or probation, 75% are for nonviolent crimes, and 25% of the total of those on parole or probation are for drug convictions. African Americans make up 30% of the supervised probation population but only 13% of the total population. Nearly one-third of those exiting probation or parole are being sent back to prison, not because of new crimes but rather because of parole violations. Prohibiting the use of cannabis or cannabinoid substances while on parole or probation is a standard practice in our current legal system and leads to many community supervised persons being sent back to prison. Rates of substance use by this population are two to three times higher than those in the general population; however, access to addiction services is generally not made readily available: 46% of all people on probation need substance use treatment, and currently, only about 18% receive treatment, whereas 42.2% of all people on parole need substance use treatment, and only 26.3% receive it (PEW, 2018).

Millions of Americans also struggle to find work and housing because they have prison records related to cannabis-related convictions. Should people convicted of cannabis-related crimes who now reside in legal cannabis states or those who previously committed those crimes in now legal cannabis states have their records expunged? Unfortunately, most states during the legalization process failed to adequately address this issue, although that tide has begun to turn as more states recognize the need for a social justice inclusion within their state-level legalization-regulation process. Illinois included cannabis-related crime record expungement in their law-making process when cannabis became legal for adult use there. Many argue that as public policy changes so does public opinion, and people should no longer be continually punished for things that society no longer views as criminal. Additionally, there may be people who are still incarcerated for cannabis possession in states where this is no longer an illegal act, but most state laws do not have provisions governing how to handle these populations, nor do they address what the end of imprisonment might look like for them.

An extreme case in cannabis social justice issues was that of Antonio Bascaro. Over 60 years ago, Bascaro was an anti-communist rebel in Cuba, and because of his flying and aviation capabilities he was recruited by the CIA to help assist in the overthrow of Cuba's leader Fidel Castro. Upon his release from the anti-communist military efforts, Bascaro found lucrative work, where he scouted landing sites for over a half-million pounds of cannabis to be brought into the country illegally. He received a lengthy sentence, in part because of his unwillingness to cooperate with prosecutors, so he was charged with conspiracy in addition to smuggling; the ring leader of the operation was released after 12 years of incarceration.

Meanwhile, the prosecutor in Bascaro's case was shocked when he learned how long the man had been incarcerated. Bascaro served the longest sentence in US history for a cannabis-related crime: After serving 39 years in prison, although he is now free, he faces fears that he will be deported back to Cuba, where he would be imprisoned for crimes against the country because of his earlier involvement with the CIA and the anti-communist efforts during the Bay of Pigs efforts (Nelson, 2019). Although harm may have come from Bascaro's actions, he certainly should not have served more time than the main instigators of the crimes.

The state of California is currently working to clear thousands of old cannabis convictions, and Los Angeles alone is reviewing more than 50,000 cases that would qualify for expungement of their criminal records (Tchekmedyian, 2019). San Francisco is likewise reviewing 9,300 cases that may be potentially cleared. The state of California aims to have all past eligible nonviolent cannabis-related convictions cleared by the end of the year 2020, and Illinois, Missouri, and New York are taking similar measures (Tchekmedyian, 2019).

Social equity is also an issue when it comes to the burgeoning legal cannabis industry, where people of color and women are grossly underrepresented, and those previously convicted of cannabis crimes are generally prohibited from entering the industry altogether. Activists groups such as the Drug Policy Alliance make an effort to ensure that social justice efforts prevail as we enter the era of cannabis regulation.

> ### ▶ APPLIED LEARNING

Social Justice

■ See if you can determine how many people are currently incarcerated for simple cannabis possession in your state and neighboring states. Is this directly related to the legal status of cannabis in these states? What organizations in your state and across the nation fight for these prisoners' release or commutation of their sentences?

■ Does your state (or another legal state) have social justice or equity provisions for supporting people of color and women to enter the cannabis industry? Has the discussion arisen in your state or another legal state?

■ What are the financial implications for people living in your area who want to access cannabis from a dispensary? This may require you to do some research on the cost of medicinal cannabis and consider how much cannabis a person might need to support their healing if they are staying within the often recommended range of no more than 15–20 mg/THC/day. How does the ability to afford cannabis medicine become an ethical issue of justice?

Totality/Integrity

The principle of totality means that all ethical decisions must encompass and prioritize the good of the entire person, inclusive of their body, mind, and spirit. This ethical concept is grounded in the works of St. Thomas of Aquinas and Aristotle, where the parts of the person are seen as unified with the entire person, with the various body systems and organs contributing to the well-being of the individual, thereby providing a basis for holistic approaches to care (Thompson, 2019). Sometimes, certain aspects of the whole are perhaps lost in the sacrifice of maintaining the rest of the integrity of the whole being (eg, amputation of a gangrenous toe for the betterment of the whole being).

When medical treatments may have both good and adverse effects, one must also consider the "double effect," as an action may have both good and bad effects. However, if the action is morally good or neutral, the bad effects are not a means to creating positive or good effects, the motivation is to achieve positive effects, and the good result is equal to or exceeds the bad effects, then the decision or action would be ethically in alignment with totality (Thompson, 2019).

When it comes to cannabis care, on occasion, a patient may have side or adverse effects that need to be managed, but for most medical cannabis patients who keep their doses of THC low, as suggested, the side effects (or "the bad") will not hamper the good that they receive by using the medicine in order to support homeostasis.

> ### CASE STUDY
> *Totality in Cannabis Care, a More Complex Case*
>
> Consider now that cannabis care nurses may indeed have contact with patient cases that are more complex and may require the application of the ethical decision-making process in consideration of the principle of totality.
>
> Xavier is a 52-year-old patient who is currently undergoing chemotherapy for invasive prostate cancer that has metastasized to the bone. He has experienced ongoing issues with back pain, nausea, sleep, and spiritual distress. He has refused opiates because he has a history of being a heroin addict for 5 years, and he has been "clean" from opiates for 10 years. However, he is now interested in using medical cannabis for palliation.
>
> * Apply the ethical decision-making process in light of the concept of totality. What information do you have, and what subjective and objective data do you need to gather?
>
> Xavier stated that he wants to try cannabis in part because he has heard that people cannot really get addicted to it in the same way they get addicted to heroin, with heroin having the potential for severe withdrawal symptoms.
>
> * What is your initial reaction to Xavier's statement? Does your initial reply to Xavier change when you consider totality? How can you use evidence to support your response?
> * How does your consideration of potential addiction and Xavier's need for palliation change if the prognosis of his illness is better (chance for a cure) or worse (terminal prognosis)?
> * Consider the potential for double effect with Xavier's case. What information do you need to best resolve a potential double-effect ethical issue?

LEGAL CONCERNS FOR NURSES: MALPRACTICE AND PERSONAL USE

As cannabis remains federally illegal and technically cannot be prescribed because it is a schedule I drug, malpractice insurance becomes concerning. For APRNs and MDs who are "recommending" or "certifying" medicinal cannabis use for qualifying patients, they may need to carry additional malpractice insurance coverage that specifically covers their cannabis care practice. However, at this time, no special insurance coverages are available for registered nurses, and the cannabis care nurses I have spoken with carry their own nursing malpractice insurance through groups like Nurse Services Organization. The cannabis care nurse focuses on education and coaching, and this should be enough to cover most nurses who are not undertaking a business opportunity or working at the APRN level of care.

Every nurse, whether working with cannabis care patients or not, should be aware that they should carry their own personal malpractice insurance for several reasons. First, while hospitals and workplaces are insured and your practice is covered under their umbrella, they are likely not to support the nurse if malpractice occurs, particularly regarding personal representation through a lawyer or days missed from work. Additionally, malpractice insurance for nurses ensures that the nurse is covered for actions taken outside of the workplace, whether that is responding in an emergent situation or educating or coaching patients or populations outside of the workplace, whether paid or unpaid in providing these services.

Because of the issues related to cannabis, including the lingering prohibition era stigma and federal-level schedule I status, nurses who work with cannabis care patients, or use cannabis themselves to support homeostasis, may become vulnerable to workplace issues and disciplinary action by state boards of nursing. Note that only about one-third of the states that have medical cannabis laws in place also have anti-discrimination protections for medical cannabis patients. Additionally, most state boards of nursing have moral turpitude requirements, which state that one's professional character may come into play with the granting of the nursing license, along with consideration of previous felony and misdemeanor convictions. Most state boards of nursing state that possessing or using a dangerous drug, mood-altering substance, or a controlled substance is a crime that is directly related to or has implications related to, the practice of nursing. In California, cannabis convictions are removed from one's record after 2 years, so the issue may become moot if somebody had a prior conviction and was applying for licensure 2 years later, although one would want to ensure that their record actually had been cleared.

The following are real-life examples of some legal and licensure issues that nurses who have used cannabis for healing have faced.

Laurel James, RN: A Nurse in Oregon

Nurse James became interested in cannabis nursing and took a cannabis nursing course offered through The Cannabis Medicine Institute and the ACNA. She noticed that in her home state of Oregon, there was a significant lack of education for patients accessing medical cannabis through dispensaries, and in 2015 she opened her own consulting business focusing on educating medical cannabis patients and prospective patients, mainly through outreach to senior citizen groups and working with medical cannabis dispensaries.

Nurse James says she made a mistake by calling (vs. writing) the Oregon State Board of Nursing (OSBN) to confirm that she could use her nursing license to educate and coach patients around the safe and effective use of cannabis. According to Nurse James, during the phone call, the OSBN agreed that this fitted within the scope of practice. Her main focus was on educating seniors and culling research findings for people who needed to know about cannabis efficacy and approaches to best manage their health issues with cannabinoid therapeutics. Nurse James also created many educational offerings and developed a poster to be displayed in cannabis dispensaries that reviewed best practices for safe and effective dosing strategies, inclusive of citations to support the approaches.

During her second year of business, Nurse James began working with a 25-year-old female client who had many health issues. At the initial meeting, the client's mother was supposed to be present but did not arrive. At the time, in Oregon, it was perfectly legal to share cannabis products; however, they could not be charged for. Nurse James shared some topical cannabis salve with the 25-year-old and referred to her other resources for obtaining her cannabis medicine. The 25-year-old client's mother became concerned with the consultation process and reported Nurse James to the OSBN. Nurse James had to get a lawyer, which cost her more than $15,000. She quit her business and began to work for a nurse registry. Nurse James was able to solicit letters of support from the nurse managers and colleagues she worked with through the registry to address her issues with the OSBN.

Her legal counsel was able to ensure she didn't lose her nursing license, although the OSBN was unsure of what to do about her case, as it had never had this issue before. The OSBN claimed that Nurse James was prescribing cannabis without a license to do so. However, they opted to treat her as if she had created an offense as a drug-impaired nurse, by placing her on a 2-year probation and forbidding her from doing things like working overtime, precepting, acting as charge nurse, or furthering her education. She met with her "probation officer" monthly to review her status, and although she was treated as if she was an impaired nurse, she, oddly, did not have to submit to drug testing.

At the time of this publication, Nurse James will have completed her probationary status, and she states that she does enjoy working in a health care facility and that in many ways, it is easier than having her own educational and consulting business. She was happy to be able to share her story with other nurses as a cautionary tale. She is hopeful that upon retiring from nursing, she can continue to be an educational resource for cannabis patients and dispensaries. Nurse James remains committed to the idea that cannabis medicine can replace many other medications and support health and well-being through the maintenance of homeostasis.

Dolores Montgomery Halbin, RN: A Nurse in Missouri

Nurse Halbin was working as a nurse in Missouri when her husband was diagnosed with acute angle glaucoma; he lost an eye because of the severity of the illness. The couple grew cannabis in their basement for personal medical use, despite Missouri not being a legal medical cannabis state at the time. Their property was raided in 2014, and Dolores and her husband spent a week in jail, at which time her husband was denied medications and medical treatment for his diabetes. His health declined while in jail, and he subsequently died related to complications from being imprisoned, suffering a silent heart attack that went untreated. Dolores was convicted of misdemeanor possession of cannabis and placed on 2 years of unsupervised probation.

Unfortunately, Nurse Halbin was also sent a letter from the Missouri State Board of Nursing charging her with moral turpitude, which put her in the same class of licensing as those nurses who have stolen controlled substances or committed even worse crimes. It took her several years to get her nursing license back, but because she still has misdemeanor charges against her, finding work is challenging, if not impossible. Nurse Halbin remains committed to ensuring that patients have access to cannabis for healing purposes and that they do not live in fear or face prosecution for choosing to use cannabis for healing.

Katelin Noffsinger: A Nurse and a Patient

Katelin Noffsinger was a registered nurse seeking employment in Connecticut in July of 2016, and she was also a medical cannabis patient for PTSD following a car accident in 2012. In Connecticut, cannabis patients are protected by their state law, known as PUMA, or the Palliative Use of Marijuana Act, which states that employers may not discriminate against medical cannabis users. However, Nurse Noffsinger was offered a job by a nursing home, which was later rescinded after she tested positive for THC. This was done even though she had revealed her medical status, had stated that she used cannabinoid medicines only for sleep and had a verified PTSD diagnosis. Ultimately, a judge ruled in her favor, holding that she had been discriminated against. They also stated that the law does not provide for attorney fees and punitive damages, but would allow for consideration of payment for Nurse Noffsinger's claim of negligent infliction of emotional distress.

Kaitlin McKeon: A Potential Nursing Student

Ms. McKeon had been accepted for enrollment in Florida's Nova Southeastern's nursing program and was required to take a drug test in 2018. She let school officials know that she would test positive for THC, as she had a Florida recommendation for cannabis use to help manage her chronic stomach pain. When she tested positive for THC, the school then gave her a letter stating they had a zero-tolerance drug policy. The Florida medical cannabis laws at the time of the incident offered no protection for medical cannabis employees or students. She was given an ultimatum to either stop using cannabis, which was the only medicine that was effectively managing her symptoms, or leave the school. Ms. McKeon, after wading through a lengthy process while school officials determined her fate, decided to try forgoing her medicinal cannabis use. Ultimately, that left her feeling so uncomfortable that she opted to leave the school and sue them for damages related to discriminatory practices instead. She has enrolled at a different school, focusing on public health, as her lawsuit winds its way through the judicial process.

An Anonymous Michigan Nurse

A nurse from Michigan was pulled over by police, who found a "large amount" of cannabis in her vehicle, and she was charged with "possession of marijuana." The nurse hired an attorney, who was able to negotiate a deal wherein she pleaded guilty to possession, but her sentence was diverted. After completing a probationary period of 8 months, requiring her to test negative for THC in her system, the charges were dismissed, and she did not have to legally report the incident to the Michigan Board of Nursing. The nurse avoided a trial, criminal conviction, and reporting of the issue to the Michigan State Board of Nursing. This is a case where having competent and knowledgeable legal representation helped to protect the nurse's license.

MORE LEGAL CONCERNS FOR NURSES: STATE PRACTICE ACTS

Every nurse should be familiar with their state practice act and the parameters of the scope of their practice. Additionally, knowing the ANA (2015) *Scope and standards of practice*, along with any specific applicable specialty scope and standards of practice, should be a prerequisite for any nurse who begins her practice either as a new grad or within a new state.

For the most part, nurses should be able to educate, coach, and advocate for cannabis care patients in every state in the nation. All education and coaching should be evidence based. However, whether or not cannabis is medically or adult-use legal may have implications for how nurses educate, coach, and advocate. For instance, we know that many oncology patients who live in nonlegal states may travel to other states to procure cannabis or may simply access it on the black market. This may become a bit of a tricky issue for nurses to finesse: We want to ensure patients are using safe, tested medicine in an effective and non-harmful way, and that may not be possible in every state at this time. Regardless, beginning to end the stigma and having open and evidence-based discussions with patients may help to ensure that they don't use cannabis in ways that put them at risk legally, physically, and financially. The more we can create open and honest discussions about cannabis care, the more we can fulfill our roles as educators, coaches, and advocates.

In the NCSBN (2018) report, it was made clear that nurses may not touch cannabis or administer it directly to patients, unless the state practice act allows for this. For instance, school nurses in Colorado in 2019 were granted the ability to administer medical cannabis to students under the following conditions: The cannabis container must be clearly labeled with dosage, time, and route of administration, as recommended by a physician. The student must have an approved written plan of cannabis use prior to being able to have cannabis administered at school, the cannabis must be kept in a locked storage area that only the nurse or their designee can access, any unused cannabis must be returned to the student's parent or caregiver, and the cannabis cannot be handled by the student at school or any school event. The full bill can be read here: https://leg.colorado.gov/bills/hb18-1286

Additionally, in Minnesota, the Medical Cannabis Law was written so that hospitals could determine whether they would allow the use of cannabinoids in the inpatient setting. The law clearly states that employees and health care facilities have protections and immunities while providing care or distributing cannabis to a patient who is on the Minnesota Medical Cannabis Patient Registry. Facilities may, of course, also opt to restrict or limit patient access, but Minnesota-licensed nurses should be ready to support, educate, and advocate for patients who are on the registry. Although, of course, cannabis remains federally illegal, the Minnesota Nurses Association (MNA, 2019) stated that with the state law protections, the potential liability and level of concern for individual nurses per their hospital policy should be minimal.

ADVOCACY: WHAT'S IT ALL ABOUT?

Being an advocate for cannabis care and cannabis policy/law reform can be a daunting undertaking. Although I have had experiences delving into creating transformative change of the current legal status of cannabis through political processes, many cannabis care nurses paved the way for us all to be able to take action. Before we get into just a few of these nurses' stories, it is important to be clear on what the advocacy process is and what you need to consider when advocating for cannabis patients and legal reforms.

Advocacy 101

Advocacy is different from activism, and the subtle differences are significant. Advocates are people who publicly support a specific cause, whereas activists are people who campaign to bring about social or political change. Many cannabis care nurses may be activists in their personal lives, and all cannabis care nurses are called to be advocates for the safe and effective use of medicinal cannabis, as well as for populations' abilities to access cannabis for their medicinal needs.

The ANA (n.d.) believes that advocacy is one of the pillars of nursing, and while advocating for patients in the workplace becomes instinctual for many nurses, nurses should also be focused on legislative and political advocacy. ANA has an online nurse advocacy tool kit that allows nurses to quickly and easily find their congressional representatives, so that they can call, send a letter, e-mail, or set up a meeting with them (see: https://www.nursingworld.org/practice-policy/advocacy/).

The ANA has also developed the American Nurses Advocacy Institute, which is designed to help nurses understand the relationship between the advocacy process and policy change, undertake a political scan, develop practical strategies for creating and sustaining policy change, and explore how networking and coalition building are necessary for effective advocacy efforts (ANA, n.d.). Nurses can apply to become an American Nurses Association Institute Fellow through their state ANA branch and they will spend a year working closely with their state-level ANA group to learn the political process. Being an ANAI (American Nurses Association Advocacy Institute) Fellow myself, I can attest to the ability of this program to open the doors for nurses' advocacy work.

An effective nurse advocate may work to influence and encourage leaders and people to make change. To be an effective advocate, one can take the following steps:

- Immerse yourself into the evidence and issues related to the topic. Being well educated, well versed, and completely clear on the issues and your purpose are prerequisites for beginning your advocacy journey. Knowledge is especially important in the cannabis care field because there is such a plethora of misinformation out there, and we can't afford to misspeak or propagate cannabis myths or stigma. Some ways to further your cannabis care knowledge include attending conferences, reading textbooks and evidence-based articles, and immersing yourself in organizations that focus on cannabis care. Even if your knowledge is still growing, you can learn a lot by volunteering, observing, and listening to what is going on within the organization.
- If an organization you are interested in joining has volunteer opportunities, sign up and be active in your role once you make the commitment. If you aren't sure if the organization currently has volunteer opportunities, then contact them to verify or to offer your skill set in service to them. Service is a wonderful opportunity for all nurses to share our knowledge, wisdom, and experiences with others.
- Whether it's via social media or in a public setting, avoid saying or implying that you speak for an organization you might be volunteering with. Although you may be an actively concerned person that is volunteering with the organization, you may not speak for the organization. (In general, it's the president or board of directors of the organization that makes official statements for the organization.)

- When you are attending conferences, rallies, information sessions, and so on, find some like-minded colleagues or friends to bring with you. There is power in numbers, and having close allies is essential. Likewise, be sure to reach out to others whom you meet at these events. Much of my advocacy efforts started by connecting with like-minded others, who were also there to support me when things got challenging.
- Use social media as a way to inform others and act as an advocate. If every post you make is about your advocacy work, it may become less impactful (unless you create an online presence that solely focuses on this work). Meanwhile, take the time to wisely use social media to educate your friends, family, and followers and correct misinformation that is bound to emerge.
- There is a trend now to turn things like birthday celebrations into opportunities to fundraise for your favorite advocacy organizations: Requesting donations in lieu of gifts can be a meaningful way to fundraise. Many nonprofit organizations rely heavily on donations, and if the work of the organization aligns with your interests, fundraising becomes a meaningful endeavor.
- Create a gathering of your own. Hosting a part of get-togethers with like-minded individuals can be a way to garner support for your cause. Showing a film or documentary related to your advocacy focus can help enlighten others and perhaps encourage them to join you.
- It is imperative that you "walk the talk" when it comes to advocacy. For cannabis care advocacy, this does not mean that you need to personally use cannabinoid medicines, rather, you need to support those who use cannabis for healing. The cannabis care nurse works on potentiating the health of his or her own ECS through diet, exercise, and lifestyle changes, so as to better role model the holistic approach to healing by creating homeostasis with the ECS.
- Know who the opposing side is. What are the relevant organizations that are in opposition to your advocacy works? What do their stakeholders believe and why? How would you counter their arguments?
- Remain humble and avoid being self-righteous. It can be difficult to avoid feeling angry when injustices occur, but as advocates we need to learn to channel that anger toward making constructive changes. Even when the other side is clearly wrong, we need to take the high road and strive to educate and call for positive change.
(Cravens, 2019).

With cannabis care, many patients and professionals change their minds once they understand the science behind medicinal cannabis and the ECS. This emphasizes the importance of remaining professional and using the evidence base to potentiate change through our advocacy efforts.

ADVOCACY STORIES

The following section depicts advocacy stories from some of the cannabis care nurses who have worked tirelessly to foster and create change from a political advocacy perspective. The idea of including them here is to inspire you to take action of your own, whether it's related to cannabis or other health care policy issues.

Carey S. Clark, PhD, RN, AHN-BC, FAAN

What got you interested in cannabis advocacy and the political process?

When I moved from California to Maine in 2010, I was surprised to see how "underground" the cannabis movement seemed to be. In California, medical cannabis dispensaries were seemingly everywhere, and in large cities like San Francisco, people were comfortable with using cannabis openly. I lived in Western Sonoma County, where most of my neighbors were growing medicinal cannabis outdoors, so come October, the terpenes were freely perfuming the neighborhood air. Once I moved to Maine in 2010, I was surprised that, with Maine having the second highest per capita use of cannabis in the United States, right behind California, there was not a more obvious cannabis-culture presence in the state. With a population of more than 1 million people, it was surprising that there were only six cannabis dispensaries in the entire state of Maine. I later learned that many people grew cannabis and that many people relied on cannabis caregivers, who grow cannabis for medical cannabis patients and often process products for patient consumption as well.

In the 2016 national election cycle, I was attending the democratic state convention, where I learned that a peoples' referendum would be on the Maine fall 2016 ballot allowing for adult-use (age 21 and over) cannabis consumption and sales in the state. The "yes on 1" campaign was being run by the MPP, and I decided to volunteer my services. My thinking at the time was that many people who could benefit from cannabis were not accessing it because they didn't have one of the 11 qualifying medical conditions or they simply couldn't afford to pay $200 out of pocket to get a medical recommendation. I also considered the social justice issues related to cannabis and the opportunity for cannabis to be used more widely as a harm reduction tool, potentially helping people to get off opiates or decrease their use of harmful substances such as alcohol or even other prescription medications.

When "yes on 1" and the MPP asked me to support the ballot measure from a health care perspective, I thought long and hard about it. Because of the ongoing issues of lack of education, stigma, and lingering reefer madness propaganda, I knew there would be plenty of opposition, particularly in the health care arena and in the setting where I was employed. Also, it remains to be seen what the overall impact of legalizing adult-use cannabis will be on medical cannabis programs. Luckily, I had just been promoted to associate professor of nursing and earned tenure, so I felt a sense of security about my employment.

I was able to work closely with "yes on 1" and MPP to craft an evidence-based message that was sent to thousands of health care providers around the state, ranging from CNAs to RNs to MDs, and the response was mostly mixed, as was to be expected. I was able to speak at press conferences, and I was featured in a television commercial. But this advocacy wasn't without its challenges and near consequences.

The downside was that my workplace was less than thrilled with my support of "yes on 1" and the legalization of cannabis in the state. The university where I was working was called and asked if my support of "yes on 1" meant that the university also supported "yes on 1." The university legal team scrutinized the letters that I wrote for MPP, only to conclude that I was exercising my right to free speech. Additionally, some colleagues made it clear that they felt I was doing the wrong thing by supporting this referendum and that it would have professional consequences later on. I was lucky that I had the support of the faculty union on my side and, of course, being tenured made it very difficult to fire me. Had I taken these actions prior to being tenured, I potentially could have lost my job or been denied tenure. It seems that over the last several years, with growing knowledge in this area, things have begun to shift in the workplace as well. We were successful in passing the referendum.

How did you learn to be an advocate?

I began teaching policy and politics related to health care in 2005, so I have a long-term interest and passion for the process of creating policy change. In 2015, I became the chair of the ANA, Maine legislative committee. I became quite active in the statewide legislative process, so a lot of time was spent reaching out to legislators and rallying the voice of nurses within the state. That year I also completed a year-long fellowship with the ANAI. The ANAI experience truly prepared me to better act as an advocate. I learned how to best approach policy makers and how to do a political environmental scan. I had the fantastic experience of visiting with legislators in Washington, DC and discussing some of ANA's political stances. I was then able to apply some of these concepts at the state level regarding cannabis law reformation. As nurses, we are listened to when we speak, but we do need to learn to harness our power.

What are some of your greatest challenges or obstacles in doing this work?

When we consider cannabis, the greatest challenges remain the federal scheduling of the medicine and the lingering reefer madness stigma. The federal government, with the "war on drugs" movement, did a smashing job of stigmatizing the cannabis plant and people who use cannabis. Although people are becoming more accepting and are growing in their understanding of the power of this plant to support healing, we still have a long way to go with education and advocacy. Helping people to understand how cannabis works in the body via the human ECS can be challenging, and I strive to bring the ECS physiology down to basic terms so people can grasp how cannabinoids help create homeostasis in the body.

Also, because I am passionate about the subject, I have to work hard to maintain my stress resilience and not burn out. In some ways, I can almost become my own obstacle if I don't take time to rest, relax, recreate, and rejuvenate my personal energy and my passion for the plant.

What do you count as successes?

Although it was a close vote, the "yes on 1" movement in Maine was successful in 2016, and cannabis became legal for adult use. That being said, it has taken another 4 years to get adult-use cannabis laws and regulations in place, but in that time, I have seen the culture shift, with far more medical cannabis dispensaries opening and people being more open about and supportive about the growth of their cannabis businesses. Some towns in Maine now have more medical dispensary storefronts than the whole state had some 9–10 years ago. Ideally, the presence of these storefronts allows for people to access safe, tested, pesticide-free cannabis medicines that are correctly labeled. As the state now has adult-use sales, I am hopeful that people can also use cannabis as a harm reduction tool.

What have you learned from advocacy "failures"?

I have grown from those times when we didn't necessarily "win" in our advocacy efforts. It's great to be able to look back and reflect on what went well, what could be improved upon, and what we might do differently. I also try and stay open to the complexity of the issues at hand and how difficult the change process can be. I have on occasion changed my stance when new evidence emerged. Having a sense of faith, or perhaps an attitude, that one is doing their best for the populations they serve is helpful. I have felt called to doing this work, and it helps to remember that calling and to strive to renew myself and my commitment on a regular basis.

How do ethical concepts (autonomy, justice, beneficence, etc.) guide your efforts?

When it comes to cannabis, I genuinely believe that just as the NCSBN (2018) stated, patients have the right to autonomously choose the healing path that best suits them. We can't stigmatize patients for this choice, and from a justice perspective, one's zip code should not determine one's ability to access cannabis for healing. I often think about what policies will best support our patients' rights to self-determination and what policies are likely to reduce or eliminate harm.

What are the pertinent social justice issues that still need to be addressed via cannabis advocacy work?

There are so many issues that we still face today, including the issue of people remaining incarcerated or having criminal records for cannabis possession for personal or medical use, lack of proper representation of women and people of color in the cannabis industry realm, and the lingering issues related to the federal Schedule I of cannabis being in direct conflict with state laws. We need to continue to focus on moving cannabis out of the DEA federal Schedule I, ensure that people of color no longer are disproportionately arrested and convicted for cannabis-related "crimes," and consider reparations for those who have served extraordinarily long prison terms for their cannabis-related crime. Additionally, I get concerned with over-regulation and over-taxation of cannabis, along with limitations on people being able to grow the plant, and the impact these actions might have on medicinal cannabis patients being able to access the medicine for healing.

What does the future look like for cannabis political advocacy in the United States and/or globally?

We need to continue to advocate for patients to have safe, legal, affordable access to cannabinoid medicines. This really should be on a global scale. There is also the need for more research to be done, including focusing on particular populations with particular cannabinoid medicines being used. We may run the risk of cannabis being viewed more as a recreational drug, and this could thwart the development of new medicines or, in some ways, impede access for patients who need high-quality medicines. Alternately, we may run the risk of cannabinoid medicines being exploited by pharmaceutical companies, and yet we also want to see cannabinoid therapeutics grow. Cannabinoid therapeutics should include more standardized medicines that are available in the inpatient setting and are covered by insurance, over-the-counter cannabinoid preparations, and the creation of new delivery systems for cannabinoid ingestion.

The social justice issues around cannabis remain of great concern, with many people remaining incarcerated or newly incarcerated for issues related to cannabis use or the sale of cannabis. There is a lot that nurses can and should be doing around social justice issues, but we need to educate and empower ourselves to take effective political action and stand up for those populations that need our support.

Ken Wolski, RN, MPA

What got you interested in cannabis advocacy and the political process?

In the early 1990s, while I was on a trip to Europe, I met an American expatriate, named James Burton, who was living in Amsterdam. He told me his story. Mr. Burton had glaucoma, and no medications were effective in controlling his disease. His eyesight was continually deteriorating. When he was in his 30s, he tried cannabis for the first time. He noticed an almost immediate improvement in his vision. He discussed this with his doctor, and his doctor recommended that he continue to use cannabis. Mr. Burton was a farmer, so he grew cannabis on his farm. The government found it growing there. They arrested him, tried him, and convicted him, despite his doctor's testimony at his trial. Mr. Burton spent a year incarcerated, part of that time in a maximum-security prison. Coincidentally, I was a supervisor of nurses at New Jersey's only maximum-security prison at the time, so I had a clear understanding of what he had gone through. While he was in prison, the government seized Mr. Burton's home and his farm. When he was released from prison, he fled America, never to return. This was one of the worst cases of social injustice I had ever encountered. I vowed I would try to stop this injustice from happening to other people.

How did you learn to be an advocate?

I came of age in the 1960s. I was an active participant in the cultural revolution of that decade. The first antiwar demonstration I participated in was at the age of 18 in 1967 in San Francisco. Over the next 4 years, I demonstrated in New Jersey, New York, and Washington, DC, while writing letters to the editor, contacting elected officials, attending teach-ins, etc., in an effort to end the American involvement in that war. I was also active in demonstrations for civil rights, women's rights, free speech, and drug policy reform. The latter issue has been a particular interest of mine, as I have been active in NORML since 1973. Additionally, I have belonged to the MPP, the Drug Policy Alliance, Students for Sensible Drug Policy, Law Enforcement Action Partnership, Patients Out of Time, and Americans for Safe Access. I have attended numerous conferences and workshops in the ensuing decades in an effort to reform drug policy. National drug policy reform organizations assisted my efforts in many ways (a one-time grant, organizational training, Capwiz, expert testimony, national conferences, assurances, etc.)

What are some of your greatest challenges or obstacles in doing this work?

It is very difficult to get the truth out about medical cannabis due to the campaign of misinformation being waged by the federal government. This decades-long propaganda campaign produced a stigma that is difficult to erase. An all-volunteer organization like Coalition for Medical Marijuana—New Jersey (CMMNJ), which depends for its survival on public donations, faces daunting odds. Moreover, our strongest supporters are often very ill, often impoverished by their illness, and often afraid to speak out about their use of an illegal substance. Many patients in New Jersey still face severe criminal penalties for the use of cannabis, despite the recommendations of their physicians, and despite the passage of the Compassionate Use Medical Marijuana Act into law.

Part of the problem has been elected officials. Despite the overwhelming popular support for medical cannabis, it still took 5 years for the bill to pass into law here in New Jersey. The legislature is, by nature, a conservative body. Moreover, elected officials do not always represent the people of their districts; they often represent their financial donors, instead. There are powerful, moneyed interests in New Jersey that are opposed to any type of drug policy reform. These opponents include the pharmaceutical industry, the alcohol industry, and the prison-industrial complex.

In my medical cannabis advocacy, I've only seen a handful of New Jersey physicians advocate strongly on a patient's behalf for it. More often, I've heard tales of doctors telling dying patients, "If you want marijuana, go find yourself another doctor." In the 8 years of Governor Christie's administration, only about 1% of the physicians in New Jersey took part in the state's MMP. The American Medical Association (AMA) still has not endorsed any of the 33 state MMPs. The AMA importantly endorsed rescheduling of cannabis in 2009 but has done nothing about the failure of the federal government to do so since then. The Pennsylvania Medical Society (PMS) testified during medical marijuana hearings that they "found that there are no state medical societies that have endorsed the use of medical marijuana." At the time, 29 states had medical cannabis programs, and not a single medical society in the country had endorsed any of these programs. Perhaps they all feel threatened that patients empowered with medical cannabis will be less dependent on the pharmaceutical preparations available only through the medical profession?

What do you count as successes? What have you learned from "failures"?

I received the support of the New Jersey State Nurses Association in 2002 when they adopted a resolution I wrote endorsing medical cannabis. About a decade later, I also got the support of the Pennsylvania State Nurses Association for a similar resolution. I was inspired to pursue these actions by the efforts of Mary Lynn Mathre, RN, with the Virginia Nurses Association. The ANA endorsed medical cannabis in 2004, mostly, I believe, through the efforts of Nurse Mathre.

The volunteers of CMMNJ were instrumental in introducing the "New Jersey Compassionate Use Medical Marijuana Act" into the state legislature in 2005 and passing it into law in 2010. CMMNJ volunteers continue to address the many barriers to patient access to medical cannabis that exist in the state's MMP.

CMMNJ established a professional board of directors, and we incorporated and became a 501(c)(3). We established a line of merchandise and became self-supporting, financially. Many board members contributed greatly in many ways: free use of corporate headquarters, including internet access, and most office expenses; business deals by a former board member on t-shirts, wristbands, etc.; free legal advice and assistance; no-interest loans; and precious time, freely given. It's true we had a miniscule budget, and if it were larger, we would have gotten our message out to greater numbers of people in more persuasive ways and perhaps helped to bring about medical cannabis sooner in New Jersey.

The strength, dedication, and generosity of our volunteers sustained us through the years. The patients, and their testimony, were remarkable and compelling. Patients stood up and spoke out about how cannabis helps them with their afflictions in individual acts of courage and selflessness. These patients waived their confidentiality rights and spoke out about the most intimate details of their suffering and how cannabis helped them. They did so at great legal risk to themselves.

The patients were remarkable; their testimony compelling.

We have had success in a number of ways. Media attention in New Jersey has generally been favorable, with much editorial support in major newspapers, on radio and TV. CMMNJ members have kept up a steady stream of letters to the editor, op-ed columns, press releases, radio, and TV appearances—none of which we had to pay for. Public support for medical cannabis has been very high, with favorable polls as high as 86%. (Though the public is generally unaware of how much support there is, and it is not a very important issue to most, unless they are directly affected.)

CMMNJ took part in a lawsuit that forced the Department of Health (DOH) to produce reports on the MMP that were required by law.

CMMNJ also taped a monthly television show, "CMMNJ TV," from the Princeton Community Television studio for about 2 years.

CMMNJ was responsible for adding PTSD as a qualifying condition to New Jersey's law. First, CMMNJ went through the regulatory process with a "Petition for Rulemaking" to the DOH in 2013. We argued that cannabis shows great promise in the management of PTSD—certainly better than any traditional pharmaceutical agent available today. Our disabled veterans—who are committing suicide at a rate of 22/day, primarily because PTSD is so poorly managed—deserve immediate access to the finest medical care available, and that includes cannabis therapy, CMMNJ said. They do *not* need to be told to wait additional decades for more studies when these studies cannot be done anyway. The DOH rejected the PTSD petition. CMMNJ then went to the legislature, found sympathetic legislators, and got a bill introduced. We then found disabled veterans to testify in legislative committee hearings. The testimony of the veterans was more compelling and more convincing than the testimony of the representatives from the New Jersey Psychiatric Association, who testified that there was not enough evidence to allow cannabis therapy for PTSD. The legislature passed the bill, and Governor Christie signed it into law in September 2016. I thanked Governor Christie, and it was the only time I ever shook hands with him.

CMMNJ's free, public meetings have been held for over a decade on the second Tuesday of each month at the Lawrence Twp. Branch of the Mercer County Library from 7:00 PM until 9:00 PM. All are welcome, and we are required to say, "Meeting at the library does not imply the county's endorsement of our program."

How do ethical concepts guide your efforts?

At a talk at the Institute of Catholic Bioethics at St. Joseph's University on November 14, 2007, I explored some of medical cannabis's intersections with bioethical concerns, namely,

- What are a health care professional's obligations when the safest and most effective therapeutic agent is an illegal substance?
- Has the federal government's handling of medical cannabis been a long series of ethical missteps?
- Have some groups had their objectivity on this issue compromised by lobbyists and financial contributions from the pharmaceutical industry or others?

As an RN, I try to adhere to the code of ethics for nurses that was developed by the International Council of Nurses in Geneva, Switzerland. This code says that nurses have four fundamental responsibilities: to promote health, to prevent illness, to restore health, and to alleviate suffering. Our primary professional responsibility is to people requiring nursing care.

It is from this ethical framework and my own practical experience that I have come out in support of medical cannabis. No one should suffer needlessly, and no one should ever go to jail for following the advice of a doctor.

What are the pertinent social justice issues that still need to be addressed via cannabis advocacy work?

It is a morally bankrupt position to forbid suffering patients to have access to the medical benefits of cannabis. This is especially true when licensed physicians are recommending cannabis for these patients and when this safe, effective, and inexpensive therapeutic agent is readily available.

The federal government's position on medical cannabis—total denial that cannabis has any medical benefits—is an embarrassment to science, to countless health care professionals and to patients nationwide. But worst of all, the federal government has blocked the path of inquiry into the benefits of medical cannabis. They refuse to allow large-scale clinical testing. They have systematically and consistently prevented the kind of studies that would lead to FDA approval, and then they—and their apologists—complain that the FDA has not approved it.

There have been calls to reschedule cannabis from its absurd Schedule I status since 1972, yet the federal government continues to insist that there are no accepted medical uses for cannabis. That's what happens when you allow federal police—the DEA—to determine what medical and scientific studies can be done. The DEA determines what is, and what is not, medicine in the United States. We must resolve as a nation to stop DEA's interference with science and medicine and never let it happen again.

What does the future look like for cannabis political advocacy in the United States and/or globally?

Expanding the MMP is the natural evolution of drug policy. We are going from reefer madness that was not based on science to ever-more sophisticated medical understandings and programs that are based on science. The mid-1980 discovery of the human ECS, showing cannabinoid receptors in every organ of the human body, goes a long way toward explaining how the components of cannabis can influence such a wide variety of diseases and symptoms. Cannabis is used to control the increased intraocular pressure of glaucoma, to control nausea and vomiting, to control pain, to control muscle spasms, to control seizures, to stimulate the appetite, and for many other therapeutic reasons. Moreover, cannabis is a remarkably safe drug that has never caused a fatal overdose.

The broader use of medical cannabis allows more people to have direct experience with the effects of cannabis. This direct experience proves that the harms of cannabis have been greatly exaggerated by the government for decades. When more and more people see cannabis helping the most fragile members of society—toddlers with seizure disorders or the sick and dying—there is growing support for a relaxation of penalties against its production and use. Cannabis is a safe and effective therapeutic agent for a wide range of diseases, symptoms, and conditions. More people are realizing that patients should not be made to suffer because of the federal government's absurd classification of cannabis as a Schedule I drug. A growing consensus has the direct experience that the federal government is completely wrong when it denies cannabis' benefits and exaggerates its dangers. This consensus believes that the government's reasons for cannabis' overall prohibition are wrong, as well.

The majority of New Jersey's 9 million residents could benefit from cannabis therapy at some time in their lives, when you consider all of cannabis' therapeutic uses. If you live in the Garden State, you have a one in three chance of having a cancer diagnosis at some time in your life. Chronic pain affects about one in four. The state is finally beginning to recognize mental and emotional conditions that qualify for cannabis therapy—and PTSD and anxiety are just the tip of the iceberg.

We all die, and cannabis improves the quality of life of the dying like no other drug.

Legalization of cannabis is the best and most efficient way to meet the needs of the numerous patients in New Jersey who could benefit from cannabis therapy. These patients need a consistent and reliable source of cannabis, in a wide variety of preparations, for illnesses that may well last a lifetime.

In addition to having cannabis commercially available at a reasonable price, patients should be allowed to grow their own medicine. Gardening itself is therapeutic. To grow a therapeutic herb is to get twice the bang for your buck. To produce your own medicine, and titrate it to control your own symptoms, is a wonderful advance in American health care. It eliminates the pharmaceutical industry and the insurance industry from the health care picture, along with their huge profits. Home cultivation is an important part of health care reform. But, sad irony, the Garden State does not permit it … No one is giving up on home cultivation, even if it is not in the current legalization or medical expansion legislation.

CMMNJ is also supportive of efforts to legalize medical cannabis regionally (especially in New York, Pennsylvania, and Delaware) and nationally, by changing federal law.

I am very hopeful for the continuing success of cannabis reform in the United States.

Globally, it is a different story. When I attended the United Nations General Assembly Special Section on Drugs (UNGASS) in New York City in 2016, I was dismayed at the resistance to drug policy reform that exists in much of the rest of the world. Despite some successes, I fear we are a long way from global drug policy reform.

Meanwhile, CMMNJ works to enlarge its coalition of individuals and organizations that support cannabis reform. We do so through a series of meetings, conferences, educational programs, regulatory proposals, legislative testimony, rallies, demonstrations, press conferences, media interviews, letters to the editor, op eds, debates, symposia, conversations, tabling at community events, and through a vibrant presence on the Internet and social media, including a website, Facebook, YouTube, and Twitter accounts. We're all in. (Interview used with permission from Ken Wolski, RN, MPA.)

Bryan Krumm, MSN, CNP, RN, BC
(Interview used with permission from Bryan Krumm, MSN, CNP, RN, BC)

What got you interested in cannabis advocacy and the political process?

My interest in changing the cannabis laws began in 1986 after I nearly failed out of the University of New Mexico (UNM) for the second time and I began self-medicating with cannabis. When I left for college in the fall of 1981, I didn't realize that I suffered from PTSD from many years of abuse by my stepfather. Like so many who suffer from PTSD, I began drinking heavily to numb the arousal symptoms and help me get to sleep. This habit led to 23 hours of Fs on my transcripts in 2 years, at which point the university asked me to take a leave of absence.

I began a full-time job in the customer service department at Sears, and I quickly realized I wanted to go back to school, so I joined the Army on a 2-year enlistment. The Army was great. I became more confident and more aware of my capabilities. After swearing on oath "to defend the Constitution of the United States against all enemies both foreign and domestic," I learned the importance of standing up for the freedoms we enjoy. I learned the importance of speaking truth to power and standing against anyone who would order illegal, unethical, or immoral actions. I also learned that I was quite capable of consuming very large quantities of alcohol on a regular basis.

I returned to UNM in the Fall of 1986 and nearly failed out a second time. That's when I began using cannabis medicinally for my "depression" and to curb my use of alcohol. I still didn't realize I suffered from PTSD, but I knew cannabis allowed me to focus on school, sleep without nightmares, and succeed in life. I also knew that cannabis was far too expensive and that I faced serious legal consequences if I got caught. It was the Reagan era of "Just Say No," and some politicians like Jeff Sessions went so far as to advocate for the death penalty for "marijuana" users. I knew I had a duty to stand up against this, and I knew the prohibition laws had to end.

Soon I found myself making the dean's list and the honor roll. I founded a NORML chapter at UNM, and then I decided to become a nurse. Nursing expanded my sense of duty to act as an advocate for my patients. I graduated with honors and went into the workforce facing the very real specter that a simple drug test could destroy everything I had worked for, so I continued to work toward legalization of cannabis. I knew that my advocacy might pose a threat to my safety and security, but I also knew that if left unchecked, the evils of prohibition would only permeate further through the fabric of our society.

In 1996, after California legalized medical cannabis, I shifted my focus from legalization to medicalization. I drafted a rudimentary Medical Cannabis Law and began seeking support from the NM Board of Nursing, NM Board of Pharmacy, NM Medical Society, and the NM Nurses Association. In 1999, I helped to draft what is now New Mexico's current Medical Cannabis Law, and in 2007 that law finally passed. Unfortunately, because cannabis is still illegal at the federal level, my fight continues. My focus is now the illegal placement of cannabis in Schedule 1 of the Controlled Substances Act.

How did you learn to be an advocate?

I learned advocacy through practical experience and through my education as a nurse. I founded UNM NORML in 1986 in order to bring together like-minded individuals, so we could collaborate, educate, and advocate for change. I began talking about medical cannabis in nursing school, doing papers and projects on the topic in order to educate both my peers and my instructors. I began reaching out to leaders in the movement like Mary Lynn Mathre in order to learn, coordinate, and strategize. Instead of waiting for someone else to tell me what to do, I learned how to be an advocate by becoming an advocate.

What are some of your greatest challenges or obstacles in doing this work?

By far the greatest challenge has been confronting the ignorance and stigma surrounding cannabis that was instilled into our society by racist, intolerant bureaucrats and perpetuated by an unethical and morally bankrupt medical system that kowtows to a corrupt law enforcement system, rather than standing up for patients. Too many politicians support ongoing prohibition out of political expediency, not because it makes us safer. Too many doctors have built careers by demonizing cannabis and now refuse to admit that they were wrong, so they simply ignore science and the truth. Too many law enforcement agencies have come to rely on money from property seized under forfeiture laws, so now they threaten and intimidate both politicians and the medical establishment in order to maintain the status quo.

My next biggest challenge has been overcoming my own fears. I was using cannabis as a medicine long before it became legal in New Mexico. I've had to worry that I could lose my job if my advocacy aroused suspicion of use by an employer. It wasn't easy going in front of my licensing board and asking them to support medical cannabis, I was afraid they might suspect "illegal drug use" and take away my license. I've feared that my door could be kicked in by overzealous law enforcement agents and I could be arrested because I've admitted to medical cannabis use in legal filings. I've feared for the safety and well-being of my family as a result of my advocacy and the attention it draws. Fear can be a tremendous obstacle, or it can be a great motivator. I've chosen to use my fear to motivate me to put an end to the prohibition, thus eliminating the fear rather than hiding from it.

What do you count as successes? What have you learned from "failures"?

There have been far too many successes to even begin to list them all. I have met so many amazing people over the decades, helping to educate some and learning from others. I played a role in bringing medical cannabis to New Mexico. I've helped thousands of patients more effectively treat their PTSD. I've spoken about medical cannabis at numerous medical conferences and patient meetings. I forced the DEA to acknowledge science and admit that cannabis is not a gateway drug, doesn't cause lung cancer, doesn't cause psychosis, and doesn't cause cognitive decline with aging. I forced the DEA to change their policy of blocking medical cannabis research and only allowing National Institute on Drug Abuse (NIDA) to supply cannabis for research purposes. I was named the *Nurse Practitioner Journal* Author of the Year for an article I wrote upon the use of cannabis for treating PTSD. I've made it to the Supreme Court in hopes that I can end federal control over cannabis.

As for failures, I'm not sure I've had any. I've had setbacks in which I made mistakes and had to learn from those mistakes. I was kicked out of college on my first try. I've made technical/procedural errors in legal filings that led to dismissal of cases. I've had times when I did everything right but things didn't go the way I hoped. However, failure doesn't come from not succeeding in everything you try. Failure comes when you stop trying. I will not stop trying! I may need to change my strategy from time to time, but I will not give up! The stakes are too high to allow for failure.

How do ethical concepts guide your efforts?

The ethical concepts fundamental to nursing and enshrined within the US Constitution drive my advocacy. All humans have a fundamental right to be treated with dignity and respect. All humans have a right to be treated fairly under the law. All humans have a right to try to avoid unwarranted suffering. Nobody has the right to impose unwarranted suffering on another. I believe that ultimately the truth will prevail and that cannabis will be legalized. I'm proud to be a part of the nursing profession. Nursing has taken the ethical high ground and is leading the way toward a better tomorrow.

CONCLUSION

This chapter has explored some of the pressing legal, ethical, and advocacy issues that cannabis care nurses face every day. It's crucial that we examine the lingering prohibition era stigma as we strive, as nurses, to be the leaders in ensuring that our patients have access to safe, quality, tested cannabis and cannabinoid therapeutics. By educating ourselves around the local, state, and federal laws and regulations related to medical cannabis, we can begin to ensure that our cannabis care practice and our efforts to educate and coach patients remain grounded in the best evidence-based and patient-informed practices and also align with state practice acts. By considering the ethical aspects of our work with cannabis care patients, we can continue to support patients as we remain the most trusted group of professionals.

For inspiration and courage, we can look to some of the brave advocate-nurses who have defined the path of cannabis care nursing and have taken on the cannabis advocacy role to establish patients' rights to access safe, effective herbal medicine that supports homeostasis. There is still much work to be done in this area, and you have the power to be part of this historical movement by ending the stigma associated with cannabis and acting as an advocate to ensure patients in your state have access to safe, affordable, tested, high-quality cannabis and cannabinoid therapeutics.

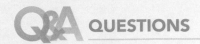 **QUESTIONS**

1. Ethics in cannabis care nursing are important because:
   A. Cannabis remains federally illegal.
   B. All nursing care should encompass ethical considerations.
   C. Nurses are viewed as the most ethical of all professions.
   D. All of the above.

2. Social justice issues abound related to cannabis, including incarceration rates and disproportionate rates of people of color being targeted for cannabis crimes. From the lens of social justice, legislation is needed to address:
   A. People who are serving prison sentences related to personal cannabis use.
   B. The expungement of cannabis convictions in states where cannabis is now legal.
   C. People of color having equal involvement within the cannabis industry.
   D. All of the above.

3. Advocacy work is important to ensure that patients around the globe have access to safe, affordable, tested cannabis and cannabinoid therapeutics. Some of the best ways for a nurse to prepare for advocacy work is:
   A. Jump right in; it's part of the nurse's role. No special training is needed.
   B. Study the topic, seek training or mentorship, and look to volunteer with organizations that are advocating for change.
   C. Call their state representative and demand change now, as our representatives are there to work for us.
   D. None of the above.

4. The best way to learn about your state MMP is to:
   A. Call the appropriate state regulating office and ask for information to be sent to you.
   B. Interview current medical patients about their experiences with accessing cannabis in the state.
   C. Do your own in-depth research, including exploring current and historical state regulations, laws, and legislation.
   D. Make an appointment with the local cannabis recommending APRN or MD to discuss the process.

5. Consider your own knowledge of your state MMP. What steps can you take to ensure that you can best support patients on their journey toward upregulating their ECS? How will you stay abreast of current local, state, and federal legislation that impacts your patients' ability to access cannabis and cannabinoid therapeutics?

ANSWERS

1. **Answer: D.** All of the above.

   Rationale: All of these answers directly relate to the need for a strong ethical foundation when providing cannabis care.

2. **Answer: D.** All of the above.

   Rationale: All of these qualify as social justice issues.

3. **Answer: B.** Study the topic, seek training or mentorship, and look to volunteer with organizations that are advocating for change.

   Rationale: Although all nurses are charged with being advocates for patients and populations, many of us lack refined skills to be effective, so seeking support and training may help us to grow in these skills as we take a hands-on approach to advocacy.

4. **Answer: C.** Do your own in-depth research, including exploring current and historical state regulations, laws, and legislation.

   Rationale: Although all of the approaches may yield helpful information, nothing can replace your own knowledge of your current state laws and legislation.

References

American Cannabis Nurses Association. (2019). *Scope and standards of practice for cannabis nurses.* https://cannabisnurses.org/Scope-of-Practice-for-Cannabis-Nurses

American Civil Liberties Union. (2013). *The war on drugs in black and white.* https://www.aclu.org/report/report-war-marijuana-black-and-white?redirect=criminal-law-reform/war-marijuana-black-and-white

American Nurses Association. (2015). *Code of ethics for nurses with interpretive statements.* Author. https://www.nursingworld.org/coe-view-only

American Nurses Association. (n.d.). *Advocacy.* https://www.nursingworld.org/practice-policy/advocacy/

Butts, J. B., & Rich, K. L. (2015). *Nursing ethics: Across the curriculum and into practice.* Jones & Bartlett.

Cannabis Control Commission, Commonwealth of Massachusetts. (2019). *Equity programs.* https://mass-cannabis-control.com/equityprograms/

Cravens, J. (2019). *How you can advocate for an issue important to you.* https://www.coyotecommunications.com/stuff/promote.shtml#credits

Cyr, C., Arboleda, M. F., Aggarwal, S. K., Belneaves, L. G., Daeninck, P., Neron, A., Prosk, E., & Vigano, A. (2018). Cannabis in palliative care: Current challenges and practical recommendations. *Annals of Palliative Medicine, 7*(4), 463–477.

Drug Policy Alliance. (2018). *Women, prison and the drug war.* http://www.drugpolicy.org/resource/women-prison-and-drug-war-englishspanish

Federal Bureau of Investigation. (2018). *Uniform crime reporting, 2017.* https://ucr.fbi.gov/crime-in-the-u.s/2017/crime-in-the-u.s.-2017/tables/table-29

Kinsinger, F. S. (2009). Beneficence and the professional's moral imperative. *Journal of Chiropractic Humanities, 16*(1), 44–46.

Kovacevich, N. (2018). *Cannabis goes global while the U.S. falls behind.* https://www.forbes.com/sites/nickkovacevich/2018/11/16/cannabis-goes-global-while-the-u-s-falls-behind/#1338eaac1783

Minnesota Nurses Association. (2019). *Are you ready to administer marijuana?* https://mnnurses.org/are-you-ready-to-administer-marijuana/

National Council of States Boards of Nursing. (2018). The NCSBN national nursing guidelines for medical marijuana. *Journal of Nursing Regulation, 9*(2), S5–S46. https://doi.org/10.1016/S2155-8256(18)30098-X

National Organization for the Reform of Marijuana Laws. (2019). *About NORML.* https://norml.org/about/intro

Nelson, S. (2019). Bay of Pigs veteran serving America's longest marijuana sentence headed to a new prison: Cuba. *Washington Examiner.* https://www.washingtonexaminer.com/policy/foreign/bay-of-pigs-veteran-serving-americas-longest-marijuana-sentence-may-be-headed-to-a-new-prison-cuba

Tchekmedyian, A. (2019, April 1). *Prosecutors move to clear 54,000 marijuana convictions in California.* https://www.latimes.com/local/lanow/la-me-ln-la-county-marijuana-convictions-20190401-story.html

The Pew Charitable Trusts. (2018). *Probation and parole systems.* https://www.pewtrusts.org/-/media/assets/2018/09/probation_and_parole_systems_marked_by_high_stakes_missed_opportunities_pew.pdf

Thompson, S. (2019). *Ethical principles of totality.* https://work.chron.com/ethical-principles-totality-4478.html

United Nations. (1961). *United Nations single convention on narcotic drugs.* https://www.unodc.org/unodc/en/treaties/single-convention.html

United Nations. (1971). *Convention on psychotropic substances.* https://www.unodc.org/pdf/convention_1971_en.pdf

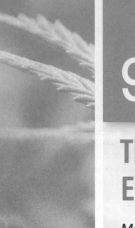

9

The Cannabis Care Nurse's Experience

Marissa Fratoni, BSN, RN, LMT, RYT, INHC,
Sherri Tutkus, BSN, RN, and Jodi Chapin, RN

CONCEPTS AND CONSIDERATIONS

This chapter discusses the current experiences of nurses involved in cannabis care practices. The authors explore how cannabis care nurses utilize their working knowledge of the endocannabinoid system (ECS), cannabis pharmacology, and current evidence to help their patients access, and safely and effectively use, cannabis as medicine. The chapter examines some of the settings in which a cannabis care nurse may provide consultations and education services, consider legal implications and career challenges faced by practicing cannabis care nurses, and explore some of the contemporary entrepreneurial endeavors and nurse-operated businesses in the cannabis industry.

Learning Outcomes

Upon completion of this chapter, the learner will:

- Understand how the nursing process is applied when providing care, coaching, and counseling of the cannabis patient in various settings.
- Observe how the National Council of State Boards of Nursing's (NCSBN, 2018) six principles of essential knowledge are applied and integrated into cannabis care nursing practice.
- Understand how state/federal marijuana laws and state nurse practice acts may shape and/or restrict cannabis care nursing practice.

THE CANNABIS CARE NURSE'S ROLE AND RESPONSIBILITIES IN VARIOUS SETTINGS

The cannabis care nurse's role is a dynamic one, consistently influenced by the laws, regulations, research, science, and business developments that encompass the legal issues related to cannabis and the burgeoning cannabis industry as a whole. Per the principles of essential knowledge set forth by the NCSBN (2018), the cannabis care nurse needs a solid working foundation of the ECS, cannabinoid receptors, and the cannabis plant, in addition to knowledge of the existing and emerging evidence for the therapeutic use of cannabis. The cannabis care nurse must be able to navigate the state's "Medical Marijuana Program" (MMP) and adult-use cannabis programs in their community to adequately care and advocate for their patients. The cannabis care nurse's primary goal is to educate and coach patients, caregivers, their support systems, and other health professionals on the ECS and how to best support its functioning to potentiate health and well-being. The cannabis care nurse is responsible for providing guidance and support as patients undergo a process of discovering how to use cannabis as medicine in the safest, most effective ways for the common goal of symptom relief, improved healing, optimal health, and wellness. The cannabis care nurse works in all settings with communities, patients, families, and their caregivers. The cannabis care nurse may act as a liaison and advocate for patients, typically bridging the gap between conventional medical practices and medical cannabis programs. Above all, the cannabis care nurse provides care that empowers patients to choose treatments that are right for them without judgment (NCSBN, 2018).

Cannabis care nurses do not give medical advice. Instead, they educate about the ECS, and how the various products available may or may not contribute to the patient's health goals. The cannabis care nurse must teach about the pros and cons that exist with each cannabinoid product and provide information about how each product may impact the ECS, both positively and negatively. The cannabis care nurse uses the evidence base to support and coach their patients toward well-being.

Cannabis care nurses are to remain within their scope of practice that includes not making false claims regarding any cannabinoid products, or regarding cannabis in general. According to the U.S. Food and Drug Administration (FDA), the only thing that can prevent, treat, or cure a disease is an approved pharmaceutical. Cannabis care nurses must remain ethically aware that their role is to provide teaching about cannabis and to provide coaching to empower their patients to make informed choices for healing and improving their quality of life. In this chapter, the learner is provided with real-world experiences of cannabis care nurses in practice who have taken care of patients across the lifespan, from the very young to the very old. Patient stories, case studies, cannabis care nurse interviews, examples of educational material, and stories from some of the pioneers in this specialty will help the learner explore the role of the cannabis care nurse in-depth.

But First, a Note About Professional Liability

There are some logistics that every cannabis care nurse has to consider before proceeding with practice. If you are reading this and thinking that you may be interested in becoming a cannabis care nurse, review Chapter 8. Please pay careful attention to the following: Nurses must understand that (at the time of this writing), *cannabis is federally illegal*. Each nurse must have a thorough understanding of the laws and regulations outlined by the state in which he/she practices. It is critical that nurses do not handle cannabis medicine (unless their state laws expressly allow this, which is currently the exception and not the rule). The cannabis care nurse's role is to teach and coach patients around how to administer their own cannabis medicine and products. It is crucial that cannabis care nurses protect their nursing licenses and, ultimately, their livelihoods from the risk associated with practicing in a new field that remains not only controversial but federally illegal.

To this end, obtaining malpractice or liability insurance may be challenging for the practicing cannabis care nurse. There are insurance corporations that will provide liability insurance coverage for cannabis care nurses, assuming that the applicant nurse's license is in good standing, the nurse is operating within the scope of his/her state's nurse practice act, and the nurse is maintaining compliance with the employer's policies and procedures (if applicable). Keep in mind that many nurses who advocate for the medical use of cannabis, teach about the ECS, or even dare to answer their patients' enquiries about cannabis in any patient-care facility may very well be out of compliance with their employer's policies, despite the NCSBN (2018) call for all nurses to be educated and competent in supporting patients using medical cannabis. The nurses endeavoring to help their patients with cannabis need to be aware of these risks and also need to be prepared for the potential (and very real) consequences of their advocacy: Until the federal laws change, the prohibition of cannabis ends, and the policies set forth by employers in healthcare facilities reflect such legal shifts, there will be potential risks related to the cannabis care nurses' license.

Bottom line, if a career in cannabis care nursing interests you, conduct your due diligence to determine what risks you may face as an employee, as a professional, and perhaps even as an entrepreneur in this up and coming, yet controversial, industry. These risks can be mitigated with proper help and guidance from liability and legal professionals.

APPLYING THE NURSING PROCESS

Cannabis care nurses utilize the nursing process while providing patient-centered, outcome-oriented care. The nursing process directs the nurse to assess the patient's needs, determine applicable nursing diagnoses, develop a plan of care, implement that plan of care, and evaluate whether the plan of care needs to be modified or continued at regular intervals (American Nurses Association [ANA], 2019). The cannabis care nurse may apply the nursing process to consultations conducted in all types of settings. The following is an exploration of how the nursing process may be applied by a practicing cannabis care nurse offering consultation services to patients who seek guidance for the use of cannabis therapy.

Assessment

The cannabis care nurse's primary concern is helping a patient safely integrate cannabis therapy into their health regimen. A detailed assessment needs to be conducted for the nurse to recognize potential risks that exist. Intake paperwork is completed before the consultation that allows the nurse to review the patient's active medical problems and symptoms, past medical history, comorbidities, lifestyle, previous treatments, current treatments, medication list, and cannabis-use history. It is also essential to determine the patient's learning style, so that time spent teaching the patient is productive and positive. The use of motivational interviewing in this phase can prove fruitful.

Diagnoses

Most patients schedule consultations with a cannabis care nurse because they do not know how to meet their wellness and healing goals with the use of cannabis. Therefore, most assessments of cannabis patients should yield the following sort of nursing diagnosis:

> *Knowledge deficit related to the use of cannabis as medicine as evidenced by the statement "There are so many different things on the menu at the dispensary, I don't even know where to start!"*

From here, the cannabis care nurse hones in on the patient's symptoms and risk factors to determine other diagnoses. Common nursing diagnoses for patients seeking symptom relief with cannabis may include:

- Anxiety
- Chronic pain
- Sleep pattern disturbed
- Sleep, readiness for enhanced
- Nausea
- Risk of injury related to knowledge deficit regarding potential interactions between cannabis, prescribed drugs, and over-the-counter medicines.

Other nursing diagnoses to consider may include:

- Spiritual distress
- Post-trauma syndrome
- Coping, readiness for enhanced
- Fatigue

Plan

In conjunction with the patient, a plan is developed. Once the cannabis care nurse has a detailed picture of the patient's condition and symptoms for which relief is sought with the help of cannabis therapy, the patient's health and wellness goals are determined, and ideal outcomes are considered. A few examples:

- Patient will have a basic understanding of the ECS.
- Patient will have a basic understanding of phytocannabinoids, chemovars, cannabis delivery methods, titration processes, and side effects.
- Patient will feel empowered to make an informed, evidence-based decision when selecting cannabis products for purchase and use.
- Patient will explore the use of holistic-integrative modalities to upregulate the ECS.

Implementation

Teaching about the ECS, cannabinoid receptors, and how cannabis interacts with the ECS is necessary for patients to maintain safety and attain their specific health improvement goals. Teaching on these topics should always be included in the care plan of the patient using cannabis. In addition to providing this necessary teaching, the following may be implemented in the care, counseling, and coaching of the patient using cannabis:

- Utilization of a shared decision-making tool to determine which applications and delivery methods of medical cannabis may help the patient reduce symptoms and attain wellness goals
- What to expect when utilizing cannabis as medicine, including potential side effects, drug interactions, and how to mitigate unwanted effects
- How to track cannabis use with a cannabis diary
- Evidence-based information regarding the titration process
- Written recommendations, journals, visual aids, and audio resources for ongoing learning
- Coaching around how to upregulate the ECS through holistic modalities and lifestyle changes to potentiate homeostasis

Evaluation

Cannabis has a wide range of therapeutic values, and every individual's ECS has different needs. Therefore, using cannabis as medicine is very personalized. It may take time for patients to discover the profile of cannabis products, delivery methods, and dosages that work best for them. It takes time to develop new healthy habits that upregulate the ECS. Most patients will need support and coaching with changing their lifestyles and taking steps toward upregulating the ECS. Therefore, some patients will need regular consultations with a cannabis care nurse over an extended period of time to attain symptom relief and other health goals. Other patients may only need one consultation before visiting a dispensary to help them determine which cannabis products and delivery methods may be most beneficial. Regardless of where the patient falls on the spectrum of need, the cannabis care nurse should always follow up with and provide an evaluation to determine whether the patient is meeting their health goals or if they could benefit from coaching or a review and modification of the original plan.

CARING FOR THE WHOLE PATIENT—OPTIMIZING THE ENDOCANNABINOID SYSTEM

The ECS is the largest neuroregulatory system that regulates other organ systems and neurotransmitters throughout the body (Sallaberry & Astern, 2018). A large number of patients who are interested in cannabinoid therapeutics have often exhausted all other treatment options. In most cases, they will have an ECS that is impaired and dysregulated. Or they may be struggling with an endocannabinoid deficiency. This means that they are not producing enough of their internal endogenous cannabinoids for homeostasis. Part of the cannabis nursing care plan must include lifestyle education and the use of holistic modalities to support biopsychosocial-spiritual aspects of healing.

Genetics, age, obesity, poor diet, smoking, chronic alcohol use, polypharmacy, chronic stress, lack of exercise, and social isolation contribute to a dysregulated ECS.

When we look at this list, we can determine what may be a contributing factor to a person's imbalanced ECS and focus on wellness tools to support them in their healing process (McPartland et al., 2014).

Many health practices will promote homeostasis of the ECS. A healthy diet, exercise, stress management, massage, yoga, meditation, acupuncture, low impact exercises, and social and intimate interactions are all practices that promote the balance of the mind, body, and spirit. All of these practices upregulate the ECS (McPartland et al., 2014).

"Let food be medicine and medicine be food" is a popular quote by Hippocrates, the Father of Medicine. Our dietary choices either support our health or they do not. Herbs, spices, and plants are part of the universal ecologic medicine that much of the world's rural population still rely on as a primary healthcare modality. There are many plants (including cannabis) that are filled with nutrients and medicinal compounds that interact directly and indirectly with the ECS. The common kitchen spice rack provides a small treasure trove of compounds that mediate the same endocannabinoid CB1 and CB2 receptors that interact with cannabis (Lee, 2016).

Eating a mainly whole food diet comprised of vegetables, fruits, herbs, spices, tea, chocolate, and essential fatty acids contribute to the optimal functioning of the ECS and enhance the effectiveness of medicinal cannabis. Sources of endocannabinoid-enhancing ω -3 fatty acids include hemp seeds, hemp oil, flax seeds, flax oil, chia seeds, walnuts, sardines, anchovies, and eggs.

Certain herbs, spices, and teas support endocannabinoid signaling because they provide terpenes (aromatic molecules that give plants their characteristic aromas) that stimulate the cannabinoid receptors. For example, β -caryophyllene is a terpene found in black pepper, lemon balm, hops, cloves, oregano, and cinnamon. β -Caryophyllene stimulates CB2 receptors, boosts immune system functioning, and helps chronic inflammatory disorders (Gertsch et al., 2008). *Echinacea* is often used during cold and flu season because of its immune-boosting properties and is also a CB2 agonist that enhances endocannabinoid tone. Turmeric is a spice in curry powder that contains curcumin, which has been known to interact with the ECS and provide multiple health benefits with its anti-inflammatory properties.

Some herbs, spices, and teas have medicinal components that prevent the breakdown of our internal endogenous endocannabinoids. This allows our circulating endocannabinoids (anandamide and 2-arachidonoylglycerol [2AG]) to stimulate CB1 and CB2 receptors independently of cannabis. Camellia sinensis, a tea from a species of the evergreen shrub, is an example of such a compound. Maca root powder and dark chocolate also inhibit enzymes from breaking down our endocannabinoids. Chocolate is rich in anandamide-like molecules, which are naturally produced in the brain; dark chocolate and raw cacao have the greatest concentrations of these molecules (Tomaso et al., 1996). Plant-derived anandamide-like molecules (such as those found in cacao) linger in the body, drawing out the joyful feeling longer than an average runner's high. Probiotics and unpasteurized fermented food can also help improve the function of the ECS by providing beneficial bacteria to the gut that supports proper ECS functioning.

In addition to food, supplements, herbs, spices, and plants, numerous lifestyle-enhancing activities can help regulate the ECS. An optimally functioning ECS protects patients from the "dis-ease"-causing effects of stress. Health-promoting activities that work in synergy with cannabis and also promote optimization of the ECS without the use of cannabis include meditation, osteopathic manipulation, acupuncture, breath-work, socializing, and enjoyable exercise or fitness routines. Hint: If you are not enjoying your activity, then you are promoting stress!

It makes sense that the cannabis care nurse would incorporate all of the ECS-enhancing activities in the care plan to support the body's ability to self-regulate with the assistance of cannabis. Remember, the goal is to help your patients live their best life!

PROVIDING CONSULTATIONS

The following sections explore some of the settings in which a cannabis care nurse may work. These pages include real-life experiences of cannabis care nurses in current practice. Protected Health Information (PHI) has been changed or removed to protect the privacy of the subjects featured. Stories, case studies, documentation examples in the form of SOAP (subjective, objective, assessment, and plan) notes, examples of educational materials, handouts, and learning aids will help the learner gain a real-life perspective of cannabis care nursing practice.

Office Consultation—Mrs. Jones' Story

The office consultation allows the patient face-to-face interaction with a nurse. This is the setting that is most familiar to patients who are seeking care from a medical professional.

Mrs. Jones, a 62-year-old Caucasian, came into the office after completing all of her paperwork with the primary complaint of arthritis in her hips and knees. Stiffness, tension, limited mobility, and pain were the symptoms she sought relief from with the use of cannabis products. She was new to cannabis, reported taking multiple pharmaceuticals, and she stated that she was afraid of getting high. Mrs. Jones' primary goal was to decrease joint pain without being impaired.

Mrs. Jones' initial consultation was focused on potentiating the ECS (Figure 9.1), using non-impairing cannabinoids such as cannabidiol (CBD), and exploring various cannabis delivery methods available for purchase inside and outside of the dispensary (Table 9.1). To bolster her learning, Mrs. Jones was provided with a patient handbook that detailed these topics with a variety of visual aids.

With guidance and teaching provided, Mrs. Jones was relieved to know that she could start with a topical cannabis product, and there were other products available that could potentially alleviate her symptoms without having to use tetrahydrocannabinol (THC). Mrs. Jones decided to start her cannabis journey by purchasing a full-spectrum CBD salve. The product's label suggested applying it topically to affected joints two to four times/day as needed. The cannabis care nurse concurred that it was best to follow the manufacturer's instructions for application. Mrs. Jones was provided a journal and agreed to record her experience to determine whether the product was effective or if she needed to make some changes to her cannabis regimen (Figure 9.2).

CANNABIS 101 (part one)

Endocannabinoid System (ECS) can be found in all vertebrate species and acts as the largest neurotransmitter signaling system to help maintain a stable internal environment within our bodies. The goal of the Endocannabinoid system is to maintain balance or homeostasis with all of our other body systems.

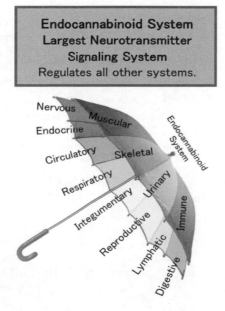

Endocannabinoids and their receptors are found throughout the body including: the brain, organs, connective tissues, glands and immune cells. They all perform different tasks but the goal is always the same which is to bring about homeostasis or balance within the body. ECS helps to auto regulate our bodies more efficiently in regards to eating, sleeping, relaxing, protecting and forgetting.

www.GreenNurseGroup.com   Call us 1(844) GNG-3882

Figure 9.1: **Cannabis 101. A page from the GreenNurse Group.** (Used with permission by Tutkus, S., & Sykes, S. (2019). *Handbook* (p. 7). GreenNurse™ Group. https://www.green-nursegroup.com/handbook)

TABLE 9.1.	Delivery methods of cannabis products			
	Options	Onset	Duration	Benefits/ disadvantages
Inhalation	Smoking, vaporization	1–15 min	2–6 h	Easy to titrate, provides quick feedback Not always discreet because of scent, short duration, greater abuse potential
Topical	Creams, salves, oils, bath bombs, sprays	Varies	Varies	Discreet, localized, nonpsychoactive effect May take an extended time to work, may have a short duration
Ingestion	Edibles such as gummies, medibles such as capsules, oils	1–2 h	6–12 h	Discreet, ideal for extended relief of symptoms Easy to take too much, may result in negative side effects such as paranoia and tachycardia
Sublingual	Tinctures, sprays, dissolvable strips	10–45 min	2–8 h	Discreet, ideal for extended relief of symptoms Easy to take too much, may result in negative side effects
Transdermal	Patches, gel pens	15 min–1 h	4–8 h	Discreet, full-body effect May take an extended time to work, may irritate the skin
Suppositories	Vaginal, rectal	Varies	Varies	Discreet, potential for use by those who cannot consume via mouth Potential for poor absorption

Adapted from Goldstein, B. (2016). *Cannabis revealed: How the world's most misunderstood plant is healing everything from chronic pain to epilepsy* (p. 91). Bonni S. Goldstein MD Inc.; Konieczny, E., & Wilson, L. (2018). *Healing with CBD: How cannabidiol can transform your health without the high* (p. 168). Ulysses Press; and Sulak, D. (2017). *Using medical cannabis: Delivery systems.* https://healer.com/using-medical-cannabis-delivery-systems/

Canna Journal

Date: 3/21   **Time:** 8am
How are you feeling today, physically? Mentally? Rate your pain level.

I am feeling very tired and stiff physically.
Mentally I am exhausted. Pain is 6/10.

STRAIN: Full-spectrum CBD salve

DOSE: Apply 2-4 times per day

METHOD OF ADMINISTRATION: topical

AROMA: fresh scent

TASTE: na

Cannabinoid Profile:
TAC: %
THC: %
THC-A: %
CBD: %
CBD-A: %
CBG: %
CBG-A: %

How are you feeling AFTER using cannabis, physically? Mentally? Rate your pain level.

30 Minutes: *I'm a little less stiff*

Pain Level:
1-Hour: 4/10

Pain Level:
2-Hours: 4/10

Pain Level:
Notes: *The salve helps, I can move better. Want to see if a tincture could help relieve my pain.*

www.GreenNurseGroup.com   Call us 1(844) GNG-3882

Figure 9.2: Canna journal. A page from patient handbook—provided by the GreenNurse Group. (Used with permission by Tutkus, S., & Sykes, S. (2019). *Handbook* (p. 25). Green-Nurse™ Group. https://www.greennursegroup.com/handbook)

Follow-up was conducted in 1 week via phone—Mrs. Jones reported a decrease in symptoms with slightly improved mobility, but she was still experiencing pain. She wanted to continue with the application of the topical product to see if she could get further relief. Two weeks later, Mrs. Jones reported that she was still experiencing some relief from her symptoms, but she wanted to try an oil tincture to see whether her symptoms would further improve.

Mrs. Jones scheduled a second office consultation for experiential, hands-on learning with tinctures. The cannabis care nurse first instructed Mrs. Jones on how to read labels of products (Figure 9.3), seeking those that were laboratory tested for confirmation of purity and potency, and to ensure the products were free of contaminants such as mold, bacteria, and heavy metals as applicable. See Figure 9.4 for an example of testing results provided by an accredited, certified laboratory that is compliant with the regulatory framework used by the pharmaceutical industry.

Once Mrs. Jones had gained confidence in choosing a quality CBD tincture product and made her purchase, the cannabis care nurse focused on how the patient could handle the product. Mrs. Jones was taught how to properly administer the tincture with the eyedropper provided. She was given a comprehensive chart regarding dosage to figure out how many drops she needed to take (Table 9.2) and instructed to start with the lowest dose of one to five drops. She would titrate her dose up, as needed, with the guidance of the cannabis care nurse every 3 to 5 days (start low and go slow). With the cannabis care nurse's help, Mrs. Jones decided to start ingesting 5 mg (about three drops) of the tincture in the morning and the evening.

Before the consultation ended, Mrs. Jones asked pertinent questions about potential interactions between her prescribed medicines and cannabis, and what to do if she experienced side effects from the tincture. The nurse reviewed drug interactions with Mrs. Jones and determined there were no significant interactions to be concerned with, but she did review potential side effects related to cannabis use that included nausea, irritability, and fatigue (Grinspoon, 2019). The cannabis care nurse recommended that Mrs. Jones contact her should she experience any side effects.

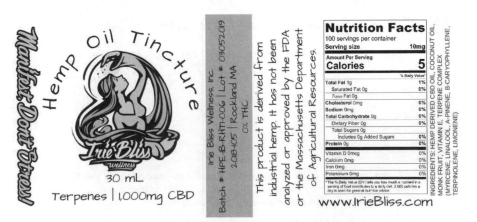

Figure 9.3: **Product label for cannabidiol (CBD) tincture.** (Used with permission by Irie Bliss Wellness, Inc. (2019). https://iriebliss.com/product/irie-bliss-drops-hemp-oil/)

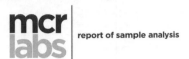

report of sample analysis

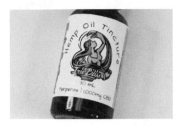

Test report: Irie Bliss 1000mg Tincture

Client:	Irie Bliss Wellness
Client contact:	
Strain:	unknown
Sample Type:	MIP
Batch:	NA
Analyst:	PS/GF/SA
Authorization:	JW
Product ID:	S19-11989
Receipt Date:	4/18/2019
Test Date:	04/19/2019

Cannabinoid Profile per Serving

Serving Size 30 mL, 27540mg

Cannabinoid	mg per serving	Weight %
THC	Not detected	Not detected
CBD	1,012.37mg	3.7%
CBN	39.38mg	0.1%
THCa	Not detected	Not detected
CBDa	Not detected	Not detected
Δ-8 THC	Not detected	Not detected
CBGa	1.10mg	0.0%
THCv	Not detected	Not detected
CBDv	10.74mg	0.0%
CBC	88.13mg	0.3%
Total	1,151.72mg	4.2%
Max THC	Not detected	Not detected
Max CBD	1,012.37mg	3.7%

■ CBD
■ CBN
■ CBGa
■ CBDv
■ CBC

■ Max THC
■ Max CBD

Figure 9.4: Laboratory testing results for cannabidiol (CBD) tincture. (Used with permission by MCR Labs, LLC. (2019). *Cannabis testing report: Report of sample analysis (Test report: Irie Blis 1000mg tincture).* https://iriebliss.com/product/irie-bliss-drops-hemp-oil/)

TABLE 9.2.	Cannabidiol tincture dosage table

CBD 450 mg/30 mL
450 mg in 1 oz or 30 mL
1 drop = 0.75 mg
5 drops = ¼ dropper = 3.75 mg
10 drops = ½ dropper = 7.5 mg
15 drops = ¾ dropper = 11.25 mg
20 drops = 1 dropper = 15 mg

CBD 2,000 mg/30 mL
2,000 mg in 1 oz or 30 mL
1 drop = 3.33 mg
5 drops = ¼ dropper = 16 mg
10 drops = ½ dropper = 32 mg
15 drops = ¾ dropper = 50 mg
20 drops = 1 dropper = 66 mg

CBD 600 mg/30 mL
600 mg in 1 oz or 30 mL
1 drop = 1 mg
5 drops = ¼ dropper = 5 mg
10 drops = ½ dropper = 10 mg
15 drops = ¾ dropper = 15 mg
20 drops = 1 dropper = 20 mg

CBD 2,400 mg/30 mL
2,400 mg in 1 oz or 30 mL
1 drop = 4 mg
5 drops = ¼ dropper = 20 mg
10 drops = ½ dropper = 40 mg
15 drops = ¾ dropper = 60 mg
20 drops = 1 dropper = 80 mg

CBD 1,000 mg /30 mL
1,000 mg in 1 oz or 30 mL
1 drop = 1.65 mg
5 drops = ¼ dropper = 8.25 mg
10 drops = ½ dropper = 16.5 mg
15 drops = ¾ dropper = 24.5 mg
20 drops = 1 dropper = 33 mg

CBD 3,000 mg/30 mL
3,000 mg in 1 oz or 30 mL
1 drop = 5 mg
5 drops = ¼ dropper = 25 mg
10 drops = ½ dropper = 50 mg
15 drops = ¾ dropper = 75 mg
20 drops = 1 dropper = 100 mg

CBD 1,500 mg/30 mL
1,500 mg in 1 oz or 30 mL
1 drop = 2.5
5 drops = ¼ dropper = 12.5 mg
10 drops = ½ dropper = 25 mg
15 drops = ¾ dropper = 37.5 mg
20 drops = 1 dropper = 50 mg

Tinctures
1 ounce (oz) = 30 mL = 30 droppers-full = 600 drops in bottle.
1 mL = 1 dropper = 20 drops.
You want to know how many milligrams are in a drop.
Divide total amount of milligrams by 600 and that will be how many milligrams per drop.
From Tutkus, S. (n.d.). *CBD tincture dosage table [chart].* GreenNurse™ Group.

Wong-Baker FACES® Pain Rating Scale

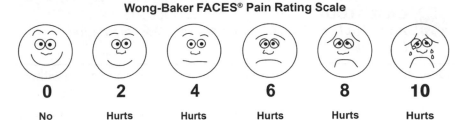

0	2	4	6	8	10
No Hurt	Hurts Little Bit	Hurts Little More	Hurts Even More	Hurts Whole Lot	Hurts Worst

©1983 Wong-Baker FACES Foundation. www.WongBakerFACES.org
Used with permission. Originally published in *Whaley & Wong's Nursing Care of Infants and Children.* ©Elsevier Inc.

Figure 9.5: **Wong-Baker FACES Pain Rating Scale.** (Used with permission from Wong-Baker FACES Foundation. (2019). *Wong-Baker FACES® Pain Rating Scale.* http://www.WongBaker-FACES.org/)

In 1 month, the cannabis care nurse followed up via phone consultation. Mrs. Jones reported a reduction in symptoms. She reported that her pain had reduced to a two on the Wong-Baker FACES Pain Rating Scale (Figure 9.5) and that she was able to come off of a nonsteroidal anti-inflammatory drug (NSAID) with the assistance of her primary care doctor. She opted to stay on the rest of her prescribed pharmaceuticals because she found that cannabis therapy complemented her conventional medicine regimen, thereby bridging the gap that existed before she started using the CBD tincture. Mrs. Jones was happy to report that she was able to successfully manage her pain, which allowed her to engage in more activities of daily living (ADLs) without assistance. As a result, her quality of life was greatly improved.

CASE STUDY
An Example of Cannabis Care Nursing Documentation

Home Consultation—Helping a Senior with Chronic Pain and Polypharmacy

Subjective	Patient complains of chronic pain from fibromyalgia and psoriatic arthritis. She also reports that she is struggling with severe anxiety. Patient states that her current pain medication regimen is inadequate for reducing her symptoms, but she has reached her limit of opioids that the pain clinic prescribes. Patient states that she needs to find alternative methods of pain control and relief. She is resistant to self-care and refuses to implement nonpharmaceutical methods of pain relief. The pain clinic doctor recommends that she try CBD. Patient states that she "doesn't want to be high."

CASE STUDY
An Example of Cannabis Care Nursing Documentation
(continued)

Objective	An 80-year-old divorced female living alone without family in the state.
	Patient's current medical diagnoses—hypertension, borderline personality disorder, fibromyalgia, severe anxiety, irritable bowel syndrome, and depression. Past medical history is significant for stage 1 adenocarcinoma of the left lung in remission after surgical removal. Surgical bowel resection of her small intestine due to a bowel obstruction. Patient had one kidney surgically removed because of benign retroperitoneal fibrosis that damaged the kidney and ureter beyond repair. As a result, the patient is unable to take NSAIDs for chronic pain. Patient also has a history of polypharmacy, substance abuse, self-medicating habits, and agoraphobia. Patient lives alone. She has assistance from a home health aide three times a week for 4 hours/day. An assistant helps with shopping, transportation, appointments, and socialization.
	Medications—Zoloft, oxycodone, Percocet, Ambien, Ativan, hydrochlorothiazide, Bentyl, Zofran, Prilosec, and losartan.
Assessment	Patient requires pain relief methods that are not pharmaceutical in nature.
	Patient is concerned about side effects related to the use of cannabis.
	Patient requires simple administration and clear visualization and instruction of dose.
Plan	Teach patient basic information about the use of CBD for potential pain reduction and relief. Example—CBD is a non-impairing cannabinoid, unlike THC.
	Emphasize that CBD will not cause her to be high, but may help reduce her symptoms of pain and, possibly, anxiety.
	Identify any potential prescribed drug and cannabinoid interactions.

(continued)

	Using sertraline together with cannabis (Schedule I substance) may increase side effects such as dizziness, drowsiness, confusion, and difficulty concentrating. Some people, especially the elderly, may also experience impairment in thinking, judgment, and motor coordination.
	Teach patient that the recommended maximum number of medicines in the "Central Nervous System (CNS) Drugs" category to be taken concurrently is usually three. Her list includes four medicines belonging to the CNS drugs category: ● Cannabis ● Zoloft (sertraline) ● Ambien (zolpidem) ● Ativan (lorazepam)
	Teach patient that the benefits of taking this combination of medicines may outweigh any risks associated with prescribing multiple medications for the same indication.
	Remind patient to check with healthcare providers to determine whether any adjustments to your medications are needed.
	Help patient select a full-spectrum CBD oil to purchase on her next outing.
Implementation	Recommend that the patient starts with a low dose of CBD on the basis of the manufacturer-suggested use instructions.
	Provide hands-on learning experience—direct patient how to properly measure tincture with eyedropper and have the patient teach-back to confirm that she understands.
	Leave easy-to-follow, written recommendations and visual aids on the fridge or other frequented locations in the patient's home for learning reinforcement. Written recommendations include information on how to calculate dosage, desired effect, and side effects that she should report.

CASE STUDY

An Example of Cannabis Care Nursing Documentation
(continued)

Recommend that the patient takes tincture with food for better absorption.

Discuss potential low-to-moderate risks:

Patient was advised that using sertraline, lorazepam, oxycodone, and Percocet independently or together with CBD may increase side effects such as dizziness, drowsiness, confusion, and difficulty concentrating. Some people, especially the elderly, may also experience impairment in thinking, judgment, and motor coordination and should be reported to the cannabis care nurse.

Teaching and coaching provided:

CBD may cause liver problems, and using it with other medications that can also affect the liver such as acetaminophen may increase that risk. Acetaminophen may be used independently, but it can also be found in combination with other prescription medications, such as Percocet.

Omeprazole may increase the blood levels of CBD. This may increase side effects such as drowsiness, diarrhea, decreased appetite, and liver problems.

Coadministration of some CBD products with antihypertensives and other hypotensive agents such as losartan and hydrochlorothiazide may result in lowered blood pressure.

Close monitoring for the development of hypotension is recommended.

Patient advised to avoid rising abruptly from a sitting or recumbent position and to notify her physician if she experiences dizziness, lightheadedness, syncope (fainting), orthostasis (decrease in blood pressure soon after standing), or tachycardia (fast heartbeat).

Patient advised that she should avoid or limit the use of alcohol while being treated with these medications.

(continued)

CASE STUDY
An Example of Cannabis Care Nursing Documentation
(continued)

	Patient should talk to her doctor regarding any questions or concerns. It is important to tell the doctor about all other medications being used, including vitamins and herbs. Do not stop using any medications without first talking to the doctor ("Drug Interaction Report," n.d.).
Evaluation	Patient reported trying 15 mg of a full-spectrum CBD tincture to start. Patient did not experience relief or adverse reactions/side effects with administration of this dose.
	Cannabis care nurse coached the patient around titrating up slowly over time until the desired effect is attained.
	Over the course of 2 months, patient discovered that 25 to 50 mg CBD prn helps her experience less painful episodes and improved mood.
	A 50-mg dose at bedtime results in better sleep and reduced use of Ambien.
	Patient also reports that she has "leftover" pain medications at the end of the month.
	Patient was able to gain adequate pain control and relief with the use of CBD.
	Patient reports that she has decreased her use of oxycodone, Percocet, Ambien, and her blood pressure medication dosages have been reduced.

Patient with Stage 4 Pancreatic Cancer Graduates from Hospice

A social worker initiated the consultation for a female patient who had just started on hospice. The patient had received her medical cannabis card and visited her local dispensary, where she purchased a variety of cannabis products. Within a few weeks of using cannabis on her own, she realized that she needed to learn how to medicate with cannabis appropriately because she was sleeping all the time from overconsumption.

Intake paperwork had been completed before the home visit that took place in the patient's living room with her husband and nephew. She had unresectable pancreatic cancer. She had failed chemotherapy and radiation and was sent home on hospice as a result. Through motivational interviewing, it was determined that the goal was to decrease pain, improve sleep, and enhance the quality of life with the use of medical cannabis.

The cannabis care nurse focused on teaching the patient about the ECS and the different products that the patient had purchased. She was coached around how to use the products and provided information about self-titration to reduce symptoms and improve the quality of her life.

Utilizing a shared decision model, the patient had wanted to continue with a Full Extract Cannabis Oil (FECO) that delivered a potent dose of THC, but she was coached to only take the FECO before bedtime to reduce pain and insomnia symptoms and help her gain restorative sleep. With the cannabis care nurse's guidance, the patient decided that it would be better to put the FECO oil in a capsule instead of pushing the oil out of the syringe. In the daytime, she used a CBD tincture oil and CBD gummies, which were adequate in managing her symptoms while allowing her to stay alert and active. She did very well with this, and her quality of life improved.

The patient checked in monthly and reported feeling much better with the implementation of her cannabis regimen. It appeared that she was not dying any longer. After 6 months, she called to report that her cancer was in complete remission, and no evidence of disease was noted. Her next life improvement goal was to wean off of her narcotics.

The cannabis care nurse contacted the patient over the phone for the next consultation. The patient reported that she was working with her doctors to come off of her narcotics. The cannabis care nurse assisted her with adjusting her cannabis doses via the shared decision model tool. Critical questions that required the patient to pay close attention to her body were asked. The cannabis care nurse recommended that she make decisions depending on how she felt mentally, emotionally, and physically—keeping track in the provided journal. Over the course of the next 4 months, she was able to come off of all of her opioids and benzodiazepines. Her next goal after graduating from hospice was to go to Italy for a month with her family. In the end, the patient felt confident in her ability to manage her health with cannabis therapy as a result of working with her team of health providers.

Opportunities for Nurses to Improve Patient Care in the Dispensary Setting

It is a common occurrence in the cannabis space—a patient using medical cannabis visits a dispensary. The product menu reads like a doctrine delivered from a foreign planet. Kush, cookies, OG, haze, Indica, Sativa, hybrids, oils, topicals, vapes, tinctures, edibles, flower, terpenes, vaporizers, water pipes, and papers. To a cannabis-naive patient, one glance at such a menu may be all things overwhelming and confusing.

Realistically, a menu such as this can be confusing for even the most experienced users, especially if they are seeking relief from symptoms.

For patients who registered with their state's MMP, they may have spent a short time with a recommending healthcare provider discussing what some of these terms mean. They may have come away from their recommending healthcare provider consultation with a brief guide to choosing cannabis products and have a few suggestions for choosing cannabis products jotted down. But then they enter a dispensary and guidance from their qualified health provider is insufficient to help them negotiate the overwhelming cannabis menu and make decisions that may benefit them.

Enter the dispensing agent, more commonly known as budtenders. Dispensing agents are dispensary staff members responsible for helping patients decipher the menu by providing information about the various cannabis products. They also fulfill the patient's order and complete the sale at the cash register. They are often not healthcare professionals; more often, they are people with retail, customer service, and sales backgrounds.

Here is where their role gets tricky—to help patients decide about which products to purchase depending on symptoms reported, dispensing agents very often give medical advice that is far out of the realm of their skill set, training, and knowledge base. It is not the dispensing agents' fault that they are in such predicaments, but the fact that the majority of dispensing agents are giving medical advice in some way, shape, or form is disconcerting from a medical and health perspective. Conveying unauthorized medical advice without a license is not only a criminal offense, but doing so may also place patients at risk for legitimate adverse events. Sometimes the adverse events and side effects of using too much cannabis product can also impact the patient's future choices around continuing to explore the use of cannabis.

In medical cannabis dispensaries, dispensing agents may have access to a very limited list of conditions from which the patient suffers. A patient's health history may be missing from intake forms completed and signed by the patient during the initial dispensary visit, which presents risks.

For one thing, cannabis does interact with other medications. Cannabis may impact the way pharmaceutical medications are metabolized in the body, in some cases speeding up the metabolism of medications, and in other cases slowing the metabolism down. Cannabis may have a synergistic effect with medications, or it may have an antagonistic effect (Project CBD, 2019). The risks to the person consuming cannabis with other medications on board may range from rendering the prescribed treatment ineffective to an experience of severe interactions or negative experiences that require emergency medical attention.

Another significant risk is that patients may erroneously believe that they can simply replace their prescribed medications with cannabis. Too often, unknowing dispensing agents relay anecdotes from other patients who have successfully weaned off of this medicine or that medicine. This is unfortunate because no patient should wean off of any medication without oversight and guidance from a qualified healthcare provider, because the effects of doing so may be very harmful.

As stated earlier, it is not entirely the fault of the dispensaries or the dispensing agents that these businesses profess medical advice. Most states have developed disjointed cannabis programs. In some cases, MMP state regulations specify that it is a conflict of interest for recommending healthcare providers to have any affiliation with the dispensary businesses. On paper, this makes sense. A recommending healthcare provider who develops a relationship with specific dispensaries has the propensity to engage in questionable business practices and vice versa. However, in practice, there are aspects of these restrictions that put patients at risk, mainly because they are provided certification, recommendation, or registration from their qualified healthcare provider, and then left to navigate the cannabis space on their own with only the help and guidance of the dispensary staff who are typically not qualified to help them in any medical capacity.

Here is an example of this scenario in action: The state cannabis laws and guidance documents established in Massachusetts specify that recommending healthcare providers are explicitly not allowed to counsel patients at dispensaries. Nor are health practitioners employed at dispensaries allowed to provide any clinical counsel. As a result of the potential conflicts of interest specified in the laws and guidelines, the dispensary staff does not contact the recommending healthcare providers on the patient's behalf.

To better understand this issue, consider this hypothetical scenario: A patient goes to the physician with a medical problem or illness. The physician writes a prescription and hands it to the patient. The patient then brings the prescription to the pharmacy to have it filled. The pharmacy staff experiences difficulty reading the physician's prescription order and requires clarification to fill the order. But the pharmacy staff cannot have any contact with the prescribing physician because the physician is not allowed to counsel patients at the pharmacy. Then the pharmacy staff guesses what the patient needs, fills the order, and wishes the patient the best. This is not something that would happen in the conventional medical system. Pharmacies regularly ask for clarifications on physician orders to maintain the patient's safety, which just makes sense. MMPs should require continuity of care for patients between recommending healthcare providers and dispensaries, but this is more the exception than the rule.

What needs to happen to improve patient safety when accessing cannabis in the dispensary setting? Perhaps the easiest solution to this problem is to require dispensaries to hire nurses to fill these gaps. Nurses are charged with the care and safety of their patients, have a well-defined and understood scope of practice, and act as the liaison between patients and their medical teams. Nurses are the perfect missing piece in the dispensary puzzle nationwide. Nurses do exist in the cannabis space and should work with dispensaries to promote patient safety, to reduce risks, and to empower patients to reach their greatest healing potential with the safe and effective use of cannabis medicine. Any other "medical" facility would be considered inoperable without nurses.

CASE STUDY
Dispensary Consultation—Parkinson's Patient Experience

Parkinson's Patient Seeking Relief with Cannabis in a Medical Marijuana Dispensary	
Subjective	"I want to eat real food. I hate these shakes because I can't get a fork to my mouth without stabbing myself. These shakes are constant. I'm exhausted. I want to get myself showered, dressed, and fed. I'm not an invalid. My pain is a 7 or 8 all the time. I don't sleep at all. I do everything my doctor tells me to except for using the stupid walker. I hate this disease. Cannabis is my last resort. My son gave me a puff the other day and I was able to eat! That's why I'm here!"
	Patient reports that his "shakes" impede his ability to go about ADLs.
	Patient calls tremors "shakes."
	Patient reports that he falls often, but refuses to use assistive devices.
	Patient states he has experienced weight loss because of severe tremors that impede his ability to feed himself. He also states that he is struggling with pain, insomnia, and dyskinesia.
Objective	Severe pill-rolling tremor.
	Pain and insomnia related to dyskinesia as evidenced by—arms and legs moving involuntarily, causing uncontrolled movement and regular occurrence of muscle spasm.
	Patient is grimacing and rocking in his chair. He can't stop grimacing despite attempting to relax his facial muscles. He can walk without assistance. He has come to the dispensary to access medical cannabis and would like to focus on reducing tremors, pain, and insomnia so that he can actively participate and complete ADLs.
Assessment (No clinical assessment is provided or allowed in dispensary setting.)	Patient is at high risk for falls r/t involuntary/uncontrolled movement and spasm of extremities.
	Knowledge deficit r/t medical cannabis AEB patient report.
	Patient is new to medical cannabis. Patient requires assistance with selecting products. Knowledge deficits.

Plan	Use motivational interviewing and coaching techniques.
	Discuss the benefit of using assistive devices for ambulation to prevent falls and injury.
	Teach about and coach around medical cannabis therapy concepts:
	Start low and go slow.
	Inhalation is easy to titrate up as needed.
	ECS 101, phytocannabinoids, terpenes, indica, sativa, neuroprotectant, antioxidant, entourage effect discussed.
	CBD mediates the effect of THC.
	Self-discovery process—use the journal to track cannabis use and symptom reduction/relief/exacerbation.
Implementation	Products selected:
	1:1 CBD to THC vape oil pen.
	Rationale—no fire element to "fiddle with"—to be used prn,
	CBD tincture—sublingual for ECS upregulation throughout the day—started at 10 mg with meals tid.
	Indica preroll to try for sleep—son will assist with using this method of administration/consumption.
Evaluation	Patient reported that symptoms were reduced significantly!
	Patient rated pain as 3/10 with 1:1 CBD to THC vape oil pen.
	Patient reported that he was able to eat because of reduced/nearly eliminated tremor and gained 10 lb in a couple of weeks!
	Patient reported that he felt less tired, anxious, and depressed.
	Patient reported that the Indica preroll promoted better sleep than did the sedatives he was prescribed.

(continued)

CASE STUDY
Dispensary Consultation—Parkinson's Patient Experience
(continued)

Patient reported that the Indica preroll made him very hungry and tired. He welcomed both side effects, had two bowls of ice cream, and went to bed.

Patient reported that his balance improved, but his wife convinced him to use his walker more often as needed.

Patient stated that his "shakes" were reduced by the vape oil pen. His face didn't feel "stuck" either (symptom of tardive dyskinesia secondary to long-term l-dopa treatment).

Patient reported he medicated with vape pen before meals along with taking his tincture. He used his tincture with meals, and he really had to focus on holding the CBD oil under his tongue for 1 minute, but he now has few challenges doing so.

Patient reported medicating with the pen a great deal. He went through it quickly and the cost was about $70 per vape oil cartridge, so he became motivated to learn how to make his own medicine. Last I heard, he grows his cannabis and he loves the process of making his medicine.

Last report from this patient—"I feel like I'm in the driver's seat. I have control of my body and my life. It's been years since I have felt this way!"

Providing Unbiased Care—Considerations for Cannabis-Use Disorder

It is believed that the use of cannabis can lead to dependence. Cannabis-use disorder (CUD) is also known as cannabis addiction or marijuana addiction. *The Diagnostic and Statistical Manual of Mental Disorders Fifth Edition* (*DSM-5*) defines CUD as a pattern of cannabis use that leads to clinically significant impairment or distress, as evidenced by the presence of at least two of the following criteria within 12 months:

- Taking more cannabis than intended
- Difficulty controlling or cutting down cannabis use
- Spending a lot of time on cannabis use
- Cannabis cravings
- Problems at work, school, and home as a result of cannabis use
- Continuing to use cannabis despite social or relationship problems
- Giving up or reducing other activities in favor of cannabis

- Taking cannabis in high-risk situations
- Continuing to use cannabis despite physical or psychological problems
- Tolerance to cannabis
- Withdrawal when discontinuing cannabis

When determining whether a patient might benefit from CUD treatment, healthcare providers should focus on two key criteria during their brief visit:

1. If cannabis use is causing the patient problems
2. If the patient is amenable to treatment

Cannabis withdrawal symptoms can occur in one-half of patients in treatment for CUDs. These symptoms include dysphoria (anxiety, irritability, depression, and restlessness), disturbed sleep, gastrointestinal symptoms, and decreased appetite. Most symptoms begin during the first week of abstinence and resolve after a few weeks (Patel, 2019).

The cannabis care nurse is responsible for assessing whether a patient may be at risk for improper use of cannabis. An initial consultation should include an adequate health history report and screening tools such as the Cannabis Use Disorder Identification Test (Figure 9.6) (Adamson et al., 2010) to determine the risk factors that would help the nurse identify whether a patient is at risk for improper use or abuse of cannabis. The cannabis care nurse is well-positioned to support the patient struggling with CUD by providing solution-oriented, nonjudgmental care that may include implementation of a desensitization protocol in which the patient ceases cannabis use for some time to reduce tolerance and need for high doses of cannabis. Once that period has elapsed, the cannabis care nurse may recommend that the patient use very small amounts of cannabis to achieve a therapeutic effect, increasing very slowly as needed. Should the patient still struggle, complete cessation of cannabis and referral to a substance abuse specialist may be necessary.

NURSE INNOVATORS AND ENTREPRENEURS IN THE CANNABIS INDUSTRY

> *Cannabis nursing is both a learned skill and a practiced art, where the cannabis care nurse builds upon expertise from previous experiences with healing and nursing while enacting reflective practices to support growth toward expertise.—American Cannabis Nurses Association—Scope and Standards of Practice for Cannabis Nurses (Clark et al., 2019).*

In the following pages, you will meet some of the nurses who have stepped out of the cannabis closet to be advocates, educators, coaches, and navigators for the patients in their communities for those who need guidance and support to integrate cannabis medicine into their lives. They have started companies, developed patient-centered care programs, and embraced entrepreneurship. They are some of the leaders in the field of cannabis care nursing, and they are striving to improve the health and well-being of patients in every community across the nation.

The Cannabis Use Disorder Identification Test - Revised (CUDIT-R)

Have you used any cannabis over the past six months?   Yes_____   No _____

If you answered "Yes" to the previous question, please answer the following questions about your cannabis use. Circle the response that is most correct for you in relation to your cannabis use over the *past six months.*

1. How often do you use cannabis?

Never	Monthly or less	2-4 times a month	2-3 times a week	4+ times a week
0	1	2	3	4

2. How many hours were you "stoned" on a typical day when you had been using cannabis?

Less than 1	1 or 2	3 or 4	5 or 6	7 or more
0	1	2	3	4

3. How often during the past 6 months did you find that you were not able to stop using cannabis once you had started?

Never	Less than monthly	Monthly	Weekly	Daily/almost daily
0	1	2	3	4

4. How often during the past 6 months did you fail to do what was normally expected from you because of using cannabis?

Never	Less than monthly	Monthly	Weekly	Daily or almost daily
0	1	2	3	4

5. How often in the past 6 months have you devoted a great deal of your time to getting, using, or recovering from cannabis?

Never	Less than monthly	Monthly	Weekly	Daily/almost daily
0	1	2	3	4

6. How often in the past 6 months have you had a problem with your memory or concentration after using cannabis?

Never	Less than monthly	Monthly	Weekly	Daily or almost daily
0	1	2	3	4

7. How often do you use cannabis in situations that could be physically hazardous, such as driving, operating machinery, or caring for children?

Never	Less than monthly	Monthly	Weekly	Daily/almost daily
0	1	2	3	4

8. Have you ever thought about cutting down, or stopping, your use of cannabis?

Never	Yes, but not in the past 6 months	Yes, during the past 6 months
0	2	4

This questionnaire was designed for self-administration and is scored by adding each of the 8 items:

Question 1-7 are scored on a 0-4 scale
Question 8 is scored 0,2, or 4

Score: _____

Scores of 8 or more indicate hazardous cannabis use, while scores of 12 or more indicate a possible cannabis use disorder for which further intervention may be required.

Figure 9.6: **The cannabis use disorders identification test-revised.** (Adamson, S. J., Kay-Lambkin, F. J., Baker, A. L., Lewin, T. J., Thornton, L., Kelly, B. J., & Sellman, J. D. (2010). An improved brief measure of cannabis misuse: The cannabis use disorders identification test-revised (CUDIT-R). *Drug and Alcohol Dependence, 110*(1–2), 137–143. https://doi.org/10.1016/j.drugalcdep.2010.02.017)

Cannabis care nurses come from all walks of life and all types of nursing specialties. We all started our careers in the conventional medical field. Very few (if any) currently practicing cannabis care nurses came into the nursing field to become a cannabis care nurse. Now you might be wondering how a nurse decides to become a cannabis care nurse. Much like the patients we care for, we may have suffered a debilitating injury or illness. We may be managing a chronic condition. We may have exhausted every treatment, intervention, and therapy available to us in the conventional medical space only to find that we had a serious gap that needed to be filled for us to heal properly, fully, and with dignity. We may have found that cannabis complements our conventional health regimens in a way that promotes great improvements in our quality of life. Or perhaps we held the hands of people who were struggling with all of these issues and realized that cannabis is necessary medicine as we witnessed the healing processes of others. Regardless of where we started, or the specifics of how we arrived on this path, most of us came into this role because we have personally experienced the healing power of cannabis.

CANNABIS CARE NURSE STORIES AND INTERVIEWS

As this chapter comes to a close, we would like to introduce you to some of the nurses who have taken the time to share their stories as patients, their successes as professionals and entrepreneurs, and their challenges as nurses who willingly push against the barriers and stigma that remain in the medical field and society as a result of cannabis prohibition. Special thanks to all of these nurses for taking the time to answer our questions and sharing their cannabis nursing experiences.

The Evolution of a GreenNurse—From Nurse to Patient to Cannabis Care Nurse

Sherri Tutkus, BSN, RN (Figure 9.7)

Founder of GreenNurse Group. https://www.greennursegroup.com/

Upon discovery that she had an ECS deficiency, which played a significant role in her disability, Sherri Tutkus, RN, founded the GreenNurse Group to bridge the gaps that exist for patients like herself.

Sherri Tutkus is no stranger to the debilitating nature of severe chronic pain. She found herself on the other side of the sickbed in 2012. She was a healthy single mother

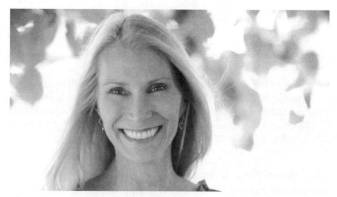

Figure 9.7: **Picture of Sherri Tutkus, RN-BSN; Founder of the GreenNurse Group.** (Photo provided by Sherri Tutkus, RN-BSN. Used with permission.)

of three working full-time as a registered nurse (RN) in the Boston Hospitals. She was also a holistic nurse who educated via multiple platforms on diet, nutrition, energy healing, and the mind-body connection. She contracted a type of acute colitis that is caused by a contagious infectious bacterium. This condition is often an adverse reaction from taking prescribed antibiotics, but in Sherri's case, she was exposed to *Clostridium difficile* bacteria while working as a nurse in the hospital. Sherri became a disabled nurse as a result and suffered immensely.

She started with flulike symptoms such as fevers, sweats, chills, and irregular bowel patterns alternating between diarrhea and constipation. She developed severe urgency, cramping, had difficulty defecating, and a feeling that she was retaining stool. The pain was so severe on admission to the hospital that they worked her up for a ruptured appendix. She was healthy before this, so no one thought she could be as sick as she was. A computed tomography (CT) scan revealed that her colon was swollen, slowly progressing to "megacolon." She was admitted to the hospital after the CT scan revealed pseudomembranous *C. difficile* colitis, and she was placed on multiple antibiotics and hospitalized in a critical condition.

Once discharged from the hospital, she did not get better. She continued with severely debilitating symptoms and started to acquire other plaguing ailments. She experienced pain upon eating, suffered from frequent unpredictable bouts of painful diarrhea. Her belly was distended and filled with air. The abdominal pain that she experienced was immense and affected every aspect of her life. She was prescribed multiple opioids, benzodiazepines, antidepressants, and steroids. As a single mother of three, she was unable to work for months. When attempting to return to work, her symptoms would worsen, and she would develop another medical problem.

Sherri was malnourished. She had a difficult time keeping weight on and was not absorbing nutrients. She then developed an autoimmune condition called polymyalgia rheumatica that led her to experience yet another type of severe chronic myofascial pain. Polymyalgia rheumatica is an inflammatory disorder that causes muscle pain and stiffness, especially in the shoulders. She described the pain as feeling like she had hot searing pokers scraping up and down the back of her neck and shoulders. She said it felt like she had on a turtleneck sweater filled with sticky glue and sharp glass. With every breath she took, she felt that sharp, hot, searing-glass tear through her neck, upper chest, back, and shoulders. The pain was so debilitating that she would vomit, and hence the cycle of ongoing malnutrition and pain.

She was prescribed over 15 medications at the same time, including different combinations of antibiotics, opioids, steroids, nonsteroidal anti-inflammatories, benzodiazepines, selective serotonin reuptake inhibitors (SSRIs), tricyclic antidepressants, neuroleptics, β-blockers, supplements, probiotics, lidocaine patches, and creams. She pursued both traditional and complementary holistic healing modalities, including acupuncture, chiropractic care, physical therapy, occupational therapy, exercise, massage, meditation, nutritionist, supplements, essential oils, aromatherapy, homeopathy, energy healing work, and trigger point injections. She was determined to get better, and yet nothing worked. Sherri had become a disabled nurse and suffered from horrible bouts of debilitating depression, anxiety, insomnia, panic disorder, and agoraphobia.

Panic, anxiety, post-traumatic stress, insomnia, and pain plagued her daily. Sherri felt isolated, depressed, and disconnected from her family and community. She was in a constant state of fight or flight and struggled with multiple side effects from taking both prescribed and over-the-counter medications. She ran out of options and exhausted conventional and holistic therapies. She describes circling the drain of despair, experiencing the dissonance of wanting to live and die at the same time. She did not want to die. She wanted the pain to stop.

That peaceful moment came when a retired nurse colleague visited her one afternoon to share cannabis education and a joint. Sherri only knew cannabis as being a recreational substance. She never thought that cannabis would work—how could it when powerful pharmaceuticals and all of the complementary therapies did not work? Sherri had nothing to lose and had tried everything else. Two puffs of the cannabis joint and she felt the pain slowly dissolve away into background noise. It worked!

Sherri describes feeling like she was pulled out of the trajectory of illness and was forced to take a more in-depth look at the big picture of her life. She became a medical cannabis patient and started to administer cannabis to treat her symptoms. Once cannabis started working for her, she was able to wean off all of the medications that were not helping and were causing side effects. She medicated with cannabis multiple ways, including smoking, vaping, tinctures, edibles, creams, lotions, and salves of different cannabinoid profiles and terpenes. She had effectively bridged the gap from what she was not receiving through conventional and holistic therapies.

Her condition greatly improved and she felt connected to her family and community again. Over time, Sherri realized that she suffered from a clinical endocannabinoid deficiency because no matter what she did, she was not getting better. It was the plant that opened the door to a signaling system within her body that started to bring about balance and make all of the other therapies that she was pursuing work. Cannabis was the tool that bridged the gap from what she was not getting from traditional and holistic therapies.

It took Sherri 2 years to figure out how to medicate with cannabis below the threshold of impairment so that she could function. She had a community of caregivers to guide her, and yet it was a situation of trial and success for her to figure out the right combinations of products and methods of administration to manage symptoms. Although she still has multiple chronic illnesses, she is not plagued with debilitating symptoms. She became a cannabis care nurse and patient advocate to educate and empower patients to optimize healing from their chronic illnesses and diseases. Sherri is living her best life and helping others do the same.

Interview with Jessie Gill, RN (Marijuana Mommy) (Figure 9.8)

(Interview used with permission from Jessie Gill, RN)
Founder of MarijuanaMommy.com. https://www.marijuanamommy.com/

Jessie Gill, RN, is a cannabis care nurse with a background in holistic health and hospice. After suffering a spinal injury, she reluctantly became a medical cannabis patient and then quickly transitioned into acting as an advocate. Her site, MarijuanaMommy.com, educates about cannabis while challenging the stigma against use. She's been featured on Viceland and her work has appeared in VICE, *Good Housekeeping*, *Cosmopolitan*, MSN, and more.

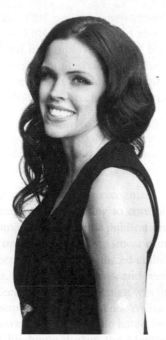

Figure 9.8: Picture of Jessie Gill, RN; Founder of MarijuanaMommy.com. (Photo provided by Jessie Gill, RN. Used with permission.)

How did you learn about cannabis?

I'd used it many times earlier in life and had a lot of negative associations with it that scared me. So when a friend suggested using medical cannabis, I was reluctant but my mother convinced me to try it.

What were you doing before you got sick or contracted your illness or condition?

I was a hospice nurse when I injured my neck at work.

What were your initial symptoms?

Pain. The night of the injury the pain in my head started and it never went away. I suffered from pain, endless muscle spasms, and dysfunction of my arm and neck.

Did you use conventional medicine?

Yes, I tried everything—injections, pharmaceuticals, and I eventually had a multi-level spinal fusion surgery, which made my condition worse.

How has this chronic debilitating disease/symptoms affected your mind, body, and spirit?

It ended my hospice career which was my passion and vocation, that alone was pretty devastating. But it also ended a lot of my independence and left me dealing with chronic pain, which also contributed to anxiety and depression.

When did you first learn about cannabis?

After a few years of suffering and using opiates, benzodiazepines like valium, and other pharmaceuticals, a friend suggested I try cannabis. He had a similar injury and had great results.

How has cannabis helped your physical body?

Immediately, I was able to stop taking valium and opiates. The pain didn't disappear but cannabis helped manage it far better than pharmaceuticals. I was able to titrate off all the other medications within a year.

How has cannabis helped you mentally and emotionally?

Just getting off the pharmaceuticals revived my mental and emotional health. Depression and fatigue are significant and devastating side effects.

How has cannabis helped you socially?

Cannabis finally managed my pain to the point where I could leave the house again. I still deal with limitations and pain, but I'm attending events and teaching classes and managing.

How has cannabis helped you spiritually?

It's allowed me the energy and motivation to meditate again. And on top of that, it greatly enhances my meditative practice. Cannabis also adds a profound introspective element to my life that allows me to connect with my spiritual self.

What are you doing now that you didn't think you would be able to do?

Touching the lives of those who are suffering. I loved hospice nursing because I relieved the suffering of others every single day. When I realized I'd never be a nurse in that capacity again, I was broken-hearted. But now, through my website MarijuanaMommy.com, I'm touching the lives of thousands of people every single day, teaching why and how to use cannabis. I've spoken at the Cannabis Science Conference and the Cannabis Nurses Network Conference. I've also done chapter events with Women Grow and Ellementa. I've spoken at a lot of events with Canna Pop-up and other local groups. I hold grassroots community-style classes in New Jersey to introduce doctors, nurses, pharmacists, and patients to cannabinoid therapeutics. I'm doing new patient consults in New Jersey, recording a course for new patients, and I'm in the process of starting up a local support group for cannabis patients.

Interview with Eloise Theisen, MSN, AGPCNP-BC (Figure 9.9)

(Interview used with permission from Eloise Theisen, MSN, AGPCNP-BC)
Board Certified Adult-Geriatric Nurse Practitioner
President of the American Cannabis Association (2020–2021). https://cannabisnurses.org/
Founder and Chief Visionary Officer of Radicle Health Clinician Network (formerly Green Health Consultants). https://www.radiclehealthcare.com/

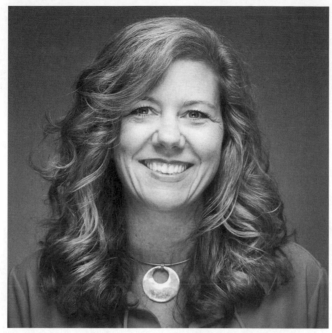

Figure 9.9: **Picture of Eloise Theisen, MSN, AGPCNP-BC; Founder of Radicle Health Clinician Network.** (Photo provided by Eloise Theisen, MSN, AGPCNP-BC. Used with permission.)

VP of Clinical Education and Integration of Illumesense. https://www.illumesense.com/

Adjunct Faculty, Pacific College of Health and Science, Medical Cannabis Certificate Program. https://www.pacificcollege.edu/medicalcannabis

Everyone has a story as to why they came into the cannabis industry, what propelled you?

It started personal, and then patients started asking me about it daily which led me to start my own clinic.

What were you doing before you got sick or contracted your illness or condition?

I was working as a hospital nurse manager, overseeing over 400 full-time employees.

How did this condition affect your mind body and spirit?

I struggled with chronic pain. I became severely depressed, and at one point I was suicidal.

Did you use conventional medicine at first?

Yes. I was on eight medications by the age of 36. I had a failed surgery, multiple injections, physical therapy, acupuncture, and massage.

When did you first learn about cannabis?

I had a relationship with cannabis at an early age, left it for a while to pursue nursing, and *reluctantly* came back to it after a car accident.

What made you decide to use cannabis?

Desperation: I felt that I had tried everything.

How has cannabis helped?

Cannabis provided pain relief. I was able to get off all meds. It also lifted my mood and allowed me to function again. Cannabis helps me to pause, stay in the moment, and think things through.

What are you doing now that you didn't think you would be able to do?

WORK. I was disabled and lost my livelihood.

How has cannabis helped you to live your best life?

It gave me my life back and allowed me to be a productive member of society—how is that for irony?!

What do you feel is most important for people to know when they are exploring cannabis as an option?

It is not a silver bullet—patience and support during the process are keys to success.

What types of services do you provide?

I provide consultations to patients who want to use cannabis as medicine. In some cases, patients reduce and/or eliminate other medications once they begin cannabis.

Radicle Health also provides solutions for the cannabis industry through education, product formulations, research and development, content/blog creation for websites, speaking engagements, and advocacy.

Interview with Janna Champagne, BSN, RN (Figure 9.10)

(Interview used with permission from Janna Champagne, BSN, RN)
Founder of Integrated Holistic Care. http://www.integratedholisticcare.com/
Mission: To educate patients about natural alternatives to pharmaceuticals and holistic wellness strategies, so patients can make fully informed decisions about their health.
Founder of Cannabis Nurse Approved. https://www.cannabisnurseapproved.com/
Mission: To highlight medical quality cannabis suppliers meeting our objective FLOW criteria, and ensure patients understand what research supports to be optimal formulations for medical cannabis use. Our process includes vetting suppliers based on FLOW criteria, to ensure any product receiving our seal of approval meets research-supported standards for optimal medical quality. This results in nurses having cannabinoid (and ideally terpene) lab information, which helps to match our client's specific needs to the most potentially optimal cannabis compounds for their situation.

What propelled you to become a cannabis care nurse?

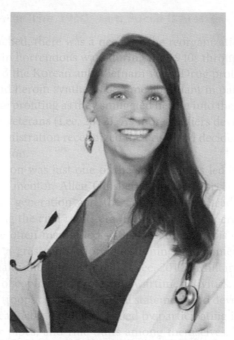

Figure 9.10: **Picture of Janna Champagne, BSN, RN; Founder of Integrated Holistic Care; Cannabis Care Nurse.** (Photo provided by Janna Champagne, BSN, RN. Used with permission.)

Like so many of my colleagues, my journey to becoming a cannabis care nurse began when I experienced a health crisis in 2012 and became a cannabis patient who happens to be a nurse. I suffered a complete health collapse, complicated further by totaling my car in a traumatic accident, so I should be the poster child for opioid addiction and polypharmacy. I ended up on disability with half a dozen diagnoses, including Lupus, chronic renal failure, hepatitis (non-viral), pancreatic insufficiency, and severe immune deficiency. After 18 months of mainstream treatment, I was disenchanted with the lack of progress offered by following the mainstream approaches and tried cannabis as an alternative to opioids for pain management. Thanks to cannabis, not only is my chronic pain well-managed without potentially harmful pharmaceuticals, but my immune function is back to optimal levels, and my autoimmune markers seroconverted (now I test negative for Lupus).

A couple of years after my health issues occurred, my teen daughter with autism entered puberty, triggering extreme-level behaviors. Puberty crisis is common to an estimated 50% of kids with autism, so most parents have heard it can be a game-changer, and I can personally attest this is true. My daughter was limited verbally at the time, so her extreme pain symptoms were expressed through self-injurious behavior, aggressive rages towards authority figures, and property destruction. As a homeschooling mom, I never considered out of home placement, but during this phase, this very scenario was nearly enforced due to safety issues. Cannabis eased our situation and spared my daughter the added trauma of being taken from her home and family. Now my daughter's behaviors are well-managed, and cannabis has been integral in improving both her quality of life and overall function. My daughter's story, including the science supporting cannabis for autism, featured on the cover of a nationwide industry magazine in December 2017, which I refer to as my "coming out of the cannabis closet" moment. These are just a few life events that fed my passion for the sacred plant and its potential to positively impact patients' lives. Now I'm able to utilize the knowledge gained through my personal experiences to help patients, giving purpose to otherwise traumatic events.

> *How did you prepare to become a cannabis care nurse? Have you taken online courses, attended seminars, attended conferences, attended conventions? Basically, can you explain how you became (and stay current) as an expert in this field in terms of education and experience?*

I was fortunate to ease into the cannabis industry by starting off as a grower. Gardening was the physical therapy that helped rebuild my muscle strength and stamina while offering the flexibility needed to recover from my health ordeal. In addition to growing for myself and my daughter, I picked up a few patient cardholders and began researching and growing strains to specifically target their situation. This led to making a variety of products to meet their preferences, adding to the knowledge base I now extend to my clients. I believe this experience is invaluable, knowing the evolution of the plant and being able to teach patients to grow and make their own, which provides quality control and is cost-effective compared with purchasing retail products. In addition to doing my research, I connected with kindred nurses through professional organizations like the American Cannabis Nurses Association (ACNA) and Cannabis Nurses Network, attending conferences, and taking the online education courses they supported. I began working for organizations with nurses providing cannabis patient education and realized the importance of transferring this support system that's expected in other areas of nursing to clinical application of cannabis. The ability to ask other nurses for a second opinion or another perspective on a client's situation is priceless. In addition, since the approach to cannabis can vary greatly depending on the patient's area of diagnosis, it's helpful to have nurse mentors and colleagues with experience in that field, to brainstorm possible considerations of cannabis therapy (including interactions with common pharmaceuticals that may be utilized). I remain current by continually learning, signing up for new research notifications, and seeking answers to the outstanding questions about cannabis and ECS science. We are still in our infancy regarding knowledge of cannabis, its mechanisms of action, and how its best applied to specific situations, so keeping an open mind and staying current on the latest information is critical to avoid knowledge becoming obsolete.

> *What type of clinical setting do you work in?*

We work out of an office and provide consultations in many formats (in person, phone, and via video conferencing).

> *Would you please share how you educate your patients about the ECS and cannabinoid therapeutics?*

Our consultation process includes a comprehensive assessment of the patient's considerations of cannabis therapy, including diagnosis(es), symptom targets, patient's priorities for cannabis therapy, pharmaceuticals and supplements, and subjective symptom marker documentation (ie, pain level 0/10). Basic education regarding cannabis science, optimal products, titration (low and slow), and the pros and cons of different forms of administration is also included. From the assessment, an individualized care plan is created, specifying which cannabis components may be most beneficial for reaching their goals, complete with the research supporting this education. Continuity of care includes availability to answer questions or clarify written materials, and availability for follow up consultations to problem-solve or consider any new situations or medications as they arise.

As cannabis care nurses, we have a duty to bridge the knowledge gap for these patients, by ensuring they understand what constitutes medical quality cannabis. My nurses and I created the FLOW criteria to educate cannabis patients on the research-supported criteria for optimal cannabis formulations to ensure they access medical quality cannabis products. Here's a breakdown:

F: Flower-derived because we know the most potent raw material for extracting the full spectrum of plant component in the cannabis flower. Trichomes in the flower produce the cannabinoid and terpene content, and the flower also contains the highest concentration of synergistic plant compounds.

L: Lab testing is the only way to verify product contents, potency, and rule out contaminants. Being a grower myself, I know how easily plant tags can get swapped, and we simply can't rely on strain name labels to verify a product's profile.

O: Organic cannabis certification isn't possible, yet many growers advertise "organically grown," and lab testing is the best way to verify that a product is free of contaminants or harmful toxin residuals. This is especially important when guiding already sick patients, who have heightened susceptibility to toxic insults.

W: Whole Plant means concentrating cannabis as nature intended, without isolating or removing any plant components. Cannabis can produce hundreds of therapeutic compounds, including cannabinoids, terpenes, bioflavonoids, antioxidants, chlorophyll, and EFA's, which in combination provide health benefits known as the "entourage effect."

What types of patients do you work with?

My areas of specialty are pediatrics (autism/seizures), autoimmune/immune disorders, chronic pain, neuro/mental health, and gastrointestinal disorders.

Will you share a case study of a patient that you have worked with and how you worked with them?

My daughter's story is repeated in many of my autism clients, and a similar case that stands out was a teenage girl with autism and cerebral palsy. Her symptoms included being legally blind and deaf, with aggression toward others and herself, necessitating she wears a helmet and arm wraps to protect from headbanging and biting herself. I consulted with her mom, who had exhausted every pharmaceutical option without seeing any improvement in her daughter's scenario, and she pleaded with me to please help improve her quality of life. This was a family in a severe crisis, losing hope that they could find answers to help their daughter. After following my care plan for 6 weeks, we connected again for a follow-up appointment. Mom reported an astounding response, including a happier child who was no longer injuring herself (helmet and wraps were off!), who was laughing, asking to dance, and treating her family with loving gestures. Her behaviors were not perfect, but they were manageable, and mom was learning to stay ahead of the pain/behavior curve with quick-onset products to avoid the crisis levels they were experiencing previously. Mom was collaborating with their physician and had begun weaning the intense pharmaceuticals they had relied upon previously, and with every weaned medication, they were seeing the little girl they knew to come back to them. In this and many more scenarios, cannabis spares families intense crisis-level situations and gives them hope of an easier existence.

What is the biggest challenge you have experienced as a nurse working in the cannabis industry?

Maneuvering the cannabis industry that's not always focused on what's best for patients has been a big frustration (hence the Cannabis Nurse Approved program). Also, fighting a decades-long stigma by other medical professionals, who may assume that because they didn't learn about the ECS during their educational experiences, the science must not be well-established. Most are surprised to learn that tens of thousands of reputable research articles exist, supporting the balancing effects on cannabis for dozens of ailments. I teach that cannabis can revolutionize our broken health care system, and I advocate for proceeding in a patient-focused manner to avoid making the profit-seeking mistakes in our current system that can result in patients falling through the cracks.

What is the greatest reward you've experienced as a nurse working in the cannabis industry?

Patient outcomes are my biggest motivating factor for pushing through adversity and fears since this work is not for the faint of heart. We lack specific regulations and policies to guide our work, and legally there's a lot of gray areas to maneuver. Accepting that we are the trailblazers in this wild west of emerging cannabis science requires compassion, a steadfast approach, collaboration with mentors/colleagues, and tireless advocacy. It's a perfect role for nurses.

Interview with Nique Pichette, MSN, RN (Figure 9.11)

(Interview used with permission from Nique Pichette, MSN, RN)
Founder of Cannabis Nurse Navigator. https://cannabisnursenavigator.com
Mission and Vision: The Cannabis Nurse Navigator is a professional registered nurse with cannabis-specific knowledge, who offers individualized assistance to patients, families, and caregivers to help overcome health care system barriers. Developed for the nursing community and their patients, the Cannabis Nurse Navigator provides

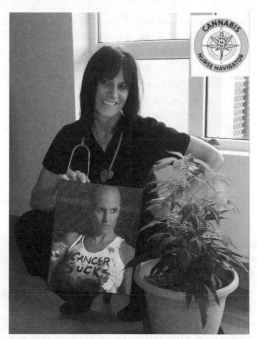

Figure 9.11: **Picture of Nique Pichette, MSN, RN; CEO, Cannabis Nurse Navigator.** (Photo provided by Nique Pichette, MSN, RN. Used with permission.)

education and resources to facilitate informed decision-making in a timely fashion to quality health care providers knowledgeable in cannabis therapeutics and psychosocial care throughout all phases of the cannabis therapeutics continuum.

What propelled you to become a cannabis care nurse?

My breast cancer returned in May of 2013, 18 months after my first diagnosis. I opted for chemotherapy and radiation this time, as my first diagnosis was treated with a total left mastectomy. I became very ill from the side effects of chemotherapy, and I was allergic to the antiemetics I was prescribed to treat nausea. I would blog almost daily as a nurse on the other side of the nurse's station in my blog, "Breast Cancer & Me." Through ongoing dialogue from absolute strangers, I decided I needed to get my medical cannabis card and try an alternative form of treatment. I was now 111 lb, frail, and afraid: afraid to lose my nursing license, afraid I would fall back into my anorexia, and afraid to die. This is ironic coming from someone who struggles with chronic suicidality.

If you are a medical cannabis patient and nurse, would you share your story?

I am both a nurse and a medical cannabis patient. I started using cannabis during my radiation treatments, and the benefits for my insomnia, anxiety, and appetite were extremely helpful. It was a difficult decision to make, as I was always in fear of losing my nursing license, but at this point in my life, and with all of the mental health issues I had overcome already I felt that I had no choice. My journey with cannabinoid therapeutics began during my second battle with breast cancer in August of 2013, and it continues today. Although my initial rationale for using cannabis as medicine was breast cancer, I continue to use it today for anxiety and depression that is the result of PTSD. Cannabis led me to develop the Cannabis Nurse Navigator role, as I had no one at Dana Farber Cancer Institute to help me. I was grateful for my cannabis caregiver for the knowledge and medicine he provided.

Understanding how to use cannabis as medicine is the key to being successful with healing. It has led me to several other forms of alternative therapy, such as cupping, float deprivation therapy, acupuncture, yoga, walking, nutrition, and, most recently, equine therapy. All of which replenish the deficiencies in the ECS naturally. I only use my inhalers for my asthma now. My daily medication regimen is cannabis only. I have never been to such a place of emotional wellness, physical health, and spiritual health. Without the journey to heal from within that cannabis has allowed me, I would not be the person I am today.

> How did you prepare to become a cannabis care nurse? Have you taken online courses, attended seminars, attended conferences, attended conventions? Basically, can you explain how you became (and stay current) as an expert in this field in terms of education and experience?

Although you may disagree, I do not think of myself as an expert. I have been researching cannabis as medicine since 2013, and there is so much more to learn. I have attended many cannabis conferences. As I searched the internet to find as much information as I could, I met a cannabis care nurse who guided me towards the Patients Out of Time Conference. I attended in 2015—that conference changed the direction of my life as well as my career.

Since that time, I have attended numerous cannabis conferences, gained CEU's for my nursing licensure, and met amazing nursing professionals from around the world who are changing the way we look at healthcare. I am a co-founding member of the Cannabis Nurses Network, the CEO of the Cannabis Nurse Navigator, and a doctoral nursing student at Salve Regina University in Newport, RI developing the research behind the Cannabis Nurse Navigator specialty. I graduated with a Bachelor of Science in Nursing from Salve Regina University in May 1995. It is an honor that this Catholic University accepted my proposal for the Cannabis Nurse Navigator role, with an expected graduation date of May 2021.

> What type of clinical setting do you work in?

I am currently a staff nurse at a behavioral health hospital that treats adolescents to geriatrics, with dual diagnoses which include addictions. I am not allowed to discuss cannabis or the ECS with my patients at the hospital.

> Would you please share how you educate your patients about the ECS and cannabinoid therapeutics?

Every patient I see is unique. I meet with them most of the time or talk over the phone and we discuss the best forms of learning for them. Each patient has an individualized teaching session based on their age, medical condition, and direction of care that they are seeking. I complete a needs assessment with my patients, and then I either work with them or navigate them to the best place of care for their condition and needs. It is important to know your scope of practice and add the appropriate medical team and resources for the best patient outcome.

What types of patients do you work with? (seniors, children, adults through lifespan, hospice, etc.?)

I work with any patient who is seeking assistance and guidance with cannabinoid therapeutics.

Will you share a case study of a patient that you have worked with and how you worked with them?

My greatest accomplishment in working with cannabinoid therapeutics was my journey with a 16-year-old girl with sarcoma-like cancer. We met at Relay for Life, and her spirit was so vibrant and beautiful. I was selling my t-shirts and other small items to raise money for patients who used cannabis as medicine, and she came to my booth. She instantly said, "you need to meet my mom, she believes in cannabis," and a connection was made. I met her mother briefly—she mentioned that her cancer was in remission. We shared some of our journeys as cancer survivors, and we parted ways.

A few months later, I received a call from this beautiful girl's mom. She asked if we could meet to start a cancer cannabis protocol for her as her cancer was back and now she was paralyzed from the waist down. I met with the family, and I navigated them to certain cannabis experts—from healers to laboratories and medical professionals who specialize in cancer—and our journey began.

I will never forget the day she came home from the hospital. She was on a stretcher as cancer had taken away her mobility, and every bump the stretcher rolled over, she screamed. The tears that rolled down her cheeks with every movement of the stretcher had me believe that her cancer had metastasized, but her family did not mention that, so I kept those feelings inside. In time the stretcher had to be put in Trendelenburg's position to get through the door. The tears and the pain I heard from this 16-year-old girl will stay with me forever.

We worked with a team of people who were knowledgeable in different forms of alternative therapy. We used cannabis transdermal patches, oils administered rectally, and topicals for the pain and to attempt to stop the tumor growth. Over time, her pain began to subside. She was able to use the trapeze over her head to sit up now, and then she was able to be transferred to her electric wheelchair. She attended football games, went to the mall, attended her fundraisers with complete joy and happiness. I had never witnessed this transition before.

I sat in treatment teams with the medical staff at the children's hospital, where she received care. I watched family and friends administer cannabis oils while she was in the hospital. I saw miracles happening every day on so many levels. She lost her fight on November 21, 2015, but her quality of life was made possible by cannabinoid therapeutics. As a nurse who has helped many patients die, I know it was cannabis that helped her have such a beautiful transition surrounded by her family and friends.

What is the biggest challenge you have experienced as a nurse working in the cannabis industry?

My biggest challenge in working as a nurse in the cannabis industry is protecting my nursing license as a medical patient. It is a very real risk to be a cannabis care nurse while working in traditional roles.

What is the greatest reward you've experienced as a nurse working in the cannabis industry?

To have found a cannabis care nurse that had the knowledge and confidence to take me under her wing and heal me without me even realizing what she was doing. That is when I realized, Nursing taught me how to treat, cannabis has taught me how to heal.

CONCLUSION

In summary, the cannabis care nurse's role is a dynamic one, consistently influenced by the laws, regulations, research, science, and business developments that encompass the legalization of cannabis, and the burgeoning cannabis industry as a whole. Any nurse endeavoring to take on the role of a cannabis care nurse must have an understanding of the ECS, cannabinoid receptors, the cannabis plant, and the existing and emerging evidence for the therapeutic use of cannabis. Nurses must also understand that at the time of this writing, cannabis remains federally illegal, a Schedule 1 substance according to the Drug Enforcement Administration (DEA) and, therefore, practicing cannabis nursing without professional and legal guidance may result in consequences that may include loss of nursing license and loss of employment. The cannabis care nurse has many responsibilities with primary goals aimed at educating patients, caregivers, their support systems, and other health professionals on the ECS and using cannabis as medicine. Above all, cannabis care nurses advocate for the safe and therapeutic use of medical cannabis for all patients across the lifespan in all settings.

Q&A QUESTIONS

1. **All of these are the role of the cannabis care nurse, *except*:**
    A. Educates patients, caregivers, their support systems, and other health professionals on the ECS
    B. Provides guidance, coaching, and support on how to administer cannabis in a safe manner
    C. Gives medical advice and specific dosing instructions
    D. Acts as a liaison and advocate for patients, bridging the gap that exists between conventional medical practices and medical cannabis programs

2. **True or False: Cannabis is a cure for *everything*!**

3. **Which of the following supports a healthy ECS?**
    A. Eating clean whole foods, herbs, spices, tea, chocolate, and essential fatty acids
    B. Massage, yoga, meditation, acupuncture, osteopathy, enjoyable aerobic exercises, and social and intimate interactions
    C. Genetics, age, obesity, poor diet, smoking, chronic alcohol use, polypharmacy, chronic stress, lack of exercise, and social isolation
    D. A and B
    E. C only

4. **A patient using cannabis who is experiencing anxiety and depression symptoms that are worsening with the use of medical cannabis should be directed to:**
    A. Increase administration of THC via inhalation tid
    B. Decrease administration of cannabis products
    C. Consider taking desensitization holiday and cease use of cannabis to see if symptoms improve without cannabis
    D. Follow both B and C

5. **Cannabis care nurses work in a variety of settings including:**
    A. Hospitals
    B. Long-term care (LTC) facilities
    C. Primary care physician offices
    D. None of these

ANSWERS

1. **Answer: C.** Cannabis care nurses do *not* give medical advice. Instead, we educate on the ECS, and how the various products available may or may not contribute to our patient's health goals.

2. **Answer: False.** According to the FDA, the only thing that can prevent, treat, or cure a disease is a pharmaceutical. Despite what they may have personally experienced or have seen, cannabis care nurses are to remain ethically aware that their role is to provide

teaching/coaching, remain within our scope of practice, and not make any false claims regarding any cannabis products, or regarding cannabis in general.

3. **Answer: D.** There are many complementary health care tools that will promote homeostasis in the ECS. Balancing the ECS requires a healthy diet, exercise, and less stress. Unfortunately, it is often difficult to change your environment and virtually impossible to change your genetics. Restoring balance will be unique to each person.

4. **Answer: D.** Overconsumption of cannabis can result in negative symptoms that impede normal and ideal functioning. The patient using cannabis who is overconsuming it must reduce cannabis use or cease its use for a period ranging from a few days to a few weeks to determine whether cannabis is causing the negative symptoms.

5. **Answer: D.** Because cannabis remains a federally illicit, Schedule 1 substance, practicing cannabis care nurses tend not to have practice privileges in conventional medical settings. Nurses who do practice in such environments and advocate for the use of cannabis may face consequences including employment termination and loss of nursing license.

References

Adamson, S. J., Kay-Lambkin, F. J., Baker, A. L., Lewin, T. J., Thornton, L., Kelly, B. J., & Sellman, J. D. (2010). An improved brief measure of cannabis misuse: The cannabis use disorders identification test-revised (CUDIT-R). *Drug and Alcohol Dependence, 110*(1–2), 137–143. https://doi.org/10.1016/j.drugalcdep.2010.02.017

American Nurses Association. (2019). *The nursing process.* https://www.nursingworld.org/practice-policy/workforce/what-is-nursing/the-nursing-process/

Clark, C. S., Bernhard, C. E., Quigley, N., Smith, K., Theisen, E., & Smith, L. D. (2019, March 22). *Scopes and standards of practice for cannabis care nurses.* American Cannabis Nurses Association. https://cannabisnurses.org

Drugs.com. (n.d.). *Drug interaction report.* https://www.drugs.com/interactions-check.php?drug_list=2333-1544,1488-899,1752-1120,1750-1118,1260-0,3919-0,2758-0,72-1135

Gertsch, J., Leonti, M., Raduner, S., Racz, I., Chen, J., Xie, X., Altmann, K., Karsak, M., & Zimmer, A. (2008). Beta-caryophyllene is a dietary cannabinoid. *Proceedings of the National Academy of Sciences, 105*(26), 9099–9104. https://doi.org/10.1073/pnas.0803601105

Goldstein, B. (2016). *Cannabis revealed: How the world's most misunderstood plant is healing everything from chronic pain to epilepsy.* Bonni S. Goldstein MD Inc.

Grinspoon, P. (2019). *Cannabidiol (CBD)—What we know and what we don't.* https://www.health.harvard.edu/blog/cannabidiol-cbd-what-we-know-and-what-we-dont-2018082414476

Konieczny, E., & Wilson, L. (2018). *Healing with CBD: How cannabidiol can transform your health without the high.* Ulysses Press.

Lee, M. A. (2016). *I'm just mad about saffron (& other kitchen spices that activate the endocannabinoid system).* https://www.projectcbd.org/wellness/spices-and-endocannabinoid-system

Mcpartland, J. M., Guy, G. W., & Marzo, V. D. (2014). Care and feeding of the endocannabinoid system: A systematic review of potential clinical interventions that upregulate the endocannabinoid system. *PLoS One, 9*(3), e89566. https://doi.org/10.1371/journal.pone.0089566

MCR Labs, LLC. (2019). *Cannabis testing report: Report of sample analysis (Test report: Irie Blis 1000mg tincture).* https://reports.mcrlabs.com/reports/irie-bliss-1000mg-tincture

National Council of State Boards of Nursing. (2018). The NCSBN national guidelines for medical marijuana. *Journal of Nursing Regulation, 9*(2), S5. https://doi.org/10.1016/S2155-8256(18)30083-8

Patel, J. (2019). *Cannabis use disorder.* https://www.ncbi.nlm.nih.gov/books/NBK538131/

Project CBD. (2019). *Project CBD releases educational primer on cannabinoid-drug interactions.* https://www.projectcbd.org/how-to/cbd-drug-interactions

Sallaberry, C. A., & Astern, L. (2018). The endocannabinoid system, our universal regulator. *Journal of Young Investigators, 34*(6), 48–55. https://doi.org/10.22186/jyi.34.5.48-55

Sulak, D. (2017). *Using medical cannabis: Delivery systems.* https://healer.com/using-medical-cannabis-delivery-systems/

Tomaso, E. D., Beltramo, M., & Piomelli, D. (1996). Brain cannabinoids in chocolate. *Nature, 382*(6593), 677–678. https://doi.org/10.1038/382677a0

Tutkus, S. (n.d.). *CBD tincture dosage table [chart].* GreenNurse™ Group.

Tutkus, S., & Sykes, S. (2019). *Handbook.* GreenNurse™ Group. https://www.greennursegroup.com/handbook

Wong-Baker FACES Foundation. (2019). *Wong-Baker FACES® Pain Rating Scale.* http://www.WongBaker FACES.org/

Picture of Alice O'Leary-Randall, LPN. (Photo provided by Alice O'Leary-Randall, LPN. Used with permission.)

Following a diagnosis of juvenile glaucoma, Robert keenly observed that his eye-sight improved after consuming cannabis. Initially, Miss O'Leary doubted him, but as his symptoms progressed, she observed his visual improvements under the influence of cannabis and supported Robert's choice to consume cannabis to improve his health despite the illicit nature of the Schedule I drug. Needing a safe and dependable method to maintain Robert's cannabis supply, the couple successfully grew their medication on their apartment balcony in Washington, DC. While away on vacation in August 1975, looking on from a neighbor's porch, police officers stumbled upon several cannabis plants growing on the Randalls' sundeck. Robert and Alice arrived home to a ransacked house and a note on the table from the authorities instructing them to turn themselves in. Thus, they began the convoluted legal processes of a series of criminal and civil proceedings, where Robert Randall was ultimately victorious and declared to be the first medical cannabis patient in the United States.

Alice O'Leary-Randall was a senior spokesperson for the medical cannabis movement beginning in 1976 with her late husband. In 1980, the Randalls founded the ACT, the first nonprofit organization dedicated solely to resolving the medical cannabis issue. They drafted national legislation that was introduced in the U.S. House of Representatives with 110 cosponsors. ACT served as the primary plaintiff in the historic DEA hearing on marijuana's medical utility in the mid-1980s. In the 1990s, Alice and Robert secured funding from a Chicago-based backer and took the medical movement to new heights, paving the way for state ballot initiatives that have secured legal medical access to cannabis for citizens of 17 states.

Ms. O'Leary-Randall has a solid background in association leadership and management. She served as director for the ACT from 1980 to 1995 and on the Society for Scholarly Publishing as Administrative Officer from 1981 to 1989. In addition, Ms. O'Leary volunteered with the NORML. She also served as coordinator for a Medical Reclassification Project from 1978 to 1980, and she was on the National Women's Health Network as membership coordinator from 1976 to 1977. In addition,

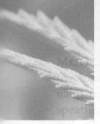

Index

Note: Page numbers followed by *f* and *t* indicates figures and tables respectively.